MENTAL HEALTH SYSTEMS COMPARED

MENTAL HEALTH SYSTEMS COMPARED

Great Britain, Norway, Canada, and the United States

Edited by

R. PAUL OLSON

Minnesota School of Professional Psychology
at
Argosy University–Twin Cities

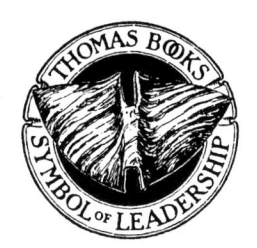

CHARLES C THOMAS • PUBLISHER, LTD.
Springfield • Illinois • U.S.A.

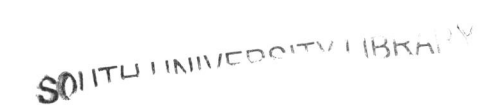

Published and Distributed Throughout the World by

CHARLES C THOMAS • PUBLISHER, LTD.
2600 South First Street
Springfield, Illinois 62704

This book is protected by copyright. No part of
it may be reproduced in any manner without written
permission from the publisher. All rights reserved.

© 2006 by CHARLES C THOMAS • PUBLISHER, LTD.

ISBN 0-398-07658-8 (hard)
ISBN 0-398-07659-6 (paper)

Library of Congress Catalog Card Number: 2006040458

With THOMAS BOOKS *careful attention is given to all details of manufacturing and design. It is the Publisher's desire to present books that are satisfactory as to their physical qualities and artistic possibilities and appropriate for their particular use.* THOMAS BOOKS *will be true to those laws of quality that assure a good name and good will.*

Printed in the United States of America
UB-R-3

Library of Congress Cataloging-in-Publication Data

Mental health systems compared : Great Britain, Norway, Canada, and the United
  States / edited by R. Paul Olson.
    p. cm.
  Includes bibliographical references and index.
  ISBN 0-398-07658-8 (hard) -- ISBN 0-398-07659-6 (pbk.)
    1. Mental health services--Great Britain. 2. Mental health services--
  Norway. 3. Mental health services--Canada. 4. Mental health services--
  United States. I. Olson, R. Paul.

RA790.7.G7M482 2006
362.2--dc22   2006040458

CONTRIBUTORS

John L. Arnett obtained his Ph.D. in clinical psychology from the University of Manitoba, Winnipeg, Manitoba, Canada. He is Professor and Head of the Department of Clinical Health Psychology, Faculty of Medicine at the University of Manitoba. His research interests and publications address professional training, clinical health psychology, neuropsychology, and psychosocial effects of various medications with seizure disorders. Dr. Arnett served as President of the Canadian Psychological Association in 2004.

Patrick DeLeon obtained his Ph.D. from Purdue University in clinical psychology and thereafter, a masters degree in public health from the University of Hawaii, and a jurisprudence degree from the Columbus School of Law at Catholic University. Following work as a staff psychologist in Hawaii, he has served since 1973 as Administrative Assistant to U.S. Senator Daniel K. Inouye. He is a former President of the American Psychological Association, and presently a member of its Board of Trustees. He has served on boards and committees with numerous other professional associations, and he is presently on the National Advisory Committee of the Institute for Public Policy Studies at Vanderbilt University. He has been a consulting editor with several professional journals and he is the recipient of several awards for distinguished service.

John N. Hall received his Ph.D. in clinical psychology from Leeds University, Leeds, England. He has worked with the British Health Service in both clinical services and as a consultant in clinical psychology to the British Government. Since 1992 he has been both part-time Specialist Adviser in Mental Health at the Health Advisory Service, and Visiting Professor in Mental Health at Oxford Brookes University. Dr. Hall is currently Chair of the Quality and Effectiveness subcommittee of the Division of Clinical Psychology within the British Psychological Society, and the head clinical psychologist for Oxfordshire. He is working presently on two projects related to mental health policy funded by the British Government Department of Health.

Haldis Hjort received her Ph.D. in psychology from the University of Oslo, with a specialization in clinical psychology. She has worked in outpatient private practice with children and adults with a variety of mental disorders, and in institutions for psychiatric and drug abusing patients. In addition, Haldis is a Senior Researcher at the Norwegian SINTEF research group (department of mental health research, Oslo), the author of three books, co-editor of another four, and author of several other chapters and articles, many of which relate to the field of psychotherapy practice. She is on the editorial staff for *Matrix*, the journal of psychotherapy for the Nordic area of Europe (Norden).

Arnulf Kolstad earned his Ph.D. from the Norwegian Institute of Technology (NTNU) and another doctorate in philosophy from the University of Bergen, Faculty of Psychology. While on the faculty of NTNU, he has been a research scientist at The Norwegian Institute for Hospital Research (UNIMED/SINTEF). He is presently a professor in social psychology at NTNU in Trondheim, and researcher with the Norwegian Research Council responsible for evaluation of Psychiatric Health Services in Norway. His expertise includes psychiatric epidemiology, planning and evaluation of mental health services, psychology of law, group conflicts and conflict resolution, and political psychology.

R. Paul Olson obtained his Ph.D. in clinical psychology from the University of Illinois at Urbana. After providing direct clinical services for several years in a private, multidisciplinary clinic and in a managed care organization, he became associate professor of clinical health psychology at the University of Wisconsin, Stevens Point. Thereafter, he served for ten years as Dean of the Minnesota School of Professional Psychology (MSPP). He is a Diplomate of the American Board of Administrative Psychology. Dr. Olson is currently a professor in clinical psychology at MSPP, a program of Argosy University-Twin Cities. His teaching interests include mental health delivery systems, professional issues and ethics, experiential psychotherapy, psychology and religion. His publications are in the areas of managed behavioral health care, graduate education, applied psychophysiology, psychology and religion, and the experience of reconciliation. Dr. Olson has provided expert testimony to both state and national committees in the area of health care policy, and he has served as co-chair of the legislative committee of the Minnesota Psychological Association.

Danny Wedding obtained his Ph.D. in clinical psychology from the University of Hawaii. He has provided clinical services in both civilian and military settings with specialties in neuropsychological assessment, behavioral medicine, and psychotherapy. He served for two years as Congressional Health Policy Fellow and Congressional Science Fellow, two programs administered respectively by the Institute of Medicine and the American Psychological Association. Since 1991 he has been Professor of Psychiatry in the Department of Psychiatry and Neurology, and Adjunct Assistant Professor of Psychology in the Department of Psychological Sciences, University of Missouri-Columbia. Dr. Wedding is the current Director of the Missouri Institute of Mental Health. His publications are in the areas of psychotherapy theory, neuropsychology, behavioral medicine, and mental health policy and services.

FOREWORD

It is a pleasure and honor to write the foreward to this book. As psychologists, as educators, and as individuals committed to the promotion of health -- captured by WHO's depiction as a "state of complete physical, mental and social well-being" (WHO, 2001) -- the authors of this volume have collectively undertaken an overview and comparison of the mental health infrastructures and services in four countries – Canada, Great Britain, Norway and the United States. Their very comprehensive, thorough and comparative approach makes this a unique volume – they address mental health services as part of a larger social service and health care delivery system, embedded in larger systems of culture, history, attitude and belief.

What you will learn from this book. The authors, psychologists from the four countries surveyed, used a common framework to organize their information on the mental health systems of Canada, Norway, the United Kingdom and the United States – countries that vary in size, wealth, population, and governmental and social services organization. Collectively, the chapters on these countries offer a trove of information that will educate readers about the current status of mental health care in a rich context from a public policy and public health perspective. Understanding mental health care in any one country requires both detailed and organized understanding of how that system is positioned within the larger health care system. This volume provides that overview by describing the many layers comprising the system. These include a snapshot of each country's social, political, demographic, geographical and economic history with an eye to capturing the context in which health and mental health are addressed; an overview of important policies and programs, and the resulting health and mental health systems, including indications of effectiveness, cost, and serving the needs of the population. No one can help emerging from this book without two things – an appreciation of the broad-ranging attention paid to health and mental health by commissions, researchers, politicians, agencies and global bodies, and a sense of awe at the extent to which an ideal world with quality health and mental health care, accessible in a timely fashion to all is still not fully realized even in those countries with a vast protective net.

Why you should read this book. As editor Paul Olson points out, the time is right for a volume that provides a common framework for looking at information across countries. Thoughtful comparative summaries concern such broad issues as access to services, mental health workforce needs, and meeting the needs of the population; a section on lessons learned provides a wealth of information and inspiration for those who want to understand and improve their country's mental health system services. We always benefit from looking beyond our own borders to see how others, with different histories, systems and expectations have approached solving common challenges. This volume contributes to that discussion.

Merry Bullock
Senior Director, Office of International Affairs
American Psychological Association

PREFACE

In September 2000 representatives from 189 countries, including 147 heads of state, met at the Millennium Summit in New York City to adopt the United Nations Millennium Declaration. The declaration set out the principles and values that should govern international relations in the twenty-first century. (WHO, 2003, p. 25)

National leaders made commitments in several areas including the development of nations and eradication of poverty. Goals prepared subsequently in this area are generally called Millennium Development Goals (MDGs). The MDGs are the collective expression of desired ends and intended outcomes, not a prescription for the means by which these ends are to be achieved.

Three of the eight MDGs, eight of the 18 targets required to achieve them, and 18 of the 48 indicators of progress are health-related (WHO, 2003, Table 2.1, p. 28). Mental health was not cited specifically or separately as one of the health-related goals, targets, or indicators. Though not mentioned explicitly, mental health is an implicit goal by virtue of the WHO definition of health as ". . . a state of complete physical, mental, and social well-being" (WHO, 2001, p. 3).

Moreover, as a component of health, the WHO has endorsed mental health as both a universal human right and a fundamental goal for the health systems of all countries irrespective of their stage of development. The right to health was affirmed in the Constitution of the WHO drafted in 1946: "The WHO Constitution identifies 'the enjoyment of the highest attainable standard of health' as 'one of the fundamental rights of every human being without distinction'" (WHO, 2003, p. xi). Health, including mental health, is viewed as a goal closely connected with two other core values to be actualized internationally in the twenty-first century – the values of security and justice. An essential aspect of justice is the promotion among nations of universal access to affordable mental health care of the highest attainable quality.

One year after the Millennium Summit, the WHO devoted an entire annual report (WHO, 2001) to a description of the mental health needs of 192 member nations. This landmark report included prevalence estimates of selected mental disorders and their contribution to the burden of disease worldwide evident in the death and disability attributable to mental disorders. Nations' health expenditures in public and private sectors were cited as indicators of how well the mental health needs were being met.

In the same report, the WHO reaffirmed that the prevalence and consequences of mental disorders have a substantial impact on health care systems generally. A large proportion of medically ill and injured individuals experience co-morbid depression, which interferes significantly with patients' adherence to recommended medical treatments (WHO, 2001, Box 1.3, p. 9).

Tragically, many individuals do not receive any health care for their mental disorders, let alone mental health services appropriate to their specific type and severity. The WHO cited two common barriers to treatment: (a) stigma and discrimination, and (b) inadequate mental health infrastructures to meet the large and increasing need for mental health services. The present volume addresses the second factor by comparing the mental health systems of four selected countries (WHO, 2003, Box 1.4, p. 19).

These four countries illustrate both strengths and limitations in the way mental health services are organized, delivered, and financed. An understanding of their commonalities and differences provides insights about both the challenges many countries face, and the possibilities for meeting them. It is the authors' hope that our respective countries might learn from one another what policies and strategies seem to work, and how the gap between mental health needs and mental health services can be bridged to reduce this form of human suffering worldwide. We believe that improvement in the mental health of countries will help to promote international security, justice, and peace, in addition to promoting the well-being of individuals.

The purpose of this book is twofold: First, to describe the mental health systems of four Western industrialized societies (Great Britain, Norway, Canada, and the United States), and second, to evaluate and compare these systems on a set of common criteria. Particular attention is given to how each society delivers and finances mental health services for their population with identified mental disorders. The authors from each country evaluate their own mental health system relative to six common criteria to facilitate comparison with the other three countries. Common criteria include access/equity, quality/efficacy, cost/efficiency, financing/fairness, and protection/participation. On the final criterion (population relevance), the authors provide a summative evaluation by addressing the degree to which their country's present mental health system meets the identified needs for mental health services. All six criteria are defined subsequently in the introductory chapter. The authors' evaluations lead to recommendations for improvement in mental health policies and in the structure and functioning of their country's system for delivering and financing mental health services. The book's final chapters address convergence and divergence among the four systems, and provide conclusions and recommendations for mental health system reform.

World Health Organization (WHO) (2001). *The World Health Report 2001: Mental health: New understanding, new hope*. Geneva, Switzerland: Author.

World Health Organization (WHO) (2003). *The World Health Report 2003: Shaping the future*. Geneva, Switzerland: Author.

CONTENTS

	Page
Contributors	v
Foreword by Merry Bullock	vii
Preface	ix
List of Illustrations	xiii

Chapter

1. INTRODUCTION 3
   R. Paul Olson

2. MENTAL HEALTH DELIVERY SYSTEMS
   IN GREAT BRITAIN 24
   John N. Hall

3. MENTAL HEALTH SERVICES IN NORWAY 81
   Arnulf Kolstad and Haldis Hjort

4. HEALTH AND MENTAL HEALTH IN CANADA 138
   John L. Arnett

5. MENTAL HEALTH CARE IN THE UNITED STATES 185
   Danny Wedding, Patrick H. DeLeon, and R. Paul Olson

6. CONVERGENCE AND DIVERGENCE
   IN MENTAL HEALTH SYSTEMS 231
   R. Paul Olson

7. MEETING THE NEEDS, CONCLUSIONS, AND
   RECOMMENDATIONS 306
   R. Paul Olson

Index 353

ILLUSTRATIONS

Figures   *Page*

Figure 2.1. The Relationship Between the NSF for Older People
             and the NSF for Adult Mental Health 44

Figure 2.2. The Relationship Between the Elements of a
             Comprehensive Mental Health Service 48

Figure 3.1. Suicide by Age and Gender, 2002. Ratios per
             100,000 Inhabitants 91

Figure 3.2. Average Number of Patients During the Year in Different
             Service Settings 100

Figure 3.3. Average Numbers of Patients in Psychiatric Nursing Homes
             in a Year 1950–2003 101

Figure 4.1. Canadian Health Care Expenditures in Current and
             Constant (1997) Dollars, 1975–2004 163

Figure 4.2. Canadian Per Capita Total Health Expenditures in Current
             and Constant (1997) Dollars 164

Figure 4.3. Total Health Expenditures as a Percentage of Gross Domestic
             Product: Canada, 1975–2004 165

Figure 4.4. Canadian Health Expenditures by Source of Finance,
             1975–2004 165

Figure 4.5. Public and Private Shares of Total Health Expenditures
             by Use of Funds, Canada 2002 166

Tables

Table 1.1.   Basic Indicators for Four Countries 2003 11
Table 1.2.   Estimated National Expenditures on Health 2002 11
Table 1.3.   Per Capita Health Expenditures 2002 13
Table 2.1.   Prevalence of Mental Disorders in Children and
             Adolescents by Gender in Rates per 1000 31
Table 2.2.   Point Prevalence of Mental Disorders in Men and Women

	in Rates per 1000	31
Table 2.3.	Prevalence of Substance Abuse in Men and Women in Percentages	32
Table 2.4.	Mortality Rates from Suicide for Men in England and Wales by Year and Age	33
Table 2.5.	Conservative Estimate of Number of Older People with Dementia by Ethnic Group	35
Table 2.6.	Examples of Current Provision of Adult Inpatient Mental Health Beds in Three PCT Areas Within One Mental Health Trust in Northern England	52
Table 2.7.	Head-Count Figures for Subgroups of Psychiatrist Consultants, 1989 to 2004	55
Table 2.8.	Mental Health Professional Groups, 1990 to 2003	56
Table 2.9.	Comparisons of Evaluation Criteria	64
Table 2.10.	Investment in Millions of Pounds for Direct Service Categories at 2004/5 Prices (US$ in parentheses)	67
Table 2.11.	Unmet Need for Mental Health Services in England as the Percent Not Receiving Full, Appropriate Treatment	72
Table 3.1.	Percentage With a Mental Disorder in Oslo	88
Table 3.2.	Self-Rated Mental Health Problems, Norwegian Population 2002 (Percentages)	89
Table 3.3.	Mortality Ratios per 100,000 in 2002	90
Table 3.4.	Deaths by Sex, Age and Underlying Cause of Death: Alcohol Abuse and Drug Dependence. The Whole Country, 2002.	91
Table 3.5.	Disability Pensions for Mental and Behavioural Disorders. Ratios per 10,000 Inhabitants Aged 16-67. End of 2003.	92
Table 3.6.	Mental Health Services 1990–2003. Key Figures	97
Table 3.7.	Use of Specialized Mental Health Services by Age Group. Ratios per 10,000 Inhabitants in 2003	98
Table 3.8.	Patients in Norwegian Adult Psychiatric Institutions (per 10,000 Inhabitants) by Year and Service Setting	99
Table 3.9.	The Distribution (Percents) of Diagnosis in Inpatient Psychiatric Institutions for Adults. November 20, 2003	103
Table 3.10.	Qualified Providers in the Specialist Health Service. Key Figures for Personnel in Man-Years 1990–2003.	107
Table 3.11.	Mental Health Services. Key Figures in Man-Years 1990–2003 ...	108
Table 3.12.	Man-Years in Psychiatric Institutions for Adults and Children and Adolescents by Category of Personnel	109
Table 3.13.	Number of Contracted Psychiatrists and Psychologists (Man-Years) by Regional Health Enterprises, 2003. Per 100,000 Inhabitants	118

Table 3.14.	WHO National Health Account Indicators: 1998, 2002	121
Table 3.15.	National Mental Health Services Expenditures for 2003	122
Table 3.16.	Expenses for Psychiatric Institutions, 1990–2000	123
Table 3.17.	Current Expenses and Current Revenue for Specialized Mental Health Services by Category of Expenses, 1990–2000	124
Table 4.1.	Estimated Prevalence of Mental Disorders in Canadian Children and Adolescents to 19 Years of Age	144
Table 4.2.	Prevalence of Mental Disorders and Substance Abuse among Canadian Adults Ages 15 Years and Older in the Past 12 Months	145
Table 4.3.	Prevalence of Mental Health Problems and Perception of Adjustment And General Health Over the Past 12 Months in Canadian Forces (CF) Regular and Reserve Members Relative to Each Other and to the Standardized Canadian General Population	146
Table 4.4.	Prevalence of Major Disorders by Gender	147
Table 4.5.	1992 Economic Costs of Alcohol and Tobacco Abuse in Canadian dollars (CDN) and US$	148
Table 4.6.	Estimated Costs of Mental Disorders 1998	150
Table 4.7.	Total Public and Private Canadian Health Expenditures and Percent of Total Expenditures by Category	166
Table 4.8.	WHO National Health Account Indicators: 1998 and 2002	176
Table 4.9.	Total and Government Per Capita Expenditures on Health, 1998 and 2002	177
Table 5.1.	Leading Sources of Disease Burden, 1990	191
Table 5.2.	Best Estimate 1-Year Prevalence Rates Based on ECA and NCS, Ages 18–54	192
Table 5.3.	Children and Adolescents Ages 9 to 17 with Mental or Addictive Disorders, Combined MECA Samples	193
Table 5.4.	Best Estimate Prevalence Rates Based on Epidemiological Catchment Area, Age 55+	193
Table 5.5.	Medication Expenditures, 1987	194
Table 5.6.	Medication Expenditures, 2001	194
Table 5.7.	Proportion of Adult Population Using Mental/Addictive Disorder Services in One Year	201
Table 5.8.	Proportion of Child/Adolescent Populations (Ages 9–17) Using Mental/Addictive Disorder Services in One Year	201
Table 5.9.	WHO National Health Account Indicators: 1998, 2002	214
Table 5.10.	Per Capita Expenditures on Health: 1998, 2002	214
Table 6.1.	WHO Rankings of Goal Attainment and System	

	Performance, 1997	234
Table 6.2.	Frequencies of Ratings	235
Table 6.3.	Goal Attainment Scale	235
Table 6.4.	Current Expert Ratings of Levels of Goal Attainment	236
Table 6.5.	Hypothesized Relationships of Present Criteria and WHO Categories	237
Table 6.6.	Practicing Physicians and Nurses per 1,000 Population in 2003	250
Table 6.7.	Estimated Ratios of All Professionals Rendering Mental Health Services in 2005	251
Table 6.8.	Rankings of Efficiency (Performance) and Goal Attainment	270
Table 6.9.	Health Expenditures 2003	271
Table 6.10.	Percentages Spent on MH and SA Care and all Health Care by Payer, Calendar year 2001	289
Table 7.1.	Changes in Percentages of Populations Age 60+ Years, 1992 to 2002	307
Table 7.2.	Population Estimates, Geographic Area, and Population Density	316
Table 7.3.	GDP Per Capita, 2003 at Current Prices in U.S. Dollars	317
Table 7.4.	Comparative Statistics	322
Table 7.5.	Mental Health Specialists Per 100,000 Population	323
Table 7.6.	Ranking of Values: Quality above Cost	337

MENTAL HEALTH SYSTEMS COMPARED

Chapter 1

INTRODUCTION

R. Paul Olson

OVERVIEW AND CONTEXT

Within the past decade mental health has received increased international attention. Stimulated by calls to action by the United Nations Secretary General (Boutrous-Ghali, 1995) and by World Health Organization (WHO) health ministers (WHO, 2001a), the WHO began a project on "nations for mental health" (Jenkins, McCallough, and Parker, 1998), and devoted its annual world health report to mental health (WHO, 2001b). "In 1999, the World Bank established positions for mental health in its Washington, DC headquarters and for the first time, considered the funding of mental health interventions within its lending program as well as including mental health in its policy dialogue with countries" (Gulbinat et al. 2004, p. 6).

Within this same period, there have been significant advances in technical knowledge and cost-effective interventions (WHO, 2001b), but the application of empirical research in mental health delivery systems has been limited, and especially in developing nations, with the result that the large majority of people with mental disorders remain untreated. Estimates of *untreated* mental and neurological disorders in developing countries (85%) is much greater than in developed countries (54%), but remains high in both (Institute of Medicine, 2001).

Among the causes for the wide treatment gaps both within and between countries, three system factors have been identified: (a) the lack of a policy on mental or neurological health; (b) the failure of professionals in the fields of mental health and neurology to engage in the economic aspects of the health and social policy dialogue; and (c) the lack of preparation and training for leadership in policy development and dialogue (Gulbinat et al. 2004, p. 6).

A fourth factor implicated in the treatment gap is the small number of international comparative studies of mental health needs and mental health systems that are more or less successful in meeting their population's needs. Gulbinat et al. (2004) observed that international comparative studies of mental health services, programs, and policies have been very limited, if not nonexistent until the late 1990s when a few studies were published (e.g., Global Forum for Health Research, 1999; Gulbinat et al. 1996; Jenkins and Knapp, 1996; Manderscheid, 1998; Sartorius, 1998). This limited research is itself one of the barriers to establishing evidence for the impact of mental health policies and mental health systems.

In recognition of the need for comparative studies, particularly on the impact of mental health policy formulation and implementation upon sector-wide reform, the International Consortium on Mental Health Policy and Services developed (a) a framework (template) identifying key domains and elements of a national mental health policy, and (b) a standardized method (mental health country profile) to assess a country's current mental health status. Additional goals of this international effort included (c) establishing a global network of expertise in mental health policy and services, (d) evaluating the cost-effectiveness of implementations of various elements of mental health policy under different conditions, and (e) generating guidelines and examples for improving mental health policy and mental health system performance appropriate to existing delivery systems and demographic, cultural, and economic factors (Gulbinat et al. 2004, p. 9).

Among mental health specialty groups, clinical psychologists have not been trained systematically, if at all, in mental health policy formulation and implementation, nor in systems theory or mental health services research. One consequence has been much less psychological research on the performance of mental health delivery systems than on the development of cost-effective, evidence-based clinical interventions. There has been a particular deficit in professional psychology curricula devoted to understanding the language of health economists, finance experts, and health policymakers and politicians. Psychologists who have contributed to systems level research on policy formulation and implementation have been those with a keen interest and practical experience in positions that require a system-wide perspective. We have found examples of these experts from the four countries that constitute the focus of the present comparative study of how countries finance, organize, and deliver mental health services to meet their population's needs.

None of our contributing authors claim to represent a consensus or official perspective on the performance of their mental health system. All of them have been immersed in the operations of these systems at clinical and/or administrative levels, in the education and training of clinical psychologists, in research, consultation or supervision related to the delivery of mental health services and/or in mental health policy formulation and implementation.

Our authors have volunteered to share their own expert views of the mental health systems operating in their own country. They have not been asked to create a complete "mental health country profile" according to the specifications of the International Consortium on Mental Health Policy and Services (Jenkins et al. 2004), but elements and domains of the guiding framework (template) have been selected to facilitate comparisons among these four developed countries (Townsend et al. 2004). To be more specific, the authors have been invited to address some, but not all of the elements of all *four domains* pertinent to mental health policy formulation: context, resources, service provision, and outcomes.

The purpose of this chapter is to provide an overview and context for the planned comparisons among the systems for delivering and financing mental health services in Great Britain, Norway, Canada, and the United States. Because this book addresses specifically the systems for treating mental disorders, the introduction begins with definitions of two central terms: "mental health systems" and "mental disorders." Thereafter, an international perspective is provided on the significance of mental disorders by citing current statistics summarized by the World Health Organization on the prevalence and the contribution to the burden of disease evident in the death and disability attributed to mental disorders (WHO, 2001b, 2004).

A mental health system does not exist as an autonomous sector within a society; rather, it functions as a subsystem within a society's overall health care system. How mental health services are delivered and financed is influenced significantly by the way in which a society organizes, delivers, and finances all health services. Consequently, to understand similarities and differences among the four mental health systems selected for this study, it is helpful to appreciate the comparative estimates of both total health expenditures and the predominant sources of public versus private financing. The World Health Organization (WHO) provides these estimates in its annual reports, though not for mental health spending separate from total health expenditures. The latter data have been reported most recently in the *Mental Health Atlas – 2005* (WHO, 2005a).

Following the report of health expenditures by each of the four countries, the domains and criteria are discussed in this chapter relevant to the twin goals of description and evaluation of the mental health system for each country. This discussion is followed by presentation of the common chapter outline adopted by the contributing authors to facilitate comparisons. The introduction concludes with comments about our authors and intended audience.

In its annual report devoted to mental health, the WHO recognized that mental health is crucial to the overall well-being of individuals, societies, and countries. The report also acknowledged the following:

> Unfortunately, in most parts of the world, mental health and mental disorders are not regarded with anything like the same importance as physical health. Instead, they have been largely ignored and neglected. Partly as a result, the world is suffering from an increasing burden of mental disorders and a widening 'treatment gap.' (WHO, 2001b, p. 3)

It was estimated that in 2001 about 450 million people worldwide suffered from a mental or behavioral disorder, but only a small minority received even the most basic treatment. There continues to be significant unmet needs for mental health services around the world. The WHO projected that the burden of disease attributable to mental disorders will increase from ten percent in 1990 to 15 percent in 2020 (WHO, 2001b, p. 19).

The annual report devoted specifically to mental health (WHO, 2001b) reflects the growing awareness within the international community of the significant impact of mental health upon the social, economic, political, and individual well-being of the world's population. Moreover, the WHO acknowledged the significance of mental health by including it as an essential component in the basic definition of health. Health is "not merely the absence of disease;" rather, health is ". . . a state of complete physical, mental, and social well-being" (WHO, 2001b, p. 3). This definition reflects a consensus about both the holistic nature of health and consequently, the integral part mental health plays in general health.

Although the present volume focuses on the ways the diagnosis and treatment of mental disorders are organized, delivered, and financed, it is important to appreciate conceptually and empirically that mental health is more than the absence of a mental disorder. Moreover, the contributing authors share the conviction that the promotion of mental health and the prevention of mental disorders are as important as their diagnosis and treatment, but it is the latter that our contributing authors have been asked to emphasize, though not exclusively.

Use of the terms "mental health" and "mental illness" would seem to imply endorsement of a medical model of these phenomena. Mental illness is a general term, which refers to all diagnosable mental disorders regardless of their etiology. While acknowledging the major advances biomedical science has brought to our understanding and treatment of mental disorders, the authors of this volume embrace a biopsychosocial model of these forms of human suffering. Appreciation for all three dimensions in the etiology, diagnosis, and treatment of mental disorders provides a more comprehensive and inclusive approach, which recognizes and invites the contributions of multiple disciplines and professions to multimodal interventions.

The preferred term for the phenomena under study will be "mental disorders" to connote the more holistic, biopsychosocial model and to appreciate the impaired (disordered) functioning that individuals suffer as a consequence of these conditions. Nevertheless, we adopt the conventional term "mental health services" utilized in the specialized area of research called health services research, of which this text is one example. More specifically, this book compares mental health systems from four countries in terms of the way they organize, deliver, and finance mental health services. Since mental health systems are the focus of this volume, it is appropriate to elaborate on the meaning of that term prior to defining mental disorders and discussing indicators of their prevalence and consequences.

Definitions

Mental Health System

Based on the WHO definition of a "health system" (WHO, 2000, p. xi; 2003, p. 105), the working definition adopted for the purposes of this study is as follows: *A mental health system comprises all organizations, institutions, and resources that produce actions whose primary purpose is to improve mental health.*

In order to describe a mental health system, one needs to ask such questions as who delivers what services to whom, when, where, how, and why. Ultimately a description of a mental health system requires researchers to attend not only to providers, patients, and payers, but also to health plan managers, regulators, and policymakers as they interact in their various roles as members of the system. One of the goals of this volume is to provide information to these constituencies to help them understand how their own and other mental health systems work, and how to work their system in order to ensure high quality mental health services at affordable cost, distributed equitably, and financed fairly.

The previous statement suggests that a performance appraisal of a mental health system involves the application of values and criteria expressed in goals and performance standards. These will be discussed subsequently in this introductory chapter and by each chapter author. Prior to that discussion, a few more comments are offered here about the definition of a mental health system.

The general definition of a mental health *system* denotes structures and functions as elements for analysis addressed in general social systems theory (e.g., Ashley and Orenstein, 1990; WHO, 2000, Chp.1; Willing, 1989). The structures are not only organizations, institutions, and resources for delivering and financing mental health services, but include the statuses and roles occupied by various individuals who perform different functions that contribute in different ways and in varying degrees to the general goal of enhancing a society's mental health. Theoretically speaking, a mental health system is an abstract concept; nevertheless, it refers ultimately to concrete relationships and interactions among its members in their various roles.

A *mental health* system includes more than the human and financial resources organized to provide diagnosis and treatment of a society's population suffering with mental disorders. The definition implies that integral components include the organizations, institutions, and resources that help to *prevent* mental disorders from developing and to *promote* mental health as an essential element to social and individual well-being. Neither prevention nor promotion can be subsumed by the diagnosis and treatment of already existing and newly developing mental disorders summarized in epidemiological studies of both prevalence and incidence. It is important to acknowledge these other vital aspects of a mental health system in a volume like this one, which emphasizes the delivery and financing of mental health services to people already manifesting mental disorders. The organization and financing of prevention/promotion activities are no less important, but do not constitute the primary focus of the present study. For a global perspective on disease prevention, the reader is referred to the WHO annual report devoted to identifying, measuring, and reducing risks to health (WHO, 2002, pp. 47–98, 79–81). Although its focus was on health in general, that report mentioned a small number of mental disorders and behaviors as risks to health, such as addictive substances and child sexual abuse.

One final comment about this working definition is in order. A mental health system is not limited to mental health services provided solely, or even primarily by mental health specialists such as psychiatrists, psychiatric nurses, clinical-counseling-health psychologists, social workers, professional counselors, case managers, or other mental health care workers. This statement recognizes both a fundamental reality and a preferred approach. The reality is that a majority of individuals with symptoms of mental disorders receive services in primary health care settings such as general hospitals and medical clinics, not in specialized mental health hospitals, psychiatric clinics, or community mental health centers. Family physicians, internists, and other medical personnel are more likely to see these patients before any of them are seen by mental health professionals, and many mental patients are seen by no mental health professional. While the latter may rightly lament this situation, there is a growing recognition that a functional mental health system must integrate mental health services into primary health care delivery systems, and that an integrated approach is preferred to a more fragmented system that segregates mental health patients from other health services and health professionals, or removes them from their local community.

Primary health care principles were reaffirmed recently by the WHO as a way to return to population health criteria upon which to base health policy decisions affecting how health care services are organized, paid for, and delivered (WHO, 2003, p. 108). This integrated approach seems consistent with the conception of the individual person as a psychosomatic unity, or more aptly, as a biopsychosocial unity. The United States Department of Health and Human Services has advocated a similar approach by recognizing "the inextricably intertwined relationship between our mental health and our physical health and well-being" (DHHS, 1999b, p. v).

Mental Disorders

In addition to the concept of a mental health system, a second term central to this work is the mental disorders these systems function to prevent, diagnose, treat, and manage. Mental disorders are generally conceptualized in contrast to mental health. The reader is referred to Secker (1998) for a summary of contemporary conceptualizations of mental health. These concepts are neither value-neutral, nor value-free; rather, they are rooted in value judgments. Because these judgments vary across cultures, any attempt to formulate a universal definition of mental health is subject to challenge (Cowen, 1994). Nevertheless, unanimity on a definition of mental health is not necessary to determine mental health service needs of a given country, nor to proceed with comparative evaluations of mental health systems (Gulbinat et al. 2004, pp. 11–13).

The contrasts drawn between mental health and mental disorders are not absolute. Distinctions are drawn on a continuum, which suggests the presence of one or the other condition in varying degrees. For the purposes of this study, mental health services are construed as services provided to people with identified mental disorders. Consequently, it is the latter term that warrants elaboration.

According to the official nomenclature used in the United States, a mental disorder is:

> ... a clinically significant behavioral or psychological syndrome or pattern that occurs in an individual and that is associated with present distress (e.g., a painful symptom) or disability (i.e., impairment in one or more important areas of functioning) or with a significantly increased risk of death, pain, disability, or an important loss of freedom. In addition, this syndrome or pattern must not be merely an expectable and culturally sanctioned response to a particular event, for example, the

death of a loved one. Whatever its original cause, it must currently be considered a manifestation of a behavioral, psychological, or biological dysfunction in the individual. Neither deviant behavior (e.g., political, religious, or sexual) nor conflicts that are primarily between the individual and society are mental disorders unless the deviance or conflict is a symptom of a dysfunction in the individual, as described above. (APA, 2000, p. xxxi)

This definition underlies and informs the current revision of the classification system of mental disorders called the *Diagnostic and Statistical Manual of Mental Disorders* (DSM-IV-TR) published by the American Psychiatric Association (APA, 2000).

Like other diagnostic classification systems, this one has both limitations and its critics. *First,* attributing a mental disorder to an individual does not allow for the fact that an individual could be a symptom bearer of a dysfunctional family system; *secondly,* by using the term "mental" disorders in contrast to "physical" disorders, this nomenclature tends to perpetuate an anachronistic mind/body dualism; and *thirdly,* some of the discrete categories and differential diagnoses lack precise boundaries, which reduce the interrater reliability of diagnoses and their validity.

Despite these and other limitations, DSM-IV-TR is the official system used in the largest country in this comparative study. It serves as a satisfactory foundation for understanding the concept of a mental disorder. Moreover, the current revision provides codes and terms fully compatible with the current edition of the *International Statistical Classification of Diseases and Related Health Problems* (ICD–10) developed by WHO and published in 1992 (as cited in APA, 2000, p. xxix).

It must be granted that mental disorders have been defined by a variety of other concepts such as maladjustment, a failure to cope with conflict, maladaptive behavior, irrational thinking, distortions in perception, emotional dysregulation, or statistical deviation from social norms. In DSM-IV-TR, a single criterion has been rejected in favor of a multidimensional definition of mental disorders. The Surgeon General of the Department of Health and Human Services, U. S. Public Health Service has endorsed a similar multidimensional definition of mental health: "Mental health refers to the successful performance of mental functions, resulting in productive activities and fulfilling relationships with other people, and the ability to adapt to change and to cope with adversity" (DHHS, 1999a, p. ix).

Where a multidimensional definition of a mental disorder is applied, it has implications for mental health policy, programs, and clinical practice. All dimensions of mental disorders (i.e., dysfunction, disability, distress, risk, and loss of freedom) are essential considerations in their etiology, diagnosis, and treatment. For example, treatment for a major depression that enables an individual to return to work (functioning) cannot be considered complete or successful if the individual's mood remains dysphoric (distressed), the person continues to be socially withdrawn, or remains at risk for suicide. Consequently, a "return to functioning" model for determining "medically necessary" mental health care cannot be considered satisfactory (Olson, 1999).

The multidimensional perspective expressed in the definition of mental disorders provides the context for the focus of the present volume. However, to provide a global perspective and to facilitate cross-cultural comparisons, researchers must rely upon international nomenclature and available data. The World Health Organization provides both definitions and global data.

The terms for mental disorders used by the WHO are "mental and behavioural disorders" and "neuropsychiatric disorders" (WHO, 2001b, pp. 10, 22). Both terms reference a set of disorders classified not by DSM-IV-TR, but by ICD-10 on the basis of international reviews of scientific literature, and on worldwide consultation and consensus in order to be applicable cross-culturally. Despite some differences between these two descriptive nomenclatures, mental disorders defined by both systems share in common some combination of abnormal thoughts, emotions, behavior, and relationships with others (WHO, 2001b, p. 10). Examples of major mental disorders include schizophrenia, depression, mental retardation, and disorders associated with alcohol and drug abuse.

A second term for mental disorders used by the WHO is "neuropsychiatric disorders." This category is also derived from ICD-10, but it is a broader term that includes disorders that are commonly considered as physical and neurological disorders (e.g., epilepsy, Parkinson's disease). The inclusion of the latter disorders is a further expression of the biopsychosocial model adopted by the WHO to encourage integrated care and in recognition of the obstacles to such care:

> The artificial separation of biological from psychological and social factors has been a formidable obstacle to a true understanding of mental and behavioural disorders. In reality, these disorders are similar to many physical illnesses in that they are the result of a complex interaction of all three factors. (WHO, 2001b, p. 10)

A comparable statement has been made by Dr. David Satcher, the Surgeon General of the U. S. Public

Health Service: "... one of the foremost contributions of contemporary mental health research is the extent to which it has mended the destructive split between 'mental' and 'physical' health" (DHHS, 1999b, Preface, p. vi.).

For cross-cultural comparisons the WHO compiles statistics from 192 member countries on a selected subset of "neuropsychiatric disorders." These disorders include unipolar depression, bipolar affective disorders, schizophrenia, epilepsy, alcohol use disorders, Alzheimer and other dementias, Parkinson's disease, multiple sclerosis, drug use disorders, post-traumatic stress disorders, obsessive-compulsive and panic disorders, primary insomnia and migraine (WHO, 2004, Annex Table 2, p. 122). The statistics on mental disorders reported by the WHO in its annual reports are based on this subset of "neuropsychiatric disorders." Utilizing the WHO categories and statistics enables us to provide a global perspective on the scope of these disorders and their consequences.

The Scope of Mental Disorders

Mental disorders are found universally in all countries, developed and underdeveloped, wealthy and poor, urbanized and rural, regardless of geographic region or political and economic systems. The scope of the challenge presented by mental disorders can be estimated by noting both their prevalence worldwide and within the four countries selected for this comparative study. Moreover, global statistics on the mortality and disability rates associated with mental disorders provide estimates of their contribution to the burden of disease. Current international data are reported for year 2002 in the annual report published by the WHO (2004). The WHO (2001b) annual report devoted specifically to mental health is also referenced here.

Prevalence Estimates

Based on the selected sample of neuropsychiatric conditions that constituted the focused study of the WHO, this subset of mental disorders had an aggregate *point prevalence* of about ten percent for adults. That is, about ten percent of the adult world population was estimated to have a mental disorder at a particular point in time (WHO, 2001b, pp. 22–23). When a broader sample of mental and behavioral disorders from the ICD-10 is included, higher point prevalence rates have been reported. Moreover, prevalence rates at any time during a period (*period prevalence*, such as within a one or five-year period), or at any time in one's lifetime (*lifetime prevalence*) yield generally higher estimates of the number of people who may require mental health services. In terms of numbers, about 450 million people worldwide in 192 countries were estimated to be suffering from neuropsychiatric conditions in the year 2000.

Surveys of developed as well as developing countries reported in 1988, 1989, and 1997 indicated that during their entire *lifetime*, more than 25 percent of individuals worldwide develop one or more mental or behavioral disorder (WHO, 2001b, p. 23). These international estimates appear in the range of period prevalence reports of about 20 percent of Americans with a mental disorder in any one year (DHHS, 1999b, p. xvii) and 28 percent when substance abuse disorders are included (DHHS, 1999a, p. 408). Using the National Institute of Mental Health Interview Schedule for Children, version 2.3, Shaffer (1996) reported a prevalence rate of 21.0 percent for child and adolescent mental disorders (as cited in WHO, 2001b, Table 2.2, p. 36). The average of three epidemiological studies conducted each decade in the United States since the 1980s for a 12-month period prevalence is 28 percent, with the most recent lifetime prevalence estimated at 46.4 percent (Insel and Fenzton, 2005; Kessler, Berglund, Demler, Jin, and Walters, 2005; Kessler, R. C., McGonagle et al., 1994; Robins, L. and Regier, D.A., 1991).

Mental and behavioral disorders are quite common among medical patients who are seen in primary health care settings, though all too often they are undiagnosed and untreated. Prevalence rates for mental disorders in cross-cultural studies reported in 1995 indicated a substantial proportion (about 24%) of all medical patients in primary care had a mental disorder (WHO, 2001b, pp. 23–24). The estimates in 14 cities worldwide ranged significantly from 7.3 percent to 52.5 percent. These estimates warrant concern because a recent analysis by Mechanic and Bilder (2004) of a nationally representative community survey in the United States indicated that contact with a primary care provider for mental health care was directly related to the seriousness of the disorder. In other words, the more serious the disorder, the more likely there would be contact with a primary health care provider.

The significant range and prevalence of mental disorders make it imperative both (a) to describe how various countries organize, deliver, and finance their mental health services to address the identified need for these services, and (b) to evaluate how effectively and efficiently they do it. Prevalence alone, however, reveals neither the need for mental health services (Mechanic, 2003), nor the costs in human suffering through premature death and disability, nor the enormous financial burdens associated with mental disorders.

Mortality Rates Associated with Mental Disorders

Based on worldwide estimates for both men and women in 2002, the subset of "neuropsychiatric disorders" accounted for about 1,112,000 deaths, which was 1.9 percent of deaths from all causes (WHO, 2004, Table 2, p. 122). The estimates for specific disorders were 177,000 deaths attributed to alcohol and drug use disorders, 23,000 to schizophrenia, 13,000 to unipolar depression, and 1,000 to bipolar affective disorders.

One of the major causes of premature death associated with mental disorders is suicide. The estimated rate for suicide worldwide in 1996 was 15.1 per 100,000, 3.5 times higher in men than in women. In 29 selected countries in the European region, including Great Britain and Norway, suicide was among the top three leading causes of death (WHO, 2001b, pp. 37–39). Rosenberg, Mercy, and Potter (1999) reported that of all persons who died from firearm injuries in the United States in 1997, a total of 54 percent died by suicide. The mortality rates suggest that premature death is one of the tragic consequences of mental disorders.

Disability Rates Associated with Mental Disorders

Estimates of premature deaths constitute one of two types of indicators used by the WHO to assess the contribution of mental disorders to the burden of disease. A second type of indicator is the estimate of disability caused by mental disorders. To quantify the burden of diseases due to disability, the WHO uses a measure of "disability-adjusted life years" (DALYs).

> The DALY is a health gap measure, which combines information on the impact of premature death and of disability and other nonfatal health outcomes. One DALY can be thought of as one lost year of "healthy life," and the burden of disease as a measurement of the gap between current health status and an ideal situation where everyone lives into old age free of disease and disability. (WHO, 2001b, p. 25)

The World Bank introduced DALYs in 1993 as a way to measure the global burden of disease and to assess the association of this burden with health and other social policies. This construct is not without its critics:

> Critics argue that DALYs lack a sound theoretical framework and are inequitable because they value years saved for the able-bodied more than for the disabled, the middle-aged more than the young or old, and the currently ill more than those who will be ill tomorrow. By introducing DALYs, the bank contends it improved analysis of international health systems. Critics remain concerned with its use in global health, and the debate continues. (Ruger, 2005, p. 165)

For both men and women in 2002, the subset of neuropsychiatric disorders was estimated to account for 193,278,000 DALYs, which was 13.0 percent of DALYs from all causes (WHO, 2004, Table 3, p. 128). For both sexes of all ages in 2000, mental disorders were among the top twenty leading causes of disability-adjusted life years. Unipolar depression disorders ranked as the 4th highest cause of disability, self-inflected injuries ranked 17th, and alcohol use disorders ranked 18th among causes (WHO, 2001b, Figure 2.2, p. 27).

Using the same measure of the burden of disease (DALYs), Murray and Lopez (1996) reported that in established market economies in 1990 all mental illnesses were the second leading cause of both disability and premature death. Among the top three leading causes were all cardiovascular conditions (18.6%), all mental illnesses (15.4%), all malignant diseases (cancers) (15.0%). The burden of disease caused by mental disorders (15.4%) exceeded the combined rates for all respiratory conditions (4.8%), all alcohol use (4.7%), all infections and parasitic disease (2.8%), and all drug use (1.5%) (cited by DHHS, 1999b, Table 1, p. ix.)

In contrast to the estimates of 13 to 15 percent of the global burden of disease caused by mental and behavioral disorders, the mental health budgets of the majority of countries constitute less than one percent of their total health expenditures. In the view of the WHO, "the relationship between disease burden and disease spending for mental disorders is clearly disproportionate" (WHO, 2001b, p. 3). Moreover, the WHO noted that 40 percent of member countries of the WHO had no mental health policy, and over 30 percent had no mental health program. More than 170 (90%) of member countries had no mental health policy that includes children and adolescents, and many health plans do not cover mental disorders at the same level as other illnesses.

The four countries selected for this comparative study possess both mental health policies and programs for children and adolescents as well as adults; however, parity in insurance and access to appropriate treatment of mental disorders is quite variable among these four countries and among mental health services provided within them. The proportion of total health expenditures allocated to mental health also varies.

The global estimates of prevalence, mortality, and disability caused by mental disorders suggest that the scope of this challenge is not specific to any particular country, though some countries address this challenge more effectively and efficiently than others. It is important to learn from other countries what seems to be working well. Discussion turns now to the four developed countries with advanced mental health systems, which are the focus of this comparative study. Discussion of population statistics is followed by presentation of WHO data on health expenditures.

Overview of the Selected Countries

The estimated world population in 2002 was 6,224,985,000 (WHO, 2004, Table 2, p. 120). The estimated population of 187 of the 191 member countries of the WHO for the following year 2003 was 6,282,436,000. (Calculated from WHO, 2005b, Table 1.1, p. 16). The four countries included in the present comparison accounted for a combined population of about 387 million in 2002 and about 389 million in 2003. Although they constitute a small sample of the global population, they are a representative sample of western industrialized countries with established democratic governments, constitutional law, market economies, national mental health policies, and relatively advanced mental health delivery systems. However, it is wrong to infer that mental disorders are found only in relatively wealthy parts of the world, which these four countries illustrate. Mental disorders are not merely the product of the fast pace of modern, developed, and largely urban societies (WHO, 2001b, p. 23).

Nor is it accurate to infer that other western industrialized societies are less advanced in their mental health services, or that they are identical with one of the four selected for this study in the way that they organize, deliver, and finance mental health services. The four countries included in this study were selected largely because they illustrate a continuum from a highly centralized and publicly financed, national health service in Great Britain (market-minimized) to a predominantly decentralized, and more privately financed market of mental health services in the United States (market-maximized) (Anderson, 1989). In between these two types are examples of national health service and insurance programs in Norway and Canada, which have both similarities and differences between them and with the other two countries. The diversity in mental health infrastructures among just these four countries provides an enlightening perspective on some of the challenges and possibilities for organizing, delivering, and financing mental health services.

Population Statistics

Based on WHO statistics reported for 2003 (WHO, 2005b, Annex Table 1, pp. 174–181) an initial comparison among these four countries can be provided on a few demographic indicators. These are summarized in Table 1.1.

The WHO statistics reported in Table 1.1 reveal a significant range in population size from about 4.5 million in Norway to about 294 million in the United States for the year 2003. That range can help to assess how the size of a society might influence the shape of its mental health system (Deber, 2003). The population growth rates in 2003 were 1.1 percent or less for all four countries, indicating relatively stable population sizes. A significant, but roughly comparable minority of their populations are elderly people. The percentages of men and women aged 60+ years ranged from 16.3 percent in the United States to 20.8 percent in Great Britain. Moreover, the rates of *life expectancy at birth* for men and women combined appear comparable, ranging from 77.0 years in the United States to 80.0 years in Canada. Finally, the rates of *healthy* life expectancy at birth for men and women combined are relatively close, ranging from 69.3 years in the United States to 72.0 years in Norway and Canada, with Great Britain in between at 70.6 years. "Healthy life expectancy" is most easily understood as ". . . the equivalent number of years in full health that a newborn can expect to live based on current rates of ill-health and mortality" (WHO, 2004, p. 96).

This comparison of demographics suggests that apart from population sizes, these four countries have significant similarities. Additional statistics from these member countries of the WHO reveal striking differences in their expenditures on health.

Health Expenditures: Total and Sector Spending

The most recent estimates of health expenditures published by the WHO are for 2002 (WHO, 2005b). Expenditures in both public and private sectors are summarized for the four countries in Table 1.2.

Table 1.1. *Basic Indicators for Four Countries 2003*

Indicator	Great Britain	Norway	Canada	United States
Total population	59,251,000	4,533,000	31,510,000	294,043,000
Annual rate (%) population growth 1993-2003	0.3	0.5	0.9	1.1
Percent of population aged 60+ years	20.8	19.8	17.4	16.3
Total fertility rate	1.6	1.8	1.5	2.1
Under 5 years mortality rate/ 1,000 both sexes	6.0 (5-7)	4.0 (4-5)	6.0 (5-6)	8.0 (7-9)
Life expectancy at birth (years) for both sexes	79.0 (78-79)	79.0 (79-80)	80.0 (79-81)	77.0 (77-78)
Healthy life expectancy at birth (years) in 2002	70.6	72.0	72.0	69.3

Note. Data are abstracted from WHO (2005b). *The World Health Report 2005: Make every mother and child count*, Annex Table 1: Basic indicators for all WHO member states, pp. 174-181. Healthy life expectancy was not recorded in the WHO (2005b) annual report, but was reported in the WHO (2004) annual report. Figures for life expectancy in parentheses represent uncertainty intervals. Adapted with permission by the WHO.

Table 1.2. *Estimated National Expenditures on Health 2002*

Expenditure Estimate	Great Britain	Norway	Canada	United States
Total expenditure on health as % of GDP	7.7	9.6	9.6	14.6
General government expenditures as % of total health expenditures	83.4	83.5	69.9	44.9
Private expenditure on health as % of total health expenditures	16.6	16.5	30.1	55.1
General government health expenditures as % of total government expenditures	15.8	18.1	15.9	23.1
Social security expenditure on health as % of general government expenditures on health	0	0	2.1	30.8
Out-of-pocket expenditures as % of private expenditure on health	55.9	97.2	50.3	25.4
Private prepaid plans as % of private health expenditures	18.6	0	42.1	65.7

Note. Figures are calculated in the national currency units. Data are abstracted from WHO (2005b), Annex Table 5, pp. 192-199. All four countries had 0% of total expenditures on health from external sources, hence that indicator is not included. Adapted with permission by the WHO.

Because these allocations generally include the expenditures for the mental health system, these indicators provide a context for more detailed descriptions and evaluations found in subsequent chapters.

Three indicators reported in Table 1.2 warrant clarification in order to interpret their meaning. These are "total expenditures on health," "general government expenditures," and "gross domestic product."

Total expenditure on health (TEH). Cited in the first three rows of Table 1.2, this indicator is defined as:

> the sum of general government expenditure on health (GGHE commonly called public expenditures on health), and private expenditures on health (PvtHE). All estimates are calculated in millions of national currency units (million NCU). The estimates are presented as ratios to gross domestic product (GDP), to total health expenditure (THE), to total government expenditure (GGE), or to private expenditure on health (PvtHE). (WHO, 2005b, pp. 160–161)

General government expenditure (GGE). Referenced in rows two, four, and five in Table 1.2, GGE is defined to include:

> . . . consolidated direct outlays and indirect outlays (for example, subsidies to producers, transfers to households), including capital of all levels of government (central, federal, provincial, regional, state, district, and municipal, local authorities), social security institutions, autonomous bodies, and other extra budgetary funds. (WHO, 2005b, p. 161)

Gross domestic product (GDP). Cited in row one of Table 1.2, GDP is:

> . . . the value of all goods and services provided in a country by residents and nonresidents without regard to their allocation among domestic and foreign claims. This (with small adjustments), corresponds to the total sum of expenditures (consumption and investment) of the private and government agents of the economy during the referenced year. (WHO, 2005b, p. 161)

The first striking difference among these four countries evident in Table 1.2 (row one) is the variability in their *total expenditures* on health as a percentage of their gross domestic product. Percentages range from a low of 7.7 percent in Great Britain to a high of 14.6 percent in the United States.[1] On this indicator, the United States is nearly double that of Great Britain. Norway at 9.6 percent and Canada at 9.6 percent are both closer to Great Britain than to the United States. The much higher percentage of expenditures on health by the United States raises a question: Does the population of the United States enjoy nearly twice as much access and utilization, or twice the quality and effectiveness of their mental health services than the population of Great Britain, and proportionately more than Norway and Canada? This type of cost/benefit question will be addressed in subsequent chapters.

A second striking difference among these four countries is the *government expenditures* on health as a percentage of the total national expenditure on health (Table 1.2, row two). Great Britain (83.4%) and Norway (83.5%) were nearly double the United States (44.9%). Canada (69.9%) was 25 percent higher than the United States, and closer to the other two countries. The statistics indicate the dominance of public expenditures over private expenditures for health in three of the four countries with the exception of the United States. How do the differences on this indicator impact access, quality, equity, and efficiency of the delivery and financing of mental health services? While none of the contributing authors are economists, their descriptions and evaluations of their own mental health system in comparisons with the other three countries will provide suggestive hypotheses as well as informed judgments.

Thirdly, the relative dominance of the private sector in the United States (55.1%) versus the other three countries is consistent with the previous indicator. *Private expenditure* on health is defined by the WHO as ". . . the sum of expenditures by four primary entities: (a) prepaid and risk-pooling arrangements, (b) corporations' expenditure on health, (c) nonprofit institutions serving mainly households, and (d) household out-of-pocket spending for all health-related goods and services" (WHO, 2004, pp. 100–101). Table 1.2 (row three) indicates that private expenditures on health as a percentage of total national expenditure on health in 2002 is about three times higher in the United States (55.1%) than in Great Britain (16.6%) and Norway (16.5%), and about 25 percent higher than Canada (30.1%).

Fourth, the *percentage of government expenditures on health* relative to total *government* expenditures were surprisingly comparable, ranging from 15.8 percent in Great Britain to 23.1 percent in the United States (Table 1.2, row four). The rates vary less than eight percent among all four countries, with Canada (15.9%) and Norway (18.1%) both closer to Great Britain.

Fifth, only the United States utilized *Social Security expenditures* on health as a significant percent (30.8%) of general government expenditures on health. Canada's was only 2.1 percent. The other two countries spent none from social security funds, or reported none. Although the United States government has discrete financial accounts for public health care programs such as Medicare and Medicaid, the state

---

1. Other data from the Organization of Economic Cooperation and Development (OECD) estimate that total health expenditures for the United States increased from 13% of GDP in 1997 to 14.6% in 2002, compared to the average 13% of all 30 member countries (OECD, 2004).

children's health insurance plan, federal employees, military personnel and veterans, the substantial use of social security funding for health care appears to be unique to the United States. Three major factors account for this expenditure: (a) Social Security disability benefits are paid to people who cannot work because they have a medical condition that is expected to last at least one year or result in death; (b) for children under 18 and adult citizens and nationals who are blind, disabled, or poor, and for poor elderly people age 65 and older, the federal Social Security Administration makes payments to supplement income (SSI) to help pay for health costs and other expenses (SSA, 2004); (c) Medicare premiums are deducted from Social Security payments. Unfortunately, surplus revenues in social security retirement funds have been used (or misused) to fund other federal government programs.

The sixth and seventh indicators refer to private expenditures on health. *Out-of-pocket expenditures* as a percent of total *private* expenditures (Table 1.2, row six) varied considerably from a high of 97.2 percent in Norway to a low of 25.4 percent in the United States. The latter was about half the percentages for Great Britain (55.9%) and Canada (50.3%). It would appear that it is much more costly for people in Great Britain, Norway, and Canada to opt out of their publicly financed health care system, or to purchase private health insurance, and to pay for health care in their private sectors. In the United States, individual employees bear about one-fourth of the cost of private expenditures for their health care. That figure would be substantially higher if employers were not paying health insurance premiums for their employees. In the private sector of the United States, a voluntary, employment-based health insurance system is the dominant system over private individual plans or other private group plans.

Seventh and finally, there is a very striking difference among these four countries in the role of *private, prepaid health plans.* Prepaid health plans (and risk-pooling arrangements) are health plans defined by the WHO to include the following:

> . . . the outlays of (a) private insurance, (b) private social insurance arrangements (with no government control over payment rates and participating providers, but with broad guidelines), (c) commercial and nonprofit [mutual] insurance plans, (d) health maintenance organizations, and (e) other agents managing prepaid medical and paramedical benefits (including the operating costs of these arrangements. (WHO, 2004, p. 100)

As a percentage of all expenditures in the private sector, the expenditures of private, prepaid plans in 2002 was 65.7 percent in the United States, 42.1 percent in Canada, and 18.6 percent in Great Britain. No data were reported for Norway, but private prepaid health plans play an insignificant role in its publicly financed health care system. As a cost-containment and risk-pooling strategy, prepaid health plans have a much more substantial presence in the private sector of health care in the United States than in private sectors in the other three countries. Prepaid plans have been adopted also by several American states to administer their Medicaid programs, which are financed jointly by both the federal government and the states, though administered by the states.

Per Capita Expenditures on Health

The differences among these four countries in their expenditures for all health goods and services become even more striking when measured levels of per capita expenditures are compared. The latter statistics for the four countries for the year 2002 are summarized in Table 1.3.

Table 1.3. *Per Capita Health Expenditures 2002*

Indicator	Great Britain	Norway	Canada	United States
Total expenditures on health per capita	2,031	4,033	2,222	5,274
Government expenditure on health per capita	1,693	3,366	1,552	2,368
Percent of total per capita expenditure spent on health by government	83.4	83.5	69.8	44.9

Note. The estimated figures are expressed at the average exchange rate in U.S. dollars. Figures from the first two rows are abstracted from *The World Health Report 2005: Make Every Mother and Child Count,* Annex Table 6, pp. 200-203 (WHO, 2005b). Adapted with permission by the WHO.

The per capita ratios in Table 1.3 were calculated by dividing the expenditure figures by population estimates for each country. The per capita figures cited are expressed in U.S. dollars at an "average exchange rate," which is defined by WHO as ". . . the observed annual average number of units at which a currency is traded in the banking system" (WHO, 2004, p. 101).

The rank order of *per capita total expenditures* on health for 2002 (Table 1.3, row one) is the United States ($5,274), Norway ($4,033), Canada ($2,222), and Great Britain ($2,031). Per capita expenditures on health in the United States were more than double that spent by Great Britain, and exceeded the other three countries by at least $1,241.[2] The striking per capita differences raise once again the question of whether Americans experience benefits, access, and quality of mental health care proportional to the significantly higher per capita expenditures on health in general. That question will be addressed subsequently by contributing authors and especially in the chapter on the U.S. system.

A second indicator in Table 1.3 (rows two and three) reveals another striking difference between the United States and the other three countries on the sources of expenditure. The rank order of *per capita governmental* expenditures on health for 2002 was Norway ($3,366), the United States ($2,368), Great Britain ($1,693) and Canada ($1,552). However, when the percentage of *total* per capita expenditures on health spent by the *governments* is calculated, the United States (44.9%) had the lowest compared to Canada (69.8%), Great Britain (83.4%) and Norway (83.5%). The differences in percentages support the conclusion that the primary source for financing health care is public, with the exception of the United States, where more than half of all health expenditures in 2002 were in the private sector.

It is unfortunate that the WHO does not routinely publish in its annual reports the same indicators just reviewed of expenditures by countries for mental health services as a separate category of all health expenditures. Mental health expenditure data have not been included in annual reports by the WHO in the years 2000 through 2004, not even in the 2001 annual report devoted specifically to mental health. The reader must rely upon the national economic indicators reported in subsequent chapters in this volume. The sixth chapter will include comparisons of data presented for the individual countries on whatever indicators they share in common. In order to make comparisons among them, contributing authors will include all expenditures expressed in their own country's currency with conversions into U. S. dollars based on the "average exchange rate" reported by the United States Federal Reserve Bank for the year the expenditures are reported.

Comparative Domains and Evaluation Criteria

The contributing authors have accepted a twofold challenge: to describe and to evaluate their country's system for delivering and financing mental health services. This is a daunting task, and the authors are to be commended for the time and expertise they have volunteered to this project in order to provide a more global, comparative perspective among a sample of developed countries with mental health policies and advanced mental health systems.

In the descriptions and evaluations of their own country's mental health system, the authors have been guided by several considerations, which might be summarized by Rudyard Kipling's phrase from his poem, *The Elephant's Child:* "I keep six honest servingmen: (they taught me all I knew). Their names are what and where and when, and how and why and who. . . ." To know who provides what mental health services to whom, how, where, when, and why is to gain a good introduction to the system presented. Nevertheless, more is required to describe and to evaluate them relative to one another. A common set of criteria has been adopted for a more comprehensive and comparative assessment.

The definition of a mental health system suggests relevant domains for its description and evaluation. Structural domains include the public and private organizations, institutions, and resources that produce actions whose primary purpose is to improve the mental health of the country's population. The country's financing system and work force plans are also essential and are discussed separately in each chapter.

In addition to these structural variables, the processes by which members of the society attain access, promote quality, contain costs, and pay for the mental health system are referenced in the common chapter outline. Evaluative judgments may be included in these discussions, though they are stated more explicitly and intentionally in Part Two of each

---

2. According to other current data, total health spending in the United States reached $5,267 per capita in 2002, almost 140% above the average of $2,144 among 30 developed countries, who constitute the membership of the Organization for Economic Cooperation and Development (OECD, 2004).

chapter according to the following evaluation criteria: access/equity, quality/efficacy, cost/efficiency, financing/fairness, protection/participation, and population relevance.

These criteria are representative of the values and standards addressed in much of the literature on health services research. The list of criteria is neither comprehensive nor exclusive of other standards or values pertinent to the performance appraisal of mental health systems. Contributing authors could apply additional criteria, which they believed important.

Although this book is an illustration of health services research (Whitener, Van Horne, and Gauthier, 2005), and the contributing authors are all social scientists, the domains and criteria selected for comparison are expressions of values. For example, universal access to high quality care at affordable cost and fairly financed are all terms that function as values by which mental health systems can be judged as relatively good or better in meeting the needs of those with identified mental disorders. These criteria function also as goals or ends, which have been construed in moral philosophy as "nonmoral values," distinguished conceptually from moral values (virtues) (Frankena, 1973). The values that underlie and guide selection of the ends and means of a mental health system are expressed in the country's culture, mental health policies, program purposes, laws and regulations, and health expenditures. An example is the list of values, which constituted the ethical foundation for the federal plan formulated by the White House Domestic Policy Council (1993) for national health care reform championed by President Clinton, but defeated by numerous private health industry interests. The values included universal access, comprehensive benefits, consumer choice, equality of care, fair distribution of costs, personal responsibility, intergenerational justice, wise allocation of resources, effectiveness, quality, effective management, professional integrity and responsibility, fair procedures, and local responsibility.

Mental health systems differ both in their ranking of ends as well as the means they adopt to achieve their selected ends. For example, a mental health system might emphasize the values (ends) of cost-containment and efficiency over quality and effectiveness, or prescribe particular strategies (means) for delivering mental health services (e.g., private managed behavioral health organizations or public, regional psychiatric centers), or specific strategies for financing these services (e.g., income, payroll, or health taxes versus premiums paid to private, prepaid health plans). The main point here is that insofar as social scientists address human problems and systems, an ethical perspective is as relevant as a functional description. Nevertheless, it is also important to provide an objective description of the mental health system and to avoid a biased presentation due to implicit value judgments.

Chapter Outline

To encourage an objective description and a separate evaluation, each chapter is divided into three major sections: Description, Evaluation, and Recommendations. To facilitate comparisons among the selected countries, the following chapter outline has been adopted by contributing authors:

Part One: Description
    A. Introduction
    B. The Need for Mental Health Services
    C. Policies and Programs
    D. Delivery System(s)
    E. Financing System(s)
Part Two: Evaluation
    A. Access and Equity
    B. Quality and Efficacy
    C. Cost and Efficiency
    D. Financing and Fairness
    E. Protection and Participation
    F. Population Relevance
Part Three: Recommendations

Part One: Description

Introduction. The chapters begin with a brief description of the country's geographic and demographic characteristics, and its political and economic system. Cultural values relevant to the purposes, policies, and mental health programs are noted. A brief history and overview of the country's health care system is provided as the context in which the mental health system resides and functions.

The Need for Mental Health Services. The second section of each chapter addresses the indicators of the need for mental health services in the population. National prevalence data are presented as point, period, and/or lifetime occurrences of all mental disorders combined, and by specific categories of major mental disorders. Where data are available, prevalence rates are cited for all males and females (separately and combined) for the following mental disorders: unipolar depression, bipolar affective disorder, schizophrenia, alcohol use disorders, drug use disorders, post-traumatic stress, obsessive-compulsive disorders, panic disorders, and primary insomnia. These are the major neuropsychiatric disorders included in the WHO prevalence data, *excluding* epilepsy, Parkinson's disease, multiple sclerosis, and migraine disorders, which are commonly construed primarily as physical-neurological disorders. Data on other mental disorders may be included by chapter authors. Our authors were asked to present prevalence data on the above mental disorders by gender and age groups: children and adolescents (0–17 years), adults (18–59), and for older adults (60+ years), and for all years combined, consistent with WHO age groupings. (Statistics from some countries may classify elderly as 65+ years and other adults as 18–64 years).

Prevalence is an ambiguous measure of the need for mental health services apart from information on the severity, distress, and disability associated with the disorders (Mechanic, 2003). The major mental disorders included in the list of neuropsychiatric disorders (e.g., schizophrenia and major affective disorders) provide an estimate of severity. As a further estimate of the burden of disease, international statistics and/or current national statistics are cited by contributing authors on the death and disability associated with mental disorders.

If available, the numbers and percentages of the population on mental health disability or workman's compensation due to a mental disorder will be cited, along with other indicators selected by authors to estimate the scope of the challenge presented by mental disorders and to document the need for mental health services in their country.

Policies and Programs. The third section in Part One of each chapter is a description of some of the primary federal policies and programs. National mental health *policies* expressed in policy documents, laws and federal regulations are germane here, both in terms of benefits (coverage) and eligibility criteria for public and private mental health programs. Examples include privacy laws, statutory definitions of "medically necessary" mental health services, parity legislation, civil commitment legislation, and patient rights and protection regulations. Policies pertinent to patient protection and participation are evaluated in a later section under that title in Part Two of each chapter. Although health policy usually includes reference to mechanisms for financing health programs, the question of how these public and private programs are funded is discussed subsequently in the section on financing systems.

The public and private *programs* designed to implement mental health policies are described in this third section of each chapter on policies and programs; they are evaluated subsequently in Part Two of each chapter according to the selected criteria. This third section helps to answer the questions about who is eligible for which benefits/services provided through what types of programs.

Program descriptions are important because programs can vary in the degree to which they actually implement stated policies and standards. For example, Medicare is a national health insurance program for elderly, disabled, and kidney dialysis patients in the United States. Medicare policy entitles all eligible beneficiaries to the same benefit package, which is supposed to include all reasonable and necessary items and services for inpatient and outpatient health care, and effective January 2006, a prescription drug benefit. Medicare policies are implemented through both fee-for-service programs and increasingly through private managed care organizations. Unfortunately, the federal reimbursement program and decentralized administration of the programs through numerous private fiscal intermediaries and carriers for inpatient and outpatient services respectively has resulted in variability in both the equity and quality of services provided throughout the country (Feenberg and Skinner, 2000; Foote, Wholey, Rockwood, and Halpern, 2004; Skinner and Elliot, 1997).

Our authors may cite a particular state/province/region/district to illustrate how federal policies and programs are implemented in a smaller geographic region of the country. For example, the editor's home state of Minnesota, with a population about the size of Norway, has the second or third highest penetration of managed care organizations (MCOs) among all states. A very small number of very large MCOs dominate the private sector of health care services, and increasingly control services provided to the state's medical assistance and general assistance population. The medical assistance program is this state's version of the federal and state funded Medicaid program for low income families and nursing home care for the elderly. States have the power to mandate which mental health benefits will be included in both governmental and commercial health insurance plans, with the exception of self-insured plans, which are being adopted at an increasing rate by private employers, partly because under another federal statute, the Employee Retirement Income Security Act of 1997 (ERISA), these employers are exempt from state mandated benefits including coverage for mental health and substance abuse services (Hellinger and Young, 2005). Moreover, the Minnesota State Department of Health has obtained waivers allowing it to require medical assistance and general assistance enrollees to receive services from private, prepaid health plans.

Delivery System. The fourth section of Part One provides organizational comparisons among mental health systems. Both structures and processes are described in this next section about how the mental health systems are organized and how services are actually delivered. This fourth section is a more complete description of what mental health services are delivered, how, when, where, and by whom. The section may be organized according to major programs listed in the previous section or across programs if they are more alike than different. A brief historical perspective may be provided on the development of mental health services in the country.

Services provided by general medical personnel in *primary care* settings are described first, followed by descriptions of the *specialized* delivery systems for diagnosis and treatment services for children and adolescents, adults, and elderly in public and in private sectors.

Two examples of publicly financed, specialized delivery systems are Norway's organization of public mental health services into district psychiatric centers with both inpatient and outpatient services, and community mental health centers in the United States.

Descriptions of the delivery of specialized mental health services includes demographic data on mental health specialists. Total numbers, ratios to total population and to mental health prevalence are presented along with comments on the regional distribution of mental health specialists. In this section, the authors also discuss educational/certification/licensure requirements for mental health professionals to participate as independent practitioners, and address any additional requirements for them to qualify for public and/or private insurance reimbursement. Examples from the United States are requirements set by managed behavioral health care organizations to certify mental health professionals as acceptable "preferred providers," whose services cost enrollees less in deductibles and co-payments than the same services provided by specialists who are not a part of the health plans' approved panel of providers. In Canada, licensed psychologists employed by hospitals participate in the national health insurance program (Medicare), but private practicing psychologists (and other non-physician mental health specialists) do not qualify for Medicare reimbursement.

For both public and private sectors, this section addresses questions about which mental health professionals are permitted to participate in the mental health system, how many do, and how these personnel are distributed throughout the country (e.g., urban versus rural areas).

Finally, where available, statistics are presented on numbers and percentages of regulatory and administrative personnel in public and private health sectors and plans, in medical clinics, general medical hospitals, and in mental health specialty facilities. Descriptions in this section provide a basis for the subsequent evaluation of how efficiently a mental health system operates to allocate limited *human* resources.

Financing Systems. The fifth section of Part One in each chapter is a description of the financing system(s). The mechanisms for financing the previously described programs and services are discussed here. Do mental health policies and mandated programs stipulate how they are funded and who pays how much for what services?

Discussion of *public* funding mechanisms precedes private financing systems. Illustrations of the former include estimates of the amounts and/or percentages of income or payroll taxes paid for public mental health services, and whether these (or other) health taxes are progressive or regressive. Thereafter, *private* sector expenditures are presented. Examples might include employer-based insurance; illustrations of other group and individual insurance plans; examples of types of private managed care plans (health maintenance organizations, preferred provider organizations, independent practice associations); estimated average amounts for insurance premiums, co-pays, and deductibles charged to patients with mental disorders compared to other medical patients; hardship funding provided by private companies and foundations; noncompensated care by private hospital emergency rooms and by mental health providers in private practice. Figures are expressed in both the national currency and converted to U.S. dollars at the current average annual exchange rate for the year data are reported.

Finally, what are the predominant *cost-containment mechanisms* applied in this country's mental health system? Examples include centralized planning and administration, budgeting, price controls and regulated fee schedules, utilization review procedures and organizations, provider discounts, user co-payments, and deductibles, and market forces of supply and demand.

Part Two: Evaluation

This second major section of each chapter is the authors' assessment of their own mental health system. Following mention of any national program evaluations conducted previously or currently, six major criteria provide the organization for this section: (a) Access and equity, (b) quality and efficacy, (c) cost and efficiency, (d) financing and fairness, (e) protection and participation, and (f) population relevance.

Access and Equity. The first criterion of access and equity is addressed with respect to both public and private sectors of the mental health system. Does the system provide access to comprehensive coverage for all types of mental disorders and for appropriate levels of service? What disorders and/or services are excluded? Is there universal access to the covered mental health services? Are mental health service centers (clinics, hospitals) located and operating conveniently for clients? Is there parity between mental health and medical patients? For example, are the criteria limiting the number of sessions of outpatient psychotherapy the same or different for treatments with patients presenting physical illnesses and injuries?

Data on *utilization* of mental health services and level of services is one source of relevant information for this assessment. Particular attention is given to the utilization of mental health services by women, children, and elderly adults (60+years), minority groups, military personnel and veterans, indigenous populations and immigrants, to help assess the degree to which there could be unintended neglect, discrimination, and/or inequitable rationing of services. Are there statistics on numbers and percentages of prison populations with mental disorders? Do these numbers suggest that "criminalization" and incarceration in jails has become an alternative to specialized mental health treatment? Are mental health services provided to incarcerated prisoners?

Since the 1990s, confronting health inequities has become a priority for health policy makers at both national and international levels. Attention focused on socioeconomic determinants of health has led to conceptual distinctions between health disparities/inequalities and health inequity/inequity (Casas-Zamora and Ibrahim, 2004). Both concepts address the question of whether people are treated fairly by their health care systems. These distinctions aside, the criterion of equity does not require that identical services be provided to all potential recipients of mental health services, but that some equivalence is evident in the type and level of service, based on actual need or type, duration, and severity of mental disorder, irrespective of the individual's racial or ethnic group, gender, sexual orientation, age, religion, or history of prior conditions and treatments (Daniels, 1982; Whitehead, 1992). Do all people with mental disorders have relatively equal access to appropriate mental health services in this country's system? Who are the underserved, underinsured, and uninsured? What are the estimates of their numbers and percentages of the total population, and of the population with identified mental disorders? A more summative assessment of unmet need is provided subsequently by contributing authors in Part Two of their chapters under the criterion of population relevance.

Quality and Efficacy. What is the quality of mental health services provided through this country's mental health system? Authors address this evaluation criterion by illustrating some of the quality assessment and quality improvement strategies adopted, and some types of measures employed – structure, process, and/or outcome measures. Since appraisals of the performance of a mental health system will depend partly upon the perspective of the respondent (WHO, 2000, p. vii), evaluations by various stakeholders in the mental health system may be illustrated: Clients, clinicians, payers, managers, regulators, and government agencies.

Practice guidelines, implementation of evidence-based practices, and professional ethical codes are structural indicators of quality, in addition to accreditation programs for mental health service organizations, and certification or licensure standards for mental health professionals.

A high quality mental health system would provide integrated services and continuity of care. Are mental health services fully integrated with primary health care services? Are community mental health centers or regional treatment centers integrated effectively with other health agencies and with primary health care professionals? Is there an easy transition from one level of service to the next? For example, is there consistent outpatient follow-up for hospitalized mental health patients discharged into the community? Are there any data on hospital recidivism rates for the severely and chronically mentally ill? What kind of support services are provided in addition to mental health services?

Cost and Efficiency. The third major criterion for evaluating mental health systems is cost and efficiency. Here the authors cite estimated expenditures for the entire health care system and for mental health/substance abuse services, percents of gross domestic product, per capita costs, estimated costs in lost productivity due to mental disorders and/or mental health disability costs. Where available, estimates will be provided of the costs to employers of both treated and untreated mental disorders, along with "medical offset" costs. Costs/expenditures are listed in both the country's currency and converted to U.S. dollars based on the average annual exchange rate for the year the data are reported.

If possible, national expenditures for outpatient, partial hospitalization, (day treatment), inpatient, and residential mental health care will be cited separately and summed, along with references to the expenditures for psychotropic medications. Further sources of estimated costs are expenditures for health insurance premiums paid by government, private employers, employees, and individuals, including estimates of out-of-pocket costs such as deductibles and co-payments by recipients of mental health services compared with patients receiving other medical services.

As an indication of efficiency, estimated *administrative personnel and costs* are cited for public and for private sector programs and entities such as general and psychiatric hospitals, public and/or private clinics, or managed behavioral health care organizations. Estimates of waste, fraud, or abuse, and mechanisms for controlling them are also relevant. The two general questions addressed by this criterion are: *First,* to what degree are mental health services affordable both to the country as a whole and to sectors of the population, and, *secondly,* how efficiently are resources being allocated and managed? Implicit in these questions is the issue of rationing of mental health resources.

Financing and Fairness. Since the criterion of efficiency relates also to the system for financing the mental health system, relevant questions addressed in this section are how the mental health system is paid for, whether there is a fair distribution of costs, and fiscally responsible allocation of resources for both current services and for research for program evaluation, quality improvement, and treatment innovation. Is there a "fiscal gap" between benefits promised and available funding? An example of the latter is the *unfunded* prescription benefit legislated in 2004 as an amendment to the federal Medicare program, which is the single-payer, national health insurance plan for about 42 million elderly (65+ years) and disabled individuals in the United States.

Protection and Participation. At the level of professional-user interactions, the *protection* criterion addresses issues of patient safety (e.g., suicide prevention) and protection from incompetent or unethical providers, or from other forms of exploitation or abuse of the mentally ill. Patient rights to informed consent and to privacy and confidentiality are germane considerations. Legislation and regulations may be cited with respect to patients' rights to access appropriate care, to appeal treatment decisions, and even to refuse treatment. Protections of individual rights in civil commitments or involuntary treatment regimens, and insanity defenses in criminal cases are cited. For mental health patients who are judged incompetent, principles and procedures for courts to appoint guardians of their personal welfare and/or conservators of their finances are also relevant in this discussion. What are the policies, procedures, and practices that protect the rights of people with mental disorders? Are protections implemented consistently and effectively?

At the level of direct services, patient *participation* refers to the degree to which a recipient of mental health services participates in the decision to seek treatment, in the development and implementation of treatment plans and strategies, and in decisions to terminate treatment. At a systems level, this criterion raises the question about the degree to which there is genuine representation of all stakeholders, democratic decision-making, and shared power and responsibility in formulating mental health policies. Are policy decisions about the allocation and administration of mental health resources made by elected representatives, appointed regulators, mental health professionals, patients, or payers? Who decides which benefits will be provided by whom, to whom, and at what cost? Are policy decisions made at a national, regional, provincial, district, state, or local level? How are mental health policies changed? Who holds and actually uses the power to effect change in the mental health system? Is the system "of the people, by the people, and for the people?"

Population Relevance. The sixth and final criterion for evaluation is an overall assessment by authors of the extent to which identified needs for mental health services are met by the present mental health system. Is the system providing sufficient and appropriate services relevant to the population's identified mental health needs? This is a summative evaluation related to the general problem of a "treatment gap" between identified needs and provided services. The authors' evaluations based on the previous five criteria are subsumed under this sixth criterion to support their concluding, general appraisal of their mental health system. All six major evaluation criteria just discussed were selected because of their frequent application in mental health services research, and because they constitute common values addressed in most mental health policies and systems.

Part Three: Recommendations

The final major section of each chapter consists of the authors' recommendations for improvement of the system through which their own country delivers and finances mental health services. These recommendations may be summarized first in terms of the six major evaluation criteria previously discussed: Access and equity, quality and efficacy, cost and efficiency, financing and fairness, protection and participation, and population relevance. Additional recommendations are offered subsequently based upon the authors' knowledge gained as a result of their own experience and research, and their review of relevant literature. The authors were invited to include international data cited by the World Health Organization or by the Organization for Economic Cooperation and Development, in addition to reports of national statistics and program evaluations. Authors' judgments may reference what they have learned from their colleagues who have written about the other three countries. The chapter concludes with a listing of references in Part Four.

Our Authors and Audience

Our Authors

Brief biographical sketches about the authors are provided at the front of this book to highlight their particular qualifications as contributors. Additional comments are provided here. The contributing authors of this work are psychologists. All of them obtained their Ph.D. from accredited universities within their own country. Collectively their professional careers have included clinical practice, supervision and consultation, research and teaching, administration, mental health policy formulation and advocacy work. None of the authors was trained initially in public health administration, nor in health economics or primarily in health services research. Most authors began as providers of mental health services in clinical settings, and moved into complementary positions and roles relevant to the present study of mental health systems. All of them have direct experience with their country's mental health system. Most have less experience and knowledge about how other countries have delivered and financed mental health services, hence each one has learned from the other contributing authors as a result of this international dialogue.

All of the contributors are published authors, and all have been active in a variety of professional and advocacy organizations in varying degrees. Two of our authors are past presidents of their national psychological associations; three have served as research consultants to their government's mental health system, and one has served as a consultant to the Australian Parliament.

Although authors from other mental health professions such as psychiatry, psychiatric nursing, and social work have not contributed to this volume, these professions are included in the discussion of mental health personnel, and in some instances, as sources for evaluation of the mental health system.

The authors share both genuine and legitimate concerns about their country's mental health system. Their concerns illustrate a population-based, public health perspective, broader in scope than the biopsychosocial model of mental disorders, which they also endorse. Although their contributions to this book have emphasized the delivery and financing of mental health services, they are also concerned about the prevention of mental disorders and the promotion of mental health as integral to the economic and social well-being of their societies.

Particular attention has been given to both a description of their mental health system, and to an evaluation based on multiple, common criteria, followed by recommendations for improved performance of their system. Their acceptance of common evaluation criteria reflect shared values, and their recommendations for improvement of their mental health systems reflect their commitments to health care reform to enhance human welfare and to advance social justice for people suffering with mental disorders. It has been a privilege to work with this group of distinguished colleagues, all of whom illustrate how the range of competent concern of professional psychologists extends beyond the consulting room with individual clients. Nevertheless, the chapters that follow reflect the authors' primary commitment to the welfare of clients who receive mental health services.

The reader will not find here any minimizing of system deficiencies by our contributing authors. While each author is rightly proud of the strengths of their own system, they are also critical of its limitations, and particularly the commonly experienced treatment gap between those who need mental health services versus the significantly smaller number who actually receive them. Nevertheless, we are optimistic that our mental health systems can be improved, and we hope that this book will inform decision-makers and clinicians to help implement needed improvements for the common good.

Our Audience

Our intended audience includes practitioners from all mental health professions, especially clinical, counseling, and health psychologists; mental health program administrators and managers; academic professionals teaching graduate level courses related to professional training and public health policy and financing; researchers in the area of mental health services; state and federal regulators; government representatives and policymakers; and mental health advocacy groups. A secondary audience is a college-educated public interested in mental health policy, delivery, and financing.

The primary objective of this book is to provide in one volume a description and evaluation of mental health systems in selected industrialized countries in terms of six primary criteria: access and equity, quality and efficacy, cost and efficiency, financing and fairness, protection and participation, and population relevance. This book is intended to educate readers about a variety of mental health systems within developed countries, and about both their relative strengths and limitations when compared with other systems on several criteria relevant to the delivery and financing of mental health systems. Evaluations provide the basis for recommendations for improvement in each system.

The book begins with a focus on a highly centralized, publicly financed mental health system in Great Britain as an integral part of its state-run National Health Service. Norway's publicly financed and centrally administered mental health system is closer to Britain's system than to Canada's decentralized, national health insurance system administered by its Provinces and Territories. Lastly, we present the most decentralized and most privately financed system in the United States. The sixth chapter notes convergence and divergence among the mental health systems described. The final chapter addresses unmet needs and offers conclusions and recommendations.

A personal note brings this introduction to a close. This book has its roots in the editor's experience as a clinician working for several years in the American mental health system, and in my subsequent roles as a dean and professor in a practitioner-oriented graduate program for doctoral level clinical psychologists. The idea for this book was precipitated by my growing awareness that our own educational system for training mental health professionals has been slow to respond to the dramatic changes that have occurred in the past decades in the nation's mental health system. Graduate curricula for mental health professionals are sometimes shaped more by past academic and professional traditions than by inspiring, but realistic visions of the future roles of professional psychologists in a reformed mental health system. As a professor, I have attempted to help my students understand how the present system works, and how to work the system for the benefit of their future clients.

Over the past decade I have become more keenly aware of the shortcomings of the American system, and I felt that I also needed to encourage the next generation to critique and reform the present system. The conclusion by the President's New Freedom Commission on Mental Health (2003) that the American mental health system is fragmented and in disarray supports the need for reform.

In my search for alternative models, I became convinced that we could learn a great deal from the way other countries organize, deliver, and finance their mental health systems. I am gratified to have found experts with a shared systems and public health perspective to write about their own mental health systems to help advance our understanding of both the convergence and divergence among them. All of our contributors have volunteered for this project because they accept as one of our professional ethical obligations the duty to promote public welfare. We hope our readers will be inspired to assume the same obligation to advance health care reforms, which will provide all those with mental disorders high quality mental health services at affordable cost, financed fairly, and delivered efficiently and effectively. Health care justice for the mentally ill is one of the major human rights issues of our time. It will remain so for decades to come. There is a great deal of work to be done. The reader will find in this book informed judgments about what work needs to be done and insights about some of the better ways to do it.

REFERENCES

American Psychiatric Association (APA) (2000). *Diagnostic and statistical manual of mental disorders* (DSM-IV-TR). 4th ed. Washington D.C.: Author.

Anderson, O. (1989). *The health services continuum in democratic states.* Ann Arbor, Michigan: Health Administration Press.

Ashley, D., & Orenstein, D. M. (1990). *Sociological theory: Classical statements.* Boston: Allyn and Bacon.

Boutros-Ghali, B. (1995). *Remarks at Launch of World Mental Health: Problems and priorities in low-income countries.* New York: United Nations.

Casas-Zamora, J. A., & Ibrahim, S. A. (2004). Confronting health inequity: The global dimension. *American Journal of Public Health, 94*(12), 2055–2058.

Cowen, E. L. (1994). The enhancement of psychological wellness: Challenges and opportunities. *American Journal of Community Psychology, 22*(2), 149–179.

Daniels, N. (1982). Equity of access to health care: Some conceptual and ethical issues. *Milbank Memorial Fund Quarterly, 60*(1), 51–81.

Deber, R. B. (2003). Health care reform: Lessons from Canada. *American Journal of Public Health, 93*(1), 20–24.

Department of Health and Human Services (DHHS) (1999a). *Mental health: A report of the surgeon general.* Rockville, Maryland: Author.

Department of Health and Human Services (DHHS) (1999b). *Mental health: A report of the surgeon general. Executive summary.* Rockville, Maryland: Author.

Feenberg, D., & Skinner, J. (2000). Federal Medicare transfers across states: Winners and losers. *National Tax Journal, 52*, 713–732.

Foote, S. B., Wholey, D., Rockwood, T., & Halpern, R. (2004). Resolving the tug-of-war between Medicare's national and local coverage. *Health Affairs, 23*(4), 108–123.

Frankena, Wm. (1973). *Ethics.* 2nd ed. Englewood Cliffs, New Jersey: Prentice Hall.

Global Forum for Health Research (1999). *Community-based interventions in neuro-psychiatry, 99.* Geneva: Author.

Gulbinat, W.H., Manderscheid, R. W., Beigel, A., Costa, E., & Silva, J. A. (1996). A multinational strategy on mental health policy and care: A WHO collaborative initiative and consultative program. In M. Moscarelli, A. Rupp, & N. Sartorius (Eds.). *Schizophrenia – Handbook of Mental Health Economics and Health Policy* (pp. 531–535). Chichester, England: John Wiley & Sons.

Gulbinat, W. H., Manderscheid, R., Baingana, F., et al. (2004). The international consortium on mental health policy and services: Objectives, design and project implementation. *International Review of Psychiatry, 16*(1–2), 5–17.

Hellinger, F. J., & Young, G. J. (2005). Health plan liability and ERISA: The expanding scope of state legislation. *American Journal of Public Health, 95*(2), 217–223.

Insel, T. R., & Fenton, W. S. (2005). Psychiatric epidemiology: It's not just about counting anymore. *Archives of General Psychiatry, 62*, 590–592.

Institute of Medicine (2001). *Neurological, psychiatric and developmental disorders: Meeting the challenge in the developing world.* Washington, DC: National Academy Press.

Jenkins, R., & Knapp, M. (1996). Use of health economic data by health administrators in national health systems. In M. Moscarelli, A. Rupp, & N. Sartorius (Eds.), *The Handbook of Mental Health Economics and Health Policy* (pp. 553–510). Chichester, England: John Wiley & Sons.

Jenkins, R., Gulbinat, W., Manderscheid, R., et al. (2004). The mental health country profile: Background, design and use of a systematic method of appraisal. *International Review of Psychiatry, 16*(1–2), 31–47.

Jenkins, R., McCulloch, A., & Parker, C. (1998). *Nations for mental health: supporting governments and policy-makers.* (WHO/MSA/NAM/97.5, 1–24). Geneva, Switzerland: World Health Organization.

Kessler, R. C., Berglund, P., Demler, O., Jin, R., & Walters, E. (2005). Lifetime prevalence and age-of-onset distributions of DSM-IV disorders in the national comorbidity survey replication. *Archives of General Psychiatry, 62*, 593–602.

Kessler, R. C., McGonagle, K.A., Zhao, S., et al., (1994). Lifetime and 12-month prevalence of DSM-III-R psychiatric disorders in the United States: results from the National Comorbity Survey. *Archives of General Psychiatry, 51*, 8–19.

Kipling, R. (na). *The Elephant's Child.* Retrieved January 20, 2005 from http://www.online-literature.com/kipling/165/

Manderscheid, R. W. (1998). From many into one: Addressing the crisis of quality in managed behavioral health care at the millennium. *Journal of Behavioral Health Services Research, 25*(2), 233–237.

Mechanic, D. (2003). Is the prevalence of mental disorders a good measure of the need for services? *Health Affairs, 22*(5), 8–20.

Mechanic, D., & Bilder, S. (2004). Treatment of people with mental illness: A decade-long perspective. *Health Affairs, 23*(4), 84–95.

Murray, C. L., & Lopez, A. D. (Eds.) (1996). *The global burden of disease. A comprehensive assessment of mortality and disability from diseases, injuries, and risk factors in 1990 and projected to 2020.* Cambridge, MA: Harvard University Press.

Olson, R. P. (1999). *A critique of Minnesota's managed mental health care with special reference to medical necessity determinations for outpatient psychotherapy.* Minneapolis: Author. White paper presented as testimony to the Minnesota Senate Subcommittee on Health, November 17, 1999.

Organization for Economic Cooperation and Development (OECD) (2004). *Health spending in most OECD countries rises, with the U.S. far outstripping all others.* Retrieved June 22, 2004 from http://www.oecd.org/document/12/0,2340,en_200118531938380_1111,00.html

President's New Freedom Commission on Mental Health (2003). *Achieving the Promise: Transforming Mental Health Care in America.* Available at http://www.mentalhealthcommission.gov/finalreport/fullreport.htm

Robins, L. N., & Regier, D.A. (Eds.) (1991). *Psychiatric disorders in America: The epidemiologic catchment area study*. New York, NY: The Free Press.

Rosenberg, M. L., Mercy, J. A., & Potter, L. B. (1999). Firearms and suicide. *New England Journal of Medicine, 341*, 1609–1611.

Ruger, J. P. (2005). The changing role of the World Bank in global health. *American Journal of Public Health, 95*(1), 160–170.

Sartorius, N. (1998). Scientific work in third world countries. *Acta Psychiatrica Scandinavica, 98*(5), 345–347.

Schilder, K., Tomov, T., Mladenova, M. et al., (2004). The appropriateness and use of focus group methodology across international mental health communities. *International Review of Psychiatry, 16*(1–2), 24–30.

Secker, J. (1998). Current conceptualizations of mental health and mental health priorities. *Health Education Research, 13*(1), 57–66.

Shaffer, D. (1996). The NIMH Diagnostic Interview Schedule for Children version 2.3 (DISC-2.3): Description acceptability, prevalence rates, and performance in the MECA study. *Journal of the American Academy of Child and Adolescent Psychiatry, 35*, 865–877.

Skinner, J., & Elliot, F. (1997). Regional disparities in Medicare expenditures: An opportunity for reform. *National Tax Journal, 50*, 413–425.

Social Security Administration (SSA) (2004, Feb.). *Supplemental Security Income* (SSI). SSA publication No. 05-11000, ICN480200.

Townsend, C., Whiteford, H., Baingana, F., et al. (2004). The mental health policy template: Domains and elements for mental health policy formulation. *International Review of Psychiatry, 16*(1–2), Feb./May, 18–23.

White House Domestic Policy Council (1993). *The President's health security plan: The Clinton blueprint*. New York: Random House.

Whitehead, M. (1992). The concepts and principles of equity and health. *International Journal of Health Services, 22*(3), 429–445.

Whitener, B. L., Van Horne, V., & Gauthier, A. K. (2005). Health services research tools for public health professionals. *American Journal of Public Health, 95*(2), 204–207.

Willing, R. D. (1989). *Handbook of industrial organization, Vols. I & II*. Amsterdam, Elsevier Science.

World Health Organization (WHO) (1992). *International statistical classification of diseases and related health problems* (ICD-10). Geneva, Switzerland: Author.

World Health Organization (WHO) (2000). *Health systems: Improving performance*. Geneva, Switzerland: Author.

World Health Organization (WHO) (2001a). *Mental health: A call for action by the world health ministers*. Geneva, Switzerland: Author.

World Health Organization (WHO) (2001b). *The world health report 2001. Mental health: New understanding, new hope*. Geneva, Switzerland: Author.

World Health Organization (WHO) (2002). *The world health report 2002: Reducing risks, promoting healthy life*. Geneva, Switzerland: Author.

World Health Organization (WHO) (2003). *The world health report 2003: Shaping the future*. Geneva, Switzerland: Author.

World Health Organization (WHO) (2004). *The world health report 2004: Changing history*. Geneva, Switzerland: Author.

World Health Organization (WHO) (2005a). *The mental health atlas–2005*. Geneva, Switzerland: Author.

World Health Organization (WHO) (2005b). *The world health report–2005: Make every mother and child count*. Geneva, Switzerland: Author.

Chapter 2

MENTAL HEALTH DELIVERY SYSTEMS IN GREAT BRITAIN

JOHN N. HALL

PART ONE: DESCRIPTION

Introduction: Understanding Britain and the British Health Care System

Understanding Britain

To give Great Britain its full title of "The United Kingdom of Great Britain and Northern Ireland" says two important things about Britain. First, Great Britain, or the British Isles or (hereafter referred to simply as Britain) includes the largest island of North-West Europe, made up of England, Scotland and Wales, and Northern Ireland, which is the Northern section of the island of Ireland, the larger and Southern section of which is the Republic of Ireland. Second, politically Britain is both a constitutional monarchy and a Parliamentary democracy, and although there is one national government and one national bicameral legislature – Parliament – there are significant variations in internal regional government among the four "home nations." This chapter will describe mental health systems in England, which is by far the largest of the four nations, and because differences in the systems are relatively minor.

To understand England's mental health system, it is important to appreciate the context in which it has developed. The context includes its geography, demographics, its political and economic system, cultural values expressed in policies and programs, and a brief history of the country's health care system in which the mental health system functions.

Geography. England lies in the central and southern part of the island of Great Britain. It covers about three-fifths of the island and has an area of 50,364 square miles, about the size of the state of Alabama in the United States. Greatest distances are North-South – 360 miles (579km); East-West- 270 miles (435km), with a coastline of about 1,150 miles (1,851km). Elevations range from 15 ft (5m) below sea level in the Fens near Ely (depending upon the tide), to 3,210 ft. (978m) above sea level at Scafell Pike (*World Book Encyclopedia*, 1980, v. 6, p. 235). An efficient, public transportation network throughout the country facilitates commerce as well as access to the sites where health care services are provided.

Demographics. The Population of Britain as a whole at the 2001 census was 60.0 million (m); the populations of the constituent countries are England 50.0m, Scotland 5.1m, Wales 2.9m, and Northern Ireland 1.7m. Britain is a relatively densely populated country, but with significant variations in population density. The British measure of population density is based on the metric unit of measure called the hectare, which is equal to 2.47 acres. The population density of England is 3.8 persons per hectare, Wales is 1.4 per hectare, and Scotland is 0.65 per hectare. Within that five-fold variation, Northern Scotland (and the Scottish Islands) and central Wales contain the least populated areas, with large metropolitan centers in southern, central, and northern England, central Scotland, and south Wales. While not as significant a factor as in the other countries represented in this book, these variations in population density affect the health care delivery system, and they are similar to the range of population densities in other North-Western European countries.

Political System. The political system of Britain has evolved steadily for over a thousand years. The earlier individual Saxon communities became the parishes that emerged from the eleventh century, and with the larger shires (counties) that emerged, the parish and shire systems remained the most important units of local administration to the nineteenth century outside London and for the handful of large cities that existed at the time. The tension between royal and parliamentary power erupted in the English civil war of the mid-seventeenth century, and the subsequent settlement at the end of that century effectively created the political institutions of present-day Britain.

The Head of State is the present Queen Elizabeth the Second, the "Crown." Although Acts of Parliament are technically approved by the Crown, the residual political powers of the Queen are now highly circumscribed. Parliament consists of two chambers: first, the nationally elected House of Commons, elected presently through universal suffrage by adults aged 18 or over, and the second chamber of the House of Lords. Previously, this second chamber has exercised considerable political power, but it functions now as a chamber whose main function is to critique and revise legislation, which the government must respond to. Most members of the House of Lords are appointed by the Crown on the nomination of the main political party leaders for life on the basis of national eminence. A residual number of hereditary peers, and a small number of Anglican Bishops and senior judges complete the membership of the House of Lords. A significant proportion of newly appointed members of the House of Lords have previous experience in the House of Commons and in government positions, and most other members have occupied posts of considerable responsibility.

England has no written constitution, but some aspects of constitutional procedures are fixed by legislation – known as *Acts of Parliament.* Other procedures are determined technically by convention, but those conventional norms are so powerful that a government minister could be forced to resign if a convention were not honored. Parliamentary general elections must take place at least every five years, but general elections may occur within a shorter interval, if the government is defeated on a major measure, or if the Prime Minister decides to do so. The electoral system is a "first-past-the-post" system, which means that the party with the largest percentage of popular vote becomes the ruling party in Parliament and the government. One consequence is that a ruling party may have received less than 50 percent of the popular vote. For example, in the 2005 General Election, the Labour party was re-elected with a majority of 61 of the total of 645 seats in the House of Commons, and with 36 percent of the popular vote, while the Conservative party gained 33 percent of the popular vote. While the Labour and Conservative parties have been the leading political parties in Parliament for the past 80 years, new parties have emerged, notably the Liberal Democrat party, and national parties in Scotland, Wales and Northern Ireland, and there is considerable volatility in adherence to political parties.

Since Britain joined the European Community (EC) in 1971, the decisions of the European Parliament and Commission impact or British legislation, with the positive consequence of convergence in standards of health care, and free movement within the EC of citizens, including health care workers. The Republic of Ireland became fully independent in 1937, but Irish citizens may vote in England, and their systems of professional education, including health care professions, are fully consistent with British standards. While there is considerable ambivalence throughout Great Britain about the level of control exercised by the European Commission and Parliament, there is broad support for closer links with Europe. British social and political values, as in the North-Western nation states of Europe particularly, strongly support some form of welfare state and public financing and delivery of health care and social services, although the mechanisms for service delivery may vary.

The National Government is selected by the Prime Minister, who is the leader of the controlling political party with the largest number of seats in the House of Commons, which currently has a total of 645 members. Government Ministers must be Members of Parliament, with the convention that senior ministers (known as Cabinet Ministers) are members of the popularly elected House of Commons. The executive function of government is thus contained within the legislature, and there is no separate election of the Prime Minister, who is necessarily a member of the current majority party.

Cabinet Ministers have defined areas of responsibility. For example, the Chancellor of the Exchequer is the Cabinet Minister who has responsibility for overall financial affairs and approval of all public expenditure. The Secretary of State for Health is the Cabinet Minister with responsibility for all health affairs in England. Like other Cabinet Ministers, the Secretary of State for Health reports directly to the Prime Minister.

The Secretary of State for Health functions as the head of the Government's Department of Health (DoH), previously titled the Ministry of Health, and subsequently the Department of Health and Social Security. Presently, there are five junior health ministers (four of whom are members of the House of Commons, and one a member of the House of Lords) to whom responsibility is delegated by the Secretary of State for Health to perform various aspects of the work of the DoH. The greatest part of public health funding actually spent is determined by the Chancellor of the Exchequer, who negotiates with the Secretary of State for Health the amount of funding for the DoH.

There are separate Secretaries of State in Parliament for Wales, Scotland, and Northern Ireland, who have responsibility for health care in those nations. There has been a gradual devolution of central government functions to the other "home nations," which means that the Parliamentary Secretaries of State must now act collaboratively with the devolved political bodies popularly elected within those countries, who will have their own lead minister for health. Two political bodies, the National Assembly for Wales and a Scottish Parliament, were first elected in 1999. The Northern Ireland Assembly had their first elections in 1998, but the Assembly has been intermittently suspended for significant periods of time, and the government of Northern Ireland has been led directly by the Secretary of State for Northern Ireland. The government of England has supported moves toward more regional powers being devolved in England to decentralize powers within England, but with the exception of London, there are no other elected regional bodies in England.

Economic system. The economic system of England is best described as a mixed economy of regulated capitalism and a welfare state. Major sectors of the economy include agriculture, fishing, manufacturing, and mining. The basic monetary unit is the pound sterling. As an advanced industrialized country, Great Britain is one of the member nations of the Organization for Economic Cooperation and Development (OECD). The Gross Domestic Product for Great Britain was £1.1 trillion in 2003, with a gross household annual income of £25k. At the 2003 exchange rate (ER) of 1.64, the figures are respectively US $.67 trillion and US $15k. England has a strong economy with a relatively low unemployment rate of 4.8 percent in 2004.

Cultural Values. The British people are both independent and egalitarian. Individual freedom is highly valued, as is the protection of human rights, yet with a strong commitment to the well-being of their society as a whole. Cardinal values expressed in their health care system are both universal contribution (everyone pays a progressive National Insurance tax to finance the National Health Service) and universal free access (NHS services are free to everyone at the point of delivery). Their practicality is evident in an insistence upon efficient organization, and high standards of integrity in the delivery of all public services.

The English democratic spirit is evident in the elected representatives both to their national legislature (the House of Commons), and in locally elected representatives who provide oversight of the social services (e.g., education, fire and police protection, housing, and public health) provided by Local Authorities to counties and municipalities. The lead employed officers of public agencies at both national and local level are permanent, and do not change with a change in the governing political party. Britain's compassion is manifest in significant international aid and their cooperation is expressed in international efforts to curb global warming and to abide by international law. Having survived devastating bombings of London in WWII, and more recent acts of suicide terrorists, the English are as resolved to establish and maintain national security and world peace as other member nations of the United Nations. Although the Church of England (Anglican) is the official state church, English people may worship as they choose. Freedom of religion, speech, and the press are fundamental principles in this parliamentary democracy.

Britain's National Health Service: An Historical Perspective

Medieval patterns of health and social care in England were similar to those in continental Europe, relying on the church for both funding and for what little formal medical treatment was available. The development of the "poor law" from Tudor times made the parish responsible for the care of the sick and destitute. From a very small number existing before the eighteenth century, charitable hospitals developed into a patchwork of public workhouses and voluntary infirmaries funded mostly by and intended for the more affluent. Medical care in the cities and larger towns was provided by surgeons and physicians, with the more rural areas depending on apothecaries. The cost of any sort of medical practitioner was in any event unaffordable by most of the population, who relied on herbalists and local lore.

The nineteenth century saw a range of both innovation and regulation to improve health care in England. These included *Factory Acts* to improve conditions in the often appalling environments of industrializing Britain; the regulation of medical practice through the 1858 *General Medical Act;* and the beginnings of legislation relating to public health, which established local Public Health Boards that had the statutory responsibility for providing a range of institutions and services. The poor state of public health was thrown into relief by the difficulty the British Army had in recruiting men physically fit for the South African Boer War in 1899, and a range of measures were taken to improve standards of nutrition and housing. By the end of the 1930s something like a national pattern of health care had developed, though very much a mixed and variable health economy of charitable, private, and public provision, funded by a mixture of national and local taxation, insurance schemes, and private expenditure.

The NHS Act of 1946. Remarkably, in the middle of WWII, the central government began planning to reform the whole system of health and social care. The Beveridge Report of 1943 set out a blueprint for a "welfare state" with a national scheme for health care as one of the main elements. One of the first priorities of the Labour Government elected in 1945 was to establish a single national, publicly funded, health service for the entire country. The authorizing legislation for this was passed by Parliament as the *National Health Service Act* of 1946, and the National Health Service (NHS) began operations in 1948, funded principally by federal taxes paid as "National Insurance," a progressive tax payment deducted at source from everyone in employment. Central principles of the NHS were that health and social services should be financed, administered, and delivered in the public sector (nonprofit), and that these services should be free to everyone at the point of delivery. These guiding principles have remained, now with some modification, in all the changes to the NHS.

The 1946 *NHS Act* created the so-called tripartite system for the administration and delivery of health care, including (a) *Local Authorities* (cities, towns and counties), which provided public health (including infection control), community and school medical services; (b) *Local Practitioner Committees* (LPCs) to fund family doctors, dentists, and pharmacists; and (c) *Hospital Management Committees* (HMCs) that managed hospitals (and Boards of Governors managing those hospitals with a medical school).

Under the Act *Regional Health Boards* were established, with responsibility for all the HMCs in their area. They had appointed members, who were responsible for the permanent officers who did the actual work of the Board. England was covered by fourteen Regional Hospital Boards, each containing at least one medical school, and each Regional Health Board appointed medical advisers, including a psychiatric adviser, invariably a senior psychiatrist. A Regional Health Board covered a population up to about five million, and typically included several counties.

A committee appointed by the Regional Board managed each Hospital Management Committees (HMC) within its region. The committees were required to include designated personnel, for example, a doctor and a nurse, and in practice they included nominees of the local councils so that elected local politicians were then directly involved. Since the Local Practitioner Committees were considered one of the three major elements of the NHS, the Regional Health Boards exercised administrative authority over the LPCs as well as the HMCs. Local Authorities at that time were independent of the Regional Boards.

Discussions during the passage of the NHS Act examined whether or not to include the mental hospital system within the NHS, under the authority of Regional Health Boards. It was included as a publicly funded and provided service, so that mental hospitals were also managed by HMCs. In most cases the mental hospital HMCs did not include any other type of hospital, although they could include the then "mental handicap" hospitals for children and adults with learning disabilities.

Commonly Managed Health Districts since 1974. The original National Health Service system remained essentially unchanged until 1974, when for the first time NHS health authorities (providing health services) and Local Authorities (providing social care, housing, and education services) were organized based on the principle of "co-terminosity," which meant that the geographical areas served by both were identical, leading to improved joint administrative decision-making and implementation. Additionally, the hitherto separate Local Practitioner Committees and Hospital Management Committees which served a particular locality were also brought together under one common management system in order to improve coordination of both health and social care functions in any one area. The resulting *Health Districts* had typically a population of between 300,000 to 500,000.

The NHS Trusts of the Early 1990s. Since the 1970s, successive governments have restructured the NHS. An important change from the early 1990s was the creation of "NHS Trusts," which now are the organizational bodies responsible for the delivery of health services within a county or major conurbation area.

The significant feature of a NHS Trust is that it is not directly managed by the Department of Health; rather, it has its own Board of Directors. Moreover, half of the Board of Directors include the senior professional managers and administrators of the services provided by the NHS Trust, including a Chief Executive, and medical, nursing, and finance directors. The other half of the Board of Directors consists of nonexecutive directors, one of whom is the Chair of the Trust, appointed directly by the Secretary of State for Health. This gives some latitude for direct political bias in appointments, although there is a national public appointments scrutiny system to minimize that bias. The Chair of the Trust is ultimately the leader of the Board of Directors, to whom the Chief Executive is accountable. This organizational structure includes relatively few lay or nonexecutive members, and no locally elected politicians among the Board members.

Since Trusts were established, many have been merged so that now the typical pattern of NHS Trusts within a county or major conurbation is that there will be one NHS Trust providing all general medical and surgical services and one separate NHS Trust providing all mental health services. A specialist Trust providing, for example, specialized rehabilitation services, and also a Trust providing ambulance services may also exist in some, but not all counties or major conurbation areas.

Local Authorities and Councils. A number of public services contributing to the overall pattern of mental health services are provided at city, town, and county levels by Local Authorities through various Councils. Cities within the larger conurbations, such as Birmingham (with a population of 980,000) and Liverpool (with a population of 439,000), are classed as Metropolitan Borough Councils. Other large cities, such as Bristol (with a population of 380,000), and sectors of some counties, are classified as *Unitary Councils.* Some *County Councils* contain within them lower-level *District Councils,* thus having a two-tier system of local government, while some counties operate on a one-tier system by being divided into a number of Unitary Authorities. With a population of about 7,465,000, London is governed uniquely by the Greater London Assembly (established in 2000), which in turn, is divided into London Boroughs with populations ranging from about 150,000 to 300,000. Throughout England, the level of Local Authority or designated Councils responsible for different categories of service (such as housing and social care) is carefully specified, and they are required to work in partnership with their local NHS Trusts.

The incoming Labour Government of 1997 initiated a number of changes to NHS procedures under a banner of "modernization." Two major changes, which are in tension with each other, include (a) increasing the autonomy of providers, while (b) setting increasingly prescriptive performance targets for providers. Moreover, there has been a fundamental shift away from control by specialist health care, represented by hospitals, towards greater control by primary health care, represented by family doctors and staff working closely with them and directly in the community.

Primary Care Trusts and Strategic Health Authorities. The new emphasis on primary health care was reified by the creation of *Primary Care NHS Trusts* (PCTs) in 2002, which now have a major role in commissioning all local nonspecialist health services, and which function as the employer of health care staff working in the community and in primary health care services. The introduction of PCTs was accompanied by the creation of 28 *Strategic Health Authorities,* which replaced the previous and more numerous District Health Authorities. The target size of a PCT was initially set at about 100,000 total population, although in practice, following mergers of smaller PCTs, their average size is about 150,000 to 200,000, with some around 300,000.

The present core structure of the NHS in England is thus a three-tier system. First, the central Department of Health (DoH) determines national priorities and strategies; establishes overall levels of funding negotiated with the Chancellor of the Exchequer; and sets performance targets as a means of monitoring access, quality, and expenditure for the delivery of health care services. The DoH is headed by the Secretary of State for Health, who serves as a Cabinet Minister and reports to the Prime Minister of the central government.

In the second tier, the DoH exercises its administrative authority through 28 Strategic Health Authorities (SHAs), which are essentially outposts of central government. Each SHA covers a population on average of about one and a half to two million. SHAs have no function in the delivery of services; rather, as the name suggests, they have strategic and monitoring functions to ensure that Primary Care Trusts (PCTs) and other Trusts commission and/or deliver services in accordance with national priorities established by the DoH of the central government.

In the third tier, acting as providers, the PCTs and other NHS Trusts, such as Mental Health Trusts, are the front-line of the NHS, managing and providing the whole range of health care services. NHS Trusts, other than PCTs, consist of a single hospital or groups of hospitals and associated specialist community services. A single medical and surgical Trust will normally provide a comprehensive range of general medical and surgical services, often with two or more major hospitals. As one type of NHS Trust delivering specialist care, *Mental Health Trusts* provide most of the range of mental health services, many including learning disability services as well. Within the past few years the number of stand-alone learning disability Trusts has been reduced to two across the whole country in 2005. There is an ongoing process of merger of Trusts and of PCTs, with the trend clearly being to reduce the number of separate Trusts.

By way of summary, the line of administrative authority for England's National Health Service begins with the elected Parliament, which provides legislative authority for the central government's Department of Health (DoH). The DoH is headed by the Secretary of State for Health, who serves as a Cabinet Minister in the central government, reporting directly to the Prime Minister. The DoH delegates its administrative authority and responsibility to 28 Strategic Health Authorities, which have oversight responsibility of the NHS Primary Care Trusts (which commission health care services and provide primary care services), and oversee the specialist NHS Trusts (e.g., Mental Health Trusts) which deliver specialist health care services.

While these arrangements may seem complex, the configuration and catchment area of local Trusts usually follows the historical pattern of services and settings of the main provider hospitals. Despite the organizational changes that have occurred over time, there tends to be stability in who provides what, so that within any one locality, GPs and other health professionals will know which Trust is responsible for which services.

Local Authorities. Complementing the NHS are Local Authorities, who are elected locally. In contrast to NHS services, the services provided by Local Authorities are managed to a greater extent by the locally elected representatives and councilors. Consequently, local political influences lead to different emphases in service elements. Moreover, unlike NHS Trusts, Local Authority services are managed by the relevant service Director, such as the Directors of Education, or of Social Services, who are directly accountable to the wholly locally elected Council via a Council subcommittee. Local communities now have the option to choose to vote for a directly elected mayor, but directly elected mayors are in the minority. Health care can be a major issue in local politics. For example, in a constituency where the local hospital was threatened with closure, in the 2001 General Election a local doctor who was not affiliated with a major political party was elected as Member of Parliament on a "save-our-hospital" ticket. Funding for the services managed and delivered by Local Authorities comes from both central government and from local taxation.

The third public set of partners in the provision of welfare services are those services provided by the central government through civil servants. The most important are the social security and disability benefits systems, administered through the *Jobcentre Plus Network*, which is the government agency responsible for social security, and for which the Secretary of State for Work and Pensions is directly accountable. It is centrally administered with no local elected input at all.

Gatekeeping Functions of General Practitioners. Despite the bewildering rate of organizational changes in the British NHS within the past decade, an enduring feature is the central role of the family doctor or general practitioner (GP). Because of the national scope of the NHS, every part of the country has reasonably convenient access to a family doctor. This has led to reliance on the GP for three separate functions: (a) for initial medical assessment and first-line treatment; (b) for referral to specialist medical care and hospital care; and (c) to authorize social security benefits.

Unlike most European countries, British medical *specialists* do not have walk-in clinics. Moreover, there is a very clear demarcation between primary care and specialist medical practice. Until the past few years the GP has been the primary route to specialist care and hospitalization except for medical and psychiatric emergencies. Consequently, GPs have had a degree of control of access probably unparalleled in other health care systems.

The key features of the British NHS are *first*, it is a single, comprehensive, federally funded delivery system, encompassing primary and specialist care, community and hospital services; *second*, it is guided by one nationally uniform set of policies and procedures; and *third*, most health care services are provided free of charge at the point of access. While there may be some geographic variations in funding and in the quality of hospital buildings, there is less variation in procedures and performance criteria than exists among states or provinces found in countries with much smaller populations (such as Australia, with six states and two territories for a population of about 20 million).

A *fourth* key feature of the NHS is that health care providers are basically public employees, so that the NHS is a nonprofit, publicly financed and *delivered* service, not merely a national health insurance program like Canada.

The Scope and Size of the Problem – Levels of Need for Mental Health Services

In common with other countries, there is a debate about how mental health problems should be categorized: (a) by formal diagnosis (with medical model implications), (b) by the nature of the problem (psychological model), or (c) by the environmental determinants or consequences (social model). A more or less explicit diagnostic system underpins most service planning and public debate, and thus the size of the problem continues to be presented in broadly conventional diagnostic categories. Nevertheless, broader biopsychosocial models (such as that of Tyrer and Steinberg, 1999) are increasingly modifying policies and service delivery. All of these formal models are vociferously challenged by the very active service users and carers movement.

Britain uses both the World Health Organization's International Classification of Disease (ICD-10), and the American Psychiatric Association's Diagnostic and Statistical Manual (DSM-IV) terminology. Because the NHS provides the overwhelming majority of mental health services, and because the government collects regular statistics covering the associated social support and disability services, the quality of prevalence data is good, and is supplemented by information from case registers. The following statistics are derived from data provided by the NHS and by the Office for National Statistics (ONS), and includes data from large-scale surveys, such as the private household psychiatric morbidity studies, last carried out in 2000.

Overall figures for Britain given in the *Choosing Health Consultation* (Department of Health 2004a) are: (a) one in ten children and young people under the age of 15 suffer from a mental disorder; (b) at any one time, one in six adults (16%) have a mental disorder – around nine million people in total; (c) up to 670,000 people have some form of dementia, five percent of people over 65, and 10 to 20 percent of people over 80; (d) approximately 500,000 people believe they were experiencing work-related stress at a level that makes them ill; (e) incapacity benefit data shows that 866,000 adults on benefit report their primary condition to be mental ill health; (f) suicide rates are falling, but young men are one of the highest risk groups; (g) up to one in four consultations with a family physician (GP) concern mental health issues.

These global figures give an indication of the overall size of the mental health problem in Britain. These figures vary between parts of the country, with differing levels of social deprivation accounting for a significant proportion of the variance. Other personal factors affecting individual risk, apart from family history of mental disorder, include age, gender, employment status, and ethnicity.

Mental Health Needs Among Children and Young People

Data on the prevalence of mental disorders in children and adolescents, provided by Meltzer et al. (2000), are listed in Table 2.1.

Children with a mental disorder are more likely to (a) live in social sector housing, (b) live with a lone parent, (c) have problems with the police, (d) have bereavement issues, (e) have poor physical health, (f) have a parent with no educational qualifications, (g) have both parents unemployed, (h) have mentally-ill parents.

Mental Health Needs Of Working Age Adults

The most authoritative current figures for psychiatric morbidity in Britain were provided by 'The Office of National Statistics' systematic survey of adults up to the age of 74 in private households in 2000 (Singleton et al. 2001). This interview-derived data was obtained from a sample of 8,800 people in Britain (excluding Northern Ireland) aged between 16 and 74. Gender-specific and age-specific (by 5-year intervals) data is reported. The disorders covered included neurotic disorders, psychotic disorders, alcohol and drug dependence, and personality disorder.

Table 2.1. *Prevalence of Mental Disorders in Children and Adolescents by Gender in Rates per 1000.*

	Boys Aged 5–10	*Girls Aged 5–10*	*Boys Aged 11–15*	*Girls Aged 11–15*	*All Children and Adolescents*
Anxiety	3.2	3.1	3.9	5.3	3.8
Depression	0.2	0.3	1.7	1.9	0.9
Conduct disorder	6.5	2.7	8.6	3.8	5.3
Hyperkinetic disorder	2.6	0.4	2.3	0.5	1.4
Less common disorders, e.g., Obsessive compulsive disorder, phobia	0.8	0.2	0.5	0.7	0.5
Any disorder	10.4	5.9	12.8	9.6	9.5

The method of data collection included mental health concerns, such as sleep problems, as well as formal mental health problems. These data give the best indicators of the need for mental health services in the population. Point prevalence of mental disorders in men and women in rates per 1,000 are presented in Table 2.2.

The most commonly reported neurotic symptoms were sleep problems (29%), fatigue (27%), irritability (20%) and worry (19%), with the lowest frequency being for panic (2%). Converting these figures into *period* prevalence data, 164 cases per 1,000 adults were assessed as having a neurotic disorder in the week before the interview. The most prevalent single disorder was a mixed anxiety and depressive disorder (88 cases per 1,000), with general anxiety disorder the next most commonly found (44 adults per 1,000). Prevalence rates were higher among women than men for all neurotic disorders except panic. The lowest rates for neurotic disorders were found among older people: the prevalence for those aged 70 to 74 was 94 cases per 1,000. The highest prevalence rates for any neurotic disorder occurred in the three age bands between 40 and 54.

Adults with a *neurotic* disorder are more likely to be women between 35 and 54 years, who are separated or divorced and live as a one-person family unit or as a lone parent. They are less likely to have formal educational qualifications, and more likely to have a predicted IQ of <90 and come from social class V (the least occupationally skilled). Moreover, they are likely to be economically inactive, tenants of Local Authorities and Housing Associations (cooperative housing schemes for those unable to buy their own home), to have moved two to three times in the last two years, live in an urban area, and also to suffer from a physical complaint.

Overall about one in 25 adults were assessed as having a personality disorder (44 cases per 1,000 adults). The prevalence was higher among men, with the most prevalent type being obsessive-compulsive personality disorder, with a rate of 19 per 1,000. No other form of personality disorder had a prevalence higher than 8 percent (for avoidant, and for schizoid).

Table 2.2. *Point Prevalence of Mental Disorders in Men and Women in Rates per 1000.*

	Men	*Women*	*Total*
All neurosis	135	194	164
Mixed anxiety and depression	68	108	88
Generalized anxiety	43	46	44
Depression	23	28	26
Phobias	13	22	18
Obsessive-compulsive disorder	9	13	11
Panic	7	7	7
Personality disorder	54	34	44
Obsessive compulsive	26	13	19
Avoidant	10	7	8
Schizoid	9	8	8
Paranoid	12	3	7
Borderline	10	4	7
Antisocial	10	2	6
Dependant	2	0	1
Schizotypal	0	1	1
Histrionic	–	–	–
Narcissistic	–	–	–
Probable psychosis	6	5	5

The prevalence rate for probable psychotic disorder was five per 1,000 for adults aged 16 to 74.

Substance Abuse Among Adults. One-quarter of informants were assessed as having a hazardous pattern of alcohol drinking during the year before interview. Data on the prevalence of substance abuse in men and women provided by Singleton et al. (2000) are listed in Table 2.3.

The period prevalence for men (38%) was over twice that for women (15%). Prevalence of hazardous drinking decreased markedly with increasing age, and it varied significantly by gender. The prevalence of alcohol dependence was 74 per 1,000 of the general population, with 119 per 1,000 for men and 29 per 1,000 for women. With respect to drug use, eight percent of men and 13 percent of women reported using illegal drugs in the previous year. Cannabis was the drug most frequently mentioned (10% overall) with amphetamines, cocaine and ecstasy the next most frequently mentioned (2% for each drug). Prevalence of drug use decreased markedly with age, so while the highest use was in the 20 to 24 age range (37% for men and 29% for women), beyond the age of 45 the proportion of adults reporting drug use was two percent or less.

This survey was an expansion of a similar survey carried out in 1993, so comparative data was available for the age groups up to 64. There were no significant changes in the overall rates for neurotic disorders or for psychotic disorders, but the figures for illicit drug dependence had doubled from two percent in 1993 to four percent in 2000 for the population aged 16 to 64.

Comparisons between those in each of the groups of disorders with those assessed as not having that disorder showed three general differences. *First,* those with *psychotic* disorders were more likely to be separated or divorced (29% compared with 8% without a disorder), living in a one-person family unit, to have lower educational qualifications, to be economically inactive, and to live in accommodation rented from a local authority or housing association. *Second,* those with *neurotic* disorders were more likely to be women (59% compared with 48% without a disorder), aged 35 to 54, separated or divorced, and living as a one-person family or as a lone parent. They were also more likely to have one or more physical complaints. *Third,* of those judged to be dependent on alcohol, only 45 percent were married or cohabiting, compared to the 69 percent without a disorder. As drug dependence is closely aged-related, it is not surprising that 57 percent of those dependent on cannabis, and 65 percent of those dependent on other drugs were single, compared to 21 percent of those not dependent on drugs. Those dependent on drugs were more likely to be unemployed (10% of those dependent on cannabis, and 10% of those dependent on other drugs) compared with three percent.

Among adults of working age, 628,000 regard mental illness as their main disability, and of these, 21 percent are employed, which is the lowest rate for any of the disabled groupings in Britain, and of those employed, over half are on a low income. (Singleton et al. 2001).

A separate study has examined the prevalence of mental disorders by *ethnic* or *national group* (Sproston & Nazroo 2002). Overall about 11 percent of the British population are from nonwhite ethnic groups. The increase in this proportion largely dates from immigration immediately after WW2, mostly from the Indian subcontinent and the Caribbean. Comparing Caucasian, Irish, Black Caribbean, Bangladeshi, Indian and Pakistani, the only overall statistical difference found was for Bangladeshi women compared with white women, but there are significant differences in service usage, of which the greater numbers of young black men who are detained in psychiatric hospitals is the most significant example.

Self-Harm, Suicide and Mental Health Problems

In the previously described mental health targets and policies developed since 1992, special attention has been paid to suicide, and a special national enquiry into suicide is maintained, with consequently excellent data quality. Although the overall rate of suicide is falling, there are more than 4,700 suicides in

Table 2.3. *Prevalence of Substance Abuse in Men and Women in Percentages*

	Men	*Women*	*Total*
Hazardous drinking (score 8 and over on audit) in the last year	38%	15%	26%
Mean audit score	7	4	5
Illicit substance use in last year of any drug.			
All ages	8%	13%	11%
20-24-year olds.	37%	29%	33%

Note. Source is Singleton et al., 2000.

England and Wales each year. Many more suicide attempts are made each year, and at least one person in every 100 appearing in a hospital after a suicide attempt will succeed within a year, and up to five per cent do so over the following decade.

Suicide rates for men are higher than for women in all age groups, and currently men are almost three times more likely than women to commit suicide. This gender gap has widened considerably over the past few decades. In 1979, the female-to-male gender ratio for suicides was 2:3 and in 2002 it was around 1:3. This difference is particularly striking for young people, with men between 25 and 34 years almost four times more likely than women to kill themselves. The group at highest risk of suicide used to be males over 65 years of age, at a rate of 24 per 100,000 population in 1979. In the past decade, the group at highest risk was males aged 25–34. However, in 2002, men aged between 35–44 had the same risk of suicide as those aged between 25–34 (22 per 100,000 population). Suicide is the most common cause of death among men between 15–44 years. In men aged 15–24 the suicide rate has risen almost 50 percent, the most over the past two decades from nine per 100,000 population in 1979 to 13 per 100,000 in 1999. Since 1999, the figures have shown a downward trend. However, for a few groups the figures have gone up; men between 35–44 and women between 25–34. The highest increase has been for older women, aged 75 years or older. For this group, the figure per 100,000 population has gone up from six suicides in 2001 to eight suicides in 2002. Young females in the 15–24 age group are at the lowest risk. The suicide rate for this group has remained fairly constant since 1979, and is now around three per 100,000 population.

The suicide rate amongst older men has been declining in recent years. In the 55–64 age range the reductions have been slight, from 18 per 100,000 population in 1989, to 16 per 100,000 population in 1999. The greatest reductions in male suicide rates have been seen in those over age 75, from 26 per 100,000 population in 1989 to 15 per 100,000 population in 2002. Mortality rates from suicide for men in England and Wales by year and age are provided in Table 2.4.

Table 2.4. *Mortality Rates from Suicide for Men in England and Wales by Year and Age.*

Year	0-14	15-24	25-34	35-44	45-54	55-64	65-74	75+	Total
1993	24	556	865	762	644	428	313	283	3875
#	*1*	*16*	*21*	*22*	*20*	*17*	*15*	*23*	*15*
1994	19	530	1000	749	622	392	305	270	3887
#	*0*	*16*	*24*	*22*	*19*	*16*	*15*	*22*	*15*
1995	10	484	977	810	606	392	283	268	3830
#	*0*	*15*	*23*	*23*	*18*	*16*	*14*	*21*	*15*
1996	14	451	956	713	628	359	274	259	3654
#	*0*	*14*	*22*	*20*	*19*	*14*	*13*	*20*	*14*
1997	14	502	929	733	645	374	244	281	3722
#	*0*	*16*	*22*	*20*	*19*	*15*	*12*	*21*	*15*
1998	15	461	1096	808	665	405	242	237	3929
#	*0*	*14*	*26*	*21*	*19*	*16*	*12*	*17*	*15*
1999	11	436	935	865	692	427	261	277	3904
#	*0*	*13*	*23*	*22*	*20*	*16*	*13*	*20*	*15*
2000	16	398	840	811	685	379	265	265	3659
#	*0*	*12*	*21*	*20*	*20*	*14*	*13*	*19*	*14*
2001	12	405	832	795	692	410	258	264	3668
#	*0*	*13*	*23*	*21*	*20*	*15*	*13*	*18*	*14*
2002	11	373	799	864	639	398	250	211	3545
#	*0*	*11*	*22*	*22*	*19*	*14*	*12*	*15*	*14*

Note. Source is the Samaritans Information Resource Packet (2004).

The figures in **bold print** are the total number of deaths by suicide within each group. The figures in *underlined and in italic print* marked # give the rate per 100,000 population. It is important to note the difference between the two figures, as a higher number of suicide in one group may indicate there are more people in this age group, rather than this age group being at higher risk for suicide. For example, in 1999 a total number of 277 men aged 75 years or older died by suicide. The total number for the group between 55 and 64 was much higher at 427. However, the numbers per 100,000 reveals that the 75 years or older group was at higher risk with 20 per 100,000 population, while the figures for the group between 55–64 was 16 per 100,000.

Safer Services (Department of Health, 1999) reported that one in four people who subsequently took their own lives – about 1,000 people each year – were found to have been in contact with specialist mental health services in the year before their death. Of these, 16 percent were inpatients at the time of their death, and 24 percent had been discharged from hospital within the previous three months. Many were not fully compliant with treatment when discharged, and in most cases staff perceived the immediate risk of suicide to be low. *Safer Services* also recorded that around half of the suicides were committed by people with a history of self-harm and either substance misuse or previous admission to hospital. Major mental health problems such as schizophrenia and manic depression occur in about 0.4 per cent of the population. People with a diagnosis of schizophrenia are at an increased risk of suicide and especially when they are young. The onset of schizophrenia tends to occur between 17–25 years of age, when many are struggling to establish an adult identity and relationships.

The arrival of distressing symptoms at this time, along with the stigma attached to the diagnosis, increases the risk of suicide. A lifetime risk of up to 10 per cent has been suggested, but even this may be an underestimate, and there is growing concern that suicide risk is increasing.

A number of studies seem to show that as many as 90 per cent of all suicides had one or more psychiatric disorders when they killed themselves, and that certain diagnosed mental illnesses have increased suicide risks *(Safer Services, 1999)*. In one research study cited in the report, of 44 disorders considered, 36 had significantly higher standardized mortality rates for suicide. The authors concluded that virtually all mental disorders increased the risk of suicide except, possibly, dementia and agoraphobia. Several research studies have suggested that between 20–40 per cent of people with a diagnosis of schizophrenia have a history of attempted suicide, which shows a considerable excess of mortality by suicide in comparison with the general population. In another report on more than 200 deaths of patients detained involuntarily in hospitals under the Mental Health Act over a period of two years, 95 deaths were identified as probable suicides. The report also shows that in 60 per cent of cases of probable suicide the individual had a diagnosis of schizophrenia.

Mental Health Needs of Older Adults

There are a number of sources for estimating the levels of mental disorder in older adults. The household morbidity survey carried out by the Office for National Statistics [ONS] (Singleton et al. 2001) already described gave information on older adults aged between 60 and 74. One in ten older people aged 60–74 years living in private households in the UK will have a common mental disorder such as anxiety, depression or phobia.

Estimates of the prevalence of depression among people 65 years and older range from between 5–13 percent for men and 8–25 percent for women. An average of 10–15 percent for all older people is often assumed as experiencing some level of depression. Anxiety is very common among older people, and about 2–4 percent are likely to need intervention by a psychiatrist. High levels of social isolation, chronic illness, poverty and poor housing are associated with a high level of mental illness in people of all ages. Decreasing household income is linked with increasing risk of experiencing a common mental disorder. Being on means-tested state benefits was associated with a greatly increased likelihood of having a mental illness.

A special concern with older adults is the rate of dementia. The ONS survey systematically examined cognitive impairment in older people and reveals that 16 percent of people aged 60–64 rising to 25 percent of those aged 70–74 were relatively impaired in standard tests of memory and concentration. The prevalence of dementia increases with age: one percent at 65 years; five percent at 75 years; 20 percent at 85 years; and 33 percent at 90 years.

While the majority will not have dementia combined with physical impairments, their ability to cope alone may be compromised. The report shows that common mental disorders are strongly associated with disability, and where there is a mental health and a physical need, the person is more likely to report difficulty with activities of daily living.

Table 2.5. *Conservative Estimate of Number of Older People with Dementia by Ethnic Group.*

Ethnic group	65–69	70–74	75–79	80–84	85–89	90+	Total
White British	26	28	138	91	233	216	732
Irish	4	3	11	6	9	4	37
White other	4	4	11	7	13	17	56
W & B Caribbean			1	1	1	2	5
W & B African					1		1
W & B Asian			1		1	1	3
Mixed other			1		1		2
Asian British Indian	1	1	2	2	2	1	9
Asian British Pakistani					1	1	2
Bangladeshi	2	1	3	1	1	2	10
Asian other			1	1	1	1	4
Black Caribbean	12	9	23	12	18	12	74
Black African	2	1	3	1	1	1	9
Chinese + other	1	1	4	2	3	5	16
Total							960

The 2002 Audit Commission report on the implementation of the recommendations in *Forget Me Not* estimated that of all the people with dementia in the country, 11 percent required one intervention per week, 50 percent required one per day, and 34 percent required continual or intermittent interventions throughout the day and night. It is uncommon for older people to develop a severe psychotic mental illness in old age. However, many of those who have had lifelong mental health problems have developed neither independent living skills nor a supportive social network. Combined with physical disability this group can become extremely isolated and neglected. The number of elderly people with severe mental illness in need of psychiatric services may increase as medication no longer compromises people physically in the way it did in the past.

Social care staff report an increasing number of older people with ongoing, "crack," cocaine and alcohol addictions, and dependence on general prescription medication. Physical and mental frailty added to problems with substance misuse can result in some of the most difficult people to support either in the community or institutional care. Meeting the needs of older people with co-morbidity will be one of the challenges facing society in the next few years.

Suicide in older people is associated with depression, physical pain or illness, and loneliness. Suicide rates in the UK have dropped considerably in the latter half of the twentieth century, but the incidence of suicide in men who are over 75 is higher than that of males of 15–24.

Mental Health Needs of Cultural Minorities in England

There are significant varieties of culture within the indigenous British population, in addition to cultural differences among different ethnic and national groups. Examples of these have already been quoted, but it is important to understand the broader pattern of cultural variety in Britain.

The general concept of *social deprivation* is now widely used to describe multidimensional variations in the resources and quality of the social environment, taking account of, for example, levels of income, levels of educational attainment, and quality of housing. Using such indices, it is possible to compare the relative degrees of social need at the level of individual electoral wards, and these are known to have a significant association with rates of mental disorder. This means that in identified areas of major British cities it is possible to target mental health resources, along with other resources, to meet those higher levels of need. However, focusing resources creates an ethical dilemma in that giving people skills and support to cope with unacceptable conditions may be seen as colluding with the continuation of those conditions.

There remain significant variations between England and the other home nations in terms of culture, which may not be apparent to those outside Britain. Bhugra and Littlewood (2001) explored issues of cultural differences in Ireland and Wales. Irish people are often not seen in England as immigrants, but they are in fact the largest single migrant minority ethnic group in England, and Irish people as a group have a social profile similar to other disadvantaged groups in England. Relative to the indigenous English population, the Irish have higher rates of unemployment, and have higher levels of suicide and self-harm, and higher levels of psychiatric admissions. Issues for Welsh people include that of language. In some rural areas of Wales, Welsh speakers form up to 80 percent of the population, but it is unlikely that psychological therapies, for example, will be available to many of them in the Welsh language.

Both the Welsh and Irish are "invisible" as immigrants because of their skin colour, and because they are native speakers of English. Their "invisibility" conceals the reality of the levels of discrimination that Irish people certainly experience. This includes the risk of misdiagnosis on the basis of stereotyping, for example the overdiagnosis of Irish women as alcoholic. There may also be cultural differences in their expression of distress, reflecting lower levels of social support in an English setting.

The most common cultural factor considered is ethnicity or race. In 2002, 89 percent of Britain's population of 59.3 million (excluding Northern Ireland), or 53 million were Caucasian. The largest subgroups within the remaining 11 percent of the population were 2.3 million of Asian origin (of whom one million are Indian), 1.8 million Black, and 500,000 people of mixed ethnicity.

For the first time, the 2001 census included a voluntary question on religion, and 92 percent of the population chose to answer the question (Office for National Statistics, 2005). Forty-two million of the population (about 70%) identified themselves as Christian, but this overall figure conceals a wide variation in individual belief and practice, and does not clarify the differences between the major denominations. Nearly 1.6 million identified themselves as Muslim, and the next three most frequently mentioned faiths were Hindus (560,000), Sikhs (336,000), and Jews (267,000). These labels also conceal variation in the personal meaning of a religious affiliation, and gloss over the extent of religious pluralism.

This ethnic and religious variation is not distributed evenly. While some rural areas (and some areas of previous heavy industry) in Britain have only about one percent of their population from ethnic minorities, other urban areas (typically sections of large cities) may have over 50 percent of their population from ethnic minorities. These differences may translate into complex local patterns linking members of individual ethnic communities to particular types of employment and to very local groupings of shops and places of worship, or they may translate into a dispersed pattern of distribution wholly assimilated into the local community. The uneven geographic distribution of ethnic groups presents a challenge to the delivery of culturally competent mental health services.

The increase in the number of refugees and asylum seekers, mostly from Asia and Eastern Europe, in Britain in recent years is still not well-documented, and local health authorities may be uncertain about the numbers of resident refugees. A significant proportion of refugees have distressing histories. They may have been subject to torture, the women raped, and apart from their own experiences, they may have seen members of their families killed, quite apart from surviving possibly years of oppression and exploitation. Understanding their needs is complicated by the fact that their English may be very poor, and they may be illiterate in their own language.

These patterns of cultural variation in both the host communities and in immigrant communities are common throughout many European countries. Most of the variation in immigrants has been due to either past colonial activity by that country or economic migration, with political refugees being a more recent group. France had extensive colonies in both Africa (with Algeria being part of metropolitan France) and the West Indies, so that eight percent of the population of France is now Muslim. Spain had South American colonies, Portugal African colonies, and the Netherlands Indonesian colonies. Just over two percent of the population of Australia are of Aboriginal and Torres Strait Islander origin, and 13 percent of the population of New Zealand are of Maori origin, with a further 5 percent from other Pacific islands.

An issue of special concern is how accessible mental health services are to members of black and minority ethnic communities. The Department of Health has focused on what needs to be done at a national level to make access to services more equitable, and a number of guidance documents now exist, such as the detailed guidance document published in 2003 (Department of Health 2003a). The documents emphasize the importance of engagement with the local communities, which will lead in turn to improvement in the information available to both commissioners and providers of services so that services can be more appropriate and responsive. Three aspects of services are highlighted as of special concern: suicide, pathways to care, and acute inpatient facilities. There are particular communities at high risk for each of these concerns. Thus, there is a particularly high risk of suicide in young women born in India and East Africa, and in Irish-born men. As far as acute inpatient services are concerned, African and African-Caribbean patients are at increased risk of admission to high secure facilities, and are more likely to perceive inpatient care negatively.

Good demographic information can help to plan services more equitably. Those providing mental health services must be aware of, and be respectful of differences both between and within cultures, including differences in social structures and intimate relationships, faith and language traditions, patterns of help-seeking behavior, as well as sexual orientation and behavior. It may indeed be foolish to assume that Western systems of formal diagnosis and classification can be applied to all the problems presented by cultural minorities.

Other Approaches to Need Assessment

There are several approaches to assessing the level of need for mental health services. The figures given above represent the epidemiological approaches, and some represent measures of service utilization. The epidemiological approach can be extended to examine variations in health and social structure. There is an empirically established link between social indicators such as the general level of social deprivation and the use made of mental health services. Consequently, knowledge of the levels of deprivation gives a proxy measure of need. Service utilization data is another estimate of need, and the North-East Public Health Observatory Report *Information about mental health and mental health service use in England* (Glover et al. 2004) is particularly valuable in setting out the range of national mental health data sources available in Britain for service planning. The latter report includes a detailed case study of the former Northern and Yorkshire Region (the North-East of England), and it gives detailed information on each Primary Care Trust area. It showed, for example, that the provision of adult acute beds within one Strategic Health Authority area varied in 2002 between 35 and 61 per 100,000 population. In addition, the report examines the relationship between measures of social deprivation, in particular the MINI2000 index, showing the predictive value of these indices in estimating both morbidity and likely inpatient bed use.

Systematic surveys constitute a second major approach to needs assessment. There is one survey of psychiatric illness rates in the community for ethnic minorities (carried out in 1999), and another survey of psychiatric morbidity among prisoners in England and Wales (carried out in 1997). There is also an Annual Health Survey of England, conducted by trained interviewers with sample sizes of about 16,000 adults and 4,000 children in households. These data include the prevalence of psychological well-being, and of long-standing mental illnesses. Moreover, since 1992 there has been a special procedure for annual recording of all suicides and homicides in Britain known as the *National Confidential Enquiry into Suicides and Homicides* (Department of Health 2001).

Indicators of underserved or unmet need include local patterns of service utilization, such as high levels of bed-occupancy or long waiting lists. The problem with this approach in mental health service planning is that the level of use of any one service element is linked to the level of use of clinically adjacent services, so it can be difficult to isolate the specific area of unmet need.

In addition to epidemiological studies and various surveys, a third approach to need assessment, more suitable for smaller identified groups, is to use specific measures of need to obtain data from groups of users or potential users. Among the measures developed for this purpose are the *Cardinal Needs Measure* of Marshall et al. (1995), and the *Camberwell Assessment of Need* (CAN) measure of Slade et al. (1999). While both of these measures are too resource-demanding for routine use with large populations, they are very useful for examining the needs of small high-risk, low-volume and high-cost service users, and for sampling with high volume groups. The CAN is of particular value, as versions designed for older people (*Camberwell Assessment of Need for the Elderly* – CANE), and for forensic settings have been developed. A shortened form of CAN (CANSAS) has been developed for use in community samples, and a recent study in Gloucester by McPherson et al. (2003) has shown how it can be used routinely with minimal additional resources.

Public Policies and Programs

British public policy is usually contained in formal documents issued by the relevant government department, and presented publicly by the responsible Cabinet Minister. Major possible shifts in policy are typically introduced simultaneously in Parliament and by public speeches and announcements, and often at major professional conferences. Policy proposals are debated in Parliament with input from pressure groups, and attention by the media. An example of a mental health issue that has received extensive media attention is the occurrence of homicides carried out by people with known previous contact with mental health services. Media coverage of these events has contributed directly to the ongoing proposals to change the existing mental health legislation (see later section).

Both detailed and secondary changes in policy normally involve a process of formal and public consultation, which embraces all the relevant professional and voluntary bodies. Legislative changes in policy and procedure require Parliamentary debate during the successive stages of a Parliamentary Bill before it receives the Royal Assent. Members of Parliament are actively lobbied both by professional groups and by dedicated mental health charities and provider agencies during the passage of a Bill. Any subsequent changes in the details of protocols and procedures included in an Act of Parliament do not require public consultation.

National mental health policies are expressed mostly in policy documents, and only to a very limited extent in formal Parliamentary legislation. Those policies that are directly contained in legislation are usually monitored more strictly than other forms of policy. Examples of the latter include regulations for the implementation of the *1983 Mental Health Act*, which permit individuals to be detained compulsorily (see later Section on the Act). The five government departments issuing policies most relevant to mental health, and services for those with mental health needs, are: (a) the Department of Health (responsible for the NHS and the regulation of health care provided by other agencies); (b) the Office of the Deputy Prime Minister (responsible for regional and local issues that cut across departmental boundaries); (c) the Department for Education and Skills (responsible for all services for children, and for education); (d) the Home Office (responsible for the prevention and detection of crime, and for the prison service); (e) and the Department for Work and Pensions (responsible for child support and social security benefits).

Groupings of these government bodies and their associated agencies also issue what is essentially mandatory guidance for both the NHS and Local Authorities. These guidelines specify, for example, the broad clinical groups of users who should receive certain categories of services. Within each of the approximately 300 Primary Care Trusts in England, a Local Implementation Team (LIT) for mental health services must be set up with members from the NHS, Local Authorities, voluntary and charitable providers, and user and caregiver representatives. This local LIT, or mental health community, is required to agree on more detailed specifications and protocols for local action. While there is thus a degree of latitude for the LITs in implementing guidelines, they are subject to periodic statutory inspection by the Department of Health.

All of these policies must be implemented to be consistent with other legislation. As there is no written British constitution, the underlying legal framework is defined both by what is known as common law and by statute law. There is no provision for a Supreme Court that provides a definitive interpretation of constitutional law, but where the law is ambiguous a ruling by the "House of Lords" constitutes the ultimate judicial authority (in statutory fact this only involves very senior judges, and not the whole Parliamentary House of Lords). Under the *Human Rights Act 1998*, which came into force in 2000, the *European Convention on Human Rights* (Council of Europe 1950) is incorporated into British law. Consequently, there are several legislative acts that together protect patients' rights, for example, minimizing the risk of discrimination on the basis of race, protecting from disclosure information given during health care consultations, and providing for compensation in case of professional negligence or malpractice.

All health care professions are required to be registered under either an Act of Parliament (such as the General Medical Council for medical practitioners, currently regulated by the *1983 Medical Act*) or under a Royal Charter (a public process not directly requiring Parliamentary time). These registration procedures must include a formal code of practice and disciplinary procedures. A major change for all health professions other than doctors and nurses has been the establishment of an *Allied Health Professions Council* in 2000, which has progressively replaced the functions of previously separate professional registration for over 50,000 health professionals. The new Council already covers occupational therapists and speech and language therapists, and clinical psychologists (previously registered under a separate Royal Charter) may be subsumed within the registration and disciplinary procedures of that Council. Together, this legislative and regulatory framework offers a range of legal remedies to both service users and service providers if the provisions of the regulations are breached. In the most serious cases, these remedies could involve any or all of the following: criminal prosecution, civil action for damages, dismissal from work, and being "struck off" the relevant professional register.

National Mental Health Policy

As far as the general public is concerned, the most obvious and contentious element of mental health policy is the protection of the public, and protection from violence or self-harm of those considered to be suffering from mental illness. This policy objective of protection is achieved legislatively by the current *1983 Mental Health Act*. This Act permits the restriction, or "sectioning" of those who are considered to be a risk to the safety or life of themselves or others by virtue of a mental illness. The Lunacy legislation of the nineteenth century up to the *Mental Illness Act* of 1930 involved lay magistrates in this process of "certification." *The Mental Health Act* of 1959 liberalized this legislation by providing for the involvement of only social care and health professions, and these changes were further modified in the current 1983 Act. At present the Act requires the involvement of certain combinations of family doctor, psychiatrist, and "Approved Social Worker" in the sectioning procedure, and also provides for a number of categories of appeal procedures. However carefully these procedures are implemented, inevitably there will be occasions when a person who has previously been sectioned commits a violent offence, and this is often associated with the high levels of media attention already cited.

A revised Draft Mental Health Bill has been produced for consultation (September 2004), which makes significant and controversial proposals regarding the treatment of those with personality disorder. The controversy centers on the proposal that a person with a mental illness, who is deemed to be a nondangerous offender, hence not posing a risk to others, could be required to receive mental health treatment in the community to reduce the risk of reoffending. The Bill would broaden significantly the range of professionals involved in statutory control (mandated treatment), for the first time giving some psychologists regulatory powers.

More generally, a number of important health and social care policy changes from the late 1980s onwards by the then Conservative governments (under Prime Ministers Thatcher and Major) preceded the more comprehensive and detailed policy initiatives by the Labour (Blair) government from 1997 onwards. A number of these broader policies set the context within which mental health policies operate and with the accompanying governmental reviews and organizational changes, these policies have affected services for all age groups. All the national health and mental health policy documents quoted in this chapter are published by the Department of Health.

The *1990 NHS and Community Care Act* laid out the framework for a shift from a clear separation between the separately budgeted and managed NHS and community services (especially local authority social services departments) to a policy objective of removing boundaries between these two divisions of services. The first moves towards a comprehensive set of national clinical priorities for health, including targets for mental health services, were outlined in *Health of the Nation* (Department of Health 1992a). These included three specific mental health targets, two of which related to suicide reduction. The Conservative government's *Mental Health Nursing Review* (Department of Health 1992b), was a development from the growth of psychiatric nurses working directly in the community, and further stimulated that growth, including a recommendation that they focus on those with severe mental illness. The central government also allowed general practices (groups of family doctors and associated staff) to become "fund-holding" practices between 1993 and 1997, and a major consequence of this loosening of control was the choice by a number of practices to directly employ counselors, making counseling more generally accessible for the first time, with a degree of public funding. These detailed policies complemented other national programes, such as the capital programe for the replacement of the large psychiatric hospitals.

A central feature of the Labour government's health policy approach since 1997 has been to promulgate a series of National Service Frameworks (NSF) that spell out in detail both the overall policy framework itself, with accompanying work streams and the supporting evidence (epidemiological and clinical). While NSFs have been developed for a number of general medical conditions, such as cancer, and coronary heart disease, three NSFs, all published by the Department of Health, provide a mental health policy framework for distinct age groups: (a) *Children, Young People and Maternity Services* (2004b); (b) *Mental Health for Adults of Working Age*

(1999b); and (c) *Older People* (2001b). Another NSF published in 2005, covering all chronic conditions, is relevant to people of all ages. The NSF for mental health for adults of working age is by far the most detailed in recommendations for mental health, and the principles underlying it are explicitly seen as applicable to the other two age groups. The problems arising from these separate NSFs will be discussed later in the chapter.

The central government set up a number of agencies with three major objectives: (a) to support the implementation of all NSFs, (b) to implement the broader agenda to "Modernise the NHS," and (c) to encourage the development of evidence-based practice. Three significant agencies are (a) The *National Institute for Mental Health for England* (NIMHE), a mental health-specific government agency with a central office and eight regional offices. Their staff, all experienced in mental health provision, management, or research, support local service providers in implementing the NSFs, and as an agency they also publish useful guidance, such as the series of *Cases for Change* documents produced in 2003. (b) *The National Institute for Clinical Excellence* (NICE) develops guidance on the effectiveness of interventions for specific conditions, in the spirit of the international movement towards the application of systematic reviews and evidence-based practice. The very detailed NICE guidance documents on the treatment of schizophrenia (2002) and of PTSD (2005) are good examples. (c) *The NHS Service Delivery and Organisation Research and Development* (SDO R&D) program both funds research programs and publishes the Briefing Papers series of guidance, some specifically on mental health issues (such as Arksey et al. 2002 and Freeman et al. 2002).

Mental Health Policies for Children and Young People

The Children, Young People and Maternity Services NSF (Department of Health 2004b) differs from the other two relevant NSFs in having been issued as a set of documents, rather than as one document. The set of documents includes the core standards document, setting out five standards for all children and young people. Part Two of this NSF document addresses children and young people who have particular needs, and one section of this covers issues concerning the mental health and psychological well-being of children and young people. According to this document, a comprehensive child and adolescent mental health service (CAMHS) is defined as (a) accessible and (b) acceptable to service users, (c) it includes health promotion and early intervention as well as specialist care (d) across all four "tiers" of service, from community services to specialized tertiary services. Provision should be made for the age range from birth to eighteen, with clear pathways into adult services when needed. It is anticipated there will be a 10 percent annual increase in CAMHS funding, demonstrated by increased capacity through additional staffing and other resources.

Apart from mental health policy content of this NSF (2004), there is a wide raft of other legislation regarding the protection of children and the provision of services for children and families. For example, since the *1980 Education Act*, children with any form of special need (including those relating to behavioral disturbance and learning difficulties) may be "statemented," which means that a teacher, doctor, and psychologist together prepare a formal statement of the child's needs. That statement then constitutes an effective requirement on local education, health and social care agencies to provide services to meet those needs, collaborating as necessary.

A consolidating Act, the *Children Act 2004*, has provided a legal framework for the "Every Child Matters" program. This program is based on an encompassing set of policies that focus on four main areas: (a) early intervention and effective protection (shifting the balance towards prevention through, for example, tackling child poverty, and improving early years education); (b) supporting parents and carers; (c) local regional and national accountability and integration; (d) reform of the work force working with children.

The Act will facilitate the integration of services for children and families at commissioner and provider levels. It creates the legislative spine for developing more effective and accessible services focused around the needs of children, young people and their families. Included in its provisions is the establishment of an independent champion (the Children's Commissioner) for the views and interests of children, who will report on how these outcomes are changing. A new integrated inspection framework is being set up to achieve better outcomes with powers to intervene in areas falling below minimum standards, and a legislative basis for better sharing of information between agencies is being pursued. The specifically health aspects of this program are covered in the 2004 *NSF for Children, Young People and Maternity Services*.

Mental Health Policies for Adults of Working Age

The *National Service Framework for Mental Health for Adults of Working Age*, (Department of Health 1999b) is arguably the most significant single development in mental health policy in Britain. The NSF emerged from a process of extensive consultation about *Modernizing Mental Health Services: Safe, Sound and Supportive,* which was published in 1998 (Department of Health). It was the first of the three relevant NSFs to be published, and as services for adults of working age are by far the largest of the age-group services, this has been the main driver for change. This framework, with a set of accompanying *Policy Implementation Guides* (PIGs) (see Department of Health 2001c, 2002a, 2002b, 2003c), and a set of highly specific prescribed service targets, now constitutes the core of national mental health policy. Alongside the policy position is the current legislation providing for compulsory detention of those perceived as at risk (the 1983 Mental Health Act), and other mandatory procedures, such as the *Care Programe Approach* (Department of Health 1999c).

The NSF sets out both a set of underlying principles, and a series of targets. The ten value-driven, *guiding principles* of the NSF are to: (a) involve service users and their carers in the planning and delivery of care; (b) deliver high quality treatment and care which is known to be effective and acceptable; (c) be well-suited to those who use them and nondiscriminatory; (d) be accessible so that help can be obtained when and where it is needed; (e) promote their safety and that of their carers, staff and the wider public; (f) offer choices which promote independence; (g) be well-coordinated between all staff and agencies; (h) deliver continuity of care for as long as this is needed; (i) empower and support their staff; (j) be properly accountable to the public service users and carers.

The NSF targets a continuum of services from mental health promotion and primary care, to care for those with severe mental illness, and support for caregivers. The NSF requires a number of actions by the NHS services (now Trusts) and Local Authorities providing mental health services in a particular locality. The NSF spells out very clearly a series of *seven general targets*, which may be grouped to cover the topics of: (a) mental health promotion (Standard 1); (b) access to services, and mental health in primary care (Standards 2 & 3); (c) effective services for those with serious mental illness (Standards 4 & 5); (d) concern for carers (Standard 6); (e) action for the reduction in the rate of suicide (Standard 7).

The Policy Implementation Guides (PIGs) already outlined supplement the core requirements of the NSF, and the specific procedures, services, and support programes they describe then become targets for which Trusts are required to report progress. One of the most important of these is the *Care Programe Approach* (CPA) already mentioned, a mandatory procedure for recording the needs of those with formally identified mental health problems, and for recording the agreed care plan and the nominated key worker for each service user.

Under the Care Programe Approach, the Department of Health requires all specialist mental health services to carry out a formal assessment of need for all users as they enter the service. This assessment includes a written statement of the needs of the individual user, including a risk assessment, and also includes their care plan. The care plan lists who is responsible for the different areas of implementation. It must be (a) updated regularly, (b) it must be given to the user, and (c) if the user is agreeable, to any involved caregiver. There are two levels of service specified: (a) the standard CPA level, which covers everyone in contact with specialist services, and (b) the enhanced level (ECPA). The ECPA is applicable to everyone who is deemed to have a serious mental disorder, which is a decision based on both the assignment of a formal diagnosis and on of the level of need, as indicated by the level of service use. For example, being admitted as a psychiatric inpatient automatically leads to an ECPA classification. The number of all of those on Enhanced CPA (ECPA) in a locality is now taken as a proxy measure of service need.

In addition to the CPA, other policy guidance covers the following:

- *Mental health services for black and minority ethnic communities* (Department of Health 2003a). The evidence suggests that statutory or mandated services may not be accessible to some members of minority ethnic groups, or conversely, that there is a significant overuse of services, most significantly in the marked overuse of Sections of the *1983 Mental Health Act* for involuntary admissions of young black males to hospitals.
- *Adult acute inpatient care provision* (Department of Health 2002a). This provision is to ensure a high standard of nursing practice, environmental design, and a meaningful pattern of day activity.

- *Women's mental health* (Department of Health 2003b). Surveys have shown that a proportion of women find it frightening to be admitted to wards that also admit men, and there is now a requirement that all services must provide separate inpatient accommodation for each gender.
- *Early intervention in psychosis services* (in Department of Health 2001c). For every one million population, a team must function to focus on the needs of younger adults on ECPA who are identified as having a high risk of severe psychosis.
- *Assertive outreach services* (in Department of Health, 2001c). A team must be set up to meet the needs of those with severe mental illness, who are at high risk of dropping out of contact with services.
- *Crisis resolution and home treatment* (in Department of Health, 2001c). These services are to be the first point of contact with specialist services for those in crisis, and to provide home-based treatments as an alternative to hospitalization.
- *Policy implementation guide for PICUs and low secure environments; and commissioning arrangements for medium secure services* (Department of Health, 2002b).

Guidance for secure services has been given both for psychiatric intensive care units (PICUs) and for low secure environments in general adult services, and separately for medium and high secure services (Department of Health 2001d). High secure mental health services for Britain are provided from four hospitals: three are in England (Rampton Hospital in Nottinghamshire, Broadmoor Hospital in Berkshire, and Moss Side Hospital in Liverpool), and one in Scotland at Carstairs State Hospital. The policy guidance for these three hospitals is not well-integrated with the more general guidance for adult services.

The NSF and the PIGS together focus local attention on a set of detailed service targets. A subset of those targets are specified each year by the Department of Health, derived from the NSF and the associated PIGs (there were 45 targets in 2003). It is the job of senior managers in both the NHS and local authorities to meet these targets, in addition to the aims and principles derived from local consultation. The mental health *Local Implementation Team* (LIT) already described is required to plan service developments and monitor their implementation within the framework of the NSF and PIGs.

Journey to Recovery (Department of Health 2001d), published in 2001, summarized the main elements of the NSF, and also indicated further proposals the government intended to make to create a single modern mental health system. Among the two new emphases of the report are (a) the use of the concept of recovery as an overall principle of service planning, and (b) enabling people with mental health difficulties to be more engaged in their communities. Associated supporting programs are linked to the NSF including, for example, the outputs from the mental health *Work force design and development work group* (Department of Health, 2003d).

Responsibility for the direct management of mental health services thus rests with both the centrally managed NHS, and local Social Services Departments managed by locally elected councilors. This responsibility for service provision is carried out in partnership with the NHS and with voluntary providers, ensuring that full use is made of nationally defined and provided benefits and additional grant income. Social support embraces a wide range of services, including support for families in crisis, support in both the provision of accommodation and support to remain independent, and support to find and retain meaningful employment. Where children are at risk as a consequence of psychological distress, social services departments have specific responsibilities with respect to child protection. The government Social Services Inspectorate report *Treated as people* (2004) covers the range of services that should be provided locally as part of social care.

Alongside the lead policies of the Department of Health, a number of policies that require collaboration between different central government departments and local bodies have been promulgated by the Office of the Deputy Prime Minister. The office of Deputy Prime Minister is relatively new to the British political scene, and the power of this post is in tension with the powers of the more well-established departments. The impact on people of exclusion from communities and work as a consequence of mental illness are elaborated in *Mental Health and Social Exclusion* (Office of the Deputy Prime Minister 2004), and they are intended to increase access for those with mental health needs to general community facilities such as education and housing. This policy stresses the importance of reducing stigma and discrimination by overcoming barriers to employment, and by supporting individuals and families in accessing community services.

However, these nationally determined targets do not necessarily match local concerns, or apparent local need, and vary in detail from year to year. For the autumn 2004 LIT assessment, the targets for the assessment were changed from those monitored in 2003. Other NSFs (for example, that for chronic physical conditions), which are currently in preparation do not have the prescriptive targets of the Adult Mental Health NSF. Beginning in 2006, only two mental health targets will be required, which focus on suicide reduction and on the numbers on the Enhanced Care Programme Approach. Consequently, it is likely that the monitoring requirements of the NSFs will be relaxed. There are, however, other monitoring procedures, which until recently have included those by the Commission for Health Improvement (CHI), and by the Social Services Inspectorate (SSI), both government inspectorates. The summary reports by CHI and by the SSI on their inspections are themselves important source documents (See, for example, *Treated as people* (SSI 2004) and the 2004 CHI report).

Mental Health Policies for Older People

Health policies for older people have a long history in Britain, and the impact of the *National Service Framework for Older People* (2001b) must be assessed relative to that history. From the beginnings of the introduction of the "welfare state" in Britain from 1945, special provision has been made for the needs of older people, beyond their health care needs. Thus, the *National Assistance Act of 1948* gave the right of access to residential accommodation for older people where necessary. This right has been successively strengthened, so there is now a mandated duty of local authorities to provide a specific range of community-based services, through the *Chronically Sick & Disabled Act 1970.* As people age there is a greater likelihood of physical illness and cognitive impairment, as well as the continuing risk of enduring mental illness. A specialist service for older people with mental health problems, based on the cumulative impact of this co-morbidity and specific mental health needs, is seen as essential if a comprehensive care package is to be developed.

Policy development in relation to older people in general has been prolific in the last few years. There is a clear intention in policy to ensure that older people are valued, and that they have the right of choice and control over their lives when they require interventions in response to physical or mental frailty. There is also a commitment to developing services in the community, in response to a clear message from older people that they prefer to be cared for in their own homes. Accessibility and consistency are central tenets of new policy guidelines.

As an example of this range of legislation, the rights of caregivers for older people have more recently been recognized, as in their rights to be involved in care planning, and to receive a separate assessment in their own right. These were laid down by the *Carers Recognition and Services Act of 1995*, that legally acknowledges caregivers as a group in their own right who are critical to maintaining people in the community. Particularly relevant is the introduction of the caregivers assessment, with an associated performance indicator to assess compliance with the standard. The difficulty can be the point at which the assessment is undertaken. People are often not in contact with local care management teams until they have reached crisis point, with needs so great that the caregiver is often at a breaking point.

A funding process called *Direct Payments* was created by the *Community Care Direct Payments Act 1996* to enable disabled persons to receive the money which they paid to the providers of services. The intent of this Act was to foster greater autonomy of service recipients. This principle of autonomy was extended in 2000 to older people. The Social Services Inspectorate 2001 report *Improving Older People's Services* outlined the progress that had been made towards goals for better services for older people already identified by the Government. A *Single Assessment Process* (SAP) for all services for older people was introduced in 2001 in the *Older Peoples NSF*, and set implementation dates, aimed at ensuring older people receive a timely and integrated assessment of their health and social care needs. The independent monitoring agency, the Audit Commission, published in 2002 guidance on coordinating services for older people, which further supported the need for all services for older people to be seen as a whole system. National minimum standards for care services for the care of older people in nursing homes have been laid down, including, for example, a national requirement to ensure staff are trained and competent.

Other policies are modifications of policies developed for adults of working age with mental health problems. The 1999 *NSF for Adult Mental Health*, although highly prescriptive in its recommendations, was supported by more funding, but the introduction of the NSF service changes has been very demanding in terms of organizational resources, and the focus for Mental Health NHS Trusts on meeting government targets for the 16–64 working age group has meant that older peoples' mental health services have been relatively neglected in some areas.

However, there have been some spin-off benefits. The Care Programme Approach (CPA) developed for adults was extended to become the *Care Programme Approach for Older People with Serious Mental Health Problems* (Department of Health. 2002c). Produced by the Department of Health in 2001, this audit tool suggested a concern about mental health services for ethnic minorities, and it led in turn to a report on developing services for older people from minority ethnic backgrounds.

Set in this context, the *National Service Framework for Older People* is a key driver for service changes for older people with mental health needs. They have the right to expect access to all the initiatives and provision associated with all the standards, but Standard Seven outlines expectations for the specific subgroup of people who have mental health needs. It is very clear that for older people with severe mental illness there should be access to the same standards of provision that are available for adults of working age.

The NSF specifies that quality mental health services for older people will include ten elements: (a) health promotion and preventative services, (b) timely access to specialist services including inpatient care; (c) comprehensive multidisciplinary assessment; (d) integrated care planning and management, including CPA for those with severe and enduring mental illness; (e) specialist services with competent staff able to offer community-based support; (f) access to physical therapies; (g) specialist intermediate care or staff within the intermediate care team with expertise in mental illness; (h) support structures for staff working in mainstream services; (i) carer's support; and (j) networking to ensure best practice is shared.

There is a danger that this vulnerable group will fall between the two Frameworks, with their respective focus being on mainstream provision for older people, and meeting the requirements of adults of working age with enduring mental illness. There are ongoing local dialogues as to whether mental health services for older people should be managed within older people's services or mental health services, and both types of arrangement are in existence. Irrespective of where they are located, the aim must be to ensure services are integrated and coordinated across health and social care, and that this group of people and their caregivers are not disadvantaged.

Eligibility for Services: Universal Access

The British NHS is broadly available to all British citizens residing in Britain, and to British nationals, who, having worked in Britain and thus paid National Insurance payments, are temporarily in Britain while now living abroad. Emergency medical treatment through an Accident and Emergency Department is available without charge to anyone. Consultations with family doctors and other linked primary care staff, and appointments with hospital specialists are all free. There are charges for prescriptions (with certain exemptions, such as all those over the age of 60, and those on family support and other benefits), and for eye examinations. The availability of dentistry in the NHS is now very limited. Individuals may, of course, choose to buy health and mental health services as an alternative to NHS provision. The private provision of mental health care has grown rapidly over the past 10 years, but it is estimated that only about 16 percent of total British health care expenditure is private.

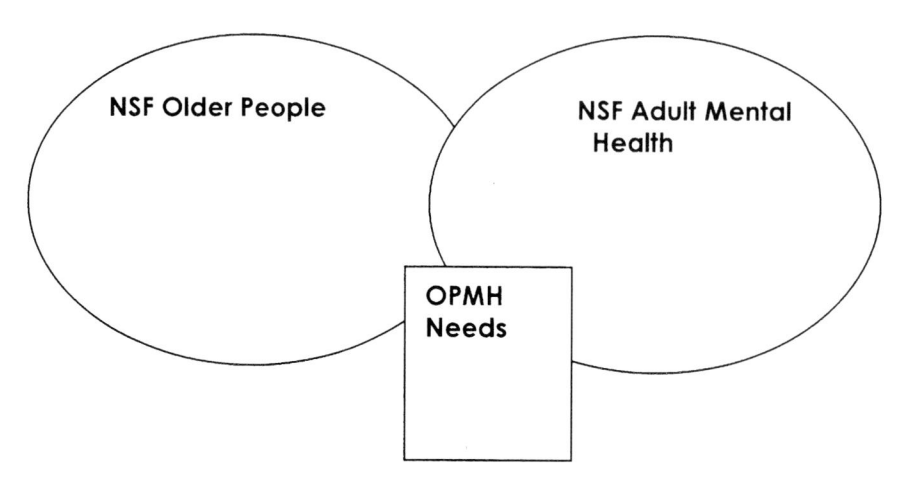

Figure 2.1. The relationship between NSF for older people and the NSF for adult mental health.

For those who are not British or European Community citizens, proof of ability to pay is required for any non-urgent treatment. There are now reciprocal arrangements with other European Community countries, so that a British citizen visiting Europe may in turn access emergency medical care by providing an E111 certificate.

Two other services that users of mental health services may require are access to the benefit system and access to supported housing of some form. The social security system is a nationally controlled and funded system, administered by local branches of the Department for Work and Pensions. Eligibility for social security payments depends on possession of a National Insurance Number, which is evidence of membership in the National Insurance scheme. Social security benefits may be payable because of short-term illness, long-term disability, unemployment, or because of responsibilities for dependents, who may include children or other sick or disabled relatives.

Short-term absence from work because of mental health problems may lead to an entitlement for sick benefits, which will be accessed after a family doctor has certified that a person is not fit for work. This "sick note" specifies both the nature of the problem and the predicted period of absence from work, and then acts as a certificate at the Benefits Office, which will pay the benefit. If a person is in employment, then the employer may continue to make full payment up to a specified time. If someone has a long-term condition, they may be eligible for disability benefit, which is payable at a number of levels depending on their needs for care.

If a person is a parent looking after their children, and if their income falls below a certain level, they may be eligible for Family Benefit. If someone is a carer for a person with a long-term condition, they may be eligible for an "attendance allowance," recognizing the loss of earning capacity because of their caring role. In all of these cases, based on their assessment of need, the social services department may authorize the delivery of services such as "home help" services for support in everyday activities of daily living.

An important recent modification to the benefits system is the introduction of *direct payments*, whereby the recipients have control of how the financial allocation is spent, thereby engaging them more actively in choosing a pattern of support that meets their needs. Benefits are means-tested, which means that an assessment of both capital and income will be made to determine initial eligibility and the level of payment. The British welfare benefits system is comprehensive, and by the standards of some other European countries, some components of it are relatively generous. This may be one reason why Britain is seen as attractive to immigrants, and why establishing the legitimacy of the claims of refugees and asylum seekers has become a political issue, which is of concern as a significant proportion of them have significant health and mental health needs.

Access to housing, with or without direct or linked personal support, is another service essential for the support of people in the community. Eligibility for these services depends on evidence of residence in the locality, evidence of financial status, and an assessment of need. If a person owns a property, or has accommodation provided by their family, they may still be eligible for personal support, according to criteria determined by the local authority. While local authorities are legally required to set criteria, the precise shape and level of the criteria will vary from authority to authority.

Local Authorities have a statutory duty to provide housing for those in need, and their housing departments may either provide accommodation directly, or make arrangements for other agencies to provide supported housing. Housing Associations are a special form of agency that provide low-cost housing for vulnerable groups, and a Housing Association itself may provide support to residents with mental health needs, or local voluntary bodies or charities may provide support. In the early days of deinstitutionalization psychiatric hospital residents were at first often accommodated in hostels, with up to 25 residents, and then increasingly in smaller "group homes," where service users lived in groups of three to six in ordinary domestic housing with day support. Younger service users now look for single accommodation units, thereby mirroring the wishes of their contemporaries.

The Delivery of Mental Health Services

The Early Development of Mental Health Delivery Systems

The first known mental hospital in England was the famous Bethlem (Bedlam) hospital. Developed from a priory in London founded in 1247, Bethlem was known to accommodate "lunatics" by the end of the fourteenth century. Thereafter, care of the mentally disturbed then followed a pattern similar to that in general medicine. By the late eighteenth century there were a number of lunatic hospitals, but most provision was made by private "madhouses." Concern about abuse in these madhouses, or asylums, led to the first attempt to create a national system of asylums through the *Asylums Act of 1808*, which permitted, but did not require, county magistrates to build asylums. The *Lunacy Act of 1845* required each county and borough to build an asylum, and created a national regulatory body, the Lunacy Commissioners. The subsequent network of some 140 asylums, largely complete by 1914, served as the institutional backbone of the mental health services until the 1960s.

While there was little change in the large hospitals, there were already by the 1920s developments in community mental health. These are illustrated both by the child guidance movement with an underlying mental hygiene philosophy, and new patterns of multidisciplinary work including social workers and educational psychologists. Outpatient clinics developed slowly, often based in nearby general hospitals.

Three Central Processes and Policies. Since the 1960s three processes have been at play in creating the existing network of mental health services for children and adolescents, adults of working age, and older adults: (a) deinstitutionalization, (b) the development of community based services, and (c) the development of a widening range of interventions by a broader range of staff.

The *first* process of deinstitutionalization began from the high point of 150,000 adult inpatients in Britain in 1955, to the present number of 34,000 NHS adult mental illness beds in 2003. The reduction in size of the hospitals has been accompanied by the steady replacement of the old buildings with new facilities that are more dispersed than previously, so that in 2004 only about 15 of the old large hospitals were still providing a significant amount of service. This replacement has improved both access and quality of services for both adults of working age and older adults. The provision of inpatient services for adults has been mostly through psychiatric units, while the provision of inpatient and residential services for older adults has been through a mixed economy of far fewer inpatient beds, and an increased range of provision through registered nursing homes and community support.

The *second* process is the development of community-based services, beginning in the 1980s with development of outpatient and day services, and since the 1990s through a comprehensive network of both generic and specialized community functions and teams, provided by statutory primary care and specialist providers, and increasingly by voluntary (charitable) and independent providers.

The *third* process is the delivery by these mental health services of a widening range of effective interventions and treatments by a widening range of professional and other staff, increasingly working from several agencies in increasingly specialized teams.

The first of these policy elements, the reduction in the number of beds in large mental hospitals, was signaled in a politically famous speech in 1961, with an overall plan for *all* NHS beds to be in multi-purpose, district general hospitals. This policy was reiterated in 1971. A more articulated government policy for mental health services was laid out in *Better Services for the Mentally Ill*, published in 1975 by the Department of Health and Social Security, which envisaged a comprehensive mental health service offering a continuum of care and a range of community services. This led to a broadening of the range of services and of the agencies and staff providing services already described, and laid the foundation for the policies and service developments dating from the early 1990s which are the substance of this chapter.

The most commonly used method in Britain to describe the delivery of mental health services is to list the service components, such as types of inpatient wards, and types of community teams. This approach confounds the vehicle for service delivery with the function of each component and the interventions offered. It also reduces the emphasis on how the components of the service relate to each other. Since mental health services depend heavily on human skills, rather than equipment or medication, another approach is to describe the skills and competencies required to deliver the service.

The Essential Components of a Comprehensive Adult Mental Health Delivery System

A comprehensive mental health service should enable access to services that meet the full range of needs in the local population. Those services should be staffed and resourced to deliver evidence-based and effective interventions, and they should enable users to move from one service to another in accordance with their changing needs.

There are a number of listings of essential service components, such as an early and influential list developed by MIND (a major British mental health charity) in *Common Concern* (1983). More recent, sophisticated lists have focused more on categories of service components. In an important book entitled, *Developing a National Mental Health Policy*, Jenkins et al. (2002) suggested the following seven "irreducible elements of care" for specialist mental health services: (a) accommodation and shelter, (b) an adequate level of income, (c) occupational and meaningful activities during the day, (d) social support, (e) physical and mental health care (which includes access to physical health care, and to medication, psychological interventions, and rehabilitation programs), (f) information and communication, and (g) assessment and triage. A similar approach has been taken by Boardman and Parsonage (2005).

Another British mental health charity, the Health and Social Care Advisory Service, has produced a "service profile," which describes for each key component the following four aspects: (a) function – the main purpose of each element; (b) essential characteristics, such as setting, access, systems, and "style" of the element; (c) interventions offered – specific interventions and treatments, and essential procedures; (d) staff skills and competencies – the knowledge and skills required, in addition to base professional competencies.

A highly influential British text by Goldberg and Huxley (1980) described "the pathway to psychiatric care" as a series of "filters" operating as an individual moves from initial identification of a mental health problem by themselves or their family, to the first contact with a family doctor who may detect a disorder, to the first contact with a psychiatrist, and on to hospital admission if warranted by their clinical condition. While this sequence should be modified to represent current British practice, the essential logic of starting from the presence of a person with mental health needs in their community of origin to successively more specialised services is attractive. Of course, this is fundamentally contradictory to the way in which mental health services developed historically in Britain, first in specialized institutions, and then *from* those institutions both to the community and to nonspecialized institutions.

A modification to the Goldberg and Huxley model, reflecting the present patterns of service delivery in Britain, would include the following seven levels or elements of service for: (a) mental disorder and distress in the community; (b) mental disorder and distress among those in contact with voluntary and self-help groups; (c) common and less severe mental disorders among primary care attenders; (d) serious mental disorders among primary care attenders; (e) serious and complex mental disorders treated in the community by specialist mental health services; (f) serious and complex mental disorders treated in inpatient settings by local specialist mental health services; and (g) serious and complex mental disorders treated in inpatient and community settings by tertiary specialist mental health services. Figure 2.2 diagrams the relationship among the elements of a comprehensive mental health service. Each of the levels of service must be appropriately staffed to provide the range of evidence-based interventions and the quality of care regime required by the needs of users.

Details of direct service personnel are given later in the chapter in that section, but the general position for all services is that some psychiatric time is likely to be assigned to most service elements. Psychiatric nurses are the largest single professional group within specialist mental health services, and while their conventional role has been as inpatient staff, their role has diversified considerably into community and other specialist functions. Clinical psychologists, occupational therapists, and social workers are the other three professions found in most service areas. Counselors work mostly in primary care settings. Other chartered professionals include physiotherapists (working, for example, with older adults, and in chronic fatigue services), and speech and language therapists (working, for example, with older adults and with children). While pharmacists may not have a hands-on function, there is an increasing proportion of pharmacists directly attached to services and accessible by users. All of these professional groups, other than doctors, may employ unqualified assistants or technicians, a proportion of whom may be very experienced in an ancillary role, and a proportion of whom are graduates qualified to acquire specific skills within an assistant role. Students or trainees in all of the professions form a significant part of the total work force.

The function of each of these professional groups is usually well-established within each local service, taking account of the skills of individuals. However, particular policy attention has been paid to the provision of psychological therapies in the NHS because this area of intervention has shown the greatest gap between demand and provision since the mid-1990s. This has led to detailed guidance by the Department of Health on the provision of psychological therapies, articulated most recently in *Organizing and Delivering Psychological Therapies* (Department of Health, 2004c). This sets out the expectation that local services will: (a) offer a range of evidence-based treatments; (b) be accessible within a reasonable time; (c) meet the psychotherapeutic needs of the range of groups and

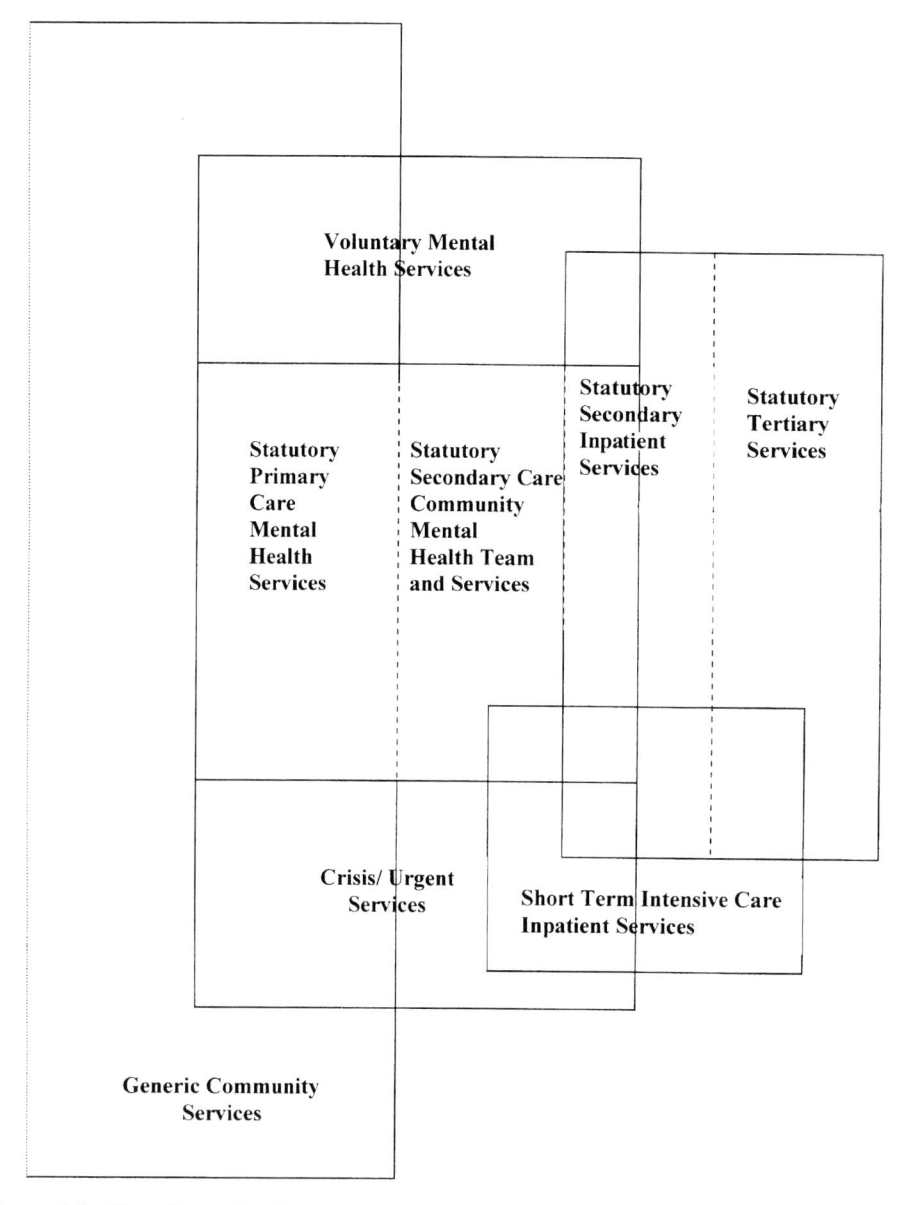

Figure 2.2. The relationship between the elements of a comprehensive mental health service.

settings in the service; (d) be coordinated across all the providing professions and agencies. Psychological therapy services should be managed so that the available staff is assigned equitably across the services, and the most skilled psychological therapists should be assigned to those patients with the most complex needs, and to supervise those working in primary care. Unfortunately, there has been no comparable guidance on the provision of a range of occupational, social, educational, work-related, or creative therapies.

The key functions and interventions to be offered by these staff at each level of service, irrespective of the age group served, are identified for five levels: support by the wider community (level 1); voluntary, self-help and independent sector provisions (level 2); primary mental health care (levels 3 & 4); generic and specialized community mental health teams (level 5).

Support by the Wider Community (Level 1)

This includes a range of generic services provided by the Local Authority and other organizations in relation to housing, employment and welfare benefits advice. It also includes community-based groups and initiatives such as *Sure Start*. Such organizations can provide support, advice and access to additional help to general members of the public and to those with mental health-related issues and to people with long-term mental health problems (whether or not they are in contact with mental health services), to promote community living, inclusion and a better quality of life. Within a whole systems approach, there is a need to raise the awareness of these organizations in relation to mental health, to build partnerships which have a specific objective in relation to people with mental health problems and to develop innovative approaches to meeting the needs of the local community through developing local resources and resilience. Specific initiatives that foster collaboration need to be developed to focus on: (a) employment: working with employment support organizations, particularly *Jobcentre Plus* (the government agency concerned with employment), pilot projects for the *Pathways to work* incapacity benefits reform; (b) promoting access to adult learning and further higher education, and (c) maximizing income through access to specialist welfare benefits advice.

Voluntary, Self-Help and Independent Sector Services (Level 2)

The voluntary sector typically provides an accessible, informal style of help which may be accessed by a range of people with greatly varying needs. They can be particularly useful when existing services are either unacceptable to potential users or unable to deliver a more informal style of help. Voluntary and independent "not for profit" agencies are capable of providing a wide range of community, day, and residential care, and of providing formal psychological and social interventions. They have a particular role to play in relation to groups in Britain who may not seek help from statutory services, such as young men from black and minority ethnic communities. These agencies have been identified also as having a key role to play in the development of community-based support for women only as alternatives to hospitalization and in the provision of advocacy, and in the development of caregiver groups and user groups. Often this provision suffers from a lack of long-term funding, and there is a need for investment in the voluntary sector to be seen as part of a local strategy for mental health provision. Some users of voluntary services may require access to tertiary specialist services but should not need to access them via statutory services if their needs would be met by that tertiary service.

Primary Mental Health Care (Levels 3 and 4)

Primary care in Britain refers to services delivered by local general practitioners (GPs) and their associated staff. Some of these family doctors practice solo (most often in inner-city areas), but over the past 20 years GP practices typically include two to five GP "partners," each partner having about 2000 patients registered on their list. Working from the same base will be a range of practice and community nurses, and there are likely to be on-site sessions available from other professionals such as podiatrists and physiotherapists. Over 70 percent of GP practices now have counselors attached to the practice. Most practices are now based in either purpose-built or adapted buildings owned by the GP partners, or in health centres owned by the Primary Care Trust, and leased to the GPs. More comprehensive Health Centres may also include a pharmacy, and other specialized community clinics, such as a paediatric assessment centre.

Primary care services deliver a spectrum of care within the context of social inclusion. A major objective of the current service changes is to resource primary care mental health services so that they can support those with severe mental health problems who do not require the full range of services provided by a Community Mental Health Team, and to provide level 4 services. It is envisaged that mental health services provided from a primary care setting will work as part of a network of community services which includes (a) generic community services (such as the Citizens Advice Bureau, and Local Authority services such as public libraries), and (b) more specialist mental health services such as local Crisis Resolution and Assertive Outreach teams. This approach of primary mental health care will be underpinned by a stepped model of care, which means that the transition to the next step is taken when needs become more complex and/or more acute, and/or there is a higher level of risk. In general the length of time (i.e., chronicity) that people have had a problem should not on its own mean that someone should be transferred to specialist services.

Gask et al. (1997) have suggested there are four common models of supporting primary care: (a) by Community Mental Health Teams (CMHTs) providing increased liaison and crisis intervention; (b) a "shifted out-patient" model, reproducing the characteristics of conventional clinics; (c) attaching mental health workers to the primary care practice; and (d) a consultation and liaison model. All of these models are essentially based on a development from secondary care service models. None of these constitute a model based on development *from* primary care, nor do they offer a model of "integrated primary care for mental health."

The emerging model of primary mental health care will be organized around single practices, or small groups of practices, and it will integrate a number of primary care services. Mental health specialist staff will work in close collaboration with primary health care team professionals, including both GPs and other primary care professionals, and social care staff. The mental health workers in primary care and based in primary care will include conventional mental health workers (e.g., psychiatric nurses), psychological therapists and counsellors, and new groups of workers, such as the new Primary Care Graduate Mental Health Workers (see section on staffing).

A broad range of people with mental health problems would receive support at this level including both people with common mental health problems, as well as those people with a longstanding, serious mental illness who do not require services provided by a Community Mental Health Team. This level of service would be available to those people currently being managed within primary care, and to those people receiving the standard level of CPA within specialized services.

Generic and Specialized Community Mental Health Teams (Level 5)

Community Mental Health Teams (CMHTs) were originally set up as generic multidisciplinary teams to provide a range of mental health services. As resources have increased, the average size of populations served by a generic adult CMHT is decreasing to between 30,000 to 50,000 people, with a primary focus on people or the Enhanced Care Programme Approach. Until very recently, CMHTs have been in most areas the primary point of access to specialist mental health services, so most people who are admitted to acute inpatient care will have been seen by a member of a CMHT before admission (unless the admission is an emergency). However, in part as a result of good practice, but also specifically stimulated by the requirements of the NSF for adults, CMHTs have become differentiated so that there is now a range of specialized teams. The specialized teams required by the Policy Implementation Guides are those offering Assertive Outreach, Crisis Resolution, and Early Intervention for Psychosis services. This section will first describe the function of generic CMHTs, and then of specialized teams.

Generic CMHTs. These teams are organized to work closely with primary care so that people whose needs cannot be met within the resources of the primary care mental health service will be referred to the CMHT, or managed jointly with the primary care mental health service. The CMHTs will: (a) integrate health and social care for people on enhanced CPA and people with complex needs who may not have a diagnosis of serious mental illness; (b) provide access to specialist assessment and effective interventions, including psychological therapies; (c) provide care management and provide a service to people whose needs are complex and/or severe.

The future of generic CMHTs, however, remains unclear, as the full impact of specialist teams, assertive outreach and crisis resolution teams, and the strengthening of primary care mental health resources has yet to be felt. CMHTs are now functioning mostly as transitional structures. It is important that in the short term CMHTs continue and operate flexibly to ensure that the people with more complex needs do not fall through potential gaps in the service. The extent to which some CMHTs may be responding to common mental health problems reflects the lack of capacity in primary care mental health services. One important function, which in practice cannot be exercised by one team only, is that of responding to crisis.

There is a wider range of interpretations on what constitutes a mental health crisis (e.g., psychiatric, social, psychological, or user definitions of crisis) and consequently a range of models exist to respond to crises. *Crisis services* need to be viewed within a whole system response to the differing degrees of crises presented by people with mental health problems and by other people living in the community. Response to a "crisis" should be the remit of all services across the spectrum of need, of which NHS and local authority services are only parties alongside the voluntary sector. To successfully respond to all forms of crisis requires closer working and ensuring that all agencies understand their role within a system of crisis response rather than to see Crisis Resolution and Home Treatment Services (or similar) as the sole response to mental health crises.

A crisis service would therefore include not only the specialist NHS crisis resolution and home treatment team working with secondary care clients, but also: (a) deliberate self-harm teams linked with Accident and Emergency Departments at acute hospitals;

(b) crisis houses (see section on acute inpatient services) and beds within rehabilitation and voluntary sector services; (c) out-of-hours GP services; (d) emergency social work duty teams; (e) help lines (e.g., Samaritans, NHS Direct, Urban area helpline); and (f) specialist mental health teams, including community mental health teams and assertive outreach teams. A broad repertoire of responses is required to meet the demand across the spectrum of need. These interventions need to be underpinned by a stepped model of care, emphasis on recovery, and an understanding that people's needs change and therefore need to be able to move through the crisis response system to access services appropriate to their level of need.

Specialist Mental Health Teams. The two other specialized community mental health teams that are required by the Policy Implementation Guides (PIGs) of the NSF are Assertive Outreach and Early Intervention in Psychosis (EIP). *Assertive Outreach Teams* have as their objective retaining contact with those individuals with severe mental disorders who are likely to drop out of contact. This will include those who remain symptomatically and behaviorally unstable after active treatment has been tried, and who may have unpredictable episodes of aggression. Typically, people in this group will have difficulty in continuing to take medication, and they are likely to have co-morbid substance misuse problems. They may not be able to support themselves in non-hospital accommodation, and may be both homeless and mobile.

Early Intervention in Psychosis (EIP) Teams are required for those aged between 16 and 35, who present with a psychotic – or probably psychotic – condition, and the probability of significant disability as a result of that condition. While for most services the population served by a team or service is not stipulated in the Policy Implementation Guide, the population to be served by a EIP team is set at one million. EIP teams are required to offer a range of effective psychological, social and medication therapies.

It is common for there to be some form of rehabilitation and community support service or team (which also contributes to the provision of meaningful daytime activity), although these are not specifically required by the NSF. These services vary in the level of active interventions they offer, and some have in effect provided Assertive Outreach and Early Intervention functions, although not labeled as such. The introduction of the Direct Payments system already described represents a significant opportunity to modernize day services and provide more individualized meaningful daytime activity, as well as a pathway into employment.

Local Specialist Inpatient and Residential Services (Level 6)

While inpatient "beds" for serious and complex mental disorders are only one component of a comprehensive service model, the variation in provision and serious underprovision of some categories of inpatient facilities mean that bed capacity is a critical factor in creating an effective model for a locality. The normal expectation is that a local service would provide acute psychiatric beds, and residential accommodation for those requiring accommodation as part of their package of community care. In addition, it is likely that each locality would have access to a small number of places in a Psychiatric Intensive Care Unit (PICU), and to some continuing-care NHS beds. Any inpatient provision over and above this would normally be seen as level 7.

Acute Inpatient Beds. A recent, key evidence-based review by Thornicroft and Tansella (2004) concludes that there is no evidence that a balanced system can be provided without acute inpatient beds. Nationally there are moves to develop a more differentiated range of acute inpatient provision, rather than provide several wards with exactly the same function. However, realistic alternative care can be provided, and they point to three options: (a) acute day hospitals, which may be suitable for about 30 percent of those who would otherwise be admitted; (b) crisis houses staffed by trained mental health professionals, which are found to be very acceptable to residents, and may offer an alternative to admission for about 25 percent of those who would otherwise be admitted. Crisis houses can operate on several different models, some of which are expensive to provide; (c) home treatment and crisis resolution services, which reduce days spent in hospital. The most recent Department of Health statistics indicate that admission rates to NHS "mental illness specialities" from 1995 to 2002 (the most recent figures) are fairly stable nationally, for adults aged between 20 and 64 at levels of between 3 to 5.5 per 1,000 for men, and between 3.0 and 4.7 for women.

Supported and Long-Stay Accommodations. The evidence for or against the effectiveness of providing different types of long-stay accommodation is weak, but essentially three categories can be identified: (a) 24-hour staffed care (high-staffed hostels), which may be provided either by the NHS or by other providers; (b) day-staffed residential places; (c) lower- or minimally-supported accommodation: the demand from service users suggests moving away from group provision to a higher proportion of single accommodation.

The Department of Health recommends approximately 25 residential places per 250,000 population, without specifying the precise mix of hospital or non-hospital places. The range of provision for those with long-standing severe mental disorders should include not only the dedicated residential provision, but also a community rehabilitation team, and provision for a range of day activities and employment opportunities. Local authorities usually have contracts with voluntary, not-for-profit, and for-profit providers, to provide nursing home, residential care and supported housing. In those parts of the country where there are very few "old long-stay" residents (who were formerly long-stay inpatients) within one Primary Care Trust (PCT), careful need-surveys reveal a wide range of clinical and social needs. This may justify three or four adjacent PCTs entering into partnership arrangements, so that each PCT provides some degree of specialization in their long-stay accommodation, to accommodate those with significant physical problems, or those who are highly treatment-resistant during continuing florid episodes.

As an example, Table 2.6 shows the current pattern of provision of adult beds in three PCTS in the North of England. One Mental Health Trust serves all three of the PCTs, one of which serves the city containing the medical school of the region. The Trust also provides in that city and elsewhere in their catchment area a range of level seven services. In the city, in addition to the acute, continuing care and PICU beds they provide, there is also a medium secure service, with 12 long-stay and 13 short-stay beds; ten new beds for personality disorder were to be provided in December 2004. The Trust also provides in the city a neuropsychiatry unit for patients with mental health and psychological problems arising from neurological conditions, such as head injury, and a research-oriented mood disorders inpatient unit. In the rural PCT there is a 5-bedded perinatal psychiatry (mother-and-baby) unit.

Tertiary Specialist Mental Health Services (Level 7)

Against the background of the reducing number of NHS inpatient beds, the general direction of change of adult mental health services in Britain over the past 20 years has been both to provide generic services more locally by dispersing the access points for services throughout the served population, and to provide more specialized, and presumably more effective, services for identified clinical subgroups. The move towards more specialized services has emerged as a consequence of *three underlying trends*.

First, improvements in psychiatric epidemiology have led to increased recognition of subgroups in the population with high levels of need that may not have been previously recognized (eating disorders being the obvious example). These subgroups may either be distributed relatively similarly across the country, or they may be very sensitive to variations in local demography, such as ethnic origin and levels of social deprivation. A *second* trend is improved research and evaluation of the range and effectiveness of clinical interventions and the modes of service delivery for these subgroups have led to the range of systematic

Table 2.6. *Examples of Current Provision of Adult Inpatient Mental Health Beds in Three PCT Areas Within One Mental Health Trust in Northern England.*

	Population	*Acute wards*	*Continuing care*	*PICU/observation*	*Low Secure*
Rural area	310,000	Three with 8, 28, and 30 beds, and access to beds for an isolated sub-locality: total 66	One with 12 beds, one with 29 "challenging behavior" beds	8 places	8 places
Mixed area with former heavy industry	153,000	Two, both with 20 beds; total 40	None	5 observation unit places	
Major city	280,000	Four, all of 18 beds: total 72	50 beds in total	8 intensive care places	

reviews, clinical practice guidelines and integrated care pathways that are now readily available. The *third* trend is the continuing subspecialization of mental health services, which are themselves partly a consequence of the above two trends, but which may be a consequence of professionally-led interests. Thus, a local specialist service may have originated on the basis of a long-standing special interest of a clinician, which does not necessarily match patterns of local need.

Tertiary services provide specialist services for those serious and complex mental disorders that are either very small in volume, or present high levels of clinical risk. The criteria for identifying specialist services recognize that some needs are best met by services serving a larger population. The largest of these tertiary specialist services in size, and the one that attracts most public attention, are high and medium secure services, which in Britain are provided by the NHS.

High, Medium and Low Secure Services. There is an important distinction between secure and forensic services. *Secure services* are provided where there is a significant risk presented by a user, usually of violence or self-harm, or of absconding. *Forensic services* are provided where a user is involved with the criminal justice system and also has mental health problems. Historically there were four "Special Hospitals" in Britain, of which Broadmoor Hospital is the most famous, providing all the high security forensic placements. Government policy over the past 25 years has been to reduce the number of places in these high secure institutions and to disperse people requiring all but the very highest level of security to a network of what were originally called regional secure units. Special national arrangements exist for commissioning these High Security Psychiatric Services (provided from Broadmoor, Rampton, Ashworth (formerly Moss Side), and Carstairs State Hospitals), and for the Medium Security Psychiatric Services that have developed from the former regional secure units (Department of Health, 1999d). These medium secure units provide both institutional secure and forensic services, and also associated community forensic services, including community-based forensic teams, or the attachment of mental health workers to probation services teams.

The policy objective of providing care in minimally restrictive settings requires *low secure accommodation* for those users who do not require any forensic input, but who present a low level of risk. This category of low secure services is not specifically covered in the NSF or in any of the PIGs, and the lack of low-secure inpatient services, and the associated community support and advice, may constitute a significant gap in provision. A number of reviews (see NIMHE 2003, *Cases for Change, Forensic Mental Health Services*) have indicated that where there is inadequate local provision of low secure accommodation, it is highly likely that there will be inappropriate placement in more secure settings than is clinically needed. Given the small size of Primary Care Trusts and the low level of need, it would be advantageous for two or three PCTs to consider planning low secure services jointly.

Arrangements for Other Tertiary Services. There are two types of arrangements for other specialist tertiary services. The Department of Health publish a number of lists of specialist clinical services for people with "serious or complex needs," including specialist cancer and neurosurgery services, for example. These are commissioned by "collaborative commissioning arrangements," which in practice means at the Specialist Consortia level (covering five or more PCTs). For mental health the list includes ten specialities: tertiary eating disorder services, neuropsychiatry, forensic services, specialised addiction services, specialist psychological therapies [for inpatients and outpatients], gender dysphoria, perinatal psychiatry, complex and treatment resistant disorders, and Aspergers syndrome) (Department of Health, 2002d).

For a very small number of even more highly specialized services there is national provision. Examples for mental health services are residential services for personality disorder at only three designated centres, and a single inpatient service for deaf children and adolescents at Springfield Hospital, London (Department of Health: National Specialist Commissioning Advisory Group, 2004). Inspection of all these different commissioning categories confirm that the criteria for specialist arrangements include: (a) low case volume in terms of either incidence or prevalence; (b) high clinical risk (in terms of either risk to others or risks to self); (c) high clinical complexity (such as gender dysphoria); and (d) high levels of skilled professional input.

Care Transitions and Total Patient Journeys

A good quality service is defined not only by the provision of services, but also by the ease with which a user can access different specific services as their needs change. In current terminology, this is the ease with which care transitions can be made. The term *Care Pathway* has been used conventionally in Britain to describe the overall sequence of service use during a clinical episode, or during a patient career. However, the introduction of the term *Integrated Care Pathway* (ICP) describes the process for a discrete element of services, and sets out evidence-based best practice and outcomes that are locally agreed, leads to confusion. Accordingly the term *total patient journey* is used here to describe the total sequence of services used (possibly more than one concurrently), and the total sequence of care transitions by a person during an episode of care and treatment. This will consist of a series of periods of use of services, measured either by length of use, or by number of treatment sessions, and the transitions between service elements.

There are three sets of care transitions to consider in the British context: (a) *age-transitions*, which include adolescent-adult transitions, and adult-older adult transitions; (b) *between-client group services transitions*, which include transitions from and to substance misuse, learning disabilities, and forensic services; (c) *within-service transitions*, such as primary care-community specialist care, community specialist care-local acute inpatient care, and acute inpatient care-local non-hospital accommodation. Given the risk of breakdown in therapeutic relationships and discontinuities in treatment, it is worth trying to minimise the impact of these transitions. In the case of age-transitions particularly, there are now several examples in Britain of young adult transition services, offering continuity of treatment across the normal 18/19 year boundary, and pilots of all-age adult services, so that adults over the age of 65 have access to all generic adult services, with an add-on service specifically for dementia.

In order for users to make the transition from one service element to another, a set of referral (or transfer) and acceptance criteria must be developed, which implies both inclusion and exclusion criteria. People and procedures must exist to ensure that these criteria are known to key staff and are applied consistently. Moreover, there should be early and continuing contact with key workers, who will retain responsibility. It may be important to distinguish between transfer of main consultant and/or key-worker responsibility, and all-age access to specialized clinical services, such as crisis services and psychological therapies.

In Britain it has often been easier to enter services from a less intensive level of service to a more intensive service than to make a transition from a more intensive level of service to a less intensive. This retention of users in services designed for higher levels of complexity or risk means that a user's needs may be exceeded, with the concurrent risk of creating dependency. Accordingly, the set of inclusion and exclusion criteria for any given service must include all possible directions of travel. Taken together, the sets of criteria for transitions from one setting to another must be (a) *exhaustive*, to include all options for transition (including possibly backwards transfer from the older adult to the adult CMHT or service); (b) *need-related*, so that the criteria include potential settings for all possible patterns of user need; and (c) *specific* to each individual setting.

Delivery of Mental Health Services in the Private Sector

All of the figures given so far relate to provision of mental health services by the NHS. It is estimated that 16 percent of the total expenditure for all health care in Britain is for private care, including private medical insurance and direct out-of-pocket payment. The percentage of mental health care delivered in the private sector is very difficult to calculate, while the provision of private mental health *inpatient* facilities is probably less than that for general medical care. The total provision for *outpatient* mental health care includes not only provision by the main mental health professions, but also provision by fully qualified psychotherapists and counsellors and by psychotherapists and counsellors undergoing training, and by other practitioners without any accepted training, as well as voluntary and charitable schemes (including those provided by churches and other faith groups).

As far as private inpatient facilities are concerned, the general market is dominated by five main organizations (other than private beds in NHS hospitals, which are not available for mental health patients). Of these other organizations, the three largest are BMI Healthcare, Nuffield Hospitals, and BUPA. The Priory Group provides mental health services only, and now has the contract with the Ministry of Defence to provide mental health inpatient facilities for the armed forces (there being no equivalent to the Veterans Administration in the United States). St Andrews Hospital, Northampton is a unique nonprofit charitable institution, dating back to 1838, which now provides a range of specialized inpatient units, and as a group employs over 2,000 staff. The general or specialist inpatient facilities run by any of these organizations may also treat a person funded by the NHS, where the person's local NHS mental health service does not have a service to meet their needs.

There are now a number of mental health private practice collaboratives or partnerships offering individual, family and group treatment. These may be single-profession or single-treatment modality agencies, or may include professionals from several disciplines. In addition, there will be individuals in solo practice. While members of any profession may do a small amount of private practice early in their careers, typically psychiatrists and clinical psychologists have worked in the NHS for a number of years at a senior level before moving into private practice full-time.

While private mental health practice is increasing in Britain, and much is of a high standard, the standard by which private practice is judged is that of the NHS, and those private practitioners from one of the main mental health professions will necessarily have trained in NHS settings. If a person is being seen privately, they retain the right of immediate access to a NHS facility if they need it.

Direct Service Personnel

Historically, the British nineteenth century asylum system employed two categories of staff – medical staff and "attendants." As the medical profession was not fully registered until the 1850s, the tradition of nonmedical or lay asylum superintendents continued until the 1846 *Lunatics Act* awarded a monopoly in running asylums to the medical profession. The attendants, or keepers were initially untrained until the then psychiatrist's organization, the Royal Medico-Psychological Association, introduced a training course leading to a certificate in the later nineteenth century. The subsequent introduction of formal registration of all nurses in 1919 created a standard of training for all branches of nursing. The first social workers were employed in British mental hospitals in the 1920s, and occupational therapists began to be employed from the 1930s. Small numbers of psychologists were working in child guidance clinics from 1927, but apart from literally a handful of psychologists working with adults before the second world war, psychologists only began to develop their work in that field in the early 1950s. Accordingly, until the 1970s the reality in many of the then large psychiatric hospitals was that there was a very restricted range of therapeutic skills available.

There has been marked growth of direct service personnel in the 30 years following *Better Services for the Mentally Ill* (Department of Health and Social Security 1975), which addressed the need for a significant improvement in key disciplines. A section of the 1999 National Service Framework was dedicated to work force planning, education and training. The Framework recognized ongoing difficulties in recruitment, and the need to build a work force that represented the local communities that are served and that has the skills and competencies to deliver modern services. Five principles for developing the work force were laid out: (a) establishing clear and collaborative inter-agency work force plans; (b) creating work forces that are culturally competent for their local areas that offer equality of opportunity for all staff; (c) ensuring that training programs are evidence-based and inter-disciplinary, stressing the value of team and inter-agency working; (d) providing opportunities for ongoing professional development; (e) enabling leadership to flourish, promoting innovation which reflects the complexity of mental health care. The implementation of these principles should lead to higher overall numbers of staff, to an enlargement in the range of professions making a significant contribution to services, and to the range of skills of those professionals.

The most recent figures for staffing numbers for England only are given for February 2005 (Hansard, 2005). Table 2.7 shows the head-count figures for subgroups of psychiatrist consultants only in the main subspecialties for five-year intervals from 1989. Table 2.8 shows the numbers in each of the other professional groups working in hospital and community mental health for approximate five-year intervals from 1990. For many parts of the country services for people with learning disabilities are provided by the same Trust that provides mental health services, so it is difficult to establish staffing levels for mental health alone for all professions.

These figures do not include unqualified staff, staff in other professions than those cited, or students and trainees, many of whom have significant relevant experience before starting their formal training.

Table 2.7. *Head-Count Figures for Subgroups of Psychiatrist Consultants, 1989 to 2004.*

Subgroups	1989	1994	1999	2004
Child and adolescent psychiatry	343	358	486	541
General psychiatry	1190	1246	1569	1911
Old age psychiatry	65	164	311	484
Forensic psychiatry	50	82	152	231
Psychotherapy	90	90	109	122
Total (for mental health, excluding learning disabilities)	1738	1940	2627	3289

Table 2.8. *Mental Health Professional Groups, 1990 to 2003.*

Professional Groups	1990	1994	1999	2003
Qualified mental health nurses	37011	34995	38999	44728
Psychotherapists	217	290	574	948
Qualified clinical psychologists	1325	2493	4572	6757
Art/music/drama therapists	389	482	646	764
Qualified occupational therapists	6241	7490	12663	15391
Qualified social services staff	n/a	n/a	n/a	241
Total	45183	45750	57454	68829

Note. Figures for groups other than mental health nurses include those working in learning disabilities.

Consequently, the numbers underrepresent the total direct care work force. However, they do indicate an overall increase of 51 percent in all categories of trained staff between 1994 and 2003. The figures also show some very interesting differences in growth between groups. For psychiatrists, the growth in consultant medical psychotherapists was only about one percent per year, while for non-medical psychotherapists, the growth was 336 percent over the whole 13-year period. For the three largest non-medical professions, the numbers of clinical psychologists grew by 410 percent over the same time. The figures for social workers underrepresent the total commitment of social work to mental health, as previously the most common mode of employment was attachment to mental health services, rather than direct employment by them.

Conventionally, there have been five main mental health professional groups – psychiatrists, psychiatric nurses, clinical psychologists, occupational therapists, and social workers. As with other medical specialties in the NHS, psychiatrists occupy a privileged position, with separate conditions of employment, and all mental health trusts are required to have a medical director. Medical practitioners in Britain qualify after five or six years with joint Bachelors degrees in medicine (M.B.) and surgery (B.S.). (The MD degree is an advanced research degree). Since 2003, two years further general training are required to enter specialist training. After three years of specialist training in psychiatry, they must obtain Membership in the Royal College of Psychiatrists (M.R.C.Psych), and to qualify for a consultant post. Counting their bacheloreate education and all subsequent general and specialty training, psychiatrists spend about ten years in training to qualify as a psychiatric consultant. While the preconsultant grades are technically training posts, both the junior and senior training grades are providing services, and make a significant contribution to services.

Psychiatric nurses in Britain are trained separately from general nurses and from nurses working with people with learning disabilities. They are the largest single professional group within specialist mental health services. While their conventional role has been to staff inpatient services, their role has diversified considerably, first by the growth of community psychiatric nursing since the 1970s, mostly in the context of community mental health teams, and secondly, by the opportunities for them to develop more specialist therapy functions. Mental health nurses train for three years, and obtain either a bachelor's degree or diploma that is accredited so they can be registered as a mental nurse (RMN).

In practice, over the past ten years clinical psychologists working in specialist mental health services have been joined by other groups of psychologists (mostly counseling, health, and forensic psychologists) and by other counselors. Collectively, these psychology specialties constitute a pooled resource to provide psychological therapies. Clinical psychologists must first obtain a three-year bachelors Honours Degree in psychology, and they must work for at least two years in a related field before proceeding to clinical training. Until 1990 post-graduate training courses were either two or three years, leading to either a Masters Degree or Diploma, but all training is now standardized at three years, leading to a doctoral degree (D.Psy. or D.Clin.Psy.) The PhD has always been retained as a research degree in Britain.

Occupational therapists are responsible for the provision of structured therapeutic regimes in both inpatient and daycare settings. As members of mental health community teams, they also facilitate the return of mental health patients to independent community living. Many OTs have developed specialist therapeutic functions. Since the mid-1990s occupational therapists have qualified with a three-year degree. Social workers in the mental health field used to be separately employed by the local authority, but increasingly joint appointments are made in conjunction with the NHS to most community mental health services. Over the years social work training has varied the most of all these groups, but full professional training is now two years after a bachelors degree.

The three separately registered groups of Art, Drama, and Music therapists are mentioned in the table above. In addition to these groups, other registered therapists also work in mental health, such as physiotherapists (working mostly with younger people, people with severe mental illness, and older adults), and speech and language therapists. Psychiatric pharmacists are also working directly in services, and teachers work in hospital schools attached to inpatient psychiatric units for children and adolescents.

A major feature of the manpower implications of the National Service Framework has been the explicit creation of totally new mental health professional groups. Target numbers for several of these were described in 2002, and they are essentially designed to enable primary care to better manage "common mental health problems." Five hundred Gateway workers were to be employed, to work with GPs and primary care teams, to strengthen access to services, and to improve community triage for people who may need urgent contact with specialist services. The most interesting group are the "graduate primary care mental health workers," one thousand of whom are to be trained to deliver "brief therapy techniques of proven effectiveness" – a carefully constructed phrase indicating they will not be using counseling techniques, but structured psychological interventions.

The development of new mental health professions illustrates the attention being paid to specific skills, irrespective of a stated profession of origin, especially where there are perceived gaps between demand and provision. Given the continued levels of vacancies in all of the five main mental health professions, detailed attention has been paid to mental health work force planning, and this topic is itself one of the major streams of work from the *National Service Framework*. *Mental Health Services – Work Force Design and Development* (2003d) aims to guide local health and social care systems to produce a local, collaborative work force plan. This approach is based on the conventional evaluation cycle, so that a review of the current work force, against expected rates of turnover and in the light of planned developments, leads to estimations of the required work force, which in turn leads to an implementation plan. The impact of new service developments on staffing demand can be difficult to ascertain. For example, from 2005 mental health services in prisons are to be provided by the general NHS, replacing the previous prison internal mental health service, but precisely how that replacement will be made has not been specified. A major component of an implementation plan will be the commissioning of numbers of training positions. Numbers of medical training positions are determined nationally, and there have been recent major expansions in the number of medical training positions, including the creation of totally new medical schools. Training numbers for all other professions are determined on a regional level through manpower and education consortia, who commission training positions from local higher education institutes (which includes universities). Upon completion of training, an individual professional is free to apply for a post in any part of the country. Consequently, for those professions where a high proportion work in the general medical field (such as occupational therapy), an increase in the number trained does not necessarily lead to a proportionate increase in those working specifically in the mental health field.

Administrative Personnel

In addition to direct service personnel, mental health services also employ managerial and support staff. Until the early 1990s there had been a recognizable profession of health service administration, but with the introduction of "general management" in the NHS under the Thatcher government, senior management posts were opened up to staff from any profession, or from backgrounds outside the health or social care fields. This led initially to a number of senior posts being filled by applicants from business and the military, for example, alongside appointments of doctors and senior nurses. The concept of general management has now been extended, so that experienced professional staff may move into middle-management posts, either as substantive posts or while retaining some clinical duties. This extension has created a far more fluid managerial field. Moreover, with the introduction of what is called *the Modern Matron* role – where senior nurses are responsible for all activities on their ward – there is now a wide range of career paths open to those who choose to enter management, up to the level of a NHS Trust Chief Executive.

With the creation of new NHS Mental Health Trusts and Primary Care Trusts around the year 2000, each with their own Trust Board of Directors, there are now in England some 400 NHS bodies, each with their Local Authority joint partners, providing NHS mental health services. Each will have a Finance Director at the Board level, with supporting staff, and a range of support functions, such as human resources and information technology (IT). Recruitment for these posts depends on the local labour market, and with salary scales fixed nationally, there can then be severe local recruitment difficulties for some grades of support staff. While figures for managers in mental health services are not available, the total number of managers employed in the NHS in 2003 was 130,000 on a head-count basis (Hansard 2005). Qualified nurses formed 30.1 percent of this figure, and all doctors constituted 8.5 percent of administrative positions. All other qualified scientific, therapeutic and technical staff were 9.5 percent of the total number of managers in the NHS. Direct support to doctors and nurses (e.g., health care assistants and medical secretaries was 23.3%), and there were several other categories of infrastructure support staff (such as catering and property staff). Managers and senior managers with a significant responsibility for budgets or manpower accounted for 2.8 percent, but this proportion, as a politically sensitive figure, conceals the significant proportion of time spent on management functions by professional clinical staff. There is no reason to suppose that these figures are not reasonably representative of the position in mental health services, except that there would be very few scientific or medical technical staff (such as biochemists or radiographers) employed. Thus, in England administrative staff account for about 10 percent of all employees in the mental health system.

The NHS is accordingly a major employer in it's own right. Many more women than are currently employed have obtained a health care professional qualification at some time in the past, and are a potential staffing resource. Britain now attracts significant numbers of health care workers from overseas, with European qualified staff now having a right of entry. Even with these potential human resources, as mental health services develop, with a demand for a new range of skills and working in new ways, the existing pool of qualified staff is simply inadequate to meet the demand for staff. Even with the major expansion in training capacity that has taken place, new patterns of working, and new ways of training staff will be required to meet public expectations.

Financing and Commissioning Systems

General Principles of Funding the Health Care System

A good account of NHS financial procedures is set out in the Healthcare Financial Management Associations's Introductory guide [HFMA] (2004). Spending on health care in Britain comes from three sources: (a) government funding – mainly, but not exclusively through the NHS; (b) funding via health insurance schemes; and (c) personal funding. Of these three sources, the first is overwhelmingly the largest, for all categories of health spending.

Government funding is primarily through general taxation, although in recent years more reliance has been placed on income from National Insurance contributions (a progressive health care tax), patient charges for certain categories of services (such as charges for prescriptions dispensed), and other sources of income. The specific figures in the following sections are taken from the Mental Health Strategies (2005) analysis of investment in mental health services. In 2003/04, at the foreign exchange rate (ER) of 1.64, the NHS spending in the UK amounted to £72.1 billion (bn) (US $44 bn), and for England the figure was £61.3 bn (US $37.4 bn). England's total health care expenditure accounted for about 7.7 percent of the Gross Domestic Product for the year 2003–04, of which about 6.5 percent was NHS spending. Health spending from the other two sources accounts for only 1.2 percent of GDP.

The system of funding has changed over the past few years and is continuing to change. In 1999, the previously separate financial allocations to the extant Health Authorities were merged to give a unified allocation, with the intention of giving commissioners of health care the greatest possible flexibility. These resources are cash-limited, in that they represent the maximum spending permitted in any one fiscal year. A recent review of the funding mechanisms of the NHS, published as the *Wanless Report* (Department of Health 2002e), concluded that public funding was a "fair and efficient" way to provide a comprehensive high quality service, based on need, and not on the ability to pay. The report also recommended an increase in funding to between 10.6 percent and 12.5 percent of national income over a 20-year period, assuming no change in private health expenditure.

This money is essentially allocated to individual Primary Care Trusts on a "weighted capitation" basis, taking account of variations in such indices as rate of births, and of older people, with the objective of producing a target fair share for each part of the country. From 2003/2004 a new formula has been used which takes better account of both social deprivation indices and unmet need. Some money is retained centrally for centrally funded initiatives, and special allocations for very specialized services (see later section). This money is then assigned by the Primary Care Trusts (PCTs) to individual provider Trusts, including the Trusts providing mental health services, on the basis of service agreements with them, which are essentially led by patterns and levels of activity, rather than by finance. The underlying principle is that money should follow work done.

The direct costs of mental illness as far as public spending is concerned in 2003/2004 were £4.8 billion (bn) (US $2.9 bn at the ER of 1.64 for 2003) for adult mental health services, £7.6 bn (US $4.6 bn) for social security and unemployment benefits, £0.8 bn (US $0.5 bn) for drug payments, and £0.7 bn (US $0.4 bn) local authority costs, totalling £13.9 bn (US $8.5 bn). But the expenditures for these public services represent only a proportion of the other costs of poor mental health, which include costs that can be calculated straightforwardly (such as working days lost) and costs that are less easy to calculate. The Sainsbury Centre for Mental Health (2003) has estimated that public service provision constitutes 34 percent of the total direct costs of mental illness, other output losses associated with missed employment being estimated at over £23 bn, (US $14 bn) and state benefits were estimated at £9.5 bn (US $5.8 bn). The total annual costs of mental health problems in England were estimated to be £77.4 bn (US $47.2 bn), the impact on quality of life accounting for well over half that figure. This figure is itself an underestimate, as it does not take account of cost for mental health services for children and young people or for older adults.

Revenue Funding

From 2003 the total funding allocation is distributed according to a complex formula, described by HFMA (2004). There are five components to the current allocation formula. The first four components are:

Hospital and Community Health Services. This is the largest single component, and accounts for 82.8 percent of the total funds allocated. The factors that combine to determine this are population, the age make-up of the population, the relative need for health care (derived itself from a combination of statistics), the market forces costs of delivering health care (reflecting differential costs of wages and housing), and the costs of ambulance services in rural areas.

Prescribing. This is 14.1 percent of the total, and funds the costs of drugs prescribed by all GPs and prescribing nurses. It covers the gross costs of drugs prescribed, and does not take account of receipts for prescriptions (which are retained centrally). In fact, charges are paid on only one in five prescriptions.

Cash-Limited, General Medical Services. This component covers payments to GPs for practice staff, premises and computer costs, and represents 2.5% of the formula. The population is age weighted to take account of longer consultation times for older patients and other vulnerable groups.

HIV/Aids. This addition to the formula represents only 0.7 percent of the formula, to take account of the very different incidence of this disease group.

These are combined to produce a unified, weighted population for each commissioner, and set a target allocation for hospital, community and family services. A *fifth component* termed "noncash limited general medical services," was first introduced in 2002/2003. They represent the cost of those primary care professionals (such as GPs themselves, and opticians and pharmacists) who are not directly employed by the NHS, but who are technically independent contractors. From April, 2004 a new contract has been introduced for GPs, and this fifth component will be wholly incorporated into the new formula.

The funding allocation formula is essentially a complex and sophisticated attempt to represent both differences in need and differences in delivery costs. In addition to the five components just discussed, PCTs have resources from centrally funded initiatives and special allocations, known as CFISSA, which provide budgets for (a) common NHS services (including statutory bodies such as the Prescription Pricing Authority), (b) funding for special initiatives that are used as agents for change (some of which can only be obtained by a bidding process), and (c) financing the costs of both medical and non-medical training (that also take account of the additional costs of providing training for undergraduate medical students).

Other sources for funding the NHS include private and paying patients. Trusts are able to charge for patients receiving services in superior facilities. This rarely occurs in mental health services, but under certain conditions, professional staff may see private outpatients on NHS premises and then pay a proportion of the fee to the Trust. Prior to the NHS, individual hospitals accumulated funds through charitable grants and bequests. The total value of these Trust funds in 2002/2003 was £1.4 bn (US$ 0.9 bn at the 2002 ER of 1.50), and now constitutes a valuable source of income that can be used by the NHS in a variety of ways, often to improve the physical environment for patients, or to pay for facilities for staff.

Capital Funding

The funding streams described so far refer only to revenue spending. Capital investment follows a different stream. For this purpose, a capital asset is defined as any individual asset with a cost of £5,000 (US $2,732 at the 2004 ER of 1.83) or more, or an asset with a life of one year or more. Capital is funded from three sources, the smallest source being charitable funds (already described). The two major sources are public capital, and private finance initiatives.

The Department of Health has a number of central capital programmes that finance medium-to-large scale schemes, which would be unreasonable to be funded from operational budgets. Examples include both major clinical equipment (such as MRI scanners) and major information technology schemes, as well as building schemes. In 2003/2004, this element of the capital budget was £1.3 bn (US $0.79 bn at the 2003 ER of 1.64). The operational capital scheme covers more routine replacement of equipment and buildings, and small scale upgrades, and this element of the capital budget was £844 m in 2003/2004. A further strategic or discretionary capital allocation covers strategic change schemes that cannot be funded from block capital, and in 2003/2004 this was £684 million (m) (US $417 m). At the 2004 ER of 1.83 for 2004, the overall capital allocations for the whole NHS in England for the successive years starting in 2004 will be £3.27 bn (US $1.79 bn) and in 2005 will be £3.95 bn (US $2.16 bn).

The second major source of capital funding is from the private finance initiative (PFI). This is a mechanism initiated in 1992 for obtaining investment from private companies to build the asset, and these are then leased back to the NHS, typically for around 30 years. The schemes must have a capital value of at least £25 m (US $13.7 million at the 2004 ER of 1.83), and typically involve the private contractor in designing, building, and operating the facility, without actually providing clinical services. The most obvious attraction of PFI is that it reduces the need for public sector capital. Less obviously, it also provides a continuing commercial incentive for efficiency. For both NHS capital funded projects and for PFI projects, the total capital assets of a NHS Trust are subject to a "capital charge," which is a levy on the total capital assets of a Trust, so that cost comparisons with private providers are realistic and encourage awareness of capital costs in day-to-day management.

Although it is estimated that about 16 percent of the total expenditure for all health care in Britain is for private care, about 12 percent of the population had some form of private health insurance by the end of the year 2000 (Laing & Buisson, 2001). A typical private insurance plan is a "package," that sets out maximum payments for different categories of health services. Private health insurance is not normally designed for particular illnesses, but there may be limits on the maximum number of treatment sessions, or maximum number of inpatient days, that are payable under the policy. Formal psychological therapy may be covered by a private policy, and counselling from a qualified practitioner adhering to a specific form of therapy, but generic counselling may not be covered.

Commissioning Processes

From the process already described, an individual PCT will be confronted with the task of how to spend their allocation. This process of determining how to spend the allocation is called *commissioning*, which in the NHS is the process of negotiating agreements with service providers to meet the health needs of a given population. While commissioning had been implicit in the NHS since it began, it became more explicit under the conservative government of the early 1990s, when an "internal market" within the NHS was created, which effectively placed adjacent hospitals in a competitive relationship to each other. This essentially destructive process has been replaced by a partnership model, but comparative costs between adjacent services still play a part in the decisions of commissioners.

Commissioning consists of a conventional cycle of (a) assessment of the needs of a given population, (b) comparing that assessment with current levels of provision to identify gaps, and (c) prioritizing desired services in the light of government priorities. Thus, effective commissioning depends on an accurate understanding both of local demography and epidemiology, and of high-need subgroups within the population. The small size of some subgroups means that their needs can be adequately understood by small scale audits of their case records, or by using a service-deliverable needs assessment such as the shortened version of the Camberwell Assessment of Need, as already mentioned. In practice, established patterns of service delivery and their associated funding cannot be changed quickly, and in any event major changes in patterns of service may require a public consultation process. Thus, the actual pattern of delivered services embodies past historical patterns of service delivery, with essentially an incremental approach to change.

Effective commissioning should also take account of the views of service users and the local community, and of available evidence on the effectiveness of specific interventions and styles of service delivery. The National Service Framework and other associated government NHS policies have increased significantly the attention paid to user's views in health and social care planning. *Acute Care Forums* are one device to ensure that attention is paid to users' views in improving the quality of care in acute psychiatric inpatient settings, for example. The central principle underlying this view is that users of services, and of the caregivers and family members of service users are the most valid commentators on the value of those services. While obtaining users' views is not easy, there is a clear policy drive to require all services, including mental health services, to obtain representative views, and this has led to the requirement in 2004 to carry out externally conducted surveys, such as those conducted by the Picker Institute for Mental Health Trusts.

Importance is increasingly being attached to the evidence-base for service practice and development. Two major, linked developments have contributed to the increased attention paid to evidence: first, the improvement in the standards of research design; and secondly, the development of systematic reviews and meta-analysis, so results from a number of studies can be pooled to give statistically stronger support for treatments. The British journal *Evidence-Based Mental Health*, for example, regularly provides succinct summaries indicating the effectiveness of different specific interventions. It is more difficult to establish the effectiveness of modes of service delivery, but research on both specific interventions and modes of service delivery are incorporated into the NICE clinical practice guidelines already described and the University of York *Effective Health Care Bulletins* (for Chronic Fatigue Syndrome, for example). All these types of research, audit and development studies direct attention to the choice of appropriate outcome measures, showing whether or not an intervention is actually effective in local conditions.

Levels of Commissioning

Commissioning is carried out at several levels, of which the most important is the Primary Care Trust (PCT), which commissions the majority of services for its local population. Mental health services are increasingly commissioned by joint commissioners at the PCT level, who pool all the funding available from both NHS and local authority sources. Each PCT area will have a commissioner for mental health services, who exercises that function together with the Local Implementation Team (LIT). Membership in the LIT includes both the PCT and Local Authority, as well as the Mental Health Trust for the locality, and representatives of local voluntary and charitable providers, as well as users and carers.

Presently, practice-based commissioning is being encouraged. Consequently, individual GP practices with populations of about 10,000 will be permitted more autonomy in their practice. Commissioning already differentiates between localities within a PCT, such as a catchment area of generic community mental health teams, or groupings of GP practices (populations between 30,000 and 50,000). This differentiation reflects awareness of variations of need down to the electoral ward and housing estate levels. There may be major differentiations between the rural and urban sections of a county, and in the most thinly populated parts of England, and even more so in thinly populated areas of Scotland and Wales, special consideration has to be paid to rural issues.

Commissioning occurs at the level of Primary Care Trusts as well as the level of GP practices. At the individual PCT level, allocations are made for populations ranging typically from 150,000 to 200,000. For some low-frequency conditions, commissioning may involve two or more neighbouring PCTs, or may cover a whole Strategic Health Authority consisting of about six to ten PCTs together with a total population of the order of 1.5 million.

The specialties that are the focus of commissioning for larger populations are determined by the *National Specialist Services Definitions* (Department of Health, 2002d), which specifies ten specialist clinical services for which commissioning arrangements must be made. These specialist services have been described earlier, and include for example, forensic services and eating disorders services. Specialist Commissioning Groups (Consortia) are set up by two or more Strategic Health Authorities, which cover up to 20 or so PCTs serving a population of three to four million.

From the inception of PCTs in their present form in 2002, there was no national guidance for mental health commissioners. This omission was rectified in 2005 with the publication of *The Commissioning Friend for Mental Health Services* (National Primary and Care

Trust Development Programme, 2005). Since only about 25 percent of the 300 or so mental health commissioners in the PCTs had previous experience as lead mental health commissioners, this guidance has been welcomed. It is extremely detailed and the layout of the guidance is instructive, with main sections on commissioning to improve mental health, working in partnership, audit and evaluation, and with appendices on, for example, using care pathways and programme and project management principles.

Each NHS Trust is required to produce an annual report, conforming to national criteria, especially in the reporting of financial information. As an example, the 2004 report for the Cambridgeshire and Peterborough Mental Health Partnership NHS Trust is analyzed below.

The Cambridgeshire and Peterborough Mental Health Partnership NHS Trust: An Illustration

This Trust is typical in providing mental health services for children and adolescents, working-age adults and the elderly, including forensic and eating disorders services and learning disability services. The Trust provides services to a population of over 800,000 people in an area of over 1,400 square miles, that includes the two major cities of Cambridge and Peterborough. Created in 2002, this Trust combined services previously provided separately by two social service departments and five NHS Trusts. The combination required considerable rational organization of different administrative systems. The financial analysis of the annual report does not separately cost the learning disability service, indicating the difficulty in establishing precise expenditures.

The Mental Health Partnership services of the Trust employed 2,166 people in 2004, consisting of 1,033 nursing staff, 373 health care assistants and support workers, 287 administrative, clerical and estates staff, 278 allied health professions (including psychologists), 138 medical staff, and 57 social care staff. Management costs were estimated as 6.4 percent of income. At the 2004 ER of 1.83, the total income of the Trust for 2004 was £99.8 m (US $54.5 m), and the total tangible assets of the Trust were calculated at £63 m (US $34 m). In order to deliver services the Trust had to develop working relationships with a number of other "related parties," including Cambridgeshire County Council, Hertfordshire County Council, Peterborough City Council, Norfolk, Suffolk and Cambridgeshire Strategic Health Authority, 13 PCTs, three other NHS Trusts (including the two general hospital Trusts serving the population), and other NHS-shared services and Authorities – a minimum of 23 different agencies.

Reports of this type put flesh on the structures and processes described earlier in the chapter. The report indicates the new services that have been started during the year, including a GP-based computerized serious mental illness (SMI) register, which enables practices to ensure that people with SMI receive regular health checks and medication reviews. A new "in-reach" team has been set up to work in one of the local prisons, providing multidisciplinary services of psychology, psychotherapy, community psychiatric nursing, and occupational therapy. Planning has begun to provide comparable services in another prison. A pilot project has been started in Peterborough to help Pakistani women with postnatal depression and at risk of depression and anxiety. A scheme in one of the localities created a mosaic at a hospital, made by clients at a vocational scheme working with an artist-in-residence. The Trust had been awarded national funding to develop a new service for people with severe and complex personality disorders (one of only eight such initiatives in the country).

All of these initiatives are additional to the 24-hour day-to-day work of the clinical teams and units and support staff. The partnerships with statutory agencies that have been listed are exceeded in number by the voluntary and charitable agencies providing information, support, accommodation, and meaningful daytime activity. Many staff will be studying for an additional qualification, or will be members of a professional organisation that will be providing ongoing educational opportunities for their members. The Trust report does not even mention the research work being carried out within the Trust by the University of Cambridge Department of Psychiatry and by other University Departments. The total range of activities carried out in Cambridgeshire (as elsewhere) to promote mental health and to support and treat those with significant mental health problems goes far beyond the scope of Department of Health policies and funding.

PART TWO: EVALUATION

EVALUATIVE AND MONITORING PROCEDURES

The performance of health and social care in general in Britain is formally regulated in a number of ways, and some of the regulatory bodies publish information that is in effect evaluative. Management bodies also provide some evaluative information. In addition, formal research and evaluative studies are funded directly by the relevant government departments, by publicly funded but independent bodies such as the Medical Research Council, and by other independent bodies large and small, such as the substantial funds of £400 million annually provided by the Wellcome Trust and the smaller Joseph Rowntree Foundation, a well-respected social policy charity. Evaluative data is thus provided from a range of sources and scrutinised by public, academic and independent organisations; in the British context much of this information may be politically sensitive.

The evaluation of the performance of publicly funded mental health and social care services in Britain is accordingly set in a context common to all health and social care, and is itself carried out publicly. All public bodies ultimately are accountable to Parliament, either directly for the performance of services through the responsible Minister, or through a body directly accountable to the House of Commons, such as the Audit Commission. For each government department there is a House of Commons "Select Committee" that scrutinises policy and performance, who have the power to require Cabinet Ministers to appear before them. Select Committees are made up of non-ministerial Members of Parliament with cross-party membership whose composition reflects the current balance of power of the main political parties. Individual Members of Parliament may ask questions relating to individual cases that are then reported in national media. As an editorial in a respected journal (Black, 2004) pointed out "there can be few countries in which the Prime Minister and Secretary of State for Health find themselves publicly involved in accounting for the care provided for a particular patient." Yet this happens not infrequently, and issues relating to the care in individuals were invoked during the general election campaign of 2005.

Responsibility for the overall monitoring of health services was carried out by the Commission for Health Improvement (CHI), which was a separate body until 2005. Among its other responsibilities, the CHI conducted on-site clinical governance reviews of 35 – half of the total – specialist mental health services in England and Wales between 2001 and 2003, and produced a detailed report summarising what was found in those visits (CHI, 2004). This report pulls few punches: it reports that while a number of Trusts are performing well, a "larger number face significant challenges" with capacity problems in management, staffing, and infrastructure. Bed capacity in many Trusts was also found to be under severe pressure, and they found that in a number of Trusts there was an inconsistent approach to the prevention and management of violence and aggression. There was also a separate Social Services Inspectorate (SSI) that similarly reviewed the mental health component of local social care services. In 2004, the SSI and CHI were merged with the Health Development Agency into one body, the Commission for Health Care Audit and Inspection (CHAI). In 2005, a new National Institute for Health and Clinical Excellence was set up, the independent organization responsible for providing national guidance on the promotion of good health and the prevention and treatment of ill health. It has now produced detailed evidence-based guidance on the treatment of many psychiatric and psychological conditions.

In addition, there is a range of both financial and non-financial performance procedures that monitor services against both standards and specific targets. A particular target that has been prominent politically is the reduction of waiting times for both outpatient and inpatient appointments. The financial regulatory framework incorporates over 30 standards, including, for example, accounting for government grants, and retirement benefits. The non-financial framework is administered by CHAI, who again specify performance targets, which have until 2005 been collated into an overall grading of each Trust, with the highest level of performance being "three-star" Trusts. Within these frameworks and other accompanying statutory and professional audit and accreditation procedures, every aspect of the six core evaluative criteria that this volume is adopting is covered.

The 2004 Appleby Evaluation

A major internal evaluation of the impact of the 1999 National Service Framework (NSF) for mental health of adults was carried out by the British National Director for Mental Health, Professor Louis Appleby, in December, 2004. While this review is by the person tasked by central government to implement the NSF, and while it focuses on adult services only, it is a comprehensive and detailed review. It is more even handed than an external review might be, and balances statements such as "an impressive range of policy initiatives has been triggered in an area of health care that was previously neglected" with "yet more is needed and some changes . . . are needed urgently." In this section comments from the Appleby review will be included under each of the six standard evaluative criteria adopted for this volume. Table 2.9 compares the main headings of the Appleby review against those criteria, indicating that all of the criteria are dealt with under one or more of the NSF standards or other sections of the review.

Equity of Access and Provision of Services

This section addresses the overall equity of the system, with respect to the comprehensiveness of the system for all types of disorders, for different levels of service, for local access, and for parity with other services.

Without question there has been increased comprehensiveness of specialist mental health services, in terms of the range of services provided and the adequacy of those services over the past 30 years or so. This has been focused on those with more serious mental health problems, where there is significant functional disruption to the individual's life. The specific targets of the NSF, requiring the creation of crisis services, assertive outreach teams, and early intervention in psychosis services, all illustrate this focus. The development of primary care mental health services has been slower, and until about the past five years much more variable in quantity. Appleby comments that a vision of mental health care in primary care is needed nationally, to include the management of long-term conditions that do not require the full involvement of a CMHT. This pattern of development of services indicates that there is a gap in provision between those being seen in primary care, who will be offered relatively short treatment, and those in specialist services with more severe problems, of those with a treatable nonpsychotic condition, who although detected do not reach the threshold for NHS treatment. Consequently, there is a paradox that this increasing comprehensiveness of the service, in terms of the range of services provided, has in some localities been accompanied by the local loss of inclusion of some types of disorder. This is because, before national prioritizing guidance was issued, local services developed their own criteria, and some local specialist services were developed, guided by the idiosyncratic interests of local clinicians rather than by local need. A good example of this would be the past availability of psychological treatment (by current standards not necessarily of high effectiveness) for relatively mild anxiety-related conditions in some localities, that would not now reach the threshold of severity to justify treatment.

However, the creation of both specialist community mental health and primary care mental health teams, with a national trend to serve increasingly smaller populations, means that geographical access to services is good. Whatever problems of distance are perceived in Britain, the maximum distance from a community mental health team of probably not

Table 2.9. *Comparisons of Evaluation Criteria.*

Criteria for this volume	Headings of the Appleby 2004 review of the NSF
Access and equity	Standard 1: promoting mental health for all: combating discrimination
	Standard 3: round-the-clock access to local services
Quality and efficacy	Standard 2: be offered effective treatments
	Chapter 13: clinical guidelines
Cost and efficiency	Chapter 9: finance
Financing and fairness	Chapter 9: finance
Protection and participation, including patient safety	Standard 7: preventing suicides
Population relevance	Chapter 15: discussion of "mental health of the whole community"

more than 25 miles in most of England pales into insignificance against distances for the other countries described in this volume. The creation of bases for those community teams in local health centres and "shop-front'" offices, and the nearing complete elimination of the old psychiatric hospitals and their replacement with new purpose-built accommodation, often on the site of a general hospital, together mean that most users of statutory mental health services access those services in non-stigmatising settings. However, Appleby admits that there are still wards that are unsuitable for the care of distressed people, and capital investment should be directed to replace the poorest wards. One function of the Strategic Health Authority (already described) is to ensure that the available resources are distributed reasonably equitably across the whole health economy, but recognising the need for prioritisation for very poor services.

Within this overall concern for equity of provision, there has been concern for provision for those deprived communities and groups where there is a recognition of either underprovision or inappropriate provision. Among the projects conducted by the National Institute for Mental Health have been those focusing on the needs of women (including ensuring the provision of single-sex wards and in-patient areas), the needs of members of black and minority ethnic groups, and of homeless people. An emerging problem during the past ten years has been the increasing numbers of illegal immigrants into the United Kingdom, among whom will be some traumatized by, for example, civil war in the Balkans or African states, where concern for their mental health needs conflicts with pressures for them to be returned to their country of origin.

Until 2005 health care for prisoners was provided by an in-house Prison Medical Service, which was recognized to be inadequate, so since then all health services are required to be provided by generic service providers, with comparable standards to that of services provided to the general population. Accordingly, local mental health trusts now provide specialist mental health services to penal institutions by seconded staff. There are particular problems in meeting the needs of some groups of prisoners. For example, in short-term or "remand" prisons a major problem is the rate of turnover, wherein the turnover of prisoners in a year may be ten or 15 times the capacity of the prison. This turnover creates a major capacity problem in the ability to rapidly assess all prisoners before some of the them move to longer-term prisons. At the other end of the scale are the five to ten percent of long-term prisoners known to have serious mental health problems.

In the absence of a dedicated national veterans agency such as the American Veterans Health Administration, the mental health needs of veterans have been partially met by a part-government funded charity known as the Ex-Servicemen's Mental Welfare Society (also known as Combat Stress). A 2005 government-funded independent review of Combat Stress has recommended, in an analagous way to the specialist commissioning arrangements already described, that mental health services for veterans should be commissioned so that they meet treatment standards, such as the NICE clinical guidelines for the treatment of PTSD, that are applicable to the general population.

Equity of access is accordingly a key – and positive – underlying principle of the British statutory services. This says nothing about the equity of access to the private for-profit sector. There has been a significant increase in the provision of private psychiatry and psychological therapies, but as this provision is guided by the ability to pay for treatment, so inevitably it is more available in larger urban centres and in more affluent parts of the country. Nonstatutory voluntary and charitable provision, often part-funded by statutory bodies, is more equitably available but the local pattern of provision of day centres and support groups varies widely.

Quality and Efficacy

The concept of the quality of mental health services is multidimensional and complex. Fundamentally, it includes both objective elements such as living arrangements and meaningful occupation or employment, and subjective elements such as the quality of interpersonal relationships that can only be assessed by self-reports and do not lend themselves to scaling approaches. A number of approaches to this issue have been taken in Britain. Rating scales have been developed, of which the *Lancashire Quality of Life Interview*, developed by Oliver et al. (1996), is probably one of the best known. Another approach has been the use of patient satisfaction surveys, and the Department of Health has required mental health trusts to carry out systematic user surveys using a questionnaire developed by the Picker Institute, the leading European agency for health surveys. A major methodological concern in quality evaluation is that users can only evaluate the treatment they have received, and so cannot evaluate a treatment procedure or mode of service delivery that may be indicated for their condition, but which they have not actually experienced.

The current Labour Government has laid emphasis on the importance of user and caregiver participation at every stage in the planning and delivery of services, exemplified by the requirement that every trust must have an Acute Patients Forum for acute inpatient settings. In applying for research grants from British statutory funding sources, an applicant is required to demonstrate how users have been involved in planning the project. For example, the government is currently funding a project concerned with the needs of carers from black and minority ethnic communities.

The effectiveness of mental health services can be assessed in a number of ways. Symptom severity measures have traditionally been the most common approach, often using scales adopted internationally, such as the *Beck Depression Inventory*. A problem with symptom measures is that they are not helpful in evaluating the effectiveness of the management of longer-term problems, when they must be supplemented by other approaches. For a number of years the Department of Health has supported the introduction of the *Health of the Nation Outcome Scale* [HoNOS] (Wing et al. 1996) as a routine outcome measure for adult services, with variants of HoNOS for other clinical groups, such as HoNOSCA for child and adolescent mental health services, being developed. HoNOS is a 12-item rating scale, covering both symptoms, and social status (such as the form of current housing). While it has apparently general validity, in fact the instrument has limited sensitivity to change, and is not applicable across the whole range of adult specialties. As far as psychological therapies are concerned, the computer-based *CORE* system (Evans et al. 2000) has been widely adopted as a generic outcome measure for all psychological therapies, and offers the advantage of access to a large national database for benchmarking local services. The development of systematic reviews and meta-analyses have meant that information from individual treatment effectiveness studies can now be combined powerfully, and information from Cochrane Collaboration Groups now informs the content of the NICE clinical practice guidelines already described. It is, of course, important to demonstrate that local services are delivering services effectively, so there is a key role for a local clinical audit, using one or more measures of demonstrated utility on at least a sample of users, and clinical audit is one responsibility of the mandatory "clinical governance" groups within each trust. Clinical cohort studies of this type are essential to ensure that the outcomes of research studies, carried out by skilled staff with carefully selected participants, are robustly replicable in more typical service settings. One gap in the mental health research literature that has been identified is the lack of evidence regarding effectiveness in primary care settings, and the lack of evaluation of preventive techniques (Cooper, 2003).

One aspect of a high quality service is the retention of service users in contact as they move from one element of service to another, and during what may be a long-term condition. This may require the coordination of a number of agencies, and draws attention to the importance of managing the transition between services well. A good example is managing the transition between adolescent and adult mental health services, when a young person with complex needs may concurrently be in contact with mental health, physical health, educational, criminal justice, and substance misuse services. They then may encounter complex changes in entitlement criteria and delivery agencies, and not least in valued personal therapeutic relationships, just because they are a few months older. While the universal British NHS system, with a single NHS number, helps to record multiservice linkage, and while the degree of "co-terminosity" between health, education, and social care bodies helps agencies to cooperate, breakdowns in community support inevitably do take place. When a "serious untoward incident" takes place involving a mental health service user, such as a homicide, an independent review must take place, the reports of the more serious of these reviews being public documents, and these are often valuable in revealing system deficiencies. Often a failure of reporting or communication between key people, maybe in the middle of the night or at a weekend, lies at the heart of the tragedy: no system can rule out human error or fatigue.

Cost and Efficiency

The general costs of mental health services, both direct and indirect, have already been described. Mental Health Strategies, an independent mental health advisory agency, has carried out (2005) a survey of investment in mental health services in England for 2004/2005 and compared it with the three previous years. While information for adult services is virtually complete, information for child and adolescent, and for older people's mental health services is less complete. The overall key findings were that investment in adult services for 2004/5 was £4.47 billion (bn) (US $2.44 bn at the 2004 ER of 1.83), or £140 (US $76) per head of weighted working age population, which represented a successive increase of £360, £420, and £564 million for each year from 2001/2. At the ER of 1.44 for 2001, the increases were respectively in U.S. currency, $250, $292, and $392. This represents a real increase in reported investment from 2001/2002 to 2004/2005 of 18.6 percent over that period. Appleby comments that the answer to the question "has the amount of money spent on mental health increased?" is not a simple yes or no. He acknowledges that some of the money that reached services was used to shore up old services, or was swallowed up in a local health economy, or that other national priorities have been seen as more important by either PCTs or SHAs.

The analysis of this expenditure for the eight largest major categories of services is shown in Table 2.10.

Table 2.10 shows that while the investment in secure and high dependency services increased by 81 percent and in access and crisis services by 79 percent, the largest increase in any of the other major categories – accommodation – was only 17 percent. A further way of analyzing the figures was to examine the variation between different Strategic Health Authorities in their mental health spending. At the 2004 ER of 1.83, against the overall national figure of £140 (US $76) per head, the lowest spend was £109 (US $60) and the highest was £189 (US $103). Interestingly, four of the five highest spenders are in London, which demonstrates that different areas attach different priorities to mental health services, compared to other services – as already noted, and which is hardly surprising. Variations in the efficiency with which services are delivered will also account for some of the variation. In a country with a long-established expectation of state funding at the national level for core mental health services, and with mental health funding mechanisms imbedded within overall health spending, it is difficult to isolate the efficiency of mental health services from the efficiency of public services generally.

Overall administration costs are difficult to estimate. A regular political ploy in Britain, as no doubt in other countries, is to criticize the number of administrators in public services, but repeated exercises in cutting administration costs are followed in monotonous regularity by the gradual increase in administration costs. The government's requirements for data are well-known, and there are signs of some

Table 2.10. *Investment in Millions of Pounds for Direct Service Categories at 2004/5 prices (US$ in parentheses).*

Service categories	*2001/2*	*2002/3*	*2003/4*	*2004/5*
CMHTs	478 (332)	511 (341)	516 (315)	542 (296)
Access & crisis services	168 (117)	197 (131)	246 (150)	300 (164)
Clinical services (including IP services)	757 (526)	732 (488)	787 (480)	834 (456)
Secure & high dependency	326 (226)	365 (243)	459 (280)	590 (322)
Continuing care	346 (240)	361 (241)	368 (224)	384 (210)
Psychological therapies	123 (85)	138 (92)	139 (85)	142 (78)
Day services	176 (122)	159 (106)	166 (101)	149 (81)
Accommodation	298 (207)	306 (204)	358 (218)	348 (190)
Total (for 15 categories)	2876 (1997)	2973 (1982)	3269 (1993)	3564 (1948)

Note: US dollars are calculated according to the foreign exchange rate for each year (e.g., for 2001/2002, the 2001 exchange rate of 1.44 was applied). Exchange rates for each year are those released from the U. S. Federal Reserve January 3, 2005 available at http://www.federalresearve.gov/releases/G5A/current/. See Tables 1.2 and 1.3 for comparisons for the year 2002, and Table 6.9 for 2003.

Note: Source is Mental Health Strategies (2005).

attempts to tackle these data collection costs systemically. For example, the Health Care Commission has supported a Concordat between all the main health regulatory bodies, including the main health professional bodies, to reconcile their regulatory requirements into a common format, and to allow the completion of one regulatory procedure to act as a proxy for other related procedures, to reduce the burden of inspection.

Financing and Fairness

The British mental health system, as part of the broader National Health Service, is essentially publicly funded, with the exception of relatively small charges for medication, which are in any event subsidized, and supplied free for those with low incomes. The national system of funding by weighted capitation formulae means that funding is, relative to many health care systems, highly equitable. The overall expenditure on mental health is monitored directly by the Department of Health, and the Secretary of State is directly accountable to Parliament for that expenditure, so fiscal responsibility for the mental health program is held at the highest political level. The 1999 *National Service Framework for Mental Health for Adults of Working Age* was accompanied by funding directly tagged to achievement of set targets. The separate funding systems for professional education, for external research and treatment innovation mean that they are to some extent protected from cash flow problems of service providers. On an international comparative basis, the financing of the British mental health system is accordingly fair and publicly accountable.

These facts do not, however, mean that the internal distribution of funding is as flexible as is wished by many service managers and professional leaders. The funding is divided into revenue and capital funding, with virtually no local opportunity for alternation between these headings. This means that where major buildings are inadequate, the procedures for rebuilding are cumbersome, and may involve the politically contentious Private Finance Initiative already described.

Although the creation of Care Trusts, which combine both health and social care provision, has helped to overcome some fiscal boundaries between NHS and local authority spending (where they have been established), the creation of dedicated pooled budgets results in a reduction in the spread of overall financial risk by both partners. Similarly, the separate funding streams for primary care and specialist mental health services mean that when structural reorganization is being considered, both parties are reluctant to make even medium-term, joint funding arrangements, for fear of losing flexibility in their spend.

The accumulation of NHS insufficient funding – or excess spending – that has been particularly apparent in 2005 has become a major public and political issue, the resolution of which is being carried out in the full glare of media attention. The fairness and accountability of the financing of the British mental health system is thus compromised by the rigidity of the funding system, which crucially limits the ability of local services to respond to locally identified high needs.

An excellent British review of the financing of mental health services (Knapp, 2005), taking account of international trends, suggests some changes to the finance system that would be beneficial. Some of these suggestions are of international and general applicability, such as the comments that mental health services are underfunded by comparison with total health expenditure, and that the process of changing services is itself costly. Two of Knapp's comments are more relevant specifically to British mental health services. *First*, he points out that some reforms to financing can promote user choice, including the use of direct payments to clients (already described) and delegating more funding responsibilities to care managers. *Secondly*, he also points out that there is an increasing economics evidence-base on the cost-effectiveness of some frequently used treatments, most obviously for depression and schizophrenia. Knapp concludes that economic evidence, unlike clinical evidence, does not travel well from country to country: the development of both locally and individually flexible funding procedures, consistent with the broader British welfare system, could be of considerable benefit to service users.

Protection and Participation, Including Patient Safety

Protection

One important criterion of a mental health service is that it is safe: safe for users, staff, and the public. *Safety* embraces a number of factors: protection from direct assault and aggression, protection from exploitation and neglect, protection from unwarranted intrusion, and protection from inappropriate security – the minimal restrictiveness factor. As protection implies passivity on the part of the protected, these factors can be turned around to assert positive rights to access to safety, rights to appropriate support, and rights to privacy.

The normal civil and criminal law of Britain potentially offer both protection and rights, but some people with mental health needs may not know how to access the law, or may lack the money to do so. Although there is a legal aid scheme in Britain for those unable to afford the full cost of legal advice, this is only available under certain circumstances, and users of mental health services do not have any protected access to legal aid. Nonetheless, if an individual who might appear a bit odd was being harassed unreasonably by a neighbour, for example, they or their relative could take out a Court Injunction preventing that harassment, and if the neighbour persisted the neighbour could be arrested for contempt of court. There are legal protections to those with mental health problems who are charged with a criminal offence, protection when someone is deemed to be incompetent to take major decisions, such as the management of money, and protection to those who may be compulsorily detained by virtue of their disorder.

Protection to those who are charged with a criminal offence takes a number of forms, which can be illustrated in two ways. There is a risk that a person with a mental health problem, if arrested and interviewed by the police, may misunderstand what is going on, to the extent they may confess to a crime they did not commit. The rules of evidence now require, under the Criminal Justice legislation, that if there is any reasonable doubt as to an individual's mental competency, they must be accompanied during interview by a chosen advocate, and indeed any evidence so obtained not in the presence of an advocate is inadmissible in court. On first appearance at a magistrates court the magistrates can ask for psychiatric reports before the case proceeds, and if a person is charged with a serious offence and it is likely that they have a major psychiatric disorder, then their fitness to plead will be established before the case proceeds in a higher court, and if found unfit to plead, they may then be dealt with under the *Mental Health Act* rather than under Criminal Justice legislation. The protection available to someone who is deemed to be incompetent to make major decisions takes several forms. Relatives may apply for right of attorney, where the individual agrees that the relatives can make major decisions on their behalf. If no relative is available, the local authority can apply for guardianship of the individual. Another remedy is through the Medical Visitors of the Lord Chancellors Department, who are distinguished psychiatrists authorised to establish the competency of individuals – typically of older people without relatives who have become cognitively impaired.

The largest field of protection is around those who may be compulsorily detained by virtue of their disorder, including those who are considered to be at risk of harming themselves. The *Mental Health Act 1983*, already described, is the main legislation in this area, with a comparable but different Act in Scotland. This establishes a number of mandatory review and optional appeal procedures, including appeal to a Mental Health Review Tribunal that involves a senior lawyer, an independent psychiatrist, and a lay member. A new *Mental Health Bill* has been proposed by the government that would bring personality disorder into the terms of the legislation, would create the possibility of community treatment orders, and would also widen the range of those who could act as "clinical supervisors" of detained patients under the Act. The *Mental Health Bill* has been seen as overly concerned with protection of the public, and the *Bill* has been opposed by a wide range of groups including the Royal College of Psychiatrists and radical user groups – an unusual coalition in British mental health politics.

The active prevention of self-harm, other than by invoking the *Mental Health Act*, has been a key target of mental health policy from the first Health of the Nation targets in 1992. Suicide prevention is now enshrined in standard seven of the NSF. This is addressed both directly, by ensuring round the clock and rapid access to services and by providing safe hospital accommodation, and indirectly by delivering high quality primary mental health, and by supporting prison staff in preventing suicides among prisoners.

Participation

Participation in decision-making by all parties, focusing on users and carers, has been encouraged by a number of related policy initiatives. The Office of the Deputy Prime Minister's report on social exclusion, already described, outlines active steps that can be taken to encourage the return to participation in the full range of community and workplace activities by the "socially excluded," who include those with severe mental health problems. Department of Health guidelines require the active involvement of service users in decisions about their care, best illustrated by the Care Programme Approach (CPA) guidance where, for example, the individual must be given a copy of his or her care plan. However, the review by the Commission for Health Improvement of CPA procedures found that the recommended procedures were not always followed, and that some users were not given copies of their care plan. The Acute Care Forums already described are another example of encouragement of participation directly in the care setting. There are a number of well-established voluntary bodies acting as advocates for improved mental health services, two of the most influential being the National Association for Mental Health (MIND) and Rethink (formerly the National Schizophrenia Fellowship) both of which have very strong user and carer memberships. Some voluntary organisations have a very specific remit, such as the Zito Trust, with a specific concern for the victims of those assaulted by people with serious mental health problems.

The extent to which there is genuine representation of all parties at all levels is variable. For example, it is possible for a vociferous past service user to be seen by service managers as the local voice for users, although the individual has not used services for several years and does not know current conditions. The professional and academic communities can make strong appeal to evidence and rational argument, and have a major influence on policy creation, since they normally are well-represented on consultation panels. A relatively new category of stakeholder is the senior manager or academic who discloses their own history of mental distress, as illustrated by Peter Beresford's (2005) account of his own journey to become a Professor of Social Policy. Rogers and Pilgrim (2001) offer a full description of the whole process of creation of mental health policy in Britain, and the contributions of different alliances and interests to that process.

Population Relevance

Whether services meet the mental health needs of the populations they are meant to serve depends on accurate knowledge of the population's need, and on the existence of sufficient resources to meet identified needs. The ability of services to meet needs also depends on whether those needs are properly construed as mental health needs.

This raises the question of how mental health problems and needs are formulated, and the extent to which formal mental health services are seen as the main means of meeting those needs. If social factors are seen as causal, then correction of social factors such as poor housing and levels of unemployment must be part of the solution. If patterns of child-rearing, such as bonding with the parents in the early months of life and the encouragement of self-esteem, are seen as important then part of the solution may lie in legislation encouraging parental leave, and in promoting parenting classes. Major life events of loss, such as the death of parents and friends, are part of normal living in families and social groups, and to construe them as abnormal is to minimize the positive value of good friendship and good, common caring in coping with these events. The major traumatic life-situations such as enduring violent civil war that are endemic in some countries – but not in any of the countries described in this volume – create levels of personal tragedy and trauma that go beyond the competence of most mental health staff.

Problems that may be seen from some points of view as mental health problems may then be seen from other perspectives as social problems, developmental problems, problems of unresolved grief, or problems of international politics. No mental health system can be asked to address all of these issues, and mental health systems are entitled to negotiate boundaries to their own responsibilities, while being willing to be partners in addressing issues beyond their capacity.

The whole of this chapter has been based on concepts and data derived from conventional Western notions of psychiatric and psychological disorder, moderated by ideas of dysfunction and disability and of differential personal and social risk, with services provided by identifiable mental health agencies. Within that framework, it is possible to address the question of the adequacy of the British mental health system.

The British mental health system has developed significantly over the past 30 years, following key policy statements in 1971 and 1975 that went beyond merely the intention to replace the old mental hospitals, with articulated policies regarding the development of community services linked to social care and primary care, and the identification of the core elements of a comprehensive service. With the establishment of a health care structure in 1974 that brought all health care resources within a locality into a single administrative unit, coterminous with local authority services, it was possible for far greater collaboration between different agencies. Since 1997 there has been an unprecedented growth in the development of mental health policy, accompanied by the production of detailed service guidance and clinical guidelines that draw on international research and best practice. Despite scepticism in the field, the development of mental health policy is a real achievement, and the implementation of that policy is supported by a national resource, the National Institute for Mental Health for England. There has been real growth in the resources available for mental health, and that increase has been clearly targeted at those adults with the most severe needs. Since *Health of the Nation* in 1992, the focus of UK policy formulation has been the severely mentally ill (SMI). Moreover, the new services funded through the 1999 *National Service Framework for Mental Health for Adults of Working Age* have been for SMI users. Clear guidance is available on the most appropriate interventions for the most common and serious conditions through the guidance issued by the National Institute for Clinical and Health Excellence, and through the policy guidance on availability of psychological therapies.

Additionally, there has been real growth in the resources available to *primary care*. For the first time primary care has been funded directly, rather than making specialist resources more available. Both the increased funding and clinical guidelines for primary mental health care are important because about 90 percent of all care and treatment of identified mental health problems in the UK takes place in the primary care sector. The most common mode of treatment is medication, but only about 54 percent of seriously mentally ill patients are fully compliant with medications.

Despite the announcement of increased funding, not all of the promised funding has gone to mental health services. This is because within a Strategic Health Authority (SHA) any overspend by one trust has to be balanced by savings from other trusts. So if a mental health trust has balanced its books, and a major general hospital within the same SHA has been unable to contain its cost pressures, the mental health trust will be required to make savings to cover the overspend. This is one consequence of mental health services being seen as an integral part of local services, rather than a totally separate budget.

Even if delivered funding matched promised funding, there would still be underprovision. There are major shortages in all mental health professions, as noted in the review by the Commission for Health Improvement, and the maintenance of adequate levels of skilled and experienced staff is essential to the delivery of services. The creation of new personnel categories, and the encouragement of new career paths, especially for those with a nursing background, have increased flexibility of deployment of staff, but still the skill shortage remains.

The recent focus on the severely mentally ill means that there are two service gaps, between those with severe mental health needs, and those who are helped by brief therapy in primary care settings. The first gap is around secondary mental health prevention and health promotion, and the second gap is around services to those with significant treatable mental health needs, who if left untreated are likely to deteriorate. Given the impact of psychiatric disorders on employment, there is also a gap in occupational health services in their ability to offer mental health services rapidly.

There is also identified underprovision for a number of known high-risk groups. The debate around the proposed Mental Health Bill is partly about whether or not serious personality disorders are treatable. Young people with complex needs and who are in contact with multiple agencies are at high risk as they encounter adult services, especially as special educational resources are then not provided. There are significant subgroups within the prison system who have severe mental health needs. While most of those who have been in the armed forces have a successful career and are successful after they leave military service, a proportion, especially young infantrymen who have seen active service, are at risk not only of PTSD but of other psychiatric problems. The historical focus on black minority groups may obscure the needs of other less visible immigrant groups: Irish people in Britain have a similar profile of needs as other minority groups, and people from Eastern Europe may have similarly high but as yet unreported levels of need. Many people with sleeping disturbance have a mental health problem.

In general, an appraisal of unmet need depends upon both the source of identification of need for mental health services and actual service take-up (utilization). There will be differences between self-identification and professional-identification, with the former picking up more psychological distress, and the latter picking up more mental disorders, which may not be self-identified. Issues of compliance, engagement, and attrition during treatment bedevil the issue.

Additionally, the utilization rates of both primary and specialty care have been found to vary by the level of severity of mental disorders. The study by Goldberg and Huxley (1980) indicated wide variations in the rates at which family doctors identify mental disorders, with less difference among mental health specialists. Thus, estimates of need vary by setting. Moreover, not all of those identified with severe

Table 2.11 *Unmet Need for Mental Health Services in England As the Percent Not Receiving Full, Appropriate Treatment.*

Level of Mental Disorder	Primary Care	Specialist Care
Severe mental disorder	50%	30%
Moderate mental disorder	80%	60%

mental disorders will accept a referral to a mental health specialist. Consequently, an estimate of unmet need in terms of the percentage of patients with identified mental disorders, who do not receive full, appropriate treatment is presented in Table 2.11 (see left) as a two-dimensional table contrasting level of severity of mental disorders and the setting in which treatment is provided.

Table 2.11 indicates that unmet need for mental health services is greater in the *primary* health care sector for people with both severe and moderate mental disorder. The percent of people with mental disorders not receiving specialty mental health services ranges from 30 percent for severe disorders to 60 percent for moderate disorders.

PART THREE: RECOMMENDATIONS

There is no shortage of recommendations for improving mental health delivery systems. Everyone from user groups, professional organizations, campaigning groups, researchers, and opportunistic journalists writing after someone's personal tragedy, call stridently for improvement in services. While more money usually comes somewhere in these calls, cash by itelf is not enough, without a more careful analysis of both the prime objectives of any improvement of services, and of the main deficiencies of services. The more thoughtful and informed calls for improvement consistently highlight similar issues. The major recommendations for the British mental health systems fall into two categories: those that are, not surprisingly, common to most developed countries; and those specific to the United Kingdom.

The World Health Organization has produced a number of reports within the past five years on international aspects of mental health. The 2001 WHO Annual Report was dedicated to mental health, and concludes with an excellent matrix of the minimum actions required for improving mental health care, given three differing levels of resources. Britain – in common with the other countries in this volume – has a high level of resources by any international comparison, so fits with the WHO scenario C. This scenario suggests that the ten main detailed recommendations would be as follows:

1. *Provide treatment in primary care*, by improving referral patterns and improving the effectiveness of management of mental disorders in primary care
2. *Provide easier access to newer psychotropic drugs*
3. *Give care in the community* by closing any remaining psychiatric hospitals and developing alternative residential and community facilities, including facilities for people with serious mental disorders
4. *Educate the public* by public campaigns
5. *Involve communities*, families and consumers by fostering advocacy initiatives
6. *Establish national policies*, programs and legislation, ensuring fairness in financing
7. *Develop human resources* by training specialists in advance treatment skills
8. *Link with other sectors*, especially by providing special facilities in schools and the workplace, and by initiating evidence-based mental health promotion programs
9. *Monitor community mental health* by developing advanced mental health monitoring systems
10. *Support more research* on the causes of mental disorders, on improving service delivery, and investigating evidence on preventing mental disorders

These recommendations have a reasonable fit with the needs of the British mental health system, but they *omit four important issues* for Britain, and some recommendations require significant amendment to be best fitted to the British situation. The single most important omission is to aim for a major shift in *national understanding* of the nature of mental health problems – implied by public education, but far broader than that. Other omissions are:

11. *Improve initial assessment* and case formulation
12. *Encourage flexibility* and appropriateness of services
13. *Stabilize organizations and funding.*

After discussion of the first omitted recommendation relating to a major shift in thinking, the ten WHO recommendations are dealt with in turn, modified in name and detail where necessary, followed by discussion of the last three recommendations (numbers 11–13).

Shift Understanding – Mental Health or Mental Illness Services?

The semantics of psychological distress are an issue. Existing mental health services are primarily a response to the actions of people who are mentally distressed, disabled, or dysfunctional, and they do not primarily promote positive mental health. This is likely to remain a problem as long as mental health services are organizationally part of a national health service, where the dominant conceptual model is a biomedical one, and where doctors, nurses, and hospitals are the dominant public images of a health service.

It is not the case that attitudes towards mental illness will automatically improve. There is some evidence that there has been a deterioration in positive attitudes towards those with mental health problems, and the whole basis of the work of the Office of the Deputy Prime Minister on social exclusion is that mental illness remains a major cause of such exclusion.

Any underlying classifactory system of psychological distress that sees problems as the manifestations of discrete diagnostic conditions, rather than as being somewhere along a continuum of problems that are mostly common to many members of a population, means that this dominance will remain. The work of Richard Bentall (2003), in his historically fascinating and challenging book on constructing new ways of thinking about mental illness, is an example of a fundamental challenge to existing psychiatric typologies.

There must therefore be a continuing campaign to see mental health problems as problems likely to affect many of us, either personally or indirectly through our relationships with families and friends, and as problems best described in terms of the mix of personal, social, and medical factors that cause them. The quality of services should be primarily determined by the priorities of those who use them.

Provide Treatment in Primary Care

The four ways in which treatment in primary care has been improved are (a) increased use of medication by GPs, and the attachment to primary teams of (b) counselors, (c) mental health specialists (particularly, social workers, psychologists, or community psychiatric nurses), and (d) the new graduate primary care mental health workers. There is more scope to support primary care further, for example, by providing mental health resource centres, with some capacity for a meaningful day program, located to support several primary care practices, and linked to local voluntary and private provision.

Provide Easier Access to Treatments

While the WHO guidelines perhaps surprisingly mention only psychotropic drugs, there is undoubtedly a treatment gap in the British system, but this has been identified most clearly in the area of psychological therapies. Not only has the Department of Health issued more guidance on this area than on other general forms of intervention, but an influential government adviser, Richard Layard, specifically recommended in 2004 the training of 10,000 more psychological therapists. User groups also specifically call for more psychological therapy to be available as the first option. What has not been identified in policy is the treatment gap for occupational and activity therapies, including the encouragement of physical exercise and activity, not only in the community but also in all residential settings (see Everett et al. 2003 and recommendation three). What is therefore needed is more comprehensive guidance on providing a balanced range of pharmacological, psychological and social interventions in all settings.

Closing this gap therefore depends on the availability of staff skilled to provide the required therapies, and thus a proper mental health work force plan (see recommendation seven), and planned provision for post-basic training in the identified therapies and interventions.

Give Accessible Care in the Community

The general goal of providing care in the community is well-recognized, and national policy has had this as a central objective for at least fifteen years. The establishment of crisis and home treatment teams has in a number of areas led to significant reduction in bed use.

However, simply placing services in the community is not enough. Mental health services should be easily accessible to all those who may want to use them. Accessibility is not simply a matter of physical accessibility, such as the location of sites of service delivery so they fit with the availability of public transport, but includes psychological accessibility, so that buildings are not prominently marked with an institutional sign or logo indicating their purpose. Access by a nonmedical route of entry may be valued by some of those with greatest need, such as young adults with co-morbid substance misuse problems, or the profoundly isolated (and possibly abused) homeless person. Non-traditional sites and routes of entry may be particularly valuable in inner-city areas with marked social deprivation and high rates of social mobility.

However much treatment is carried out in the community, there is likely to be a continuing need for treatment in some residential setting, for reasons of observation, safety or availability of treatment, quite apart from the potential value of asylum in the original sense – the removal from what may be a toxic family milieu. However, it is also true that some of the greatest concerns in the United Kingdom mental health system relate to the poor quality of current patterns of inpatient care. One of the most important recommendations to make is therefore to improve the quality of residential care by improving staffing levels, improving the range of meaningful activities available during the waking day, and improving the intensity of impact of individual care packages. These residential facilities do not all need to be in hospitals. The provision of alternative settings, such as a respite center, that may be run by voluntary agencies, can improve acceptability to those who would not return to a ward/which they did not experience as being therapeutic. Increasing the range of types of residential setting is thus a key recommendation.

Given that the most acceptable first form of help may not be a formal mental health intervention, access to other services that may be valued by the person with a psychological problem is equally important. These services include further and higher education, finding a way through the complex benefits system, such as establishing eligibility for incapacity benefit, and creating pathways back to work, including negotiating the barriers of perverse financial incentives. All of these are community interventions in the sense that they either take place away from a mental health institutional setting, or use agencies also accessed by the general public.

Educate the Public – Better Information and Understanding

When mental health problems arise, they are often misunderstood both by those they affect, and by those around them. People with the problems need information about the nature of the problems confronting them, about the courses of action open to them, and how to make the choices about which course to follow. If that problem arises suddenly, and they are confused by the problem, they are at risk of control of their life being taken over by someone else, and they may find themselves suddenly in a strange or threatening place – of which a busy Accident and Emergency Department or a Police Station are only two examples. In those circumstances they may require an advocate in the original non-technical sense – someone empowered to speak for them on their behalf.

This means that information about mental health problems should be readily available in nonstigmatising places, such as public libraries and information centres, so it can be accessed without having to go a place that already implies the existence of a problem. The information should be available in a number of formats, including not only normal written form, but in Large Type format, and in audiotape, CD and electronic forms, and in the languages of at least the most common of the language communities of an area. That information will be better understood if there is also an easily accessible centre with someone to talk to, which may either be specially for those with mental health problems, such as a Mental Health Resource Centre, or for a wider range of groups, such as a Carers Centre for those caring with a range of disabilities.

Involve Communities

The involvement of communities, familes and users in all aspects of service planning, delivery, and monitoring is already a central aspect of policy. In many areas of the country there are excellent traditions of voluntary agencies supporting users and campaigning for better services, often working closer with the statutory providers. These agencies may be stand-alone local charities, or more commonly they are branches of a national organization, gaining support and back-up from a national head office that often has a lobbying function with Government, Parliament and with local authorities.

Many users have a need for social support equal to their need for formal interventions. The National

Service Frameworks specifically recognise the needs of carers for support, and all new guidance requires or recommends the involvement of service users and carers in various ways. For example, the major research funding bodies stipulate that research proposals must show evidence of consultation with representatives of the patient group that are identified as research participants.

Establish National Policies

The last thing that needs to be recommended for Britain is more mental health policies. As already commented, the years from 1999 have seen an unprecedented flow of mental health policy with associated implementation guidance. Most of the policy initiatives are clear, and they are often evidence-based. There are two problems with these policies, however. The policies are too complex, and they are too inflexible. The major limitation of current policies is the prescriptive way in which targets are set nationally, with little scope for modifying policy to fit both local patterns of need and pre-existing patterns of service delivery where they already achieve the required outcomes. For a busy service manager it is impossible to keep abreast of the unending flow of paper, and there is a case for putting a moratorium on any new policies, and concentrating on rationalizing and prioritizing around existing policies. Accordingly, a recommendation would be that existing policies should be able to be modified and prioritized to fit local patterns of need.

Develop Human Resources

There are continuing shortages in all mental health professions, but the scope for addressing these is different for each professional group, because of the different ways in which career choices can be made within each profession. Psychiatry is not one of the most popular career options for doctors, and guidelines for improving their working conditions have been prepared. While accepting the desirability of community-based work, for psychiatric nurses this has been achieved at the cost of the most experienced nurses leaving inpatient care settings, so there remains an agenda to improve working conditions for them, as the staff group who have the highest levels of face-to-face contact with seriously disturbed service users.

Developing human resources may involve a more radical shift in the professional mix than simply adding graduate mental health workers. The logic of the arguments already discussed around the need for education and health promotion mean that those with teaching and educational skills could have skills transferable to mental health settings, for example.

Link With Other Sectors

Compared with other countries, links between mental health services and other statutory services may be easier to achieve in Britain, because of the co-terminosity between the boundaries of health, education, social care, and local government (including housing) agencies, and because of the national policies on benefits and employment. The Office of the Deputy Prime Minister has responsibility for improving inter-agency linkage, and there have been real improvements in this area.

The greatest remaining difficulties are around improving and coordinating work with young people, especially as they make the transition between children's services and adult services. A number of organizational changes have been introduced to try to solve some of these problems (see recommendation 13), but there remain major boundary problems in terms of the sudden reduction of funding for, and hence access to, specialized services around the age of 18. These problems are greatest for those young adults, perhaps with single parents, with the most complex problems who may individually have concurrent contact with the health, social care and youth justice systems, who live in areas of high social deprivation. Recommending a focus on young adults with the highest level of individual and community need would be a very positive step.

Monitor Community Mental Health

The NHS has made massive investments in information technology to improve both service management and service monitoring, as described in the earlier section on finance and commissioning systems. The cost of the IT system currently being introduced is estimated at between £19 bn and £32 bn, between three to five times the original cost. The autumn assessment process already described provides plentiful data on community mental health services, including the existence (but not the effectiveness) of health promotion programs.

What is needed is some simplification of these systems as far as front-line staff are concerned, so they are regularly provided with feedback on selected subsets of data on the most important areas of practice in the services in which they work. Most monitoring information is for management purposes, which is of little interest to front-line staff.

Support More Research

Since the expansion of University departments of psychiatry in the 1960s, and the more recent creation of research departments in mental health and clinical psychology, the volume of good quality mental health research in Britain has grown significantly. However, the largest research grants continue to be in the biomedical field, around neuroscience and drug trials. A new Mental Health Research Network was created by the government in 2004, to determine research priorities through wide-scale consultation, and to further support evidence-based best practice. The production of NICE guidance on a range of mental health conditions has given a significant boost to increasing the availability of the results of secondary research. The Service Delivery and Organization R&D program is paying some attention to mental health topics. There is therefore emerging a strategic approach to research in mental health, to make the best use of the available research resource.

It remains the case, however, that there is still relatively little mental health research in primary care and in social care. An important recommendation is that more research should be conducted into improving methods of service delivery, relevant to the staff who do the delivering.

Improve Initial Assessment and Case Formulation

The initial contact between a potential service user and a practitioner with mental health expertise is crucial. Existing national targets to reduce waiting list times have not applied to mental health services. The present care pathways, apart from those presenitng to services because of a crisis, typically follow a route through primary care (usually a doctor) with the first assessments usually carried out by a GP or a counsellor. Failure to carry out a timely, full and skilled initial assessment then means that a user may be retained too long in an inappropriate service, with medication being seen as the first treatment of choice.

Improving the speed of access to a skilled practitioner, with the early provision of information to both the user and their family about both the condition and the possible interventions, and the early routing to the most appropriate service then become recommendations. The careful negotiation of a formulation of their needs with a user is therapeutic in its own right, and increases therapeutic engagement, apart from laying the foundation for future work.

Encourage Flexibility and Appropriateness of Services

The needs of individuals with mental health problems usually change through an episode of care. Not only may some additional resources be helpful, but equally some other resources, provided early on, may no longer be needed. For people who have a comorbid condition, either medical or related to their psychological functioning, sometimes one service or practitioner will need to lead, and sometimes another. Simply because a person has become a couple of years older – most significantly around the ages of 17 to 19, and 64 to 66 in the British care system, their needs will not have changed, and nor will the relevance of the skills of their key-worker with whom they may have formed a very effective therapeutic relationship.

It is therefore important that individual care plans are not prejudiced by constraints of funding or managment policy, so that individuals can move through their care pathway and make service transitions with minimal disruption to them. This requires local services to have the power to be flexible in the assignment of staff, facilitating users equally in moving to less supportive or to more supportive regimes as they require, taking a life span approach to service delivery. The uptake of direct payments, already described, whereby the user themself takes reponsibility for the choice of how best to use benefit monies, has been low for people with mental health problems, but this offers more autonomy to users. All of this means more local and personal control of funding, and the resultant fuzziness around the edges of some statitisical returns would be a price well worth paying.

Stabilize Organizations and Funding

The structure and size of any organization is meant to be derived from the aims of that organization. This simple principle appears to have been lost by the British government with respect to the structure of health agencies. Within the eight-year life of the current Labour government, there have been multiple changes in the size and responsibilities of all levels of statutory agency, some changes reversing earlier changes.

The most obvious single example are the changes in relationship and size between the organization of primary care, and the two next higher levels of management. The former District Health Authorities were dissolved to create about 300 Primary Care Trusts PCTs), and 28 Strategic Health Authorities. As soon as they were formed some Primary Care Trusts began to merge, as they were manifestly too small to provide the range of functions laid upon them. The PCTs began to directly employ a range of community staff – such as physiotherapists and psychologists – and deployed them in often imaginative community schemes. Within the space of one year the Secretary of State for Health had proposed that PCTs should lose all their recently acquired provider functions, and then reversed that decision.

Meanwhile, the size and role of Strategic Health Authorities has been revised, so their size will again resemble closely the size of the Regional Health Authorities they replaced. The cost of these reorganizations is two-fold: not only are there the direct costs of the reorganization, but at every change experienced and skilled senior front-line staff and managers think that this is one change too many, and they retire or change jobs, thus losing invaluable skill and usually local networking knowledge. One most useful recommendations would thus be that the structure of both strategic and provider bodies be stabilized.

Maintaining stability of funding is a closely related issue. The big – and difficult to control – spenders in the British health economy are the large general hospitals, with their effective but expensive medical and surgical specialities. Because a Strategic Health Authority is responsible for balancing the books across a whole local health economy, an overspend in one sector has to be balanced by savings in another. As already noted, at the national level the Audit Commission commented on the unprecedented financial challenges facing local NHS bodies, and that there are deficits accumulated from previous years, as well as deficits to achieve current financial balance. The Audit Commission has identified increased transparency of financial reporting as a major theme in improving financial management.

The impact of this national picture locally is illustrated by figures from the Thames Valley SHA, responsible for health care for 1.9 million people. At the end of the 2005 financial year only four of the 28 NHS organizations in the SHA area had reported approval of their budgets, and there was an accumulated deficit of between £40 m and £60 m, depending on how it was calculated. (At the 2004 exchange rate of 1.83, the figures are respectively US $28 m and US $33 m.) Even though the Oxfordshire Mental Health Trust had finished the financial year in balance, they have been required to contribute to a levy of £9 m from all the other Oxfordshire Trusts, which means that mental health day and other services may need to be closed, and recruitment placed on hold.

This is the downside of a nationally funded comprehensive health care system. Elements of the system that have received additional funding – as mental health services undoubtedly have since the publication of the adult Mental Health NSF in 1999 – are vulnerable to overspends elsewhere in the system. Funding of mental health services is thus shown to be absolutely dependent on central government with no firewall to protect it from other elements. This raises the question of separating off the mental health funding in a protected budget.

SUMMARY

In the three years that this book has been in the writing, many changes have occurred in the British mental health delivery system. Many key elements have remained the same. The commitments to a service free at the point of delivery to all, funded equitably across the country, with additional support to those disabled by their condition, remain more or less intact. This commitment should not be undervalued.

The changes mostly derive from the comprehensive set of national policies that have been promulgated since 1999, with associated performance targets, implementation guidance, and financial incentives to achieve those targets. There is strong encouragement of practice based on the best available evidence for effective interventions. The shift to community-based services has continued, with new buildings steadily replacing the now very small number of old mental hospital sites still providing services. There has been investment in training, with more flexibility in the use of professionals skills, and improvement in the numbers of staff in training and in post. In most parts of the country there are strong partnerships with voluntary bodies and stronger involvement of users and carers in all aspects of the service.

But the change agenda remains massive, and signs of improvement are balanced by the loss of (usually the best) staff from established services to newer ones, leaving inpatient services especially still poor in the quality of the therapeutic environment they offer. There is still a treatment gap between the demand for services and the capacity of the system to meet that demand.

Most important of all, the government has not found ways to balance more sensitively meeting national priorities against meeting clearly identified local need priorities. Nor has it found ways to ensure that monies intended for mental health stay there, without being diverted to politically more popular services.

On coming into power in 1997 the present government said that change in public services was a long-term venture. It may be more honest if they were in reality to accept the long-term character of the changes that are required, and to look for sustainable change rather than setting short-term and changing targets.

REFERENCES

Acts of Parliament

Note: All public Acts of Parliament since 1988 are available through the Office of Public Sector Information (OPSI), which is a branch of the Cabinet Office (see www.opsi.gov.uk/acts.htm)

Asylums Act 1808
Lunatics Act 1846
General Medical Act 1858
National Health Service Act 1946
National Assistance Act 1946
Mental Health Act 1959
Chronically Sick & Disabled Act 1970
Education Act 1980
Medical Act 1983
Mental Health Act 1983
NHS and Community Care Act 1990
Carers Recognition and Services Act 1995
Community Care Direct Payments Act 1996
Human Rights Act 1998
Children Act 2004

Government Reports and Other References

Appleby, L. (2004). *The national service framework for mental health – five years on.* London: Department of Health.

Arksey, H., O'Malley, L., & Baldwin, S., et al. (2002). *Services to support carers of people with mental health problems.* NHS Service Delivery and Organisation Research and Development (SDO R&D) briefing paper. London: Department of Health.

Audit Commission (2002). *Forget-me-not: Developing mental health services for older people.* London: Audit Commission.

Audit Commission (2005). The balancing act. Newsletter, issue 2, 4 *Financial Health News.*

Bentall, R. (2003). *Madness explained: Psychosis and human nature.* London: Penguin.

Beresford, P. (2005). The changing role of professor: Including everyone's knowledge and experience. *Mental Health Review, 10,* 3–6.

Beveridge, W. (1943). *The Beveridge Report.* London: Public Record Office.

Bhugra, D., & Littlewood, R. (2001). *Colonialism and psychiatry.* Oxford: Oxford University Press.

Black, N. (2004). Should the English National Health Service be freed from political control? *Journal of Health Service Research and Policy, 9,* 1–2.

Boardman, J., & Parsonage, M. (2005). *Defining a good mental health service: A discussion paper.* London: the Sainsbury Centre for Mental Health.

Cambridgeshire and Peterborough Mental Health Partnership NHS Trust (2004). *Annual Report 2004.* Huntingdon, Cambridgeshire and Peterborough Mental Health Partnership NHS Trust.

Commission for Health Improvement (2004). *What CHI has found in: Mental health trusts: Sector report.* London: Commission for Health Improvement.

Cooper, B. (2003). Evidence-based mental health policy: A critical appraisal. *British Journal of Psychiatry, 183,* 105–113.

Council of Europe (1950). *European convention on human rights.* Strasbourg: Council of Europe.

Department of Health (1992a). *Health of the nation.* London: Department of Health.

Department of Health (1992b). *Mental health nursing review.* London: Department of Health.

Department of Health (1998). *Modernising mental health services: Safe, sound and supportive.* London: Department of Health.

Department of Health (1999a). *Safer services.* London: Department of Health.

Department of Health (1999b). *National service framework for mental health: Modern standards and service models.* London: Department of Health.

Department of Health (1999c). *Effective care co-ordination in mental health services: Modernising the care programme approach – a policy booklet.* London: Department of Health.

Department of Health (1999d). *Medium security psychiatric services.* London: Department of Health.

Department of Health (2001a). *Safety first: Five-year report of the National Confidential Enquiry into suicide and homicide by people with mental illness.* London: Department of Health.

Department of Health (2001b). *National service framework for older people.* London: Department of Health.

Department of Health (2001c). *The mental health policy implementation guide.* London: Department of Health.

Department of Health (2001d). *The journey to recovery – the government's vision for mental health care.* London: Department of Health.

Department of Health (2002a). *Mental health policy implementation guide: Adult acute inpatient care.* London: Department of Health.

Department of Health (2002b). *Mental health policy implementation guide: National minimum standards for general adult services in PICUs and low secure environments.* London: Department of Health.

Department of Health (2002c). *Care programme approach for older people with serious mental health problems.* London: Department of Health.

Department of Health (2002d). *Specialist services national definitions set: Specialised mental health services (adult) definition No 22.* London: Department of Health.

Department of Health (2002e). *The Wanless Report.* London: Department of Health.

Department of Health (2003a). *Improving mental health services for black and minority ethnic communities in England.* London: Department of Health.

Department of Health (2003b). *Womens mental health strategy.* London: Department of Health.

Department of Health (2003c). *Mental health policy implementation guide: Support, time and recovery (STR) workers.* London: Department of Health.

Department of Health (2003d). *Mental health services work force design and development best practice guidance.* London: Department of Health.

Department of Health (2004a). *Choosing health consultation.* London: Department of Health.

Department of Health (2004b). *National service framework for children, young people and maternity services.* London: Department of Health.

Department of Health (2004c). *Organizing and delivering psychological therapies.* London: Department of Health.

Department of Health: National Specialist Commissioning Advisory Group (2004d). *Current NSCAG designated services: Mental health services included are personality disorder; mental health services for deaf children and adolescents (inpatient); secure forensic mental health services for young people.* London. London: Department of Health.

Department of Health (2005). *Securing better mental health services for older adults.* London: Department of Health.

Department of Health and Social Security (1975). *Better Services for the Mentally Ill.* London: HMSO.

Evans, C., Mellor-Clark, J., Margison, F., Barkham, M., McGrath, G., Connell, J., & Audin, K. (2000). Clinical Outcomes in Routine Evaluation: the CORE-OM. *Journal of Mental Health, 9,* 247–255.

Everett, T., Donaghy, M., & Feaver, S. (2003). *Interventions for mental health: An evidence-based approach for physiotherapists and occupational therapists.* Edinburgh: Butterworth Heinemann.

Freeman, G., Weaver, T., & Low, J., et al. (2002). *Promoting continuity of care for people with severe mental illness.* NHS Service Delivery and Organisation Research and Development (SDO R&D) briefing paper. London: Department of Health.

Gask, L., Sibbald. B., & Creed, F. (1997). Evaluating models of working at the interface between mental health services and primary care. *British Journal of Psychiatry, 170,* 6–11.

Glover, G., Barnes, D., & Darlington, A. S. (2004). *Information about mental health and mental health service use in England.* Durham: North-East Public Health Observatory.

Goldberg D., & Huxley P. (1980). *Mental illness in the community.* Tavistock: London.

Hansard [official record of proceedings of the House of Commons] (2005). Mental health staffing numbers for England 1986-2004. *Written Answers,* 22 February 2005, column 499–502.

Healthcare Financial Management Association [HFMA] (2004). *Introductory guide to NHS finance in the UK.* Bristol: Healthcare Financial Management Association.

Jenkins, R., McCulloch, A., Friedli, L., & Parker, C. (2002). Developing a national mental health policy. *Maudsley Monograph,* No 43. Hove: Psychology Press.

Knapp, M. (2005). Money talks: Nine things to remember about mental health financing. *Journal of Mental Health, 14,* 89–93.

Laing, W., & Buisson, M. (2001). *Private medical insurance – UK market sector report 2001.* London: Laing and Buisson Publications.

Layard, R. (2004). *Mental Health: Britain's biggest social problem?* London: Prime Ministers Strategy Unit Paper.

Marshall M., Hogg, L.L., Gath, D.H., & Lockwood, A. (1995). The cardinal needs schedule – modified version of the MRC needs for care assessment schedule. *Psychological Medicine, 25,* 605–617.

McCulloch, A., Glover, G., & St John, T. (2003). The national service framework for mental health: past present and future. *Mental Health Review, 8,* 7–17.

McPherson, R., Varah, M., & Summerfield, L. (2003). Staff and patient assessments of need in an epidemiologically representative sample of patients with psychosis. *Social Psychiatry and Psychiatric Epidemiology, 38,* 662–667.

Meltzer, H., Gatward, R., Goodman, R., & Ford, T. (2000). *Mental health of children and adolescents in Great Britain.* London: The Stationery Office.

Mental Health Strategies, for the Department of Health (2005). *The 2004/2005 National Survey of Investment in Mental Health Services.* London: Department of Health.

MIND (1983). *Common concern.* London: Author.

National Primary and Care Trust Development Programme (2005). *The commissioning friend for mental health services: A resource guide for health and social care commissioners.* London: National Institute for Mental Health.

National Institute for Clinical Excellence [NICE]. *Mental health clinical guidelines: Anxiety (2004), depression (2004), depression in children and young people (2005), eating disorders (2004), obsessive-compulsive disorder (2005), post-traumatic stress disorder (2005), schizophrenia (2002), self-harm (2004).* London: The National Institute for Clinical Excellence.

NHS (2004). *NHS knowledge and skills framework.* London: Department of Health.

National Institute for Mental Health in England [NIMHE] (2003). *Cases for change booklets: Anti-discriminatory practice, community services, emerging areas of service provision, forensic mental health services, hospital services, introduction, partnership across health and social care, policy context, primary care, user involvement.* London: National Institute for Mental Health in England.

Office of the Deputy Prime Minister (2004). *Mental Health and Social Exclusion.* London: Office of the Deputy Prime Minister Social Exclusion Unit Report.

Oliver, J., Huxley, P., Bridges, K., & Mohamad, H. (1996). *Quality of life and mental health services.* London: Routledge.

Office for National Statistics (2005). *Census 2001: General report for England and Wales.* London: Office for National Statistics.

Rogers, A., & Pilgrim, D. (2001). *Mental health policy in Britain.* London: Palgrave.

Sainsbury Centre for Mental Health (2000). *Implications of the NHS plan for mental health services.* Briefing Paper no 11, Sainsbury Centre for Mental Health.

Samaritans (2005). *Information Resource Pack.* Ewell: Samaritans.

Slade, M., Loftus, L., Phelan, M., Thornicroft, G., & Wykes, T (1999). *The Camberwell assessment of need.* Gaskell, London.

Social Services Inspectorate (2004). *Treated as people: An overview of mental health services from a social care perspective 2002–2004.* London: Department of Health.

Social Services Inspectorate (2001). *Improving older people's services.* London: Department of Health.

Singleton, N., Bumpstead, R., O'Brien, M., et al. (2001). *Psychiatric morbidity among adults living in private households 2000.* London: Office of National Statistics.

Sproston, K., & Nazroo, J. (2002). *Ethnic minority psychiatric illness rates in the community (EMPIRIC).* London: The Stationery Office.

Thornicroft, G., & Tansella. M. (2004). Components of a modern mental health service: A pragmatic balance of community and hospital care. *British Journal of Psychiatry, 185,* 283–290.

Tyrer, P., & Steinberg, D. (1999). *Models for mental disorder: Conceptual models in psychiatry.* Chichester: Wiley.

World Book Encyclopedia (1980). *Entry for: England,* volume 6, page 235. Chicago: World Book-Childcraft International, Inc.

World Health Organization (2001). *The world health report 2001. Mental health: New understanding, new hope.* Geneva, Switzerland: World Health Organization.

Wing, J.K., Curtis, R.H., & Beevor, A.S. (1996). *HoNOS: Health of the nation outcome scales: Report on research and development, July 1993–December 1995.* London: Royal College of Psychiatrists.

Useful British Non-Clinical Mental Health Journals

Evidence-Based Mental Health
Journal of Mental Health
Mental Health Research
Mental Health Review
Effective Health Care Bulletins, University of York

Useful Web Sites

Audit Office: www.nao.org.uk
Department of Health: www.dh.gov.uk
Healthcare Commission: www.healthcarecommission.org.uk
National Institute for Clinical Excellence (NICE): www.nice.org.uk
National Institute for Mental Health for England (NIMHE): www.nimhe.csip.org.uk
Office of National Statistics (ONS): www.statistics.gov.uk
Service Delivery Organisation (SDO): www.sdo.lshtm.ac.uk
Social Service Inspectorate: www.dhsspsni.gov.uk
Centre for Public Mental Health, Durham University: www.nepho.org.uk

Chapter 3

MENTAL HEALTH SERVICES IN NORWAY

Arnulf Kolstad and Haldis Hjort

PART ONE: DESCRIPTION OF THE MENTAL HEALTH SYSTEM

Introduction

Geography and Demographics

Norway is located in the northernmost part of Europe, stretching 1770 km from north to south. For much of the distance it is very narrow, exceeding 160 km of breadth only in the south. Its population just reached 4.5 million inhabitants at the end of September, 2000. On January 1, 2004 the population was 4,577,000. The total area of 324,000 square kilometers (sq. km.) or 125,096 square miles, is roughly comparable in size to Germany (357,000 sq. km.) and Italy (301,000 sq. km.). Next to Iceland and Russia, Norway has the lowest population density in Europe (14 per sq. km.). If the mainland were divided equally among all inhabitants, there would be some 80,000 square meters for each Norwegian. Approximately three-fourths of the population lives in urban settlements; the remainder inhabits rural districts.

Norway's long, craggy coast forms the western margin of the Scandinavian Peninsula and fronts the Atlantic Ocean and the North Sea (sometimes known as the Norwegian Sea). The North Sea separates Norway from the British Isles in the southwest, and directly to the south the Skagerrak separates it from Denmark. Norway shares an extensive eastern border with Sweden and a shorter border with Finland and Russia in the north. The extensive coastline offers plenty of natural resources such as fish and oil. Coastal cliffs drop dramatically to the sea, forming the fjords which are among the most striking features of Norwegian geography. About 150,000 offshore islands serve as a barrier that helps to protect Norway's coast from Atlantic storms. The inland consists mostly of high plateaus and forests. Characteristic of the terrain are rugged mountains interrupted by fertile valleys that cut into the land. Only about three percent of Norway is arable land, and for this reason Norway's main source of livelihood has traditionally been fishing and timber. The highest mountains inland rise to about 2,500 meters and are not populated at all.

Due to the mountains and the fiords, transportation in Norway is difficult. Travel from north to south or from east to west requires crossing several mountains and/or fjords. In some districts on the west coast and in the north it is impossible to go by car without using ferries and it takes hours to travel 100 km.

Despite its northern location, Norway has a temperate climate provided by the North Atlantic current, especially in the southern and western parts of the country. To the north, about one-third of the country lies within the Arctic Circle, where the sun shines 24 hours at the height of the summer. In the winter months the sun does not rise north of the same latitude, and the sun cannot be seen at all for a couple of months. In most parts of Norway snow starts falling in November and covers the ground until April. Temperatures can go down to minus 40 degrees Celsius in the winter.

Population and Urban Settlements. Of the 4.6 millions inhabitants, 26 percent is below 20 years of age, 40 percent is 45 years or more, and 4.6 percent is over 80 years. Demographically, Norway is growing older. In particular, the oldest segment of the population is expanding, and this represents an extra burden for the health care system. Nursing and care for the aged must be given more priority. The fertility rate decreased from 2.94 in 1961–1965 to 1.85 in the period 1996–2000.

Only four urban settlements in Norway have more than 100,000 inhabitants. Nearly 1,330,000 inhabitants live in these four urban settlements altogether, which make up 29 percent of the Norwegian population. During 2003, the number of inhabitants increased by 10,000 in these four urban settlements, and accounted for almost half of the growth in the entire country that year.

The capital and the largest city is Oslo. Situated in the south, its population is 521,000 as of January 1, 2004. The next largest cities are Bergen (212,000) and Stavanger/Sandnes (172,000) on the southwest coast, and Trondheim (146,000) situated 500 km north of Oslo at the Trondheimsfjord. Only 10 percent of the population lives in the northern half of the country where the largest town is Tromsø (62,000).

Except for the larger cities, the country is extremely scarcely populated, and people in the countryside and along the coast are accustomed to living apart. In the northern most country, with a population of 73,000, the population density is 1.5 persons per s. km. The sparse population and complicated transportation also mean that accessibility to health services takes time and significant effort. In many places, especially in the north and west, people cannot reach their general practitioner or other primary health care facilities without traveling for hours. The specialized mental health services are even farther away, and for about five percent of the population, services cannot be reached the same day, except by plane or helicopter. The accessibility is much better in the cities and urban centers where three-fourths of the population is settled.

The Sámi People. The Sámi are the indigenous people in Norway. There are believed to be between 40,000 and 45,000 Sámi, largely concentrated in Finmark, the northernmost county, where there are some 25,000. Official policy is now based on the principle that although the Sámi are Norwegian subjects, they constitute an ethnic minority and a separate people. A Sámi is a person who: (a) has Sámi as his/her first language, or whose father, mother or one of whose grandparents has Sámi as their first language, or (b) considers himself/herself a Sámi and lives in entire accordance with the rules of the Sámi society, and who is recognized by the representative Sámi body as a Sámi, or (c) has a father or mother who satisfies the above-mentioned conditions for being a Sámi.

Thus, the everyday use of the Sámi language is decisive in determining a person's right to be classified as a Sámi and his or her right to vote for representatives to the Sámi Parliament (Sametinget). The Act concerning the Sámi Parliament and other legal matters pertaining to the Sámi (the Sámi Act) was approved by the Norwegian Parliament (Storting) in 1987 and Sametinget was opened by the late King Olav V in 1989. The Sámi Assembly is a national body, subordinate to the general regulations of public administration. Its sphere of activity, right of recommendation, and authority are laid down in the Sámi Act. The Sámi Parliament deals with all matters considered to be of special importance to the Sámi people. Sámi language and culture are different from the non-Aboriginal Norwegians. Actually there are three distinct languages: East Sámi, Central Sámi and South Sámi. In Norway, about 20,000 people speak the Sámi language. Mental health services for the aboriginals must be a significant factor in the health care.

The Immigrant Population. As of January 1, 2004 the immigrant population in Norway was 349,000 and accounted for 7.6 percent of the total population. The immigrant population increased by 16,100 (4.9%) in 2003. In comparison, the entire Norwegian population increased by 25,200. The immigrant population has changed significantly the last 25 years. The western immigrant population has increased from 65,000 in 1980 to 99,300 in 2004, while the non-western immigrant population has increased from 29,500 in 1980 to 249,600 in 2004. In 1980, people with non-western backgrounds made up 31 percent of the immigrant population. At the beginning of 2004, 72 percent of the immigrant population is of non-western origins. The majority of immigrants are from Asia (40%), followed by people from Eastern Europe (16%), other Nordic countries (15%), Africa (12%) and Western Europe (10%). Approximately 114,000 of the people that belong to the immigrant population live in Oslo. This accounts for 22 percent of the population in the capital.

State Religion. The official state-religion is Evangelical-Lutheran. Nearly 90 percent of the population has membership in the state church, but they seldom attend religious ceremonies, with the exception of baptisms, weddings, and funerals, that is, when they are ready to "hatch, match, or dispatch."

The Political System

Norway is a hereditary constitutional monarchy. The constitution, which was approved May 17, 1814, gives broad powers to the king, but the council of ministers, headed by the Prime Minister, generally exercise this royal power in council. The 169 members of the *Storting* (Parliament) are elected for a fixed term of four years by all Norwegians 18 years of age or older.

Although Norway had its own constitution since 1814, from 1814 to 1905 Norway and Sweden constituted a political union. Prior to 1814, Norway was part of Denmark for about four hundred years. Norway has been an independent monarchy since 1905. The King of Norway is presently Harald V.

Unlike America's two-party system, Norway has a parliamentarian system with several political parties represented in the Parliament. The majority in the Parliament designates the prime minister who selects the other members of the Government. The whole Government is approved by the Parliament. Seven major political parties are represented in the Parliament: the Labour party *(Arbeiderpartiet)*, which is the largest single party, the Progress party *(FrP)*, the Conservative party *(Høyre)*, the Socialist Left *(SV)*, the Centre Party *(Senterpartiet)*, the Christian Democrats *(KrF)* and the Liberals *(Venstre)*. The Labour party, which was responsible for creating the *welfare state*, headed the government for a period of 37 years from 1935 to 1981. During those years Norway followed a pragmatic social democratic policy, with a mixed economy, relatively high public spending and investment, and an established *welfare state*, which provided free education, free health services and social care, disability pensions, old-age pensions, and unemployment payments to everybody in need. In the last two decades the welfare policy of public spending and care has been under attack especially from conservative political parties, which have held the majority in Parliament since the 1980s and until the election in 2005, except for two years. As of 2005, Norway has a Left-Center ("Red-Green") coalition government.

During World War II, Norway was occupied by the Nazis for five years (1940–1945). That experience reinforced Norway's commitments to peace, expressed in both the annual Nobel Peace Prize ceremonies and Independence Day celebrations featuring children rather than military parades. Reconstruction following the war years also accelerated Norway's development of social welfare policies and its participation in international affairs including a strong support for the United Nations.

The Economic System

Industrial and Economic Activity. Norway emerged as an industrial nation at the beginning of the twentieth century, partly due to local elites investing money in shipbuilding, timber and pulp production, and partly because it's electrochemical industry thrived upon cheap hydroelectric power from the numerous waterfalls and rapids. The major exporting industries today include crude oil and natural gas, metallurgical and chemical industries based on hydroelectric power, shipping and fisheries, timber and hydropower.

Timber and fish were one of the foremost natural resources; however, with the discovery of offshore fields in about 1970, the production of petroleum and gas has become the principal industry. Norway has tremendous resources in its offshore oil and gas fields in the North Sea. The financial surplus resulting from the export of oil and gas especially has created a positive balance of trade with other countries. Consequently, oil and gas production is an important economic and political factor in Norwegian recent history. The export value of crude oil and natural gas was 258 billion NOK (US$ 36 billion at the 2003 exchange rate of 7.080), making Norway the third largest oil exporter after Saudi Arabia and Russia. Oil and gas accounted for 36 percent of all exports from Norway in 2003. Oil revenues are invested for the future in the country's *Petroleum Fund*. By June, 2004 revenues had reached a total of US $135 billion, increasing by tens of billion dollars each year. According to current estimates, Norway has oil for the next 50 years and gas for at least 100 years.

Freight shipping services are Norway's most important export within the service sector, and the second largest export industry after oil and gas. Norwegian shipping companies control around 10 percent of the world's shipping fleet. Measured in tonnage, the Norwegian merchant fleet is the world's third largest. Norway is also one of the world's biggest exporters of seafood, and the aquaculture industry enjoys continued growth.

At the beginning of the twentieth century, Norway was one of the poorest countries in Western Europe. Presently, among member nations in the international Organization for Economic Cooperation and Development (OECD), Norway has the world's second highest per capita Gross Domestic Product (GDP) (48,000 US$ per capita based on the average annual exchange rate for 2004). Oil and gas revenues, combined with a strong dollar, have contributed to making Norway one of the world's richest countries. At 13.9 percent of GDP, the current national surplus is one of the highest figures ever recorded in the OECD.

The Economy and the Welfare State. Norwegians enjoy a generally high standard of living. The gap between rich and poor is small compared to most other countries, but it is widening. Norway does not have a numerically large, lower class of unemployed people living on the streets, except for a few hundred in the capital city of Oslo. The unemployment rates have been low (between 3 and 5%), the second lowest among OECD countries, except for a few years in the 1970s and in the beginning of the 1990s. In 2004, 107,000 (4.5%) inhabitants were registered as unemployed. The youth unemployment rate is higher, about 10 percent in the last ten years. All who have been previously employed and made a certain minimum income have earned the right to unemployment benefits from the National Insurance. Benefits amount to a certain share of prior earnings. The maximum of such benefits is well under the average industrial worker's salary and payment is limited to 78 or 156 weeks. Applicants for unemployment benefits are required to register themselves at a job centre as jobseekers and they must take any jobs given them.

The *Law on Universal Social Welfare Insurance (Folketrygden)*, which was passed by Parliament in 1966, states that all persons who are either residents or working as employees in Norway are insured under the compulsory *National Insurance Scheme*. Persons insured are entitled to old-age and disability pensions, basic benefit and attendance benefit in case of disability, rehabilitation benefits, occupational injury benefits, benefits to single parents, cash benefits in case of sickness, maternity, adoption and unemployment, medical benefits in case of sickness and maternity, and funeral grant.

Primary Welfare Services Run by the Municipalities and Counties. Though unified by a national constitution, locally elected bodies in both the local municipalities and the county municipalities have run the primary welfare and health services. There are 434 *local* municipalities with a population ranging from 200 to 500,000; half of them have a population of less than 4,500. There are 19 *county* municipalities, with a population ranging from 75,000 to 500,000. One-half of the counties have a population of less than 210,000. Services are financed through local taxes, based mainly on income, government block grants, special government reimbursements and grants, plus fees.

Growth of the Market Economy since the 1980s. The transformation of the Norwegian economy into a market economy with increased privatization was accelerated in the past two decades. The central government also pursued a policy of privatizing major state holdings, and the society has developed away from a highly state-regulated and centrally planned economy toward more of a market economy. The new liberalism and deregulation of the capitalistic economy in Norway, like that in the United Kingdom and United States, has led recently to larger economic differences and social problems, such as slightly increased crime, alcohol and drug abuse and the number of poor people is increasing.

Impact on Health Services Reform. The changes in economy and politics, from a planned economy and a welfare state with high public spending, towards privatization and competition have also impacted the health care system. In 2002, the ownership structure of the specialized health services were changed. While owned by the central government, all the hospitals and the specialized services are to be operated as *health enterprises*. They are to compete for patients, and the patients are free to choose among hospitals all over the country. A new leadership model, the *New Public Management*, was also introduced, inspired by private enterprises and based to a large extent on competition. However, only a few of the hospitals or medical centres are privately owned and run for profit. Some health specialists have a private practice, working on an individual basis, but they are integrated in the dominantly public health system. The central government still owns the main part of the health system, especially the mental health system, but runs it in a revised manner since 2002.

Cultural Values Expressed in Purposes, Policies, and Programs

In Norway, the welfare of the entire population has been regarded for a long time as a responsibility of the society as a whole. National policy for the health system continues to be based on the values of the welfare state: equality, justice and solidarity. Persons who become ill in Norway are guaranteed medical treatment. The health service is a cornerstone of the Norwegian welfare state. Universal access to quality public health care is the Norwegian authorities' goal. As a basic principle, health services are to be distributed according to need – not according to ability to pay. Users' fees are limited – no one pays more than NOK 1,350 per year for public services (US $191 at the 2003 exchange rate of 7.080). Equal access to health services is a nationally shared concern and a central aim of the government's health policy. The major objective is to deliver health care services of high quality and equitably to anyone in need, independent of age, sex, area of living, economy, or ethnic origin, as stated in § 1 in *Act on Health Enterprises*. In Norway, it has been regarded unethical to make a profit on ill persons in need of medical treatment. It has been looked upon as a duty of a civilized society to pay attention to the poor and distressed. This is the basis for the welfare state. The state redistributes the wealth so it becomes more equally distributed.

There are few private services or hospitals separated from or competing with the public health services. Most of the private institutions and practitioners are however, integrated into, and part of the same public health care system. No *mental health* institution is run as a for-profit organization to provide services for particular or exclusive groups of patients. Private practitioners are to a certain degree the exemption, though the majority is part of the public services, generally through operative arrangements (contracts) with the Regional Health Authorities, but not very well integrated in the mental health services at the moment.

Main goals in the *Act on Health Enterprises* are: strengthen user (= patient) involvement; update professional skills through lifelong learning; coordinate procurement within and between regions; improve cooperation among services in the health and social sectors; increase competition *and* cooperation (regionally and locally); improve effectiveness and increase productivity; emphasize and develop treatment and care in the local community; increase accessibility; reduce waiting times; reduce compulsory admissions and use of force (http://www.nordic telemed.org/papers/1).

An Overview of Norway's Health Care System

Organization of Health Services. Through legislation and the budgeting process, the central government assumes responsibility for policy design, overall capacity, quality assurance and quality improvement of health care in Norway. According to *The Municipal Health Services Act*, which took effect in 1984, the locally elected municipalities are given responsibility for primary health activities and social services. The municipal services provided include promotion of health and prevention of illness and injuries, organizing and running school health services, health centres, child health care provided by health visitors, midwives and general practitioner services, support for families, home nursing and home help services, residences providing continuous care (ordinary nursing homes etc), long-term services for the elderly, and day-centres for training and work. These services are part of the "practical assistance" that covers all kinds of help for the performance of daily-life tasks in households with persons in need of such help.

The municipal health service is the foundation of the Norwegian health care system. For most ailments, patients should be able to visit their local health station or general practitioners (GP) and receive treatment. The task of GPs is to arrive at a diagnosis at an early stage, treat simple everyday problems and refer patients to the specialised services when necessary.

From 2002, the responsibility for providing specialized health services were transferred from 19 locally elected county municipalities to five *Regional Health Authorities* (RHAs), owned by the central government. Through ownership of the RHAs, the central government, especially the Ministry of Health, follows the activity carefully and critically by written instructions and yearly meetings with the RHAs. In this way the central government can direct activities of specialized services, but this is not to include day-to-day interference in the running and organization of services. Within the limits set by legislation and available economic resources, the RHAs and the municipalities are otherwise formally free to plan and run public health services and social services. However, in practice, their freedom to act independently is limited by instructions from the Ministry of Health and available resources, decided by the Parliament.

Specialized Services and The Act on Health Enterprises. On January 1, 2002, the ownership of the specialized health services including all public hospitals was transferred from the 19 locally elected county municipalities to the state. Even though the reform is often called a hospital reform, it comprises most specialized health services, including all specialized mental health services. Norway was divided into five *Regional Health Authorities (RHAs)*[1], responsible for ensuring the provision of specialized health services to the inhabitants in their region.[2] Within the five RHAs, the specialized

---

1. The population of the five regions varied between 0.5 and 1.6 million people.
2. Already in 1974, Norway was divided into the five health regions for highly specialized functions in an attempt to ensure better co-operation among the counties, and to reflect the fact that as far as specialist medicine was concerned one needed a large catchment area in order to secure high-quality services at an acceptable cost.

health services are organized and delivered through a total of 31 *Health Enterprises*[3] owned by the RHAs and through contracts ("operative agreements") with private service providers. Each enterprise is wholly owned by the central government (through the RHAs), but each is also a separate legal and administrative entity, rather than an integral part of the central government administration. Principal health policy objectives and frameworks are determined by the central government and form the basis for management and administration of the health enterprises. A major reason for transferring responsibility from the 19 county municipalities to the central government was to coordinate procurement within and between regions; give patients the right to choose where to be treated, and reduce queues and waiting times.

For its 4.5 million inhabitants, Norway has 85 publicly owned general hospitals and a few private, nonprofit hospitals, in addition to some very small, for-profit private hospitals. A total of about 350 institutions providing specialist health services, including mental health institutions, were transferred to central government ownership in 2002. The *Act on Health Enterprises* did not change the responsibility for the *primary health care system*. The 434 municipalities are still responsible for preventive efforts and for providing primary health care and social services.

Health Regions and Health Enterprises. The role of the health enterprise is to ensure the best possible running of its own activities to meet the health policy objectives within the financial framework determined by the health enterprise owners and the Parliament *(Stortinget)*. Each RHA has an executive board and a general manager designated by the Ministry of Health[4] with powers of authority stipulated in the 2002 legislation. The governing board of health enterprises consists of persons designated by the RHAs. Board meetings in health enterprises are to be open to the press and the public. A significant challenge in this system is finding the right balance between local autonomy for the local health enterprises and the necessary oversight by the central government.

To ensure the involvement of patients and the public, all health enterprises have a *user's council*.[5] A user's council consists of civic representatives, patients and representatives from patient and other organizations. The user's council associated with all health enterprises may be consulted by the board prior to any major health decision, and the council may also take initiatives on their own.

The Reform of Specialized Services. The new model for specialized health services (*The Specialized Health Care Act* from 2001) leaves no room for doubt that the central Government has full and complete responsibility, and that it has access to direct information and to the entire range of relevant policy instruments. In formal terms, there are no restrictions to the Government's right of control as owner of all health enterprises in the public sector. Through the *Ministry of Health*, the central Government has a greater opportunity now to intervene in the health care system than previously when owned and run by the counties. There are however, limits on how the *Ministry of Health* may exercise its power of control. Direct intervention in the day-to-day running of the enterprises would undermine the responsibility of the general manager and the executive boards of both RHAs and health enterprises. The philosophy is that the *Ministry of Health* may not exercise detailed control, but shall give the health enterprises genuine administrative responsibility. The policy prohibits micromanagement of health enterprises by the central *Ministry of Health*.

In addition to centralizing formal and political authority, the *Act on Health Enterprises* from 2002 clarifies local responsibility by giving the health enterprises a higher degree of freedom regarding investments, flexibility in the planning and provision of health services, and freedom to organize and use resources across their organization. The enterprises are economically responsible and must focus on cost control, but must also address the quality challenges. In short, they must operate in a cost-effective manner.

Former Organization. When it assumed responsibility for the specialized services in 2002, the central government ended a more than 30-year tradition. The

---

3. Due to the restructuring of 2003, the number of health enterprises was reduced from 43 at the end of 2002 to 31 at the end of 2003. Consequently there are fewer and larger health enterprises.
4. "Ministry of Health" is used as an abbreviation for "Ministry of Health and Care Services."

5. In Norway the term "user" is preferred over "patient" and "client by some professionals and receivers of services." The term, "consumer" is seldom applied in Norway's health service, which is predominantly public. Because the services are financed and owned by the State, Norwegians do not perceive themselves as consumers in a health care market.

counties had been assigned responsibility for planning, investment and running of the hospitals and other specialist services by the *Hospital Act* on January 1, 1970. By the end of the 1980s, the justifications for county ownership had been challenged and a public committee evaluated the issue of takeover by the central government. A majority of the committee, and later the Norwegian Parliament, voted in favour of continuation of county ownership. In 2001, the majority had changed, and the Parliament voted for transferring power to the central government.

Health Legislation in the 1990s. In July 1999, the Norwegian Parliament passed four new Acts that addressed different aspects of the country's health system: the *Specialized Health Care Act*; the *Mental Health Act*; the *Patient Rights Act*; and the *Health Personnel Act*. These new Acts became effective January 1, 2001. Mental health services are regulated together with other specialized medical disciplines in the *Specialized Health Care Act*. However, mental health services provided in primary care settings within local municipalities are regulated by the *Municipal Health Act*.

The new legislation on patients' rights is intended to give patients better quality health services and to ensure patients' trust and confidence in such services. These are the goals and reasons for granting (a) essential health assistance from the specialist health service, (b) the right to a medical examination within 30 days, (c) the right to a second opinion and (d) the right to choose the hospital they will use.

The General Practitioner Scheme. Of importance is also the adoption of "the list patient system," providing all citizens with a personal, regular General Practitioner (GP). In 2000, everyone in the country was invited to choose a GP. Those who did not choose themselves were assigned to a GP. Patients are allowed to change GPs according to specific regulations if they are dissatisfied with the choice. The GP are not expected to treat other patients on a regular basis than those assigned on the list. The purpose of *The General Practitioner Scheme* is to encourage better doctor/patient communication and to ensure every inhabitant access to an easily accessible medical service. The reform also gives improved continuity in the doctor-patient relationship and a more rational utilization of the country's total medical resources. Patients contact their GP frequently because of mental health problem. The GPs often become the patients' first contact with the mental health services. They therefore play an important role in the chain of services. But the GPs are not very well integrated in the mental health system at the moment.

The Need for Mental Health Services in Norway

Generally speaking, mental health services in Norway are meant to treat and take care of people with severe mental disorders, including diagnoses like schizophrenia, bipolar disorders, severe depressions and anxiety and other mental health problems. Those who suffer with such mental disorders, are dysfunctional because of their irrational thoughts, unregulated emotions or maladaptive behavior or are deviant in such a way that they become a threat to themselves or others, have the right to be provided appropriate care through public mental health services in Norway.

An increasing share of the population in Norway asks for mental health assistance, help, care and treatment. That does not necessarily mean that the mental health of the population has deteriorated during recent decades. The increased number of people asking for help, or actually referred, is partly a result of increased supply of these services. When there are no private practitioners, no psychiatric hospitals or outpatient clinics, there are also reduced demands for such services and fewer identified patients, even if the suffering and prevalence of disorders are the same. By establishing and expanding services, demands are also created.

In principle it is difficult to state what will be a "correct" or even sufficient amount of services such as the quantity of beds, staff, or other resources. Demands will always be partly a function of what is offered, not only because the beds are there to be occupied, but because establishing health services informs people in general and certain groups in particular, about how to deal with the problems of mood disorders, anxiety, deviant behavior, and other problems of living as well.

Who Needs Professional Mental Health Care? It is therefore difficult to draw the line between those in need of mental health services, and those who can deal with their problems, sadness, anxiety, or deviant behavior without being treated by a mental health professional. Yet an important and necessary task for the health authorities is to distinguish between those in need of psychiatric treatment from those who need support and assistance by other agencies, or can deal with their condition by themselves, helped by friends or relatives. To plan for, and to allocate resources to mental health services, it is important to know the approximate needs or actual demands for treatment in the population served. Such rates are estimated in epidemiological studies. However, in Norway there has been very limited use of epidemiological data for planning the allocation of resources in the mental health sector, due partly to a limited number of nation-wide studies.

Estimated Prevalence of Psychiatric Disorders. There are no epidemiological studies for the Norwegian population as a whole. Some studies give rates for groups defined by residence, age or diagnosis.[6] International studies reveal that about 50 percent acquire a mental disorder through their lifetime, and between 20 percent and 30 percent have had such a disorder within the last 12 months (Dalgard, Kringlen & Dahl, 2002). A study which compared the psychiatric morbidity of Oslo with a western region of the country *(Sogn og Fjordane)* in 1994–1997 (Kringlen, Torgersen & Cramer, 2001) confirmed these results regarding Oslo (Table 3.1). The study was based on a sample of 2000 in Oslo and 1000 in *Sogn og Fjordane* in the age group 18–65 years, using the Composite International Diagnostic Interview (CIDI) (World Health Organization, 1993) and additional instruments. The life-time prevalence of mental disorders in Oslo was 52.4 percent and annual prevalence was 32.8 percent. The lifetime prevalence outside the capital is expected to be much lower than in Oslo, probably about half.

Lifetime prevalence in the capital Oslo for some selected disorders was also given by Kringlen, Torgersen & Cramer (2001): Major depression (7.3%); Simple phobia (11.1%); Social phobia (7.9%); Panic anxiety (2–3%); Personality disorders (13.4%); Alcohol abuse/dependence (10.6%). For most of these diagnoses the referred prevalence in the capital are much higher than in the rest of the country.

It has been estimated that 15–20 percent of the population at any point in time have some psychological distress. Three percent have severe mental disorders and 0.8 percent to one percent has a serious mental illness that requires much sustained care and coordination of services. The most *prevalent* disorders are anxieties, depression, personality disorders, alcohol and drug abuse, while the most *severe* are schizophrenia and bipolar disorders.

Based on a total population of 4,577,000 in January 1, 2004, and a conservative estimate of 15 percent of the population with psychological distress, an estimated 687,000 inhabitants have a reduced mental health. An increasing share is asking for treatment and care. Approximately 180,000 people were actually in contact with the specialized mental health services in 2003, that is four percent of the total population, and about 25 percent of those with some sort of psychological distress or disorders. What follows is a sample of recent epidemiological studies first with adults, then with children and adolescents.

Studies of Prevalence Among Adults in Norway. As an estimate of *period prevalence*, during four years ending in 1955, Bentsen (1970) found a prevalence rate of psychiatric disorders at 21.7 percent in the southeast area of Norway, with 0.8 percent classified as severe cases, 6.0 percent as moderate, and 14.9 percent as mild. Andersen (1978) studied two very different communities in the north of Norway. One consisted of Sámi people (aboriginals) and the other was a traditional Norwegian agriculture and fishing municipality. The *lifetime* prevalence was 20.7 percent in the Norwegian community and 15.7 percent in the Sámi community (Dalgard, 2002). Dalgard (1980) did a survey in Oslo in the 1970s. The total *point-prevalence* of psychiatric disorders and distress was 19.9 percent, consisting mainly of anxiety and depression. *Lifetime* prevalence was estimated to 25.6 percent.

Sandanger et al. (1999) compared communities in Lofoten Peninsula in the north of Norway with the eastern district of Oslo that has many multicultural inhabitants. The subjects were first screened with the abbreviated Hopkins Symptom Checklist (HSCL-25) (Derogatis, et al. 1974). Those who scored high and low on the instrument were interviewed subsequently using the *Composite International Diagnostic Interview* (CIDI) (World Health Organization, 1993). Preliminary data from the follow-up study 1990–2001, based

Table 3.1. *Percentage With a Mental Disorder in Oslo.*

	Lifetime prevalence	Prevalence the past year
Female	54.8	35.9
Male	49.4	28.8
Total	52.4	32.8

---

6. Epidemiological results are dependent on the indicators and how disorders are operationalized. There are no neutral figures representing the frequency or rates of mental disorders in an objective way. Disorders are social constructions, dependent on types of knowledge, ideology, power and cultural values. Consequently, estimates of prevalence and incidence vary according to methods, instruments and diagnostic criteria used.

Table 3.2. *Self-Rated Mental Health Problems, Norwegian Population 2002 (Percentages).*

	Age				
	All	16–24	25–44	45–66	67+
Anxiety or phobia*	5	2	4	7	5
Tired or limp*	22	24	25	20	20
Concentration problems*	9	12	9	9	8
Sleeping problems*	18	13	15	19	26
Mildly depressed*	10	11	9	12	9
Irritable or aggressive*	9	12	10	7	5
Scores 10 or higher on a scale from 5–20 for mental health	8	8	8	9	7
Bothered by at least three psychiatric symptoms	15	16	14	15	17
Used medication for falling in sleep last week	3	0	1	4	10
Used sedatives last week	3	1	1	4	4
Used anti-depressive medication last week	4	1	3	5	4
"Nervous disorder"	5	4	4	6	5

Note: Source is Statistics Norway, 2004.
* Worries last three months.

on 2,015 and 1,691 respondents in Oslo and the Lofoten Peninsula respectively, gave the following one year prevalence in 2001: Depressions (F 32.00-F34.10 + F06.32)[7]: 8.4 percent; Anxiety disorders (F40.00-F43.99): 18.8 percent (male: 13.0%, female: 24.7%) (Sandanger, 2003). The one-week period prevalence of psychiatric cases by HSCL-25 was 13.8 percent in 2001 (male 11.2%, female 16.0%). Using the Structured Interview for DSM-III Personality Disorder (SIDP-R) with approximately 2000 adults, the two-week period prevalence of personality disorders was 13.4 percent.

Depression is presently one of the most common mental disorders in Norway, more frequent in urban than rural settlements. Depression also seems to appear at earlier ages than previously. Studies from Oslo reveal that 10 percent of all men and 24 percent of all women have a major depression during their lifetime. Six percent of men and 13 percent of women had a milder depression lasting for a minimum of two years (Kringlen, Torgersen & Cramer, 2001). In a multicentre epidemiological study conducted in five European countries from 1996–1997, using the Beck Depression Inventory (BDI) (Beck, Steer & Garbin, 1988) and the Schedule for Clinical Assessment in Neuropsychiatry (SCAN II) (World Health Organization, 1994), the four-week *period prevalence* rate for *depression* in Oslo was overall 8.8 percent (12.0% for women and 5.6% for men) (Ayuso-Mateos, et al. 2001). The rates were the same as in Turku (Finland), higher than Santander (Spain) (2.6%) and lower than Dublin (12.3%) and Liverpool (17.1%).

Self-rated mental health problems. In 1985, 1998 and 2002, *Statistics Norway* surveyed a representative sample of the Norwegian population, using the self-rating Hopkins Symptom Checklist -25 HSCL-25) (Derogatis, et al. 1974). Common rules for scoring and cut-off points were used to estimate so-called *cases* in the population (Moum, et al. 1991). In 1998, the self rated prevalence for psychological distress was 8.4 percent for men and 13.6 percent for women and in 2002, 8.9 percent and 12.2 percent respectively. The prevalence increases slightly with the age. Self-rating studies do not include the severely mentally ill population. Estimates are therefore conservative. Selected results from the 2002 survey using the self rating HSCL-25 on a representative sample of the population are shown above in Table 3.2.

---

7. The symbols in brackets refer to the International Statistical Classification of Diseases and Related Health Problems, ICD-10, Volume 1 (World Health Organization, Geneva 1992), and its revision in 1996.

Studies of Substance Abuse and Dual Diagnoses Among Adults. With increasing alcohol consumption and drug abuse in society, psychotic patients, particularly in the larger cities, have to deal with a dual problem. Many of the new schizophrenic patients from urban areas have alcohol and/or drug problems in addition to mental disorders. In 2001, 4,000 people (9 per 10,000) were in need of treatment because of a combination of severe mental disorders and extensive substance abuse. Half of them were alcohol abusers, 1,200 had a schizophrenic-like or bipolar disorder, 800 had a severe depression or anxiety or other disorder with severe dysfunctions, 1,700 had a severe personality disorder, and 300 had severe cognitive dysfunctions, were unstable or asocial (Hordvin, 2004). In 2001, more than 20,000 alcohol and drug abusers were referred to treatment, and nearly 18,000 started treatment (Hordvin, 2004).

Prevalence Among Children and Adolescents (C&A). Lavik (1976) surveyed 15 and 16 year-olds living in Oslo and in a rural municipality in the 1970s. Psychiatric symptoms and behaviour disorders were more frequent in the capital, especially among the boys (*point prevalence* 23.1%) than in the rural area (7.7%). For girls the point prevalence was 15.9 percent and 8.2 percent, respectively. Kolstad (1983) studied children and adolescents from four to sixteen years old. The average point-prevalence in the communities in the west coast of Norway was 4.3 percent. No big cities were included. The most unstable, "turbulent" and fast-growing communities had the highest prevalence, especially for behaviour disorders. In general, the rates were low due to the stable, rural communities and a feeling of belongingness to the local culture.

Today, it is assumed that approximately five percent of all youths below 18 are in need of specialized mental health care (Lavigne, Gibbons, Christoffel, et al. 1996). The National Mental Health Programme (NMHP) refers to this rate. Based on this figure it was estimated in 1996 that as much as 60 percent of Norwegian youths who were in need of specialized mental health care did not receive such care (Halsteinli, 1998).

Mortality and Disability Rates

Mental and Behavioral Disorders as Cause of Death. In 2002, 44,401 deaths were recorded in Norway. Of these, 42,114 died of diseases and 2,287 of external causes. Table 3.3 summarizes the mortality rates for selected causes of death.

Table 3.3. *Mortality Ratios per 100,000 in 2002.*

	Per 100,000 inhabitants		
	All	Female	Male
All causes	978.4	961.2	995.3
All mental and behavioural disorders (F00-99)*	28.9	26.3	31.6
Organic, including symptomatic, mental disorders (F00-F09)	17.4	8.6	26.1
Mental and behavioural disorders due to psychoactive substance use (F10-F19)	10.2	16.7	3.8
Other mental and behavioural disorders (F20-99)	1.3	1.0	1.7
Suicide	10.9	16.1	5.8

Note: Source is "Mental Health Services in Norway. Prevention – Treatment – Care." Norwegian Ministry of Health and Care Services, Oslo, 2005.
* The symbols in brackets refer to the International Statistical Classification of Diseases and Related Health Problems, ICD-10, Volume 1 (World Health Organization, Geneva 1992), and its revision in 1996.

In 2002, 1,310 deaths (28.9 per 100,000, and 3% of all deaths) were due to mental and behavioral disorders, Table 3.3. This cause of death is slightly more common among females (31.6) than males (26.3), and increases with age.

Suicide as Cause of Death. In 2002, 494 persons committed suicide (10.9 per 100,000 and 1% of all deaths that year), Table 3.3. The rate of suicide in Norway is fairly low in comparison with other Northern European countries and has been declining since the 1980s in all age groups. Still, suicide is one of the most important causes of death for people under 45 years of age, responsible for 13 percent of all deaths in this age group. The ratio was much higher among men (16.1%) than among women (5.8%). For women the rate increases with age, for men it does not vary with age over 20 years, Figure 3.1.

Deaths Caused by Substance Abuse. The number of intravenous drug abusers in Norway in 2002 was estimated between 11,000 and 15,000 people (Hordvin, 2004). It is worrisome that the mortality from alcohol and drug addiction is particularly high in Norway,

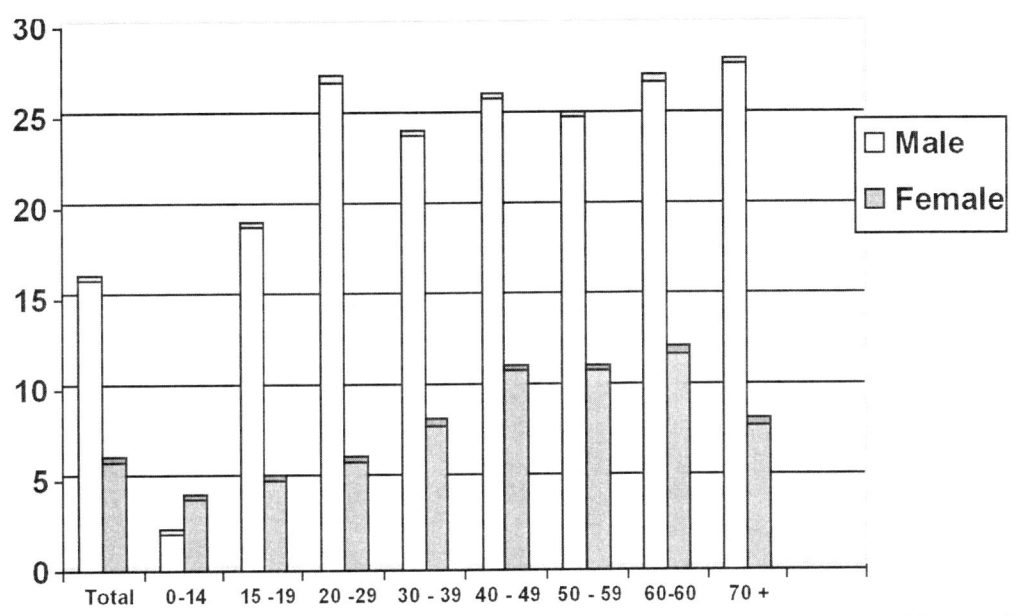

Note: Soure is "Mental Health Services in Norway. Prevention – Treatment – Care" Norwegian Ministry of Health and Care Services, Oslo, 2005.

Figure 3.1. Suicide by age and gender. Ratios per 100,000 inhabitants.

especially in the capital, compared with other European countries. The *total number* of deaths caused by alcohol, narcotics and medication amounted to 810 in 2000 and 780 in 2002 (14 per 100,000 inhabitants), or about 1.8 percent of all deaths. The number of alcohol and alcohol-related deaths has been stable the last years. In 2000, totally 392 (9 per 100,000) died of alcohol and alcohol-related diseases. The most frequent causes of deaths are liver diseases and alcoholism, 178 and 154 respectively. The mortality rates from alcohol abuse and drug dependence is shown in Table 3.4 by sex and ages.

The total number of deaths related to drugs (e.g., heroin and morphine) range from 200 to 300 per year, and has increased significantly in the last ten-year period. Drug dependence caused 272 deaths (6

Table 3.4. *Deaths by Sex, Age and Underlying Cause of Death: Alcohol Abuse and Drug Dependence. The Whole Country, 2002.*

	Per 100,000	N total	Age −24	Age 25–64	Age 65+
Alcohol abuse (including alcohol psychosis) (F10)*					
Total	4.2	190	0	124	66
Males	7.1	160	0	107	53
Females	1.3	30	0	17	13
Drug dependence, toxicmania (F11–F16, F18–F19)*					
Total	6.0	272	38	233	1
Males	9.6	215	29	185	1
Females	2.5	57	9	48	–

* The symbols in brackets refer to the International Statistical Classification of Diseases and Related Health Problems, ICD-10, Volume 1 (World Health Organization, Geneva 1992), and its revision in 1996.

Table 3.5. *Disability Pensions for Mental and Behavioural Disorders. Ratios per 10,000 Inhabitants Aged 16–67. End of 2003.*

	Males	*Females*	*Total*
All mental and behavioural disorders (F00-99) *	329	279	300
Schizophrenia, schizotypal and delusional disorders (F20-29)	59	32	44
Mental and behavioural disorders due to psychoactive substance use (F10–19)	33	6	18
Mood disorders (F30–39)	40	49	45
Mental retardation (F70–79)	52	34	42
Other mental disorders (F40–69, F80–99)	145	158	152

* The symbols in brackets refer to the International Statistical Classification of Diseases and Related Health Problems, ICD-10, Volume 1 (World Health Organization, Geneva 1992), and its revision in 1996. Source: "Mental Health Services in Norway. Prevention – Treatment – Care" Norwegian Ministry of Health and Care Services, Oslo, 2005.

pr 100,000) in 2002. In 1998, opiates caused 243 deaths, mainly men. In 1989, there were 34 deaths from opiates.

Deaths due to AIDS. From 1984 to 2002, 2,555 persons with HIV and 773 AIDS cases were registered in Norway (Hordvin, 2004); 472 of the 2,555 seropositives (18.5%) were recognized as drug users. The number of AIDS deaths has decreased since 1993, when 69 persons died. In 1998, 27 died from AIDS, 20 men and 7 women. 12 persons (0.3 pr 100,000) died from AIDS in 2002, 10 men and 2 women.

Number and Percent of Population on Mental Health Disability. Ten percent of the work force between the age of 16 and 67 have disability pension, more than 300,000 people. About one-third of these, or three percent of the population aged 16–67, receive disability pension based on a primary psychiatric diagnosis.[8] An additional 0.6 percent is on long-term sickness leave due to their mental health. Table 3.5 gives the rates for the mental and behavioural disorders in the population with disability pensions.

In 2003, the cost of psychiatric disorders because of disability pensions, sickness leave and treatment was estimated to NOK 40 billion, or 6.25 billion U.S. dollars. Loss in productivity due to psychiatric disorders is not included (*Helse-og omsorgsdepartementet, Statsbudsjettet, St.prp.1*, 2005). The cost for schizophrenia alone has also been estimated:

> The human suffering associated with schizophrenia is enormous – for patients, families, and in society at large.

---

8. To get a disability pension the person in question has to be diagnosed by an illness.

Ten percent of all disabled citizens in Norway have schizophrenia, although the yearly incidence is low (about 7–15 per 100,000). In Norway, the total cost per year for schizophrenia is estimated at 4 billion NOK (1995). In western countries costs are estimated to exceed one percent of the national budget. There is no other disorder with comparable costs. Schizophrenia alone costs more than all types of cancer and more than all cardiovascular diseases. (Johannessen, 2002)

Norway's Mental Health Policies and Programs

Mental health services in Norway are public and financed by the central Government and the locally elected municipalities. National mental health policies assert the principle that all inhabitants are to be treated on an equal level, having the same rights independent of income, private insurance, social status, place of living. Treatment and care provided are only dependent on the individual's disorders, and how the qualified providers in the primary care and specialist care sectors evaluate the need for treatment. In theory, all inhabitants have access to the same services, and can choose where to be treated. There is no discrimination on the basis of income, work, or insurance – at least not in principle.

There are no mental health services provided in a private sector independent of the public system in Norway. Most of the private practitioners are incorporated into the public system, often through an operative agreement as contracted providers, and reimbursed by the publicly financed system. Consequently, it would not be really accurate to present a public and a private sector of mental health services in Norway as if they were separate. The few "private" mental institutions and nursing homes, established and managed for a long time by religious or humanitarian organizations, are run mostly on a charitable basis, and not as for-profit corporations. Patients admitted to these "private" institutions are paid for in the same way as in the public health enterprises, by the Government, the municipalities and the National Insurance Scheme. The financing and functioning of mental health services in Norway are therefore simple to understand and analyze: there is only one "sector" – the public one – financed by State revenues and by taxes and contributions from employees, self-employed persons and employers.

Norway's Mental Health Programs: An Historical Overview

The history of Norwegian mental health services before 1850 is mainly the history of care for the poor and "unfit." Mentally disturbed people were not really identified as a distinct and separate group. The local counties had, since the 1740s, the responsibility for the deprived populations and this was also stated in the *Law on Poverty* from 1845. Counties were allowed to place the poor and deviant with designated farmers, in workhouses, or to auction them off. Beginning in the early 1800s some of the deviant, irresponsible and insane people were gradually categorized by medical doctors as people with illnesses, who should be taken care of by the medical profession. To a certain degree, the medical doctors themselves promoted this new social construction of madness and deviant behavior as "*illness.*"

A law for the mental health services was drafted in 1848 *(Sinnssykeloven)*. With minor alterations this law was at work in Norway until 1961. The law was written to secure control of the treatment of the insane within *asylums*. The head of the asylum had to be a physician with public authorization. Governmental commissions were to survey these institutions. Admission to the asylum required that (a) the individual was diagnosed as insane and (b) the doctor determined that admission was best for the patient or necessary for the public order and safety.

The first purpose-built state psychiatric hospital in Norway, Gaustad asylum in Oslo, opened in 1855 with 270 beds. During the last part of the nineteenth century, three other asylums were erected: in Trondheim in the middle of Norway, in Kristiansand in the south, and in Bergen at the southwest coast. At the onset of the twentieth century eleven new asylums were established, the majority funded by the counties. By 1930 most counties had their asylum, except for the most northern region which obtained a mental hospital in 1961. By 1921 Norway had 21 psychiatric asylums. There were hardly any other facilities established. Traditionally the church and the poor-law authorities had been involved. But their involvement diminished after "the mentally ill" were separated as a particular group of people, and confined in asylums.

In 1961, a new *Act of Mental Health Care (Lov om Psykisk helsevern)* was approved. The government aimed at opening up mental health care to new groups of patients, in new kinds of institutions, based on modern principles. The indications for treatment were widened, and psychotherapy of less serious disorders, such as neuroses, was recommended. Psychiatric wards were established in some general hospitals by the counties. The nineteen regions (county councils) were also encouraged to establish new facilities for children and adolescents. The legislation also mentioned behavioral disorders, "bad behavior in schools," and "family psychiatry" (Ot. prp. nr. 69, (1959–1960). These latter groups had not previously been provided mental health care. Among the new institutions advocated in the Act, the "outpatient" clinics were to become the most important. By using the phrase "other psychiatric institutions," the legislation also allowed for new kinds of institutions in the future (Seip, 2004). The *mental hospitals*, owned and run by the state until then, were to be transferred to the counties in which they were situated.

A new *Hospital Act* approved in 1970 also made recommendations concerning mental health services. Psychiatric hospitals should concentrate on "active" treatment. The long-stay patients should be referred to psychiatric nursing homes or their own home. The differences between the mental hospitals and the psychiatric wards in general hospitals (psychiatric clinics) were to fade away. Each psychiatric hospital or ward became responsible for a catchment area. For every 10,000 inhabitants there were to be 30 beds in a mental hospital/ward. This ratio was reduced later to 23 beds per 10,000.

In actuality, both the type and capacities of treatment facilities varied throughout the country and access to services was dependent upon the location of one's residence. Since the counties and not the central government were responsible, there were great variations in the number of beds and other resources allocated to mental health services in different counties.

Mental Health Services Are Given Priority. Recently in Norway there has been a growing political awareness and an increasing political will and commitment to improve the mental health services. Particularly during the 1990s criticisms about the capacity and quality of mental health services increased, and politicians agreed that mental health services should be given priority within national health policy.

A *Government White Paper* dealing with mental health issues, published in 1997 *(Sosial-og helsedepartementet, 1997)*, provided a clear picture of the deficiencies of the services. Though funding for mental health services had increased, the capacity and quality had not increased as much as expected prior to 1997. There were still severe shortcomings, and the complaints from patients' organizations had increased. The White Paper stated explicitly that the mental health system had severe shortcomings. The service facilities were imperfect and insufficient, the thresholds for getting treatment were too high, the after-care was lacking, and the cooperation between the primary health care and the specialist mental health services was inadequate. The productivity and efficiency, especially at the outpatient clinics needed improvement, and the use of compulsory admission and force should be reduced. A far-reaching restructuring and strengthening of the mental health services, its accessibility and quality, was considered necessary.

Based on this White Paper, Parliament ordered the central government to present a binding plan for improved mental health services, focusing particularly on local remedial measures. The former way of organizing the help and treatment as a psychiatric service delivered primarily through specialized psychiatric hospitals and wards in general hospitals did not seem to be adequate to the demands of most patients, and it was expensive. In response to this national report, the central government instigated in the spring of 1998 the plan for a mandatory investment to improve all aspects of mental health services.

Norway's Current National Mental Health Programme, 1999–2008

The legislation led to action schemes and the *National Mental Health Programme* (NMHP) for the period 1999 to 2006 (*Sosial-og helsedepartementet*, 1998). The period was later extended to 2008.

NMHP was approved by Parliament in 1998. The Programme aims at correcting the deficiencies and to restructure and develop services according to the principles recommended in the White Paper by improving accessibility, quality, organization and treatment on all levels for adults as well as children and adolescents. A central idea of the Programme is to promote further deinstitutionalization, with considerable emphasis on community-based services and treatment facilities closer to, and more integrated with primary health care services provided in areas where the patients are living. The principal aims of the NMHP are to: (a) develop more user-oriented services; (b) strengthen municipal services, preventive care and early help; (c) reorganize mental health services for adults; (d) establish more places for round-the-clock treatment and acute admission; (e) expand *District Psychiatric Centres* and outpatient clinics; (f) develop child and youth mental health services; (g) promote skill, development, education and research.

The Programme is comprehensive, covering all the different settings. It also links the different parts of the services, and combines (among other things) *primary health care, specialized health services*, the educational system, social services, and employment agencies. The following quotation from the Programme gives an idea of the new trend and ideology for the services in the beginning of 2000:

> A person with psychiatric disorders should not be looked upon solely as a patient, but as a human being with a body, a soul and spirit. Due consideration has to be taken to the human being's spiritual and cultural needs, not only to its biological and social needs. Psychiatric disorders also comprehend existential questions. The patients' needs should always be the point of departure for all treatment, and the core for all nursing. This has to be emphasised in the organisation, in practice and the leadership in all mental health services. *(Sosial-og helsedepartementet, 1998)*

One major goal is to integrate the community-based, mental health services provided by general practitioners, nurses and local outpatient clinics with the specialized mental health services. The mental hospitals have differentiated wards: acute, intermediate, long-term, psychogeriatric, etc., and they are expected to operate in close cooperation with the general services outside the hospitals. The primary services in the local community become more important than in the "old" hospital-based system. Treatment and care are to be given closer to the patient's daily environment and in connection to primary-health care and social services.

The implementation of the NMHP is the dual responsibility of the *Regional Health Authorities* (RHAs) and State authorities, i.e., the *Ministry of Health.* Established

January 1, 2002, each of the five RHAs is responsible for the development of the schedules and schemes in its region, according to the limits and goals set by the Programme and the budget.

Emphasis on the User's Perspective. Fundamental to the reform is the emphasis placed on the user's view and perspectives. The Programme states that the experience and knowledge possessed by users and their relatives is unique and necessary in improving and optimizing services and treatment. Participation is also vital for empowerment and for the ability to master one's own life, both of which are central to the vision of the NMHP.

The aim of this policy is that users and close relatives should participate at all levels. This requires involvement and cooperation both on a system level and individual level. At the *system* level this implies organized user/relative participation in planning processes, legislation, treatment procedures, etc. It is of major importance that these policies are implemented in all service sectors including political, administrative and professional leaders – the central Health Ministry, Regional Health Authorities, counties, municipalities and health enterprises. Accordingly, central as well as local authorities should be cooperating with user organizations and unions in these matters. At the *individual* level the user/relative perspective implies legally established rights of participation in arranging daily life activities, the meeting between patient/user and staff, information and consent, etc.

The *Act of Patients' Rights*, passed by Parliament in 1999, aims to improve the rights of patients, including the right to take part in the planning and coordination of the services, and the right to decide where to receive treatment. Specialized services are now required by law to establish systems for obtaining reports by patients of their experiences with, and views about services. Participation by users and relatives is equally essential for children and adolescents. The NMHP stipulates that if possible, treatment shall be provided on a voluntary basis, in open and normalized settings, and preferably on a daytime basis. Services shall promote independence, improved living conditions, quality of life and participation in ordinary life. Regarding adults, special focus is being placed on (a) satisfactory housing with sufficient assistance, (b) the possibility of participation in labour market activities or other meaningful activities, and (c) the possibility of social contact and integration, cultural and physical activities.

Individual Plans. Making individual plans that coordinate necessary services has become a mandatory task for the service providers, the health enterprises, and a legal right for the patients. In this respect, NMHP pays special attention to patients with severe or major disorders, such as schizophrenia, suicidality, and severe eating disorders, as well as especially vulnerable groups, including the mentally handicapped with severe mental disorders, children, refugees and traumatized groups.

District Psychiatric Centres (DPCs). The establishment of a new category of institutions, *District Psychiatric Centre (DPC) (Distriktspsykiatrisk Senter – DPS* in Norwegian), is a core element in the Programme and expected to play a major role. The DPCs are supposed to improve access to the specialized services and to enhance the quality of treatment and care in general. The planned 83 DPCs[9] described in the White Paper serve an important link in the new differentiated "chain" comprising both the primary care and the specialized services. The new service setting represents a comprehensive and integrated unit with responsibility for a substantial part of the general mental health services in a geographically defined catchments area. The Centres are expected to perform the following functions: (a) Out-patient clinic services, including an ambulant treatment team; (b) day care and day centre; (c) beds for crisis intervention and observation; (d) a short-term 24-hour ward; (e) wards for long-term treatment and rehabilitation; (f) counselling, supervision and consultation with the primary mental health care sector and (g) cooperation with the social services in the municipalities and psychiatric hospitals and wards.

The DPCs are expected to leave to the psychiatric hospitals and wards the more specialized treatment. Nevertheless, the DPCs are intended to have a "total responsibility" for psychiatric treatment and supervision in their catchments area. This will increase the access and reduce the distance to mental health services provided through all general facilities. Since 1998 there has been a considerable expansion of these institutions. In 2003, 71 DPCs covering 86 percent of the population were established. Not all of them cover all kinds of expected services yet. Twelve more centres covering the remaining population will be established over the coming years. Unfortunately, other institutions have been closed down at a much

---

9. The number of planned DPCs has varied during the Programme period and has fluctuated around 80.

faster rate than planned, reducing the total number of beds available for mental health patients.

Psychiatric Nursing Homes. In addition to establishing new DPCs, the NMHP stated that psychiatric nursing homes should be either transformed to active treatment units as DPCs, or be closed down gradually as other caring facilities in the municipalities were established.

Mental Health Professionals. In general, mental health services deal with complex problems related to multiple social, environmental, biological and psychological factors. A broad and multidisciplinary approach, implemented through teamwork is necessary to deal with the patients' often multifaceted problems. Consequently, another goal of the NMHP is to increase the number of mental health professionals other than psychologists and psychiatrists, with at least a three-year university college education,[10] and then make the staff better trained with more adequate knowledge for the new tasks.

Mental Health Services for Children and Adolescents (C&A). The first psychiatric institution for children in Norway, a Child Guidance Clinic, was established in Oslo in 1947. The clinic was set up as an outpatient service, with a clinical psychologist, a psychiatrist, and a social worker. The initiative came from Dr. Nic Waal, a radical physician, who was interested in public health and psychoanalysis, and who had studied and practiced child psychiatry in the United States. By 1955, the Clinic included 30 full-time therapists and 10 more working part-time (Seip, 2004). The public regulation of mental health services for C&A started with the Mental Health Act in 1961. A new Act was introduced in 1999. The NMHP recognized that mental health services for C&A needed a considerable expansion and strengthening as well, and especially the capacity of the outpatient clinics and the number of beds in small and adjusted institutions. New ways of working in the preventive field and better cooperation with the social services were also considered necessary. The Programme stated that five percent of the population below 18 years of age should have treatment offered in 2008.

Financing of the NMHP. The major reform and expansion of services has required extensive grants and subsidies from the central government, which set aside a total of NOK 6.3 billion (US$ 834 million, or US$ 19 per capita)[11] to investments to achieve the goals of the NMHP. In addition, NOK 376 million per year is allocated to other expenses like sheltered employment, and education of personnel. The national subsidies earmarked for mental health operations will be increased by NOK 4.6 billion (US$ 609 million) through 2008 compared with 1998 levels, and will not require any financing by municipal or county authorities. Earmarked grants from the central government have been supplied for expansion of services provided by the municipalities.

Expenditures and Financing for Specialized Services under the NMHP. Excluding investment and capital expenditures, the total per capita expenditure in 2003 for specialized mental health services, consumed 0.7 percent of the GDP, and amounted to NOK 2,445 (US$ 345 at the 2003 exchange rate of 7.080). This represents a 16 percent real growth in expenditures since 1998. The running costs for the specialized mental health services increases by 2.1 billion per year in relation to the 1996 level. Over the period 1999–2006, annual running cost of the specialized services is projected to increase by NOK 500 per capita (US$ 64 per capita at the 1999 exchange rate of 7.807). Expenditures are mainly channelled through publicly-run institutions and services. Services for adults account for 85 percent of the total costs. The distribution of expenditures in 2003, were as follows: inpatient (80%); outpatient (14%); daypatient services (4%) and private practice (2%). For children and adolescents in 2003, 45 percent of expenditures are for inpatient services, 47 percent outpatient services, and 8 percent daypatient services.

Expenditures are financed through (a) general (block) grants[12] from the central government to the Regional Health Authorities (78%),(b) special government grants for mental health services (12%), (c) central government reimbursements for outpatient treatment (7%), and (d) other income (4%). A new financing system is under development, which is expected to be more related to diagnosis and patients actually treated.

---

10. The institution responsible for the three years education is called "Høgskole" in Norwegian. The equivalent in English is "University college." Students enrolling in the university college are about 18 years old, and the institution provides a three-year professional education for nurses, physiotherapists, social workers, physiotherapists, etc.

11. The average annual exchange rate for 1998 is 7.5521 NOK to one US$.

12. A system of financing in which a fixed amount (or a "bulk" amount) of money is set aside for each fiscal year, making up the "income framework," which the health enterprises are to follow while producing the services.

Table 3.6. *Mental Health Services 1990–2003. Key Figures.*

Services	1990	1995	2000	2003
Beds in psychiatric institutions All	8,011	6,667	6,091	5,633
Adults	7,745	6,384	5,781	5,296
Children and adolescents	266	283	310	337
Bed-days*	2,603	2,148	1,942	1,792
Discharges	21,242	26,113	34,969	42,295
Bed-days per discharge of patients	123	82	56	42
Outpatient consultations All*	396	611	696	982
Adults*	272	429	528	710
Children and adolescents*	124	181	169	272
Outpatient consultations per 1000 inhabitants	92	140	156	215

* Numbers are in thousands (e.g., 2,603 = 2,603,000).

For the projected eight-year period of the NMHP ending 2008, the increase in gross operating costs was stipulated at NOK 2.6 billion per year (US$ 326 million at the 2002 average annual exchange rate of 7.984). Within the first four years ending in 2002, the running costs per year increased by NOK 1.1 billion (US$ 138 million), or by about NOK 275 million (US$ 34 million) (based on the average annual exchange rate for 2002).

Primary Care, Municipalities Costs. The yearly average increase in costs for primary mental health care in the municipalities is estimated to 2.1 billion, or nearly NOK 500 per inhabitant.

Mental Health Services, Key Figures 2003. Table 3.6 gives key figures for the mental health services in the period 1990 to 2003.

The number of beds decreased by 30 percent from 1990 to 2003. In 2003, there were 123 beds per 100,000 inhabitants, or one bed per 809 Norwegians. Beds in institutions for adults decreased by 32 percent, while beds for C&A increased 27 percent, from 266 to 337. As a result of the reduction in total number of beds since 1990, the bed-days were also reduced, by 31 percent, to 1,792,000 in 2003. The average bed-days per 1,000 inhabitants 18+ years of age were 487 in 2003, varying between 375 in the North Health Region and 585 in the Western Health Region. In 2003, the bed-days for C&A were 89,600 for the whole country. The average bed-days per 1,000 inhabitants 0–17 years were 83 in 2003, varying between 50 in the North Health Region and 119 in the Western Region.

The Duration of Stay. The duration of stay is reduced considerably in recent years, especially in the psychiatric hospitals. In 2003, the average duration of stay was 42 overnight stays per discharge, compared to 56 overnight stays in 2000 and 123 in 1990. The number of patients discharged from all bed institutions was doubled to 42,295 (92 per 10,000) in 2003, compared to 21,242 (50 per 10,000) in 1990, in spite of a 30 percent reduction in beds. Today, more patients are admitted to mental health institutions than ever before, and they stay for a much shorter time. Reductions in the inpatient population have been accompanied by an increase in the number of inpatients stay.

More Outpatient Consultations and More Patients. A strong growth in *outpatient* consultations has also been evident in recent years. There was a 148 percent increase from 1990 to 2003. Almost one million outpatient consultations were provided in specialized psychiatric services in 2003, an increase of more than 17 percent from the year before. With an average of seven consultations per patient, 140,000 persons (about 3% of the total population) visited the outpatient clinics during 2003. The increase in consultations from 2002 to 2003 took place both in out-patient clinics for adults (15%) and in clinics for C&A (24%). Outpatient services for adults registered 91,000 more consultations, and services for C&A almost 53,000 more consultations in 2003 than in 2002. In 2003 there were 710,000 outpatient consultations for *adults*, correspondingly 215 consultations, or 30 outpatients per 1,000 inhabitants 18 years and over. The rates varied between 190 consultations/27 patients in the North Region to 228 consultations/33 patients in the South Region.

Table 3.7. *Use of Specialized Mental Health Services by Age Group*
Ratios per 10,000 Inhabitants in 2003

Type of mental health service	Children and adolescents (0–17 years)	Adults (18 years or older)	All services
Inpatient days	828	4,788	3,852
Discharges	17	115	92
Day-patient days	299	474	432
Outpatient consultations	2,797	2,031	2,212

Source: Mental health Services in Norway. Prevention –Treatment – Care" Norwegian Ministry of Health and Care Services, Oslo, 2005.

Totally, about 180,000 patients were treated and cared for in the specialized mental health services in 2003. The distribution on in- and out-patient services for C&A and for adults per 10,000 inhabitants is shown in Table 3.7.

In 2003, there were 3,852 inpatient days and 432 day-patient days per 10,000 inhabitants. In the population 17 years and younger the rate of inpatient days was only 828. The rates of outpatient consultations were higher for C&A (2,797) than for adults (2,031). The combined rate of discharges/admissions to the bed institutions was 92 per 10,000 inhabitants, much lower for C&A (17) than for adults (115). The figures illustrate that the services for C&A are concentrated on outpatient treatment and day services, while the adult services are still based heavily on bed institutions, even if there is an increasing amount of outpatient consultations as well, Table 3.6.

More Qualified Personnel. The number of qualified man-years (full-time equivalent employers) in the specialized services has risen in recent years to 18,293 in 2003. The term, "qualified personnel" refers to physicians, psychiatrists, psychologists and qualified nurses in psychiatric institutions. The professional qualifications of personnel have also risen considerably: Thirteen percent of all personnel had a university degree, and an additional 44 percent had a university college degree in 2003. In 2003, personnel by profession in adult mental health services were distributed as follows: Regional psychiatric nurses – 21 percent, other regional nurses – 14 percent, psychologists – 6 percent, psychiatrists – 4 percent, other physicians – 3 percent, other therapists with a college education – 9 percent, other health personnel – 26 percent, other personnel – 16 percent.

Recently, the number of so-called "psychotherapists" has increased in Norway. This is a title not protected by law. Consequently, anyone can call themselves "psychotherapist" without formal approval or regulation. Especially in the larger cities psychologists without a clinical specialty and people with a three-year education from a university college, for instance, a nurse or social worker, can open an unregulated private practice as a psychotherapist. The patients pay the total cost themselves to these private practicing psychotherapists.

Compulsory Admission, Legal Requirements. Until January 1, 2001, the legal basis for compulsory admissions in Norway was regulated by the 1961 *Mental Health Act (Lov om psykisk helsevern).* Two sections in the law regulated compulsory admissions (Hatling, Krogen and Ulleberg, 2002). According to the *Observational section* a person could be kept in custody in a psychiatric hospital for up to three weeks for observation to determine whether the person met the requirements for compulsory treatment. Patients who did not meet these criteria were to be discharged. It was not permitted to start compulsory treatment under this section.

According to the *Treatment section,* a person could be admitted involuntarily and treated if he/she had a "severe mental disorder" (not restricted to psychosis), and met at least one of the following additional criteria: (a) a danger to oneself or others (the danger criteria); (b) the prospects of cure or considerable improvement would be otherwise lost or forfeited (the treatment criteria); and (c) the individual suffers harm (subject to substantial physical or mental strain).

The first criterion was sharpened and the second one abandoned in the recent modification of the legislation in *The Mental Health Act* of January, 2001. Compulsory admissions are used only in psychiatric hospitals or psychiatric wards in general hospitals. Only the chief physician with a speciality in psychiatry, or a senior doctor to whom this authority is delegated, can make this decision. The decision requires a request for admission from either someone close to the patient, from public authorities, and from an initial assessment from a qualified provider outside the admitting institution, usually a GP or a psychologist, whose conclusion has to be a request for a section specific, compulsory admission (i.e., for either observation or treatment). After receiving the request, the chief physician makes the formal commitment decision within 24 hours.

Compulsory Admissions on a National Scale. Norway has a long tradition of extensive use of compulsory admissions. In 1994, 46.5 percent of the patients were involuntary admissions to the psychiatric hospitals and 64.2 percent to wards in general hospitals. In 1998, the percentages were 47.9 percent and 58.1 percent, respectively. In 1996, the rate of compulsory admissions was 147 per 100,000 inhabitants, 66 under the observational section and 81 under the treatment section. In 2002, approximately 40 percent of the patients were involuntary admitted to psychiatric wards and hospitals. Patients suffering from psychosis, (organic psychosis, schizophrenia, affective psychosis and other psychoses) were more likely to be admitted involuntarily (61%) than nonpsychotic patients (30%); however, the proportion of compulsory admissions among the latter group was also rather high. Of the 4,200 patients in psychiatric institutions November 20, 2003, 35 percent was compulsory admission. At the psychiatric hospitals 47 percent was admitted involuntarily (Hagen and Ruud, 2004).

The rates are higher than in most other countries. In Denmark for instance, the rate of compulsory admissions is less than 10 percent (Hatling, Krogen and Ulleberg, 2002). The legal regulations are the most important factor for explaining international differences. A substantial proportion of the involuntary admissions in Norway are based on criteria not permitting such admissions in other countries. The legality of the criteria according to European human rights conventions has been questioned.

Norway's Mental Health Delivery System

Mental Health Services 1950–2003

To understand why the delivery system is modelled or configured like it is today, it is necessary to recognize the recent development. The period 1950 to 2005 also tells what has been tried out in the near past, what has been successful, and what is changed or dismantled. The services in Norway have gone through the same stages as in most other Western countries: from high thresholds for being admitted as well as for being discharged, to more easy access to the services; from huge deinstitutionalization to community care; from long duration of stay, to very short; from custodial care to active treatment. New kinds of services, institutions and delivery systems have been established. Some still exists, some has vanished. The delivery system today is based on experiences from the last fifty years.

Patients and Capacity in Different Service Settings. The mental health services up to the 1950s consisted primarily of mental hospitals (asylums) and private care. The number of registered patients increased from about 1,000 at the turn of the century to about 6,000 in 1930. The majority (85%) stayed for a long time in psychiatric hospitals. After 1930 severely disordered patients were commonly placed in private care, mostly boarded in farms, paid for by the government, and supervised from the nearest asylum. The absolute number and relative distribution of patients in different service settings in the period 1950–2003 is illustrated in Figure 3.2 (see next page). The number of inhabitants has also changed during this period. Table 3.8 displays the number of patients per 10,000 inhabitants 18 years and older for each setting in the same period.

Number of Patients. In the *psychiatric institutions*, the average number of patients increased until the mid-1970s,

Table 3.8. *Patients in Norwegian Adult Psychiatric Institutions (per 10,000 Inhabitants) by Year and Service Settings.*

Service Setting	1950	1960	1970	1980	1990	2000	2003
Psychiatric hospitals	24.4	23.4	20.8	13.6	5.5	4.0	5.8*
Psychiatric wards in general hosp	0.8	1.7	2.9	1.9	1.7	2.1	–
Psych nursing homes, etc.	3.9	8.6	8.5	10.5	9.0	2.0	0.9
District Psychiatric Centre	–	–	–	–	–	2.9	3.2
All adult psychiatric institutions	29.1	33.8	32.2	26.0	16.2	11.0	9.9
Private care	22.7	16.1	10.1	4.2	1.5	0.4	na
In-patients and private care total	51.8	49.9	42.3	30.2	17.7	11.4	9.9

Note: All figures are based on average number of patients in the institution during the year.
* Psychiatric wards in general hospitals are included.

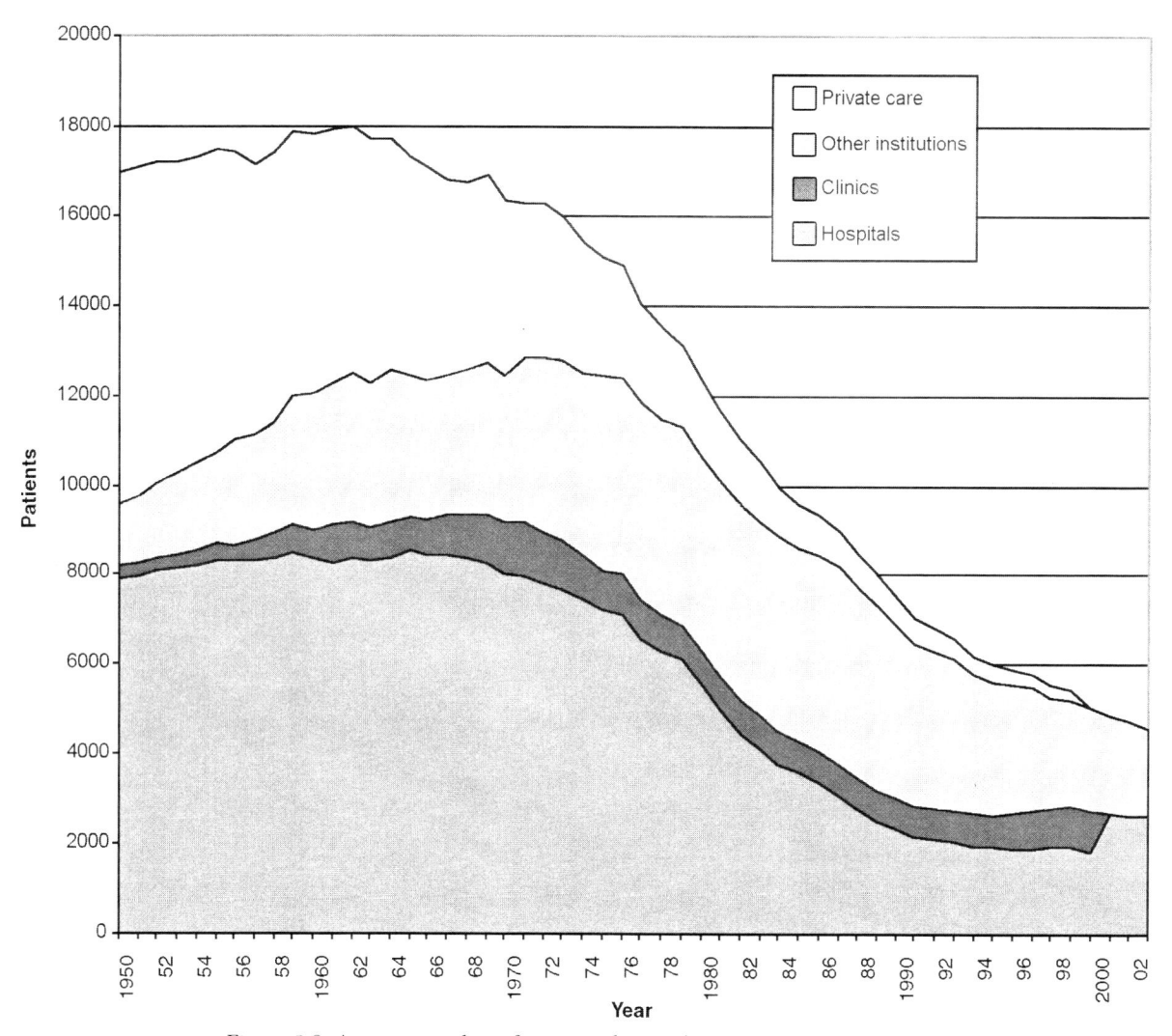

Figure 3.2. Average number of patients during the year in different settings.

but at a slower pace than the years prior to the 1960s. The inpatient population peaked in 1973, followed by a significant reduction from 1980 onwards, and it was halved between 1980 and 1995. In the mental hospitals only, it was reduced by almost two-thirds, in psychiatric nursing homes by one-third. In the decade from 1980 to 1990, the average number of institutionalized patients (including home care) was reduced by 4,800 patients (39%) from about 12,300 (30 per 10,000) to about 7,500 patients (18 per 10,000). There was a clear-cut deinstitutionalization of both hospital services and other institutionalized services during this period.[13] This decline was due mainly to a reduced capacity at the psychiatric hospitals. The number of inpatients at psychiatric hospitals peaked in the mid-60s. Since then the number of inpatients has been reduced by 5,704 (67%), from 8,515 (23 per 10,000) in 1965 to 1,811 patients (4 per 10,000) in 2000. Between 1970 and the 1990s, older patients who had stayed for a long time at the hospitals were discharged and the number of younger patients with shorter duration of stay increased. Hardly any hospitals

---

13. Studies of the process have often focused on the mental hospitals. De-hospitalization does not necessarily mean de-institutionalization. The process has often been one of trans-institutionalization (moving patients to other institutionalized settings) rather than de-institutionalization (moving patients to noninstitutionalized settings). Until 1975 de-hospitalization would be a more suitable concept than de-institutionalization for the situation in Norway as well.

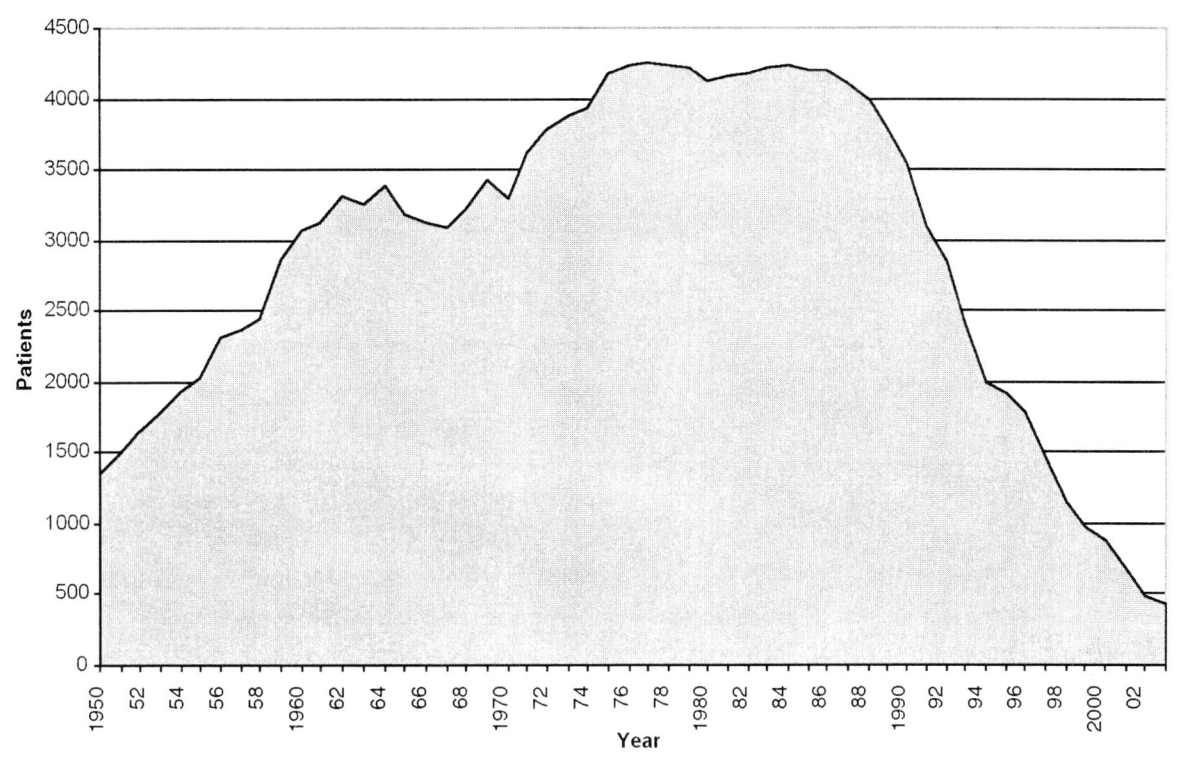

Figure 3.3. Average numbers of patients in psychiatric nursing homes in a year 1950–2003.

have been closed down; instead, they have been modernized to accommodate fewer patients. Most patients today stay in single rooms. The number of patients in psychiatric nursing homes, which constitute the major part of "other institutions," increased rapidly after 1950, Figure 3.2.

The "capacity" of the mental health services increased in the 1990s. More patients were admitted and treated than ever before, whereas the duration of stay was much shorter (Hagen and Ruud, 2004). Patients were treated outside the hospitals to a much greater extent. Services also became more "effective" and "productive," measured by the number of patients treated in a time span. Fewer patients than before had the hospital as their lifelong residence. Psychiatric hospitals and wards focused increasingly on short-term treatment. Nevertheless, low staffed custodial care dominated many wards in the mental hospitals.

Figure 3.2 and Table 3.8 indicate that the number of patients in private care declined gradually from more than 7,000 (22.7 per 10,000) in 1950 to less than 2,000 (4.2 per 10,000) in 1975, with further reduction the following years. From being a dominant caring option, with 44 percent of the patients in 1950, private care has nearly vanished.

Psychiatric Nursing Homes. A new kind of institution was introduced in the 1950s.[14] It was to play an important role in the mental health services in Norway the next 40 years. The "rise and fall" of psychiatric nursing homes illustrates the change in thinking about the services over the last fifty years and warrants comment. Psychiatric nursing homes were relatively small and low-staffed institutions built in large numbers between 1950 and 1975,[15] Table 3.8. The number peaked in the late 1970s, Figure 3.3. The explicit goal was to take care of so-called chronic patients discharged

---

14. Before 1955 there were also nursing homes taking care of disabled and elderly, but they did not exist solely for patients with mental disorders. The majority of the nursing homes before 1955 were run by humanitarian or religious organisations, but they were looked after by the public health services. From the beginning of 1950s nursing homes for *psychiatric patients* were established.
15. The inpatient population in psychiatric nursing homes increased with 86%, from 1,350 in 1950 to 4,189 in 1975.

from psychiatric hospitals and private care, or directly referred from the primary care sector. Overcrowded hospitals were a recurrent problem in Norway for many years and reached a climax at the end of the 1940s. Twenty-five percent more patients than beds was the norm in this period. Many patients stayed in the hospitals for their entire life. Psychiatric nursing homes were established to compensate for the pressure on the hospitals. The new institution was evaluated as the most suitable and adequate care facility for patients discharged from the hospitals as well as for other patients with severe or chronic disorders. Consequently, the psychiatric nursing homes came to be the last terminus for large groups of former hospital patients.

By the late 1980s there were more patients in psychiatric nursing homes than in psychiatric hospitals. Since 1984 the absolute number of patients has decreased, see Figure 3.3. However, the low-staffed custodial care continued to dominate mental health institutions, and as late as in 1989 the 117 nursing homes represented more than half of all inpatient days in the mental health services in Norway.

Gradually there were, however, fewer patients remaining in psychiatric hospitals and private care who required the kind of care that has traditionally been provided by psychiatric nursing homes. Hence, the psychiatric nursing homes have in one way fulfilled their original historical task, namely to take care of those who were said to need to stay for a long time in an institution, or those who were used to staying there after decades in a psychiatric hospital, most of the time without receiving any treatment except for medication. The psychiatric nursing homes took over the function of custodial care and provided no treatment. They were cheaper to run with a nursing staff generally lacking professionally trained therapists.

From the beginning of the 1980s some nursing homes were restructured as *Living and Treatment Centres* (*"Bo- and Behandlingssenter"* or *BOB* in Norwegian). Since the 1990s psychiatric nursing homes and BOBs were reorganized into *District Psychiatric Centres* (DPCs), established in order to meet the actual demand for more *active treatment* facilities. The number of beds in these new institutions was 313 in 1991 and increased to 1,463 in 2003, an increase of 367 percent. The number of beds in psychiatric nursing homes was reduced by 86 percent, from 3,096 to 430 in the same period. That also meant that the total number of beds in psychiatric institutions still decreased in the period from 1990 to 2003 by 19 percent, from 7,225 (17 per 10,000) to 5,828 (13 per 10,000).

The Reasons for Deinstitutionalization. The process of dehospitalization is partly a result of increased awareness of the patients' needs and desires. In the 1960s, a number of studies (Goffman, 1961; Løchen, 1965; Scheff, 1966) portrayed the hospitals as authoritarian, dehumanizing, and unresponsive to patients' needs. Surveys among inpatients also exposed that a majority preferred to stay in their own home and being supported by the mental health services (Øgar, 1981; Øgar, Kolstad and Kindseth, 1984; Hagen, 1992; Hagen, 1997; Hagen, 2001; Hagen and Ruud, 2004). November 1, 1999, 33 percent of the 5,084 inpatients preferred to be treated and cared for outside institutions and in their local community. They wanted to stay in their own home or in a sheltered accommodation (Hagen, 2001). The staff at the institutions also indicated that the ideal settings for many institutionalized patients would be in community care. In 1999, 24 percent of the inpatient population was expected to have a better offer in the community care. In 2003, 40 percent of the 4,200 inpatients would, according to the staff, be better off if treated and cared for in the community (Hagen, 2001; Hagen and Ruud, 2004).

There were other contributing factors to the dehospitalization as well: the pharmacological revolution, external economic factors (the fiscal crises of the welfare state), ideological changes within the professions, political-administrative structures and processes. The expensive mental hospitals became less attractive to the government as well as to patients.

In Norway the social security, the National Insurance Scheme, and the general welfare state system were major prerequisites for the process of deinstitutionalization. Disability pensions, old-age pensions, unemployment payments, public housing, and universal health insurance made it possible for people with mental disorders to be cared for in their own home. Patients and their relatives also wanted to have an impact on the type and location of the services. Consequently, it became more attractive to patients (and cheaper to decision-makers) to provide community-based services rather than hospital-based services (Pedersen, 1999).

The deinstitutionalization also represented a change in focus from long-term institutional care of the "chronically" ill to *immediate* and *active treatment* of many. The patients were to be *cared for* outside the institutions, in their local communities, and in their own home, and *treated actively* when occupying beds in institutions. This change in focus took place in Norway in the early 1980s; however, the living arrangements, care and treatment possibilities provided in the community were very limited until the end of the 1980s, and there continues to be severe shortcomings. The discharge of patients especially from the hospital, has been more effective than the establishing of both primary care and treatment facilities in the municipalities and decentralized specialized services with immediate access.

The Inpatient Population. Who are the patients in the mental health services in Norway? How many are treated, and what care and treatment do they receive? What would be an ideal offer to the patients according to their own preferences and according to the evaluation of the staff? These are some of the questions answered in surveys comprising all inpatients in Norway. Since 1979 the inpatient population has been surveyed on a particular day each fifth year (Øgar, 1981; Øgar, Kolstad and Kindseth, 1984; Hagen, 1992; Hagen, 1997; Hagen, 2001; Hagen and Ruud, 2004). A questionnaire has been filled in for each patient stating their age, sex, education, social class, duration of stay, diagnosis and information about referral, earlier and actual treatment.

On November 20, 2003, the inpatient population at the psychiatric institutions for adults was 4,200, (120 per 100,000 inhabitants +18). The number of patients in psychiatric hospitals and wards was 2,371; in DPCs 1,440, and in psychiatric nursing homes 389.

Sociodemographic Characteristics. In the 1970s and 1980s the inpatient prevalence rate was much higher in older adults than among the younger generations, due to the long stay. People settled for years and became old in the institutions. In the 1990s the prevalence of the inpatient did not vary with age. On November 1, 1999, the inpatient prevalence was 139 per 100,000 inhabitants in the age group 18–29 years, 136 in the age group 50–59, and 131 in 80 years or over. The mean age of the inpatients in *psychiatric hospitals* has been reduced from 56 years in 1984, to 44 years in 1994 and to 41 years in 2003 (Hagen and Ruud, 2004). The mean age is slightly higher in other institutions, especially on the remaining psychiatric nursing homes. During the first four years of the NMHP the percentage of patients below 50 years increased from 62 percent to 68 percent.

There has been for a long time slightly more women than men in the inpatient population. In 2003, 51 percent were women. The point prevalence for men and women was 119 and 121 per 100,000 respectively. Many female patients between 40 and 59 years visit the outpatient clinics and specialists in private practice.

Few patients admitted to psychiatric institutions in Norway have a regular job. In 2003, only 4 percent of the inpatient population worked for ordinary salary. Fifty percent was on disability pension, 23 percent on age pension or other pensions, and 9 percent on sick leave (Hagen and Ruud, 2004). The inpatient population also has less education and is less integrated in families and close social networks than the general population. Only 19 percent are married or cohabit, compared to 50 percent of the population 18+ (Hagen and Ruud, 2004).

Distribution of Diagnoses in the Inpatient Population. In the period between 1979 and 1989, 80 percent of the inpatient population was diagnosed with a psychosis. Nearly half of the patients were diagnosed with schizophrenia in the same period. Schizophrenia is still the dominating diagnosis for inpatients. In November 2003, 2000 patients (52 out of 100,000 inhabitants 18+) were institutionalized all day and night due to a diagnosis of schizophrenia. Affective psychoses and personality disorders have become relatively more frequent among the inpatients over the last 20 years. The number of patients with alcohol, substance and medication abuse, and patients diagnosed with neurotic disorders have increased since the 1990s. The distribution of diagnosis for the inpatient population on November 20, 2003 is displayed in Table 3.9.

The inpatient point prevalence for the main diagnoses for men and women respectively November 20, 2003 was: Schizophrenia: 64 and 41 per 100,000; Mood disorders: 21 and 33 per 100,000; Personality

Table 3.9. *The Distribution (Percents) of Diagnosis in Inpatient Psychiatric Institutions for Adults. November 20, 2003.*

Diagnosis	All institutions	Psychiatric hospitals
Schizophrenia	47	40
Mood disorders	24	28
Neurotic disorders	8	7
Personality disorders	7	7
Alcohol/substance abuse	5	6
Organic disorders	2	3
Other disorders	7	9
Total	100	100
N	4200	2371

Note: Source is Hagen and Ruud (2004).

disorders: 5 and 11 per 100,000. More men were diagnosed with schizophrenia and more women with mood disorders and personality disorders.

The most severe disorders are treated at the DPCs and at the psychiatric hospitals. At the hospitals only eight percent of the patients were diagnosed with neurosis in 1999 (Hagen, 2001). At the outpatient clinics 27 percent had this diagnosis. Among patients treated by private psychiatrists and psychologists, the percentages diagnosed with neurosis were 33 and 40 respectively. The private practitioners had four percent and two percent, respectively, treated for schizophrenia while at psychiatric hospitals, 45 percent had this diagnosis in 1999. At the DPCs the percentage with schizophrenia was 27 in 1999 (Hagen, 2001).

Referrals to the Psychiatric Institutions. On November 1, 1999, the majority (57%) of the patients in the psychiatric institutions were referred from another psychiatric institution, 28 percent from a general practitioner, and 15 percent from an out-patient clinic. The majority of the inpatient population (87%) had been admitted before. At the *psychiatric hospitals* approximately 20 percent of the inpatient population November, 2003 was admitted for the first time.

Psychotherapeutic Traditions and Treatment Ideology

An interesting issue in regard to clinical psychology in Norway is the strong position assigned to *psychoanalytic/psychodynamic theories* since early in the 20th century. At the University of Oslo researchers from different departments were interested in the same theories and problems as Freud. The first Norwegian professor in psychiatry, Ragnar-vogt who wrote a textbook in 1911, mentioned Freud's psychoanalysis (Alnæs, 1996). Freud's ideas and theories also became influential in art, literature and pedagogy in Norway at the end of 1920s. Psychoanalysis was a popular trend and Norwegian authors particularly were inspired by Freudian theory.

The most influential exponent and advocate for psychoanalysis in the 1920s was Harald Schjelderup, who became the first psychology professor in 1928 at the University of Oslo. He referred to the theories of Freud and other authors (Reich, Fenichel, Pfister, Abraham), and he wrote numerous articles on the subject.

Several people with a psychoanalytic education fled from the Nazi regime in Germany in the 1930s. In 1934, Wilhelm Reich migrated to Oslo on an invitation from Schjelderup. Norway was the only Nordic country where Reich obtained permission to work. He had a strong impact on several practicing psychotherapists and also in literary circles. His early method of *character analysis* has been inspiring in Norwegian body-oriented psychotherapy ever since. Nevertheless, a number of physicians expressed reservations about Reich's approach, preferring therapeutic methods and measures that they evaluated as more scientific (Alnæs, 1996). Moreover, when Reich developed his theory of so-called *orgon therapy*, most of his adherents became distant to him. The Norwegian public was also shocked by his practice, which seemed oriented towards sexuality in a dubious way.

Prior to World War II, the "talking cure" of Freud and elements of psychoanalytic theory and practice were only used to some extent in private practice and treatment with children, though not at all in the mental hospitals. The focus of inpatient mental health services in the period up to 1960 was long-term custodial care rather than psychotherapy. Somatic methods were predominant in mental hospitals, including insulin-coma treatment and electroconvulsive therapy. Lobotomy was also introduced and widely practiced by some of the leading psychiatrists at the mental hospitals. In the 1940s and 1950s, approximately 2,500 persons (8 per 10,000 inhabitants) were lobotomized in Norway (Tranøy and Blomberg, 2005). In the United States, approximately 40,000 persons were lobotomized (3 per 10,000 inhabitants). Lobotomies in Norway were usually performed in psychiatric hospitals rather than in the neurosurgical wards of general hospitals. Patient mortality was especially high in the early years: 18 of the first 35 lobotomies on women resulted in death (Tranøy, 1990; 1992). In 1996, the Parliament passed a temporary act of compensation that intended to offer the victims some restitution. This resolution came after a public debate following the publication of *Forfalskningen av lobotomiens historie på Gaustad sykehus* [The falsification of the history of lobotomy at Gaustad hospital] by the Department of Criminology, University of Oslo (Tranøy, 1990).

A biological view of psychiatric disorders was dominant in the mental health services until the end of the 1960s. According to this view, psychiatric disorders were considered as brain dysfunctions and abnormalities in neurotransmitters. Hjort (2000/2003) points out that the spirit of the times in the 1970s and 1980s seemed to be more influenced by theories accepting psychosocial factors, the same "zeitgeist" as in the whole western world. This psychosocial model stimulated the development of various psychotherapeutic remedies which developed and flourished in Norway more than in many other countries due significantly to payment for the psychotherapy by the welfare state.

Psychotherapy Approach. In a study of Norwegian psychotherapeutic ideologies during the period 1970–2000, Hjort (2000/2003) observed that psychoanalytic or psychodynamic therapy was the dominant orientation during the whole period for both psychiatrists and clinical psychologists. At the universities, the psychoanalytic approach is still a significant theme in theoretical lectures and practical clinical training. It has also stimulated intellectual and academic discussions in general. However, clinical psychologists have been much more eclectic than the psychodynamically-oriented psychiatrists. Psychologists have incorporated elements from the schools of thought that reached the Norwegian coasts in the beginning of the 1970s, such as behavioural, cognitive, systemic, gestalt, existential or other therapy orientations. Moreover, the influence of psychoanalytic theory diminished sharply among psychologists from the middle of the 1970s, partly because they could choose among a range of educational alternatives to become a clinical specialist. Psychiatrists, on the other hand, did not have such alternatives. Until the middle of the 1990s, psychiatrists' education depended on supervision by specialists in psychoanalysis. So, both professions seem to have chosen psychotherapy approaches that could certify them as specialists.

In the last decade, "a cognitive wind" has been blowing through mental health services, among both psychiatrists and psychologists. Cognitive and behavioral approaches based on quantitative, straightforward documentation appear to offer greater promise of cost-effective care to reduce psychiatric symptoms more rapidly than for example, psychodynamic and systemic approaches. The so-called evidence-based treatments appear therefore appealing to health authorities charged with controlling costs, (Ekeland, 1999).

In addition to the cognitive-behavioral trend, beginning in the 1990s, new biological approaches have been implemented, including psychotropic medications. Technological interventions like Electro Convulsive Shock Therapy (ECT) have also been reimplemented and are applied frequently in the hospitals. These approaches have been encouraged by promises of more cost-effective treatments. Attendant to the rise of both biological and cognitive-behavioral approaches is the risk that confidence in "talking cure" will wane due to pressures to provide efficient, evidence-based, "manualized" psychotherapy, with a context-less, "drug-metaphoric" theory of therapy (Ekeland, 1999; Lambert, 1992; Wampold, 2001).

Another trend today in Norwegian health services seems more promising and ethical for psychotherapeutic professions is the interest in focusing on the rights and participation of the *users* in treatment and research. A number of studies have shown that the *relation* between therapist and user is the most potent intratherapeutic factor (Hubble, Duncan and Miller, 1999; Wampold, 2001; Lambert, 1992). Several practitioners have started varied treatment projects in which user participation is central.

Mental Health Services in Primary Care

The mental health providers of primary mental health care are (a) general practitioners, (b) psychiatric nurses, (c) general nurses, (d) school psychologists, (e) school nurses, (f) municipality psychologists, (g) social workers, (h) family practitioners and (i) offices for family advice. However, all of these services are not available in the smaller municipalities.

The General Practitioner. Patients contact their personal General Practitioner frequently because of mental health problems. The GPs often become the patient's first contact with the mental health services. They refer the majority of the patients treated in the specialist mental health services and also subscribe most of the medication for minor psychiatric disorders like anxiety and depression. The GPs therefore have an important role to play in the chain of services. The GPs are however, not very well integrated in the mental health system for the time being, and they are hardly mentioned in the National Mental Health Programme. It is expected that the health authorities will make efforts to improve the coordination between the GPs and the mental health services in the future.

Child and Adolescent Services. Most municipalities have their *"Office for counselling in school psychology and pedagogy"* serviced by "school psychologists." The office cooperates with primary health and social services as well as offices for family support. In 2003, approximately 400 psychologists were employed by the municipalities working in the education system and in the health services. The majority was employed as "school psychologists," dealing with learning difficulties. School psychologists assess, test, and counsel students with learning difficulties as well as psychological problems and deviant behaviour occurring in the school situation, and also refer students to the specialized mental health services.

Adult Mental Health Services: Municipality Psychologists. Some few municipalities have employed a "community" or "municipality" psychologist as a generalist, and to serve as a liaison between the specialized services and the primary care in the municipality. They use their time for psychotherapy (about 45% of their time), for consultation (15%), and administration (15%). Other tasks are planning and lecturing (Christiansen, Iversen, and Stephansen, 1983). The community psychologists are also intended to participate when discharged patients are integrated into the local community, and to teach and train relatives in taking care of mental health patients. The municipal psychologists are expected to work more on the system level and with the social networks to advocate for patients, and to do primary prevention work, rather than providing traditional individual psychotherapy. Nevertheless, few municipalities have established a position for community psychologists in recent years, due partly to the lack of clinical psychologists in the specialized services, and because most psychologists prefer to provide psychotherapy full time rather than providing prevention, supervision, case management and after-care.

Specialized Mental Health Services

For all Ages. People who are in need of assessment or treatment for psychiatric disorders are referred (often by their GP), either to a private practitioner, a *District Psychiatric Centre* (DPC), a psychiatric hospital, or a psychiatric ward in a general hospital. The DPCs have a few beds, a day-centre and an outpatient clinic. From 2006 all DPCs are expected to have established an assertive outreach team. It is a policy that the services are external and based on outreach work. Some patients use only the day-center, or visit the outpatient clinic; others stay for a shorter time as inpatients. They often maintain contact with the DPC after being discharged from the inpatient unit.

Other patients are referred to the more specialized psychiatric hospitals or wards in general hospitals for examination and treatment. The hospitals/wards cooperate with the DPCs when patients are discharged and return to their local communities. Patients also can remain in contact with the more specialized services in the hospitals through the DPCs. After-care is often provided by the DPCs in cooperation with primary health care providers in the municipalities. The Individual Plan (see p. 128) is an important tool for improved coordination between settings, especially between primary care and specialized services.

Private Practitioners. The specialized services at DPCs and at hospitals are supplemented by specialists in psychiatry and clinical psychology conducting a "private" practice. Some of them have entered into contracts called an *operative agreement* with the Regional Health Authorities. Particularly in the larger cities the number of private practitioners with an agreement has increased recently.[16] An agreement implies an obligation to participate in the mental health services. The sources of income for the specialists with agreements are (a) national insurance reimbursements, (b) patient co-payments (see p. 123 for the out-of-pocket payment for households visiting the private practitioners), and (c) a fixed amount (operating grant) from the regional health authorities/enterprises.

A practitioner with an operative agreement is analogous to a "participating provider" in the U.S. mental health system under governmental Medicare and Medicaid. Patients pay less out-of-pocket to providers with an operative agreement. Specialists lacking an agreement may, with certain limitations, take as high a co-payment as the patient is willing to pay. Since people prefer to pay less, the waiting lists for specialists *with* an agreement is longer than for those without an agreement. The most experienced therapists with longer seniority have agreements more often than the younger and newly educated ones. In principle, however, the quality of treatment offered by practitioners with or without agreements is the same.

The number of private practitioners has increased steadily since the 1970s. In 2003, 293 private psychiatrists (3.7 per 100,000) had operating agreements with the health enterprises.[17] Nearly twice as many, 570 psychologists, (8.9 per 100,000) had an agree-

---

16. There is also an increasing number of specialists practising without agreements. Some of them are approved clinical psychologists or psychiatrists, others call themselves "psychotherapists" a title not protected by law. The "psychotherapists" often have three years of education from a university college, or they are psychologists without a speciality in clinical psychology.

17. http://www.ssb.no/english/subjects/03/02/speshelsefydrift_en/

ment. The number of operative agreements with clinical psychologists continues to grow moderately, while the numbers has stabilized for psychiatrists in recent years.

Education and approval of psychologists. The number of clinical psychologists in Norway has boosted over the last 40 years due to the increase in demand for treatment. The Government has given priority to establishing schools of Clinical Psychology at all four universities, in Oslo, Bergen, Tromsø and Trondheim. Approximately 220 students begin training every year to become approved (licensed) psychologists, and more than 90 percent finish their professional education in about six years at the universities. The majority specialize in clinical psychology. Until the mid-1970s everyone could call themselves a "psychologist." Under a 1973 law, the title of "psychologist" became restricted to approved (licensed) psychologists. To be approved it is necessary to prove one has obtained both a specific theoretical education and supervised practical training.

By January 1, 2004, there were 4,459 psychologists licensed in Norway, or 98 per 100,000 inhabitants. Clinical psychologists dominate in number. Most of them are working in the health services sector. Including private practitioners (about 20% of the clinical psychologists), approximately 2,800 psychologists worked in mental health services (primary and specialized care); equivalent to approximately 62 clinical psychologists per 100,000 inhabitants, or about one clinical psychologist per 1,625 inhabitants. Comparable figures for psychiatrists are 713 psychiatrists, 15 per 100,000, or one per 6,400 inhabitants.

Specialized Mental Health Services for Children and Adolescents. At the beginning of the 1960s, an increased demand for mental health services for C&A was identified. Each county was expected to establish at least one outpatient clinic. C&A services developed separately from adult services.[18] Another way of understanding disorders and behaviour problems among youth was developed among the mental health professionals working in the C&A services. The cause of illness was not to be sought primarily in the body or the brain, but rather outside, in the individual's environment. This brought multiprofessional teamwork into the C&A services and opened up the field of treatment to professions other than medical. Psychologists have dominated this segment in Norway more than in mental health services for adults (Seip, 2004). The professional qualifications of personnel in these services are generally high. Twenty-seven percent have a university degree, most of them are psychologists and an additional 53 percent have a university college degree.

Outpatient treatment is the norm for C&A. As much as 95 percent of all mental health care for C&A is delivered in outpatient settings. At the end of 2003, the number of beds in C&A institutions was 336 (2.8 per 10,000 inhabitants 18 years and below). The number of beds for C&A has traditionally been low, and has barely increased in recent years.

Personnel Providing Specialized Health Services

As noted in Table 3.10, the number of providers in the specialized health services (somatic and mental health services combined) was 87,897 man-years (193 per 10,000) in 2003.

The man-years of psychologists in the specialized *health services* were 2,134 (50 per 100,000), (a 100% increase since 1995) in 2003. Of these 1,937 man-years (42 per 100,000) were employed in the specialized *mental health services*. (Private practitioners without an operative agreement are not included in these figures.)

The total number qualified man-years in specialized *mental health services* increased from 14,469 in

Table 3.10. *Qualified Providers in the Specialist Health Service Key Figures for Personnel in Man-Years 1990–2003.*

Providers (man-years)	1990	1995	2003
All	63,062	67,098	87,897
Physicians	5,680	6,700	9,690
Psychologists	766	1,074	2,134
Nurses and midwives	19,237	23,996	30,115
Auxiliary nursing personnel	10,327	9,107	8,142
Other therapists	8,049	8,645	15,842
Administration and service	19,002	18,890	21,974

Note: "Man-years" is the number of full-time employees and part-time employees (converted to full-time employees), at the end of the year.

---

18. The C&A services is called *"BUP"* in Norwegian, and abbreviation for "Children and youth mental health services." It refers particularly to outpatient clinics.

Table 3.11. *Mental Health Services. Key Figures in Man-Years 1990–2003.*

Qualified personnel (man-years)	1990	1995	2000	2003
Psychiatric institutions (All)	14,469	14,806	16,554	18,293
Psychiatric institutions (Adults)	12,980	13,010	14,147	15,325
Psychiatric institutions (C&A)	1,490	1,796	2,407	2,968
Physicians, psychiatrists	741	886	1,141	1,292
Psychologists	606	834	1,182	1,525
Qualified nurses	3,309	3,857	4,660	5,316

Note: "Man-years" is the number of full-time employees and part-time employees (converted to full-time employees) at the end of the year. Overtime is not included.

1990 to 18,293 (40 per 10,000) in 2003 (Table 3.11). The growth in the number of qualified providers[19] has been particularly strong for psychologists in recent years.

The man-years of psychiatrists and other medical doctors in the specialized mental health services have increased by 551 (74%) from 1990 to 2003, when it reached 1,292 man-years (28 per 100,000). The man-years of psychologists have increased by 916 (151%) to 1,525 (33 per 100,000) in the same period.

Today, there are more psychologists than psychiatrists employed in both adult mental health services and in the services for children and adolescents. There are about 8,400 qualified nurses (5,316 man-years) with three years education from a university college and 7,000 other treatment personnel. Man-years in psychiatric institutions and wards for *adults* were 15,325 in 2003. The man-years in services for adults were 4.4 per 1,000 inhabitants in 2003, varying from 3.8 in the South health region to 4.7 in the Eastern health region. Man-years in mental health services for C&A were 2,968 in 2003, or 2.7 per 1,000 inhabitants, varying from 2.3 in the West and Mid regions to 3.3 in the Eastern region.

Administrative Personnel in the Mental Health System. In the specialist health services (both somatic and psychiatric) there were 21,974 man-years (48 per 10,000) in administration and service in 2003 (Table 3.10). Man-years had increased by about 3,000 (16%) from 1995. The total number of man-years in the *specialist mental health institutions* in 2003 was 18,293 (Table 3.11). Of these, 3,009 (16%) were "other personnel," that is, not providing therapeutic services. Most of them were administrative and service personnel. This number had decreased from 3,546 in 1990, due to the deinstitutionalization. In *psychiatric hospitals, clinics for adults*, and *psychiatric wards in general hospital*, the "other personnel" category represented 1,612 man-years in 2000, 1,740 in 1995, and 2,245 in 1990, a reduction of 28% in ten years. The man-years for administration and service in all psychiatric institutions for adults and C&A separately are displayed in Table 3.12.

Adults. The number of man years in institutions for adults were 15,329 in 2003. Of these 1,325 (9%) were personnel in administration and office, and 1,196 (8%) were personnel in service, technical, and/or operating functions.

Children and Adolescents. The number of man-years in mental institutions for C&A was 2,968 in 2003. Of these 365 (12%) were personnel in administration and office, and 123 (4%) were personnel in service, technical, and/or operating functions. The increase from 2000 to 2003 is due to higher activity and more patients treated.

Financing Strategies

The policies and programs for mental health services in Norway are publicly funded and administered by the public, that is, by the Government, health authorities, and the municipalities. Financing is stipulated in detail in national policy and legislation, and administered by the central health authorities, namely The Ministry of Health, and The Directorate

---

19. "Qualified personnel" includes physicians, psychiatrists, psychologists, qualified nurses and other professions with at least three years education from a college university. They are licensed by the Ministry of Health to treat medically and/or mentally ill patients.

Table 3.12. *Man-Years in Psychiatric Institutions for Adults and C&A by Category of Personnel.*

Category of personnel	Adults 2000	Adults 2003	C&A 2000	C&A 2003
All Personnel	14,147	15,325	2,407	2,968
Administration and office	1,192	1,325	283	365
Service-, technical- and/or operating functions	1,283	1,196	112	123

Note: "Man-years" are full-time employees plus part-time employees (converted into full-time employees) at 31 December.

of Health and Social Welfare.[20] The distribution of block grants, reimbursements and out-of-the pocket fees is decided by the Government and approved by the Parliament. The Ministry of Health, the Directorate of Health, and the Regional Health Enterprises determine the rates of reimbursement for mental health services.

Public Sector Financing Mechanisms. Services are financed mainly through government block grants, special government reimbursements and earmarked grants, national insurance, plus fees. Block grants are supplemented with itemized allocations – earmarked funds to priority problems or fields. These are intended to stimulate the local health service to adopt such priorities, including top financing of the running costs of hospitals, mental health services, cancer treatment and hospital equipment.

The financing system in Norway is not an insurance-based system. Only a small amount of the expenses is covered by the National Insurance Scheme or by private/voluntary insurances. The public health services are financed in the same way as other State activities, by revenues for instance, from the oil production, taxation on income, and VAT. Most providers serve as paid employees of the government-financed system. User fees, or out-of-the pocket money, play a marginal role. Private/voluntary insurance also plays a very limited role for mental health care. All mental health services are therefore in principle public services financed primarily by the Government and the municipalities.

---

20. The Directorate of Health and Social Welfare is a professional body which has legal authority within this field. The Directorate also contributes to the implementation of national health- and social policy, and it serves as an advisory board to central authorities, municipalities, Regional Health Authorities, and voluntary organizations. In the following "Directorate of Health" is used as an abbreviation.

The municipalities are responsible for providing *primary health care* and social services, including primary mental health services. These services are financed in the same way as other expenditures, through local income taxes, government block grants, special government reimbursement grants, and fees.

Expenditures in the *specialized services* are financed mainly through general (block) grants from the central government to the Regional Health Authorities (RHAs) (78%), special government grants for mental health services (12%), central government reimbursements for outpatient treatment (7%), and through other income (4%). A new financing system is under development, which places more emphasis on the activity and the number of patients treated.

The earmarked grant in 2003 for strengthening the mental health services was NOK 1.2 billion (US$ 169 million at the 2003 exchange rate of 7.080), which is two percent of the aggregate grants to the RHA.

Financing of the NMHP. According to national legislation, the National Mental Health Programme is financed mainly by earmarked grants distributed according to some objective criteria. The RHAs are not expected to change the priorities of their resources to finance the NMHP. The Programme should, according to the original plan, be financed entirely by the supply of "new money." However, the health enterprises in recent years been told by the Ministry of Health and Directorate of Health to increase the expenditures to the mental health services more than the earmarked grants for NMHP.

National Insurance Scheme. By law, all persons who are either resident or working as employees in Norway are insured under the National Insurance Scheme. All insured persons are entitled to cash benefits in case of sickness and are granted free accommodation and treatment, including free medications in hospitals. This follows from the provisions of the *Act on*

Specialist Health Care and the *Act on Mental Health Care*. In the case of treatment given outside hospitals, the provisions of the *Act on Municipal Health Care* and the *National Insurance Act* apply. Consequently, all are entitled to old-age and disability pensions, cash benefits in case of sickness and unemployment, and medical[21] benefits in case of sickness.

Predominant Cost Containment Mechanisms. Centralized planning and public control are a key terms also when dealing with cost containment. The government is the owner and operates the health enterprises through the five Regional Health Authorities (RHAs). The government allocates funds as block grants to each RHA, based primarily on the number of inhabitants in the region. The Ministry of Health and the Directorate of Health are following the activity carefully and compare the costs and activity for different enterprises and regions.

There is no utilization of review procedures employed to contain costs by requiring prior and/or continual authorization by a third-party payer or management procedures directed at providing cost-effective care. There are not established procedures implemented by people other than the professional who provides the service and the public authorities responsible. The Government and the Ministry of Health execute control by allocation of grants every year and the Directorate of Health follows the activity, quality and efficiency carefully throughout the year by, for instance, regular meetings with the boards of the RHAs. At the moment the focus of the cost-containment strategy is on price and efficiency, rather than limiting the volume of services provided.

The Health Enterprises are introducing some *market mechanisms* based on supply and demand. For instance, users are granted free choice of hospitals and other specialist services. The patient can choose to be treated at a hospital outside the region of residence. This is not expected to influence the financing or costs as much as the quality of the treatment and care and the allocation of the total resources. The Health Enterprises are encouraged to compete on quality and efficacy as well as efficiency and productivity. Competition is expected to have impact on the expenses in the long run. There is no empirical evidence for this postulate and a public system as the one in Norway is running the services efficiently and with high quality.

Increased productivity is a concern for the present government and politicians in general, also related to the mental health services, and especially the outpatient clinics. It is expected that the cost per unit can be reduced by increasing the efficiency of service delivery. In this way more patients can be treated. The main strategy at the moment is not to cut the total costs in the mental health sector, but to cut the cost per patient and in this way increase the capacity of services available and if necessary to increase the total funding to the mental health services due to the increased demand.

There are no incentives or regulations for patients to contain cost, except for their small out-of-pocket payment. The fee the patients pay themselves is marginal compared with the total cost, and is not either intended or justified as a contribution to cost containment.

PART TWO: EVALUATION OF NORWAY'S MENTAL HEALTH SYSTEM

Introduction

Prior to addressing the evaluation criteria selected for this comparative study, an overview is provided here based on the attainment of goals specified in *Norway's National Mental Health Programme (NMHP)*.

A major effort has been made in Norway to replace the traditional institutionalized psychiatric services by new and more differentiated health and social services for people with weakened mental health. The intention has been to reduce the former dominance of the psychiatric hospitals and other bed-institutions, and also to develop another care ideology or philosophy focusing on community treatment and more active treatment in smaller institutions. Consequently, *primary mental health care* facilities like sheltered accommodation in the community, and *specialized services* like outpatient clinics and *District Psychiatric Centres (DPCs)* have been given priority. A network, or a *chain* of services, composed of community health centres, daycare facilities, sheltered accommodations, short- and long-stay residences, vocational training programs, DPCs and psychiatric wards in general hospitals were intended to coordinate care and to

---

21. Total expenses of the National Insurance Scheme in 2002 were NOK 192,490 million (US$ 24,109 million, or about 24 billion dollars at the 2002 exchange rate of 7.984). The amount represents approximately 34.2% of the combined State and National Insurance budgets and 12.6% of the Gross Domestic Product. In 2002, the state grants to the National Insurance Scheme were NOK 53,391 million (US$ 6,687 million, or about 6.7 billion dollars), equal to 27.7% of the National Insurance Scheme's total expenses.

reduce the shortcomings of the traditional psychiatric hospitals and the psychiatric nursing homes giving custody but no treatment.

Prior to the 1970s, many patients with chronic and severe mental disorders stayed in psychiatric hospitals and nursing homes for most of their life. They were hidden in closed institutions. To have a psychiatric disorder was a disgrace for oneself and one's family. A veil of shame resulted in many patients suffering in silence. People did not want to admit that they were in need of mental treatment or care.

The situation is different today. Now people talk about mental disorders more freely, and some even boast about being a patient in the mental health services. The former Prime Minister of Norway, Kjell Magne Bondevik, other members of his cabinet, the vice president of the Parliament, sports heroes, popular artists and businessmen – all talk openly about their need for, and experience with treatment in the mental health services. To become a patient because of reduced mental health, psychological distress, a "depressive reaction," being "burned-out" or anxious has become something very natural and normal, almost a sort of fashion and totally different from 20 years ago. This acceptance of being treated by mental health services for life crises and (minor) disorders explains to some extent the dramatic increase in demand for mental health services. Severe disorders like schizophrenia and bipolar depression have not become more prevalent.

In addition to the reduced stigma concerning the milder disorders and distress, the increased availability of services has contributed to the increased demand. By establishing treatment and care facilities in the neighborhood without fences or walls, and by welcoming everybody with "problems," in crisis, or with a reduced "life quality," a huge proportion of the population have accepted to seek help.

Norway's National Mental Health Programme (1999–2008)

The mental health services in Norway are better adapted to the patients' demands and to professionals' recommendations than 20 years ago. But there are still serious shortcomings if 15 percent to 20 percent of the population are potential patients. The services for the severely disordered have not been developed to the same degree as decentralized settings for general treatment and care. Services remain fragmented. Overlapping services and significant gaps in coverage remain. The chains of the community care system have many weak and even missing links. There is still a substantial lack of facilities outside the psychiatric institutions: after-care facilities, sheltered accommodation, rehabilitation units and daycentres. The optimal mode of cooperation and the division of tasks between the service settings, especially between community settings and inpatient units have not been established satisfactorily. The "treatment gap" between those who are said to be in need and those who are actually treated has never been larger, although the number of patients treated throughout a year has nearly tripled the last ten years (see Table 3.6).

There is a shortage of hospital beds due first and foremost to the shortcomings in the community services. Psychiatric institutions therefore retain their patients longer than the patients themselves prefer and the staff believes is ideal. As a result, there are too few beds, especially in the acute wards. And some patients are still in institutions without being treated. The psychiatric nursing homes have taken over the task of the old mental hospitals: custodial care without active treatment. This institutional care will, however, disappear in a few years.

Every country which has discharged massive numbers of patients from psychiatric institutions has experienced the same problems of establishing alternative and adequate services outside the hospitals. In Norway, the *National Mental Health Programme (NMHP)* was designed to deal with this task, and the services have improved since the *Programme* commenced in 1999. Nevertheless, there is still a long way to go to establish the services in accordance with patients' demands and unique needs, and to implement practices supported by experiences and knowledge. Also lacking is a consensus on a coherent and comprehensive rationale or ideology for the new kind of all-embracing community services.

The NMHP was predicated upon a Governmental *White Paper* written between 1996 and 1997 (*Sosial- og helsedepartementet*, 1997). In the *White Paper*, the mental health services were characterized in this way: "Patients do not feel they get what they need; the staff does not feel they do a good job, and the authorities are not able to give the population satisfactory services." The *White Paper* further concluded: (a) primary prevention is too weak; (b) in many municipalities and communities the patients do not get what they deserve; (c) there are too few beds in security wards and in psychiatric hospitals; (d) the admission thresholds for the patients are too high, making it difficult to be admitted; (e) the time span from the first symptoms of a disorder to initiated treatment is too long;

(f) too many patients are discharged from the hospital too early; (g) the discharge of patients is not properly planned; (h) the aftercare or follow-up after being discharged do not function properly.

The NMHP Goals. Based on this critical evaluation, the NMHP stated ten national goals for the adult services and four goals for the services for children and adolescents for the Programme period (Hagen, 2003).

Goals for the Adult Services

1. Increase man-years (full-time equivalent providers) by 2,300 during the 10-year period ending 2008;
2. Educate more medical doctors, psychiatrists, psychologists and other personnel with at least 3 years of professional education;
3. Increase the number of staff at the District Psychiatric Centres (DPCs);
4. Increase by 50% private practicing psychiatrists and psychologists with "operative agreements" (i.e., contracts to provide services covered by the national health insurance);
5. Reduce compulsory admissions and the use of coercive treatment, and improve quality assurance of both when implemented;
6. Maintain the number of beds in the hospitals at the 1996 level, and make available 160 new beds for people who are sentenced to treatment in the mental health services;
7. Increase the number of DPCs to provide 1,025 new places for active treatment compared to the level in 1996, and reduce the number of beds in psychiatric nursing homes accordingly;
8. Increase the total capacity at the outpatient clinics by 220,000 consultations (a 50% increase from 1996);
9. Increase by 50% productivity of outpatient clinics for adults;
10. Increase the number of day-stays at the DPCs by 90,000 (a 50% increase from 1996).

Goals for the Children and Adolescent Services

1. Add 205 more places (beds) for adolescents and change treatment homes into clinics with more active treatment regimens;
2. Educate and place 400 more professionals for outpatient treatment;
3. Increase by 50% the productivity of outpatients clinics;
4. Increase the system's capacity to provide treatment for 5% of the population up to 18 years of age.

Evaluation of Goal Attainment. An evaluation in 2002 of the NMHP goals revealed that some of the goals were achieved, and that mental health services were developed in the direction prescribed by the *Programme*. Hagen (2003) reported that in 2002:

1. 1,404 more man-years in the services has been achieved, an average of 350 per year, exceeding the goal for the first five years.
2. During the period 1998 to 2002, the personnel with university or college education has increased by 37%, while the personnel without college education has decreased by 108 (2%). The number of psychologists has increased by 259 (42%) to 874 in 2002, medical doctors/psychiatrists increased by 124 (14%) to 995, and nurses and other college educated treatment personnel increased by 1,130 (21%) to 5,316. Mental health personnel have more education and a better formal education than previously.
3. In 1998, there were 2,763 man-years (full-time equivalent personnel) in the DPCs, or 1.9 man-years per bed. In 2002, there were 6,682 man-years at the centres, or 2.5 man-years per bed. Man-years for personnel with university or college education have increased more than other personnel.
4. In 1997, the number of psychiatrists and psychologists with an operational agreement was 56 and 98 respectively. In 2002, the numbers have increased to 163 and 403 respectively. Goal attainment exceeded the targeted 50% increase.
5. Compulsory admissions to hospitals and the use of coercive treatments have stabilized. About 40% are involuntary admissions, a significant decrease from 1997. These numbers were unchanged from 2001 to 2002; however, the differences among hospitals on this objective are considerable. Also the use of mechanical coercive means (e.g., straight jackets) varies considerably among hospitals.
6. In 1996, there were 2,940 beds for involuntary adult admissions in mental health hospitals. The number increased to 2,984 in 2002. There were still too few beds for patients sentenced to receive mental health treatment.
7. The establishment of the DPCs is the most comprehensive innovation. In 2002, 64 of the planned 83 DPCs were established. Not all are fully staffed, and only 29 DPCs are finished. The remainder needs to be rebuilt, renovated or developed with new functions or more personnel. The number of beds available in the DPCs is projected to be 2,040 in 2008. From 1996 to 2002 the number of beds increased by 831 to 1,845. According to existing plans there will be an additional 620 beds at the DPCs before 2008. The DPCs are either in new buildings or in older institutions like psychiatric nursing homes. The number of beds in nursing homes has been reduced considerably recently, in accordance with the *Programme*. Between 1996 and 2002 the number was reduced by 74% from 2,058 to 544,

and it is estimated that these institutions will disappear before 2008.

8. From 1996 to 2002, the number of outpatient *consultations* increased by 177,000 (40%). This is 80% of the increase planned for the whole period from 1996 to 2008. The goal is expected to be attained by 2004. The average number of outpatient sessions received by clients was seven consultations, and the number of *patients* treated at the out-patient clinics increased 40% from 63,000 in 1998 to 88,000 in 2002.

9. The increase in the number of consultations and patients at outpatient clinics is a result of more man-years. The productivity, measured by number of consultations per man-years per day at work, has not increased as intended. The productivity was stable the first three years of the period, and decreased in 2001 from 1.67 to 1.54. Instead of an assumed and planned 50% increase, productivity has decreased by 10%. The treatment staff increased by 43% in the period 1998 to 2002, and the number of consultations increased by 29%. The productivity in outpatient clinics for adults is about double the productivity in the clinics for C&A. Much time is used on other tasks than direct patient treatment, such as coordination with bed units and hospitals and cooperation and advice to the primary health services in the municipalities for both adult and C&A.

10. To date, reliable numbers for the day service activity do not exist.

11. The goal of increasing the number of beds in institutions for C&A has not been achieved. The net number has increased by only 16 beds (5%) from 296 in 1996 to 312 in 2002. The planned increase for the period 1996 to 2008 was 205 beds. The variations among health regions are considerable, from 2.0 beds per 10,000 inhabitants below 18 years in the South region, to 4.2 in the East region. As a result of changed models for treating C&A, the planned number of beds in 2008 is not looked upon as relevant any longer. The Regional Health Authority will evaluate number of beds in relation to capacity of the outpatient clinics and other up-to-date facilities.

12. The number of full-time equivalent personnel (man-years) in outpatient clinics for C&A has increased by 434 (60%) from 1996 to 2002, exceeding the goal. Man-years for psychologists increased by 164 (62%), psychiatrists and medical doctors increased by 52 (50%).

13. The indicator for productivity in the outpatient clinics for C&A is the number of "work units" per man-year per day. A work unit is, for example, a consultation, a meeting, supervision provided to the primary care, etc. In 1998, the productivity was 1.12; in 2002 it had increased by 26% to 1.41.

14. In 2002, 31,000 C&A were treated in the mental health services. Of those treated, 29,000 (93%) received outpatient treatment. Since 1998 the number of C&A patients increased by 10,000 (51%). The percentage of the population 18 years and below who received mental health treatment increased from 2.0 in 1998 to 2.9 in 2002. Even with the increased productivity of C&A services, it does not seem realistic that the goal of providing treatment to five percent of the C&A population will be achieved by 2008.

Four years into the implementation of the Mental Health Programme, important improvements in services have been achieved. More people seek treatment, and more people get the help they ask for. The capacity of the services has increased. Decentralized services are being developed and services have become more readily available. There has been a growth in qualified, employed personnel devoted to the mental health services, and the running expenses have increased.

Still, services are lacking in several respects. Community-based services provided by the municipality are not sufficiently developed to meet requirements. Cooperation between services and coordination of services on the individual level are also lacking in several respects. As a result, the pressure on specialized services, especially acute services, becomes unnecessary high, leading to waiting and to misplacement of patients in institutions. Despite the development of community-based services and a policy of deinstitutionalisation, 80 percent of the resources in specialised services for adults are still spent on inpatient treatment, in many cases providing services to patients primarily in need of community-based services. To meet this challenge, the government is reconsidering the distribution of resources between hospitals, DPCs and services provided by the local councils (municipalities), and will propose further expansion of the community-based services, including supported or sheltered housing. During 2005 and 2006 ambulatory teams will also be organised at all DPCs.

More Places for Long-Term Patients Are Needed. There is great pressure on acute wards in the psychiatric hospitals, and there continues to be a problem transferring patients into intermediate and long-term units, and to services outside the hospitals. Consequently, some patients stay in the acute wards too long. Several patients in the acute wards are in need of mental health services for a long period: 80 percent are expected to need care at least five years ahead, and 30 percent are in need of 24-hour support over many years. There is a need for more space in the intermediate wards and long-term services in and outside the hospitals, especially in the communities (Husby, Østberg and Hartvig, 2003).

Not all service providers have adapted to the challenges raised by the user perspective on services. Cooperation with users and relatives on an equal basis has still to be considerably improved.

A further evaluation of Norway's mental health system is provided below according to the criteria adopted for this book: Access and equity, quality and efficacy, cost and efficiency, financing and fairness, protection and participation, population relevance, and other optional criteria.

Access and Equity

This section begins with discussion of the "treatment gap," followed by discussion of problems in access by severity of mental disorders, by age (the elderly), and by the immigrant population. Thereafter, we discuss the problems of inpatient readmissions, delayed access, comments on demand and supply, and regional variations in access.

The Treatment Gap

There is a great "gap" between the number of patients in demand of treatment estimated from epidemiological studies, and the number actually treated in Norway. Though more people than ever before are treated, the "gap" has widened in recent years due to increased acceptance and demand.[22] Treatment criteria have been widened as well and consequently new dysfunctions and mood states are accepted as symptoms of psychiatric disorders in need of treatment. These days 15–20 percent of the population, or approximately 700,000 Norwegians are said to have some sort of psychological distress.[23] About 180,000 (4% of the population and 25% of the distressed) were actually treated during 2003.[24] This figure suggests that more than 10 percent of the total population in Norway, or about 500,000 people, do not receive the treatment they should benefit from, according to epidemiological studies and the service providers.

The NMHP states that five percent of the population below 18 years is in need of specialist mental health care. In 2003, specialist services were delivered to three percent of the population below 18 years.

Access to services can be improved by increasing capacity, but also by increasing the utilization of *existing* capacity (Halsteinli, Magnussen and Kittelsen, 2001). Increased accessibility to services has been observed for the last few years in outpatient clinics for children and adolescents as well as in the specialized mental health services for adults. The number of patients admitted to institutional treatment (adult plus C&A) increased by 62 percent, and the number of outpatient consultations increased by 61 percent in the period 1995–2003 (Table 3.6). Mental health services for C&A treated 33,000 patients in 2003, increased by 60 percent since 1998, and the outpatient clinic for adults increased their activity by 49 percent in the same period (*Helse og omsorgsdepartementet, Statsbudsjettet*, 2005).

Access by Mental Disorder

Another relevant question is this: What types of disorders are given priority in the services to increase the productivity? In the outpatient clinics there are more patients with minor disorders. The same happens at the DPCs. In recent years the policy for the services has been to treat patients actively, not to give them custodial care only, as happened in the asylums and also in the psychiatric nursing homes. Patients are expected to stay for shorter duration in the psychiatric institutions. This is important for people with minor disorders, but does not necessarily satisfy those with severe disorders.

When the demand for treatment increases and the service settings can choose their patients, there is a risk that some focus on high productivity, i.e., number of patients treated, and avoid the "unproductive" patients, such as the elderly and those with severe disorders such as schizophrenia and bipolar illness, often complicated with alcohol and drug abuse. Private practitioners prefer treating patients who recover and are pleasant to deal with.

For some groups of patients the services are still inadequate, the accessibility insufficient, and they therefore do not get the treatment and care they need and deserve. Especially for patients with severe disorders, the elderly, and the immigration population, there are

---

22. The prevalence of severe psychiatric disorders like schizophrenia and mood disorders do not increase.
23. The prevalence estimated by epidemiologists is higher than peoples' own judgment of their treatment needs. Studies on self-rated mental health tell that about 10% of the population is psychologically distressed, Table 3.2.
24. During any two-week period, 0.5–0.7% of the adult population visits an outpatient clinic or a private practitioner. About 0.6% receives inpatient treatment at least once a year.

shortcomings that are illustrated by the conclusion in a study among patients diagnosed with schizophrenia:

> There are reasons to believe that not all patients with schizophrenia are given treatment that is in accordance with good clinical practice. The time-lag from onset of manifest psychosis to appropriate treatment is often long – in most western countries up to 2–3 years. Early detection and treatment of schizophrenia is an important challenge. (Johannessen, 2002)

By design, the NMHP focuses in theory especially on patients with severe disorders. But it is too early in the program's implementation to decide if this group has been given the highest priority, and whether the community-based care and the focus on active treatment will suit patients with severe disorders best.

The government also focuses on the prevention and treatment of different forms of traumas. Groups exposed include children and adults having experienced violence (domestic or otherwise), sexual abuse, rape and/or torture, refugees, asylum-seekers, veterans from UN/NATO operations and personnel having taken part in international relief work (Norwegian Ministry of Health and Care Services, 2005).

Access by Age

The elderly mental disorders like senile dementia increase with age, and these disorders become more common as the expected average duration of life increases, and the total population becomes older. Moreover, elderly patients in somatic wards in the general hospitals frequently have psychiatric disorders that need care and treatment. Elderly patients are more inclined to have multiple disorders, and experience a general decay in mental as well as physical functioning, including the sensory and brain function. Alzheimers' and other memory deficit disorders have become more common. Dementia is one of the most prevalent conditions in the elderly in Norway, with a total prevalence of about 60,000 (Engedal, 2002). Depressive disorders, including major depression, are common among the elderly. For depression in hospitals and nursing homes, Rosenvinge and Rosenvinge (2003) reported an average prevalence estimate of 31 percent (range 5–58%). The prevalence of major depression in hospitals averaged 14 percent (4–26%) for patients over 60 years.

Unfortunately, there are no specialized services for the elderly, except for a few wards in hospitals and nursing homes. Moreover, there is an insufficient number of medical and other professionals who know the specific problems and disorders related to old age. Very few psychiatrists and psychologists specialize in mental disorders among the elderly in Norway. The old-age group is not very attractive to practitioners, and private practitioners are free to select from a large number of patients referred to them or asking for treatment. Private practitioners often prefer patients who recover or improve in the short run, and not patients with chronic, multiple or severe conditions, which often characterize the elderly.

Access by the Immigrant Population

The mental health services for the rapidly increasing non-Western immigrant population are insufficient as well. Immigrants from very unique cultures do not speak either Norwegian or English. They need particular attention and successful treatment requires an understanding of their cultural background. This knowledge is lacking in many service settings. It is a challenge for the services to improve their ability and knowledge to serve the immigrant population in the same way as the Norwegian-born population. Immigrants from non-Western countries occupy up to a fifth of the acute psychiatric beds (Berg and Johnsen, 2004). There is a prevailing clinical impression that they have higher morbidity than the traditional Norwegian population. Significantly more of the immigrants are men, who are diagnosed more frequently as psychotic, but they seem to have relatively fewer substance abuse problems (Berg and Johnsen, 2004).

The Norwegian Health Services Research Centre has studied the need for psychiatric treatment among immigrants seeking asylum in Norway. They are in a more uncertain situation than expatriated refugees, and in greater need for support and mental health services. However, not all asylum seekers are victims of mass violence or persecution, and among these the need for mental health services could be lower. Presently, there is insufficient help available for psychiatric problems that have been recognized among this population. The systematic identification of further unmet needs for psychiatric help will put greater pressure on the mental health system.

Inpatient Readmissions

Approximately 50 percent of the patients admitted to psychiatric institutions have been admitted before; many are treated and admitted several times, some of them very soon after their discharge. Among the 4,200 inpatients in psychiatric institutions November

20, 2003, 83 percent had been admitted at least one time before, and in the psychiatric hospitals only 21 percent was admitted for the first time (Hagen and Ruud, 2004). More readmissions are said to be a consequence of the reduced duration of stay at the psychiatric hospitals and wards. The reduction in the length of inpatient care was to be replaced by treatment and care in the community, but this plan has had some unforeseen side effects.

The readmission (recidivism) rate is one indicator of the problems in access to community-based services. A literature review to ascertain whether readmission rates differ among different service systems was conducted by Lien (2002). The results confirmed that approximately 50 percent of all patients admitted to psychiatric hospitals are previously admitted patients.[25] Longer length of stay, appropriate discharge planning, and follow-up visits after discharge predicted fewer readmissions, whereas the quantity and quality of community care did not seem to have any impact on readmission rates. Lien (2002) concluded that "readmission rates are not a suitable indicator of quality of care in psychiatric hospitals. Readmission rates may, however, be an important tool in planning access to appropriate mental health services."

Delayed Access: Waiting Lists

Another way to evaluate access is to look at the waiting lists or *queues* for treatment. One problem with this indicator is that not all patients who are in need of treatment and who would like to be treated are actually referred, especially if the waiting lists are very long. Consequently, this indicator overestimates the accessibility when waiting lists are long, since referral is perceived to be in vain, and other options outside the services are tried.

The waiting lists in the mental health services increased in the 1990s, especially for admissions to hospital wards, which suggests that accessibility to the services has decreased, even if more patients than ever before are treated. The waiting list for treatment has, however, diminished recently as a result of the increased productivity. Waiting time for C&A was reduced from about 90 to about 75 days and the waiting time for adults from about three to two months in the period from 2002 to 2004 (*Helse og omsorgsdepartementet, Statsbudsjettet*, 2005). In most of the outpatient clinics there are waiting lists, and the clinics have to choose between different types of patients. Patients are often treated on a first-come first-served basis. Waiting lists are regarded by the outpatient clinics as a consequence of scarce resources and not as a result of low productivity (Halsteinli, Magnussen and Kittelsen, 2003).

Demand and Supply Interactions

The demand for treatment seems to increase to a still larger extent than the supply. This is more or less a general law: the request for (mental) health services increases with the supply and the offer always lags behind the demand. There are several reasons for this. The supply seems to generate demand. People become aware of the possibility of getting help and treatment, the beds have to be occupied, the resources need to be used, and the services are marketed more to the public. Hospitalization rates therefore depend not only on "objective" needs or demands from patients, but to a certain degree on the facilities available.

Limited Supply of Placements

An insufficient supply of intermediate and long-term services for patients following acute psychiatric care is a factor limiting access to the mental health system in general. The acute wards have been reported to be the bottlenecks in the service chain for a long time. All beds are filled most of the time, and the acute psychiatric wards do not have available space for new patients. That does not mean, however, that the most appropriate solution is more beds in the acute wards. The hospitals often keep patients in the acute wards too long because there are no alternatives either in the hospitals or in the community. Another reason the acute wards are crowded is that patients are discharged prematurely, before adequate treatment has finished, resulting in increased readmission rates. The best solution to this problem, according to the NMHP, is not to establish more beds in the acute wards, but to establish more places in other institutional wards and in the community for patients who have completed treatment at the hospital.

The Norwegian Board of Health made a survey of the capacity in acute wards during one week in the autumn of 2002. All acute wards in the mental health

---

25. The 50% readmission rate is related to the number of inpatient stays, about 41,000 in 2003, not the inpatient population on a particular day, which was 4,200 November 20, 2003. Those who stay for a long time in an institution have more often been institutionalised before than those staying for a shorter time.

services responded. The results provide a picture of the relationship between the number of admitted patients and the capacity for all inpatients in acute wards during the survey week. There were too many patients who had completed their treatment, who could have been discharged, but remained in the hospital because they were waiting to be offered a place, for example, in a sheltered accommodation. The occupancy rate in the acute departments was 98 percent. This means that there was little free capacity to allow for situations requiring reallocation of beds or rooms. Some departments also reported that patients had to be discharged too early, or had to be sent home temporarily in order to make room for other patients. (*Report from the Norwegian Board of Health* June, 2003)

Thus, the main problem is a lack of flow of patients from the acute wards to intermediate and long-term facilities, and that patients cannot be discharged from the acute ward when treatment there is finished (Husby, Østberg and Hartvig, 2003). The insufficient number of beds in the acute wards is therefore a result of the lack of places in long-term units or rehabilitation wards, and a lack of sheltered accommodations or other adequate services in the community. The *DPCs* are meant to offer services to discharged patients, and also to assume part of the responsibility for acute mental health care. It is easier to get access to the decentralized DPCs, and they are expected to be the first offer for patients in need of institutionalization. But they are not adequately established in all regions at the moment. Consequently, the length of waiting lists for the acute wards, for adults as well as children and adolescents, vary with the health region and county (Hagen, 2003). An unintended result is de facto inequity in access to acute inpatient mental health services throughout the country in spite of the one-ownership model and free choice of hospitals. The situation has improved, but the problem is not solved.

Regional Variations

Regional disparities in the supply of mental health resources is a cause of unequal access. In the past there were considerable regional disparities with regard to the beds and other mental health services offered in the regions and counties. The highest inpatient prevalence is found in the capital, Oslo (141% of the national average in the 1990s). The lowest inpatient prevalence is in periphery counties in the north (65–71% of the national average). The disparities among the counties appear to follow certain geographical patterns: The coastal counties in the north and northwest have lower inpatient ratios than do the southeast and southern areas. A probable cause for the documented variance could be different age-distributions in the counties; however, there is no strong relationship generally between the proportion of elderly people in the counties and the inpatient rates. Regions with the highest inpatient rates are also the regions with the highest density of private practitioners. Therefore, access to the mental health services is easier in the most densely populated areas in the east, including the capital Oslo.

The national ownership of the Health Enterprises is expected to reduce the differences among counties, and consequently, to offer more equal service to the population irrespective of place of living. The centralization of ownership and control meant, however, that the local politicians representing the inhabitants at the county level was not in charge of the services any more. The idea was to make the specialized services more effective by centralization and to reduce the power of the local democratic assemblies. Within a small country like Norway, the central government through its Ministry of Health can develop several coordinated, strategic approaches to achieve more universal health-related goals. Patients are to understand that the hospitals belong to one national service, regardless of geographical location.

The former regional variations in the inpatient population were to a great extent a function of differences in bed capacity, which itself was heavily influenced by socioeconomic level and urban location. A high degree of urbanization and a higher income standard tend to increase the number of beds and the utilization of inpatient services. When the (local) society grows richer, more facilities become available, the inpatient population grows and more patients are treated at the outpatient clinics and in private practice as well.

Psychiatrists and psychologists prefer to practice in the big cities, and especially in the eastern region, close to the capital city. On the countryside and in scarcely populated municipalities far from the big cities, there are comparatively few psychologists (and psychiatrists) (Table 3.13).

In the northern region there are only 3.0 private practising psychologists (man-years) with operative agreements per 100,000 inhabitants, while in the more densely populated eastern region, including the capital of Oslo, there are 13.3 per 100,000 inhabitants. These variations between regions are large for psychiatrists as well (Table 3.13) and the uneven distribution of mental health specialists makes the access

Table 3.13. *Number of Contracted Psychiatrists and Psychologists (Man-Years) by Regional Health Enterprises, 2003. Per 100,000 Inhabitants.*

Regional health enterprises	Psychiatrists	Psychologists
The whole country	3.7	8.9
Health region East	6.0	13.3
Health region South	3.4	6.2
Health region West	3.0	9.8
Health region Mid-Norway	1.0	4.7
Health region North	1.4	3.0

Note: "Man-year" is the number of full-time employees and part-time employees (converted to full-time employees) at the end of the year.

to these services unequal throughout the country. Even though the health enterprises are state owned, market mechanisms of supply and demand play a part in the distribution of service settings and services providers, especially for private practitioners. Prevalence data seem to support however, the view that the unmet need for mental health services is probably greater in Oslo (Eastern region) than in other parts of the country (Dalgard, 1980; Kringlen, Torgersen and Cramer, 2001; Lavik, 1976).

Quality and Efficacy

Following discussion of several structural indicators of quality, we discuss strategies for quality assessment and quality improvement (QA/QI), and published evaluations of the quality of mental health services on structural and process measures.

Structural Indicators of Quality

Structural indicators include mental health practice guidelines, professional codes of conduct, certification, licensure of the mental health professionals, and the integration of mental health services.

In reorganizing the structure and administration of mental health services in Norway, enhanced funding as well as increased productivity and efficacy have been given high priority. To change ownership from the counties to the central government, establish new corporations and enterprises, and generally concentrate on the structure and frames for treatment seem to have been the more essential tasks for the government and the health authorities. The crucial question is, however, if these changes also improve the quality of the services.

Considerations of quality need to address the *content* of the services. Has care and treatment improved the mental health of the patients? What are the satisfactory outcome measures for deciding if treatment and care have a higher quality? How does one decide if the treatment has reduced patients' suffering and improved their functioning in the short and long run? And what are the relationships among quality, efficacy and efficiency in the mental health sector? Such questions are relevant for outcome studies and quality considerations. They are not easy to answer in the mental health field because there are few studies focusing on the quality of the services and the outcome of treatment and care.

Good treatment, that is, high quality psychotherapy takes time. Increased productivity and higher activity often means the opposite, namely, giving less time to each patient. Most productivity indicators are based solely on the number of patients treated per time-period or per man-year, not on the outcome or result of the treatment.

The evaluation criteria of quality and efficacy address the following questions: What is the quality of the mental health services provided throughout this country's mental health system? How effective are the mental health interventions in producing clinically significant, sustained improvement in treated patients? Structural, process, and outcome indicators of quality and efficacy are cited below.

Treatment Guidelines. The Government White Paper (*Sosial- og helsedepartementet*, 1997) indicated the need to raise the general level of competence among the personnel and to increase quality assurance activity. The Ministry of Health also initiated quality improvement by encouraging publication of *"Guidelines recommending good treatment."* The *Norwegian Board of Health* was instructed to publish guidelines for treatment of *anxiety disorders, mood disorders* and *schizophrenia.* These three guidelines for "evidence-based practices" have been issued and were implemented in 2001. They are intended only as guidelines and not made compulsory. Whether evidence-based practices are suitable in the mental health services in the same way as in somatic medicine has been a topic for discussion in the services recently, and the conclusions are uncertain.

Professional Ethical Codes of Conduct. The Ministry of Health has established a consulting group with representatives from five major user organizations. All major issues of the mental health programme are discussed in this group. Secondly, State funding has been earmarked for the organizations of users of mental health, which were traditionally weak and needed strengthening to become vital.

Certification/Licensure Standards for Mental Health Professionals. To be accepted as a therapist in the mental health services in Norway the provider has to be approved by the *Directorate of Health*. The standards for becoming an approved therapist are high, and the patients in the public mental health system are seldom treated in an incompetent or unethical way with respect to evidence-based, mainstream therapy.

Integration of Mental Health Services. An important task for the health enterprises is to justify and integrate the *private practitioners* into the remaining services, and to utilize the professional resources represented by the specialists in an even more effective manner. The private practitioners should to a larger extent work in cooperation with the DPCs and other service settings. So far, this has not been the case. The private practitioners and the GPs are not very well-integrated with the institutional mental health services.

Quality Assessment and Quality Improvement Strategies Employed

The Norwegian Board of Health (NBH) is a national supervisory authority with responsibility for general supervision of health and social services. The NBH oversees the population's need for health services and for social services, and ensures that services are provided in accordance with adequate professional standards. The Board also collaborates in activities to prevent failures and mistakes within the health care system. Patients are generally protected in an acceptable manner when admitted to the service settings, and they are seldom injured as a result of being patients in the mental health services. Locally, supervision is carried out by the Governmental Regional Boards. In matters of health and social affairs, the Regional Boards report to the Norwegian Board of Health.

Up to now, there has not been any systematic or regular quality assurance of the mental health services. A research group has for some years been involved in developing quality indicators, and an instrument for measuring the patients' experiences with the mental health services, for adults as well as for C&A, has been proposed. The new system for quality assurance is being implemented presently (2005) in the specialized services. This system strongly emphasizes indicators measuring users' experience and satisfaction with services. Specialized services are now required by law to establish systems for obtaining patients' and users' experiences with mental health services, and their evaluations of these services. A similar system will be developed for community-based services.

The evaluation of the National Mental Health Program (NMHP) is in progress through fifteen research projects financed by the Ministry of Health. The results from a preliminary evaluation were presented previously (pp. 112–113 this chapter). The results from the research evaluation will be applied to correct shortcomings and to improve the quality and functionality of the services.

The mental health services in Norway are surveyed thoroughly and monitored closely. Results from *structural and process measures* are made public regularly. Statistics Norway and *SINTEF Health Research* publish reports that summarize estimates of the activity (e.g., number of patients treated, number of staff), cost, and productivity. The Samdata reports are prepared by *SINTEF Health Research* and are financed by the Directorate of Health. These reports provide information about the specialized health services (for instance SAMDATA Mental Health Services, Bjørngaard, 2002, 2003). Several reports every year present data about structural and process indicators. The aim is to develop and exhibit data for improved control, planning, evaluation and management, and also to compare the results from different entities and service settings to make decisions concerning efficiency and productivity addressed as primary goals of the national health policy. The SAMDATA/Mental Health Services is also published on the net:

http://www.samdata.sintef.no/?p=psykisk_helsevern/sektorrapport_psyk_helse.htm

Systems for measuring the *outcomes* or *efficacy* of patient treatment in an objective way are not established to the same degree. Few empirical studies have dealt with outcomes to answer the question of whether the mental health services provided are efficacious in producing clinically significant and sustained improvement in the mental health of those who receive the treatment. There are some few studies in selected groups. There are however, expert groups working on these tasks, and the caregivers are expected to have a systematic reporting system for outcome measures in the near future.

One way to ensure quality is through regulatory guidelines such as appeals procedures for users to follow if they are dissatisfied with the services. In Norway, these regulatory and appeal processes are secured by a special institution, the Ombudsmann, see p.128. The Patient Ombudsmann is established to meet patients' needs and protect their interests and legal rights in respect to the health services. Any person may contact the Patient Ombudsman and request that a case be taken up for consideration.

Published Evaluations on Quality

The quality of mental health services has been assessed by various stakeholders: Clients, clinicians, managers, regulators, and governmental agency evaluations. Sample surveys of selected groups are provided here, beginning with patient satisfaction surveys of inpatient and outpatient services, followed by discussion of the cooperation among service units, and providers' knowledge of new laws and regulations related to quality assessment and quality improvement.

Patient Satisfaction with Inpatient Psychiatric Services. Most studies concerning the quality of mental health services have focused on patients in specific groups, or on local services in one region. There are few studies including the whole patient population. However, every fifth year since 1979 all *inpatients* in adult psychiatric institutions have been asked to state their preferred residence and treatment setting in six months (Øgar 1981, Øgar, Kolstad and Kindseth, 1986, Hagen 1992, Hagen 1997, Hagen 2001, Hagen and Ruud, 2004). The survey in 2003 comprised 4,200 inpatients.[26] The survey emphasizes that it is the patient's own opinion that shall be recorded, whether or not this is deemed realistic or ideal from the staff's point of view. For each patient, a member of the staff also gives a professional opinion about both "ideal" and "realistic" settings of services in six months. When recording "ideal" setting, actual capacity and availability should *not* be taken into account, while "realistic" settings should reflect these factors. The census also includes data on diagnosis, level of functioning in activities of daily living, patients' career, and social and demographic factors.

Survey results indicate that most patients prefer living in their own home or apartment, despite the problems often associated with life outside of the institutions (such as loneliness, poor housing quality, poor economy, and unemployment). Most patients appreciate sheltered accommodation, supportive services (preferably being able to reach staff on a 24-hour basis), but not on a live-in basis.

Given that the actual deinstitutionalization of services is supported by the patients, it was expected that the services would become better adapted to the patients' preferences. However, this has not always been the case. Patients who themselves preferred to stay in their home were not always the ones to be discharged, and elderly patients who wanted to remain, were often transferred to another setting. Patients' preferences for living in their own home seem to have changed at an even faster pace than the downsizing of the institutions. Many patients, who do not want to stay in the institutions, nevertheless continue to stay there. Several of these patients are involuntary admits.

Patient Satisfaction with Outpatient Mental Health Services. In September, 2004, the *Norwegian Health Services Research Centre*[27] carried out a study comprising 6,700 outpatients, focusing on their satisfaction with services at outpatient clinics in Norway. The research and program evaluation was financed by the Ministry of Health. Most of the patients were satisfied with the treatment provided and with their relationship with the therapist. They were least satisfied with the information given. The elderly were more satisfied than the young. Those who experienced a sort of involuntary treatment were not as satisfied as other patients. Patients who got the therapist they wanted are much more satisfied than those who did not. Codetermination of treatment seems to be important for most patients at the outpatient clinics.

Research and quality evaluation on mental health services and treatment effects also takes place at the universities.[28] The Government does not finance this research activity directly, but indirectly by financing the universities, the Norwegian Research Council, and with grants to specific research programs. Some research projects dealing with the effects and results

---

26. The registrations cover 99% of *all* patients in adult psychiatric institutions and departments. A number of patients were not able to state any preferences.
27. The *Norwegian Health Services Research Centre* commenced January 1, 2004. The Centre is scientifically and professionally independent and organised under the *Directorate for Health and Social Affairs.* The Centre has no authority to develop health policy or responsibility to implement policies but is accomplishing research and development, also related to quality assurance.
28. All universities in Norway are public, financed totally by the Government.

of the NMHP are also examples of quality evaluations. Beginning in 1999, 15 research projects are being financed by the Ministry of Health by an annual spending of NOK 5 million (US$662,000 at the 1999 exchange rate of 7.552). The evaluation research is accomplished by independent research institutions. The Regional Health Authorities are also expected to use some of their grants to conduct research and program evaluation.

Cooperation Among Service Units. A prerequisite for a comprehensive service to patients is a clear distribution of tasks and well-functioning routines for cooperation among the primary care, the "local" DPCs, the acute wards and other wards at the mental hospitals. Even if the availability of services and the cooperation between acute departments and the DPCs have improved in recent years, there are still serious shortcomings. The primary care in the municipalities is an important link in the service chain and the NMHP gives high priority to develop the primary mental health care. So far the services in the municipalities have not been established satisfactorily and the cooperation in the chain is still too weak.

In 2003, the *Norwegian Board of Health* in the counties carried out supervision of some specialist mental health institutions: DPCs and acute psychiatric wards in general hospitals. The internal cooperation within the specialist health services was inadequate in as many as half of the institutions, according to the survey. This is serious because it increases the risk that patients will not receive the treatment that they require, appropriate to their condition. The cooperation between the links in the service chain has to be improved. All providers in the public services are required to contribute to improvement in coordination, but so far only a few institutions have made plans or contribute to them (*Norwegian Board of Health*, 2003).

Knowledge About New Laws and Regulations. According to the *Norwegian Board of Health* the mental health sector seems to have inadequate knowledge and understanding of current laws and regulations, including those related to quality assessment and quality improvement. The Board regards the situation as serious, and there is a great need for better comprehension, in order to ensure that the patient rights are met and that everyone in the population receives adequate health services. The Board also points out that it is the responsibility of leadership at Regional Health Authorities and Health Enterprises to ensure that the requirements that apply to specialist health services are met and followed up.

Cost and Efficiency

The following presentation gives expenditure data for *all* health care in Norway reported by the World Health Organization (2005). Additional data is provided on expenditures for mental health services in Norway. Comparative statistics on *all* health expenditures from national health authorities are reported annually by the World Health Organization. How these estimates are standardized is discussed in the World Health report (2004, pp. 97–101). The data reported for Norway are presented in Table 3.14 below.

Increasing amounts of public resources are spent on the health sector. The total expenditures on health as a percent of GDP have continued to rise after 2002. At the average annual exchange rate of 7.080 for 2003, the expenditures increased by NOK 4.7 billion (US$ 664 million), or eight percent, from 2002 to

Table 3.14. *WHO National Health Account Indicators: 1998, 2002.*

Indicator	1998	2002
Total expenditures on health as a % of GDP	8.5	9.6
General govt. expenditure as a % of total health expenditure	84.7	83.5
Private expenditure on health as a % of total expenditure on health	15.3	16.5
General govt. expenditure on health as a % of total govt. expenditure	15.6	18.1
External resources for health as a % of total expenditure on health	0	0
Social security exp. on health as a % of general govt. exp. on health	0	0
Out-of-pocket expenditure as a % of private expenditure on health	96.6	97.2
Private prepaid plans as % of private expenditure on health	0	0

Note: Source is the WHO Report, 2005, Table 5, pp 196-197.
Note: See Tables 1.2 and 1.3 for comparisons for the year 2002, and Table 6.9 for the year 2003.

2003. In 2003, Norway spends NOK 61 billion (US$ 8.62 billion) on all specialized health services, making it *one* of the European countries – and *the* Nordic country – with the highest level of public spending on the health services per capita: and corresponds to NOK 13,400 (US$ 1,893) per inhabitant in 2003, and NOK 12,500 per inhabitant in 2002 (US$ 1,566 at the 2002 exchange rate of 7.984). Most of the expenditures are general governmental expenditures due to the dominance of the public services. In Table 3.14 the percentage of private expenditure on health as a percent of total expenditure is 16.5 percent. This percentage is higher than expected, and the reason could be that private, nonprofit institutions owned by humanitarian organizations like the Red Cross are included in the "private sector" by WHO. Private/voluntary health insurances are not common, every inhabitant is covered by the public and involuntary National Insurance Scheme. The out-of-the pocket fees have increased in recent years, but are still low. The inhabitants contribute to the expenditures on the public health services by paying tax and the special National Insurance Scheme. The inhabitants contribute to the health services according to their income and profit irrespective if they are in need of or use the services or not.

Specialized Mental Health Services. Estimates of expenditures in specialized mental health services only are provided in Table 3.15 and 3.16.

Excluding investment and capital expenditures, the total per capita expenditure in 2003 for specialized mental health services amounted to NOK 2,445 (US$ 345), which consumed 0.7 percent of the GDP. This represents a 16 percent real growth in expenditures since 1998. Over the period 1999–2006, annual cost of the services is projected to increase by NOK 500 per capita (US$ 66 at the 1999 exchange rate of 7.552). The distribution of expenditures in 2003, were as follows: inpatient (80%); outpatient (14%); daypatient services (4%) and private practice (2%). For children and adolescents in 2003, 45 percent of expenditures are for inpatient services, 4 percent outpatient services, and 8 percent daypatient services.

An increasing share of the total health costs is spent on mental health services. For the first time in several years the growth in costs of mental health services from 2002 to 2003 was larger than the growth in costs of general hospitals and institutions. NOK 11.1 billion (US$ 1.6 billion) were spent on the *specialist mental health services* in Norway in 2003.

Table 3.15. *National Mental Health Services Expenditures for 2003.*

Indicator	2003 NOK	US$	%
Total expenditure (exp.) for mental health services (mhs) only	11.1**	1.6**	
Total exp. for mhs as a % of GDP			0.7
General govt. exp. on mhs only	11.1**	1.6**	
General govt. exp. on mhs as a % of total exp. on all mhs			99.6
Private exp. on mhs as a % of total exp on all mhs			0.4
General govt. exp. on mhs as a % of total govt. exp.			2.7
External funding resources for mhs as a % of total exp. on mhs			na
Social security exp. on mhs as % of general govt. exp on mhs			na
Out-of-pocket exp. for mhs as a % of private exp. on mhs			100
Private prepaid plans for mhs as % of private exp. on mhs			na
Estimated exp. for mhs/substance abuse services as % of total health care exp.			18
Per capita exp. for mhs	2,445	345	
Estimated costs of lost productivity due to mental disorders	na		
Estimated exp./costs for mental health disabilities/sick leaves	29**	4.1**	
Costs to employers of both treated and untreated mental disorders	na		
"Medical offset" costs/savings	na		

Note: Specialist mental health services only, primary care not included.
** In billions. US$ are based on the 2003 exchange rate of 7.080.

Table 3.16. *Expenses for Psychiatric Institutions, 1990–2000.*

	Gross current expenses. NOK billion			
Institutions	1990	1995	2000	2003
All	6.1	6.4	8.5	10.4
Adults	5.4	5.7	7.4	8.6
C&A	0.6	1.9	1.1	1.8

Note: The expenses are adjusted to the prices in 2000. The Consumer price index increased by 34.8% from 1990 to 2003.

A greater than ever share of the total costs of the mental health services went to services for C&A. From 1990 to 2001, this share rose from 10 percent to 13 percent, and the rise continues. In 2003, 17 percent of the costs of the mental health services went to C&A. Services for adults account for 83 percent of the total costs.

Table 3.16 indicates the total price adjusted expenses for the mental health institutions in the period 1990 to 2003 for all institutions and for adults and C&A separately.

The expenses in the specialized mental health institutions increased by nearly 40 percent in ten years period 1990 to 2000, both for adults and C&A. There has been a further increase in the next years. In the three years period 2000 to 2003 the expenditures increased by 16 percent in the services for adults and by 64 percent for C&A.

Disability Pensions and Sick Leaves. In 2003, the cost for treatment, disability pensions and sick leaves due to psychiatric disorders was estimated to NOK 40 billion (or 6.25 billion dollars). Costs in lost productivity are not included (*Helse og omsorgsdepartementet. Statsbudsjettet,* St.prp.nr. 1, 2005). For schizophrenia alone the total cost has been estimated to NOK 4 billion in 2002 (US$ 501 million at the 2002 exchange rate of 7.984). There is no other disorder with comparable cost, and schizophrenia alone costs more than all types of cancer and cardiovascular diseases (Johannessen, 2002).

For the specialized mental health services only, expenses and revenues for selected years are provided in Table 3.17. Most of the expenditures, approximately 80 percent, are wages and social expenses.

Households Out-of-Pocket Spending. Patients do not pay for their stay in hospitals or other bed institutions, but they have to pay a *share of the cost* (a) when visiting a general practitioner, an outpatient clinic, or a specialist in private practice, (b) for prescriptions of important drugs, and (c) for transportation expenses in connection with examination or treatment. Patients receiving treatment in mental health services do not pay higher co-pay than patients receiving other medical services.

The out-of-pocket payment for visiting an outpatient clinic or a specialist (psychiatrist or psychologist) depends on the specialist's contract with the Regional Health Authorities. If the private practitioner has an operative agreement the patient pays only part of the actual cost for the visit. The specialist is reimbursed by the National Insurance Scheme which covers the main part of the expenses. For example, the cost-sharing amount for the year 2003 in connection with treatment by a general practitioner or a specialist in the psychiatric services with an agreement is NOK 114 (US$ 16 at the 2003 exchange rate of 7.080) for each consultation, and 36 percent of the expenses of important medications (maximum NOK 400 or US$ 56 per prescription). For reiterated prescriptions a new cost-sharing amount shall be paid when a supply equal to three months' consumption has been received.

The households total out-of-pocket spending for outpatient care was in year 2000 about NOK 38 million or about NOK 8 per inhabitant. (Based on the average annual exchange rate of 8.813 for 2000, the equivalent figures in US dollars are 4.31 million and 0.91 respectively.) Even if the out-of-pocket spending for specialized services has increased recently, the percentage of the total expenses is still marginal: 0.1 percent in 1990, and about 0.4 percent of the total expenses in 2003. If the specialist does *not* have an operative agreement, the patient pays the *whole* cost for the consultation, and the specialist may receive as high a fee as the client is willing to pay. This system makes it easy for rich people to get treatment from private practitioners who have no operative agreement, while ordinary and poor people cannot afford paying for long-term treatment.

There are certain exemptions from the cost-sharing provisions for special diseases and groups of people. Children under the age of 18 are exempted from cost-sharing for mental health services and dental treatment. From January 1, 2003, those who receive minimum old-age or disability pensions are exempt from cost-sharing on important medications and nursing articles.

In 1984, a cost-sharing ceiling was introduced. This cost-sharing arrangement includes coverage of expenses related to treatment by physicians and psychologists

Table 3.17. *Current Expenses and Current Revenue for Specialized Mental Health Services by Category of Expenses, 1990–2000. mill. NOK (mill US$).* *

Category of expenses	1990 NOK mill.	1990 US$ mill.	1995 NOK mill.	1995 US$ mill.	2000 NOK mill.	2000 US$ mill.
Gross current expenses	4,792	(767)	5,740	(906)	8,523	(968)
Wages and social expenses	3,894	(623)	4,549	(718)	6,874	(781)
Medical equipment	2.8	(0.4)	3.0	(0.5)	1.8	(0.2)
Other equipment and maintenance	164	(26)	179	(28)	191	(22)
Med. consump.:articles/medicine	52	(8)	57	(9)	106	(12)
Other current expenses	638	(102)	669	(106)	938	(106)
Transfers	41	(7)	283	(45)	412	(47)
Revenue Sources						
Gross current revenue	548	(88)	848	(134)	1,588	(180)
Sales and rental income	104	(17)	79	(13)	94	(11)
Reimbursement from NIA**	122	(20)	288	(45)	496	(56)
User fee for out-patient care	5	(1)	23	(4)	38	(4)
Reimbursement: paid sick leave	175	(28)	208	(33)	365	(41)
Earmarked grants: central govt.	84	(13)	188	(30)	508	(58)
Transfers	58	(9)	61	(10)	88	(10)

Note: The expenses and revenues are not price adjusted. The expenses in 1990 adjusted for the inflation rate (26% between 1990 and 2000) was, for instance, NOK 6.05 billion in 2000-prices, and the increase between 1990 and 2000 in constant prices is therefore 40%.

* Numbers in parentheses are equivalents in US$ based on the average annual exchange rate for the same year (1990–6.250, 1995–6.336, 2000–8.813) obtained from the U. S. Federal Reserve Board.
** NIA=National Insurance Administration

in private practice, important drugs, and transportation expenses related to examination and treatment. After the ceiling has been reached, a card is issued giving entitlement to free treatment and benefits as mentioned for the rest of the calendar year. The ceiling is fixed by Parliament for one year at a time, and for 2003 it is fixed to NOK 1,350 (US$ 191 at the 2003 exchange rate of 7.080). Nobody pays more than this amount out-of-pocket per year for visiting a specialist with an operative agreement. Cost-sharing amounts for children under the age of 16 are added to those of a parent in order to reach the ceiling. In US dollars, the maximum annual co-payment in 2003 was $191 for mental health services provided by professionals with an operative agreement with the RHA and/or Health Enterprises.

Are Mental Health Services Affordable? Norway is an extremely wealthy country due to the oil and gas production, and has a very high GDP. Only a minor part of the surplus from the oil and gas production is invested or consumed in Norway, for instance by financing the health services. The majority of the surplus is invested at the stock markets abroad in order to reduce the inflation rate in Norway. The public spending in Norway is however, comparatively high and there is no public deficit. The mental health services are affordable for most of the Norwegians since the maximum yearly out-of-pocket expenses for the year 2003 were NOK 1,350 (US$ 191). The employees contribute to the health services and pensions by paying taxes in general and by paying 7.8 percent of their pensionable income to the *National Insurance Scheme.* Employers contribution is assessed as a percentage of paid-out wages, and also depending on the regional zone in which the employers reside. Everybody is equally entitled to the same health services even if they cannot afford to pay for the services, either through taxes or the out-of-pocket fee. That is stated by law.

Productivity/Efficiency of the Mental Health Services. The public system is efficient and the quality is high. There is generally little waste and no profit to the owners as in private systems. A main problem at the moment seems to be however, that too many are told that their worries and perceived low "life quality" can be solved by the mental health services; consequently, the demands from people with less serious disorders rise dramatically.

The answer from the Norwegian government is to enhance the supply of psychiatric services by increasing the number of personnel, establishing new service settings and also by raising *productivity* in all services, especially at the outpatient clinics. The Government White Paper from 1997 affirmed both an increase in capacity and an increase in productivity as central political goals for the mental health care sector. The Norwegian policy for productivity growth is a strategy of combined resource growth and "mild coercion" (Halsteinli, Magnussen and Kittelsen, 2001). This is stated with explicit and quantitative measures in the NMHP.

Measuring productivity in mental health services is difficult and controversial. Calculated in a traditional way, as the number of patients treated per man-years, the health authorities in Norway suppose there still is considerable room for improved performance in the services, especially at the outpatient clinics. In 1996, the number of consultations per therapist day in psychiatric outpatient clinics for C&A was 1.1 (Ministry of Health, 1997). Thus, at this time, it was concluded that the mental health services in general seemed to be characterized by insufficient capacity as well as a low level of productivity, and the ministry stipulated that productivity at the outpatient clinics should increase by as much as 50 percent. These issues are being debated in Norway (Halsteinli, Magnussen and Kittelsen, 2001).

The number of treated patients has however, increased dramatically since 1996 along with the resources, especially the number of professional staff. Measured as the number of patients treated per full-time equivalent personnel (man-years), productivity has also increased for C&A. There was a substantial growth in productivity in the period 1996 to 2001 and it continued in the first five years of 2000. Average level of productivity in 2001 was more than 25 percent higher than it was in 1996 due first and foremost to shorter duration of stay. This implies an average annual growth in productivity of 4.5 percent. There are, however, substantial variations in capacity and "productivity" among different health regions (Halsteinli, Magnussen and Kittelsen, 2003). The health authorities still assert that there is considerable room for improved activity. Both overall increase in capacity and a more even geographical distribution is a goal for the National Mental Health Programme.

Increased Capacity. The strongest, current incentive provided by the services' financing system is to increase the number of employees. The chosen strategy contains two elements; a strong public and political focus on low levels of productivity and a growth in the amount of resources invested in the sector in order to increase capacity. Suspecting that variations in efficiency could be attributed to variations in organizational models of service delivery, in 1998 the *National Board of Health* initiated a project to review the working processes of psychiatric outpatient clinics. This project received much attention within the sector, and the resulting report suggested several areas where changes might lead to improved productivity (Halsteinli, Magnussen and Kittelsen, 2001).

The health authorities do not seem to give high priority to a revision of the financing system in the mental health services. This strategy is in stark contrast to the somatic sector where the ends (goals) of increased activity and productivity were pursued mainly by the means of changing the financing system. One explanation for the difference in financing systems is the lack of patient classification systems for psychiatric patients like the Diagnosis Related Group (DRG) system for somatic patients (Halsteinli, Magnussen and Kittelsen, 2001), and the recognition that disorders in emotions, cognitions and behaviour are different from somatic illnesses.

Financing and Fairness

Mental health services in Norway are funded by public mechanisms. The private sector plays a marginal role. The public (the Government and the municipalities) allocate financial resources to the current services, through a combination of general and separate taxation and other revenues. Employers contribute by means of a payroll tax to the central government and the municipalities, assessed as a percentage of wages paid by the employer. Non-working spouses, unemployed, students and others without wages are exempted from social security tax, but they still qualify for social security benefits. They have the same right to medical treatment as those with salaries. The national insurance, or social security which also contribute to the financing, is a collective insurance scheme to which all in Norway belong.

Financing of the National Insurance Scheme

The National Insurance Scheme is financed by contributions from employees, self-employed persons, employers' contributions, and contributions from the central government. Contribution rates and government grants are decided by the Parliament. Figures given below are for 2003 at the exchange rate of 7.080.

Contributions from employees and self-employed persons are calculated on the basis of their pensionable income. Contributions are not paid on annual, gross income less than NOK 23,000 (US$3,249). The contributions shall not exceed 25 percent of income greater than NOK 23,000. Cash benefits in the case of sickness, maternity and unemployment are taken into account as pensionable income. The same applies to the rehabilitation allowance and vocational rehabilitation allowance. The contribution rate of employees is 7.8 percent of pensionable income (gross wage income). The rate of a self-employed person's contribution is 10.7 percent of pensionable income (income from self-employment) up to 12 times the basic amount[29] (12B.a.), and the percentage is gradually reduced with higher incomes. The contribution rate for other kinds of personal benefits (pensions, etc.) is 3.0 percent.

The employers' contribution is assessed as a percentage of paid out wages. The contributions are differentiated according to the regional zone in which the employees reside. There are five regional zones distinguished by geographical situation and level of economic development. The employers' contributions vary according to the zones: 14.1 percent, 10.6 percent, 6.4 percent, 5.1 percent and 0 percent. For employees who have attained the age of 62, reduced employer's contribution rates apply.

Human Resource Strategies

For some time there has been a lack of professional manpower rather than a shortage of funding for the mental health services in Norway. The current challenge in Norway is to persuade the services to function according to the NMHP objectives and policies. The new institutions and centres have not been utilized to their full extent recently due to a lack of qualified health professionals. The capacity at the universities and colleges for education and training of mental health providers has been expanded. The NMHP goal is to get 2,300 *more* professional man-years during the Programme period ending 2008. A goal for the services for C&A is 400 more professionals for outpatient treatment. The resources for educating these professionals are available and the service settings are already or will be established before 2008.

More integrated services and extended cooperation with other professions is another aim in the new Programme. The patient can be transferred to the outpatient clinic, to the hospital or ward, or to a DPC, and back, depending on the patients' condition. This can happen more easily today than previously. Different service settings have become more appropriate to that particular person and tailored to the condition or phase of their disorders. Referral of the patient to different agencies and service settings should be based on an *Individual plan* for treatment and care (see p. 128). For most patients the increased diversity of the levels of services has been an advantage. Those in need of long-term care and treatment in stable surroundings inside an institution are however, not looked upon as the most coveted patients. These patients also reduce the overall "productivity" in a service setting.

Protection and Participation

Patient Protection Policies

We begin this section with discussion of patient protections at both the clinical and policy levels, followed by discussion of participation of users in policy formulation.

At the clinical level, the typical patient in the mental health services is treated and protected in an acceptable manner when admitted to the services. Patients are very seldom hurt or injured in the mental health services in an unintended way. In general, the institutions are a safe place to stay. At the level of provider-patient interactions patients are protected from incompetent, unethical care, or other forms of exploitation or abuse. There are occasional exceptions, which are given considerable attention in the media. Patient safety procedures (suicide prevention) are also well-established in the health care settings.

---

29. Many benefits from the National Insurance Scheme are determined in relation to a *Basic amount* (B.a). This amount is adjusted by the Parliament one or more times each year, in accordance with changes in the general income level. The main adjustment takes place on May 1 each year. In 2002, the average *basic amount* was NOK 53,233 (US$ 6,667), and the basic amount as of January 1, 2003 is NOK 54,170 (US$ 7,651).

Every patient with a suicide risk will be especially protected and taken care of. The Personnel Act has standards for professional conduct for health personnel.

More than 50 *Control commissions*, surveying the services and the way patients are cared for, are established by the Ministry of Health and Care Services. The aim of the commission is to deal with concern from the patients due to restrictions and involuntary admission. The commission is also controlling the welfare of all patients. The Directorate of Health is responsible for surveying and evaluating the reports from the 57 Control Commissions.

At a policy level, Norway has extensive legislation and regulation of patient rights to access appropriate care, to appeal treatment decisions, and to refuse mental health treatment. Examples of mandated patient rights are discussed below.

The patients' rights have been strengthened in Norway recently by a new Act. The object of the *Patients' Rights Act* is to help ensure that all citizens have equal access to good quality health care by granting patients rights in their relations with the health service. The Act is meant to protect the patient by giving information about the treatment planned, including potential risks and side effects. The provisions of this Act shall help to promote a relationship of trust between the patient and the health service and safeguard respect for the life, integrity and human dignity of each patient.

To make it easier to influence their treatment, patients were also given the right to participate more actively, to demand information, and to review their medical record. The new law also contains rules concerning complaint procedures, patient representatives, and provisions governing the special rights of children. The patient is entitled to emergency care and to receive necessary health care from the municipal health service and from the specialist health service.

The Patient's Right to Information. The patient shall have the information that is necessary to obtain an insight into his or her health condition and the content of the health care. The patient shall also be informed of possible risks and side effects. If injury or serious complications are inflicted upon the patient, the patient shall be informed of this. If, after the treatment has been concluded, it is discovered that the patient may have suffered considerable injury as a result of the health care, the patient shall be informed of this if possible.

Patient Rights to Informed Consent, Privacy and Confidentiality. The patients' right to informed consent, privacy and confidentiality is also protected by the law. But not always realised in practice.

Access to Medical Records. According to the *Act of Patients' Rights,* the patient is entitled to have access to his or her medical records with enclosures, and a copy upon special request. Upon request, the patient is entitled to a brief and simple explanation of medical terms, etc. The patient may be denied access to information in his or her medical records if this is absolutely necessary in order to avoid endangering the patient's life or serious damage to the patient's health, or if access is clearly inadvisable out of consideration for the welfare of persons close to the patient. A representative of the patient is entitled to have access to the information to which the patient is denied access, unless the representative is considered to be unfit for this. A physician or lawyer may not be denied access, unless special reasons so dictate.

The Right to Evaluation and Care. A patient who is referred to the mental health specialist services is entitled to have his or her health condition evaluated within 30 working days of receipt of the referral. An evaluation shall be made of whether health care is necessary, and information shall be provided as to when treatment may be expected to be provided. The waiting period for treatment following assessment was about two months in 2004 (see p. 85). If the Regional Health Enterprise has not ensured that a patient who is entitled to necessary health care from the specialist health service receives such care, the patient has the right to receive necessary health care immediately, if necessary from a service provider in another region or outside Norway.

The Right to Choose the Specialist Service Setting. According to the *Patients' Rights Act*, the patient has the right to choose the hospital or district psychiatric centre, or treatment unit in such an institution, in which the treatment shall be carried out. The patient may not choose the level of treatment.

In order to exercise their legal rights, such as their right to freely choose a hospital, patients need relevant, timely, and accurate information about the quality of health services provided through different service providers. Efforts have been made to develop quality indicators nationwide, in addition to a quality register, which is easily accessible on the internet and gives information about each provider's or settings' scores on the quality indicators. This goal of developing relevant quality indicators and registers has not been achieved, and in the mental health sector few patients choose specialized services outside their region. Perhaps the most important element of "free choice" is to give the patients the feeling they are allowed to choose and to have more control, whether they exercise it or not. One argument allowing free choice of services was to reduce the waiting time for treatment (two to three months). The queues have been a problem for a long time and systematic efforts designed to reduce waiting times have been given priority for many years.

The Right to an Individualized Care Plan. According to the *Act of Patients Rights,* any patient who requires long-term, coordinated health services is entitled to have an individual plan drawn up in accordance with the provisions of the *Municipal Health Service Act,* the *Specialist Health Service Act* and the *Act on the Provision and Implementation of Mental Health Care.* The principle of an "individual plan" is the result of accepting that people are different and that the diagnosis does not provide a complete picture of the patient's disorder and needs. Everybody is entitled to be treated and cared for according to individual demands. The individual plan is also expected to improve coordination between service settings in the chain and between the primary care and the specialized services. The individual plan is stated in a partly formalized manner, on a scheme, but also with individual comments from patients and the professionals. A formalized and extended individual plan for all patients is something new in the mental health services in Norway. It takes time to establish the routines for making the plan, and presently the majority of patients do not have an individual plan. The authorities are however, following the situation carefully and make efforts to increase the number of patients with a tailored plan for treatment and care.

The Patient's Right to Participation. The patient is entitled to participate in the implementation of his or her health care. This includes the patient's right to participate in choosing between available and medically sound methods of examination and treatment. The form of participation shall be adapted to the individual patient's ability to give and receive information. If the patient is not competent to give consent, the patient's next of kin is entitled to participate together with the patient. If the patient wishes other persons to be present when health care is provided, his or her wishes shall be accommodated as far as possible.

The Patient Ombudsman. The central government shall ensure that there is a Patient Ombudsman in every county. The Patient Ombudsman has oversight of public, specialist health services. The Patient Ombudsman shall perform his or her functions independently and autonomously. According to the *Act of Patients' Rights,* The Patient Ombudsman shall work to meet patients' needs and protect their interests and legal rights in respect of the health service, and to improve the quality of the health service. The Patient Ombudsman may consider cases involving matters in the public specialist health service, either on the basis of an oral or written request, or upon his or her initiative. Any person may contact the Patient Ombudsman and request that a case be considered. Public authorities and other bodies that perform services for the public administration shall give the Patient Ombudsman the information required for the Ombudsman to carry out his or her duties. The Patient Ombudsman shall have free access to all premises in which public specialist health services are provided.

Consent to Health Care Services. According to the *Patients' Rights Act,* health care may be provided only with the patient's consent. In order for the consent to be valid, the patient must have received the necessary information concerning his health condition and the content of the health care. The patient may withdraw his consent. The following persons have the right to consent to health care: (a) persons of full legal age and legal capacity, unless special provisions dictate otherwise, and (b) minors over 16 years of age, unless special provisions or the nature of the measure dictate otherwise.

The health care provider shall decide whether the patient lacks competence to give consent pursuant to the second paragraph. Based on the patient's age, mental state, maturity and experience, health personnel shall do their best to enable the patient himself or herself to consent to health care. The parents or other persons with parental responsibility are entitled to consent to health care for patients less than 16 years of age. When the child has reached 12 years of age, he or she shall be allowed to give his or her opinion on all questions concerning his or her own health. If a patient who is of full legal age and legal capacity is not competent to give consent, the health care provider may make decisions concerning health care that is not of a highly invasive nature with regard to its extent and duration. A patient who has been declared legally incapacitated shall, to the greatest possible extent, consent to health care himself or herself. If this is not possible, the guardian may give consent on behalf of the legally incapacitated person. Even if the principle of patient's consent is stated in the

Patients' Rights Act, there are still many patients in Norway who are admitted involuntarily to the psychiatric hospitals.

Compulsory Detention and Treatment. In 2002, approximately 40 percent of the patients in psychiatric hospitals and wards were admitted without giving their consent. In 2003, 75 percent of the overnight stays (42,197 stays at all) in the mental hospitals were voluntary, 4,940 overnight stays (12%) of the totals) were due to forced observation, and 4,489 (11%) were forced mental health treatment with overnight stay. Thirty patients were sentenced to mental health care with overnight stay in 2003, and 441 were admitted pursuant to other laws and not distributed admittances.

The high number and rates of involuntary admissions have been a concern for the health authorities for many years. It has also raised public debates several times in recent years. A new law covering the use of compulsory admission, treatment and other forms of coercion was implemented in 2001. Presently, compulsory admission and treatment require that patients have a serious mental illness and that at least one of two additional criteria is met: (a) the possibility of cure or considerable improvement will be lost, or (b) the patient represents a considerable danger to himself or to others. Patients can also be admitted involuntarily for observation, lasting up to ten days. The law specifies acceptable types of coercive treatment and expands the patients' rights of appeal to a supervising commission or to the courts. According to the Ministry of Health (2005), the results of these reforms are so far inconclusive.

Generally, there has been, and still is a strong paternalistic tradition in the mental health services. Professionals often think they know better than the patients themselves what would benefit or harm patients, not only in relation to treatment, but also in their general life outside the institutions. Patients' own viewpoints and attitudes are looked upon with suspicion and skepticism especially if they do not agree with professional evidence, which has changed dramatically through history. Those in charge of the institutions sometimes remain skeptical about accepting patients' reports and evaluations of their own experiences with treatment, and with patient views of adequate help.

Traditionally, mental health services have been based on the view that health professionals effect changes within a person with psychiatric problems via a range of treatment methods. Service users have had little opportunity to speak for themselves about their view of professional help or about what supports their recovery process.

Offenders with Psychiatric Disorders. Forensic psychiatry has a long tradition in Norway. In criminal cases suspecting a psychiatric disorder, the offender is often evaluated by psychiatrists or psychologists. Offenders with severe mental disorders are not responsible for their acts, and they are referred to treatment in the mental health services and not to the prisons. Again, this is how the system is expected to work. In practice it is different. Presently, too many offenders with severe disorders are kept in the prisons without adequate treatment and care. This has lasted for years. And still offenders do not receive acceptable treatment from the mental health services. Services for offenders with psychiatric disorders do not function properly, and health and prison authorities have expressed concern about the situation for years.

Surveys of serious mental disorders in prisons in the western world reveal high prevalence; on average four percent with psychosis, 10 percent with major depression, and 65 percent with personality disorders among male inmates. A few investigations in Norwegian prisons indicate a similar tendency (Hartvig and Østberg, 2004). The prevalence and severity of psychiatric illnesses, other behavioural disorders, and treatment facilities available during the prison term served were recorded from 2,850 prison inmates (95% of a national total of 3,000 prisoners). About 24 percent of inmates received some kind of treatment for psychiatric disorders.

The prevalence of psychiatric disorders, drug problems and personality disorders has been studied in a prison population in the western health region in Norway. The methods used were structured clinical interviews, self-reports and reviews of medical case notes. Psychiatric disorders in need of treatment were found in 18 out of 40 interviewed inmates (45%). Thirteen received treatment with psychoactive medication. Criteria for alcohol and drug addiction or misuse were met by over 90 percent of this sample. Personality disorders were found in 80 percent and antisocial personality disorder in more than 60 percent (Langeveld and Melhus, 2004).

Participation in Policy Decisions at National, Regional, Provincial, District, State, and Local Levels

The Norwegian health care system is democratic. Elected bodies make the decisions about the mental health budgets and programs, either in the Parliament or in local councils. Professionals and "users" have an impact on decision-making through boards and advisory groups. The Directorate of Health, the professional body, also has an impact on the decision-making as a legal authority and an advisory body to central authorities, municipalities, Regional Health Authorities and voluntary organizations.

Policy decisions are made on different levels. The Government makes proposals concerning the country's mental health policy, sets and administers the overall budget. New policies, general principles and laws for the services are passed to the Parliament for approval. The Regional Health Authorities implement policy decisions at the regional level through the health enterprises within the limits set by law, regulations, and the budget. The health enterprises and the Regional Health Authorities also have boards, consisting of professionals, elected representatives and the authorities on different levels.

The elected bodies in the municipalities responsible for the primary care and for making the decisions decide about the budget and how much resources/ money is allocated to the mental health services. The municipality council is the local "parliament." There are also elected boards for the services in the municipality, made up of patients, professionals and representatives elected by the inhabitants. The politicians in the Parliament and in the local council have the formal power to change the policy and programs for the mental health system. Nevertheless, their decisions and legislation are influenced by professionals, patients, patients' organizations and the general discussion regarding mental health services.

Population Relevance: Meeting the Needs

Whether the mental health system is providing sufficient and appropriate services to decrease the "treatment gap" between identified needs and patients actually treated is not an easy question to answer in a straightforward way. Needs are influenced by both the prevalence of mental disorders and by the capacity of the services and their marketing themselves. Demands increase as a function of the increased supply of mental health services.

A crucial question related to meeting population needs is how many people with mental disorders should ideally be given care and treatment by the primary care sector versus the specialized services? No such number or percentage has been given in Norway, and therefore questions about sufficient or appropriate capacity in total are hard to answer.

More important is the question if the services are adequate for special groups of patients, and especially for the one percent to two percent of the population with severe disorders. These patients are given high priority in all written documents affirming the aims of the National Mental Health Program (NMHP). However, the Programme has been criticized for paying most attention to people with mild disorders and who can be treated either in outpatient clinics or with a short inpatient stay in the DPC or a hospital. The severely disordered patients who need to be treated for years have not received improved services to the same degree. They need a lot of attention and more personnel and other resources outside and inside the institutions, for long periods of time, and they do not fit into the modern services preoccupied with enhanced productivity. In fact, these patients often reduce "productivity" when the criteria is the number of patients treated per time-unit or man-year, or when the criteria of successful treatment is increased functionality and reduced symptoms in a short run.

Other Optional Criteria

We have addressed the six major evaluation criteria that provide the structure for this evaluation section: Access and equity, quality and efficacy, cost and efficiency, financing and fairness, protection and participation, and population relevance. We wish to add a few more criteria of a good mental health system: (a) it provides a theoretical foundation for community-based, psychosocial services, (b) it is based upon the psychosocial processes of "turning points" in patients' lives and in the process of recovery; (c) it expresses an inclusive vision of mental health work versus a more exclusive neurobiological practice of medical psychiatry; and (d) it encourages psychologists and other mental health specialists to function as general mental health practitioners in the primary health care system.

A Theoretical Foundation for Community-Based, Psychosocial Services

Establishing mental health services tells people something about how to deal with their problems and how to conceive the causes of their distress, suffering, and reduced life quality: it has something to do with their own way of behaving, their emotions, cognitions, body or brain. Contemporary mental health systems give high priority to the diagnosis of individuals with an emphasis upon dysfunctions in the person's brain or body. Even social or living problems are personalized and conceptualized as a failure of the biological body. Consequently, the services communicate directly and indirectly that to get rid of the suffering, disorders and problems, people have to be treated individually. They must be given a diagnosis, and obtain medication, or individual psychotherapy for their distress which is construed as a psychiatric disorder or even a mental illness. This medical model has been the treatment ideology in psychiatry for several decades.

Moreover, the indications for treatment and care have been extended. Today, the great majority of those demanding care and treatment do not have severe disorders like schizophrenia; rather, they suffer from depression, anxiety, neurosis, eating disorders, posttraumatic stress disorders, or phobias. Many patients are also diagnosed with personality disorders.

The mental health system itself has therefore *constructed* a specific way to comprehend life problems, mood disorders, mood states, cognitive dysfunctions and deviant behavior in general. Even normal mood swings and existential concerns are constructed as mental disorders inside the individual, a dysfunction of the brain, or even as an illness.

The mental health services have contributed to the view that psychological dysfunction or distress are disorders or illnesses in need of (medical) treatment. Ordinary life problems have been relabeled as "abnormal" or "illnesses," hence they need professional treatment. The professions themselves have been eager to promote such perceptions and attitudes, for obvious self-serving reasons: they make their living by providing services to people who ask for help. Malfunctioning and mood swings are, however, normal occurrences for everybody at some times in their life, and do not necessarily constitute an illness that can be cured by medication or psychotherapy.

A society marked by increased competition also places heavy burdens on every single individual, and also produces increasing numbers of outsiders that are pressed away from the productive spheres. The number of people on disability pension has increased dramatically in recent years. Today about 10 percent of the labour force between 17 and 67 years of age receive disability pension because of an illness, and about one-third or 100,000 of these are diagnosed with a psychiatric illness.

In western societies, including Norway, people have become more socially isolated and even lonely as a result of cultural and social developments. Most people do not live in an extended family as was common a hundred years ago. The stability of the society also made people stable: they lived in the same neighborhood, in the same house, had the same job, the same wife or husband all their life. Today this is not the rule, but the exception. People do not have the same stability in their lives. They are moving geographically and socially, changing jobs and careers. They do not live with their extended family, and a significant percentage divorce and/or remarry. Peoples' lives are, in general, more unstable and the feeling of a social identity, of a "we," a sense of belongingness to other people, has been disrupted.

A consequence of this increased isolation is that people do not have close relatives or people with whom to talk, or to take care of them when emotions and mood disorders become difficult and disturbing. The mental health services have become a substitute for extended family and close relationships. By offering and promoting the services in the neighborhood, with easy access for everybody, the professional services become the obvious and acceptable surrogate for progressively more people having problems in their daily life. When people suffer psychological distress and ask for help more frequently than previously observed, it is therefore partly a result of changed sociocultural and living conditions, and partly a result of the increased treatment supplied with a particular content.

A vital question is where to draw the demarcation line between the health service's responsibilities and those of other sectors and institutions in the welfare system. Wage inequality, unemployment, poverty, increased job demands, and an inadequate social network comprise risk factors which increase the incidence of sickness, injuries and social problems. The issue is whether dealing with everyday problems and crises is a responsibility of the mental health service, whether other sectors should be better equipped to prevent the development of these problems and how far the responsibility of the public sector should extend.

When patients are no longer treated and cared for in bed-institutions, but cared for and treated in the community, there is need for another theoretical basis for the mental health services than the one established in the institutions and based on medical psychiatry. The professional staff is not always accustomed to practice in a new kind of community and cooperative services, outside the institutions. There is a general lack of "ideology" or theory for this new kind of mental health services in the community. Increased funding is not sufficient to deal with this issue. It is essential that the new structures, services and facilities are accompanied and supported by a coherent, comprehensive and suitable treatment and care ideology, representing and defining the new kind of services.

The psychiatric hospital or asylum was formerly the definitive centre for patient care and treatment. Services were concentrated in the institutions, especially the hospitals, and hospitals were the settings for administration, treatment, training and research. This was at least a coherent organizational form. The treatment ideology was based on a medical perspective and a diagnostic culture. The patient had a psychiatric *illness*, which could be diagnosed and treated by *the medical profession*. The mental hospital was a closed institution with unmistakable borders. Those inside were ill or disordered, and those outside were healthy and not in need of treatment, at least not for the time being. This has changed dramatically. Presently, 15–20 percent of the population is considered as actual or potential patients, and very few of them are hospitalized. The "patients" reside throughout Norway, and the majority does not want to stay in an institution. They prefer to live in the community, in their own home while they are patients in the mental health services. According to the patients' rights to be heard and participate, most of them should be given this opportunity.

Disagreements and different views among professionals within the services as to how the treatment process should be organized have to be assumed. The medical doctors and psychiatrists are *not* expected to have the same leading role as they did in the hospitals. The community services are characterized by a fluidity of structure, different from that of the hospital. The looser structure and paucity of rigid rules give the staff the freedom to focus on clients' needs and to realize a major NMHP aim: user participation. Yet, many of the professionals working within the new kind of services developed their expertise within the old institutions. Mental health professionals have typically been trained to function in well-established, structured agencies, not in innovative, loosely structured organizations that are still in the process of defining their purposes and groping for realistic means to accomplish their idealistic aims. Consequently, some mental health specialists have difficulty adapting to another model of service delivery.

The complicated process of establishing a professional identity is made more difficult by the fact that the whole ideology of community mental health care has gained recognition only recently, and is meaningfully incorporated by only a few. The contrast between the experience developed in the mental hospitals dealing with severe and "chronic" disorders and the demands emanating from the open chain system with other groups of patients has contributed to confusion with respect to the roles the staff is expected to perform. This has been particularly difficult for the psychiatrists. A concept of mental disorders that includes a wide variety of social and psychological causes automatically challenges specialized professions. This conflict is among others described in several autobiographical narratives written by psychiatrists and other physicians (Pollock, 2000).

The development of psychotropic drugs in the 1950s opened new opportunities for the medical professions in the area of psychiatric health care, and did not threaten the hegemony of physicians and medical doctors. On the contrary, those professionals were responsible for the introduction and application of this treatment. Community psychiatry and the psychosocial paradigm were however, met by skepticism and even resistance from fractions within the psychiatric establishment. The physician's educational background differs from that of the psychologist and social worker, a factor that works to the detriment of effective cooperation in areas of overlapping concern. The change from a medical to a social and psychological perspective on treatment and care make psychiatrists question their qualification to perform in the new services. It takes them into areas they do not know as professionals, and where their medical knowledge is of little use. Community care involves a fundamental shift from treating "illness" in medical institutions to develop chains of activities and different functions in the communities, in a fluid structure, an open system without definite borders.

Today, medical doctors and psychiatrists feel threatened in a mental health service that treats patients outside the hospitals, in cooperation with other health professionals, social workers and community agencies. The patients themselves do not necessarily ask for treatment of an illness, but for a better life, a strengthened self, to acquire the ability to "realize themselves," and also a job, a home for themselves with service from the community and help to establish a better social network.

The NMHP describes the person with psychiatric disorders not solely as a patient, but as a human being with a body, a soul and spirit, also comprehending existential questions. The patients' own needs should be the point of departure for all treatment, and the core for all nursing. The paternalism in psychiatry does not work any more. The content of the mental health services has changed and broadened through recruiting new groups of patients who demand to be heard and who want to tell the professionals what they need to increase their "quality of life." The professional ideology and the theoretical platform has to be changed accordingly. Community care has to be taken as a point of departure, based in a radical way on "user participation," the new slogan in mental health services. But at the universities and in the academia the wind seems to blow in the opposite direction.

It is a paradox that when the mental health services are moving into the community and the patients as well as the professionals are aware of the importance of the patient's everyday life and their social relationships, psychiatric medicine and also clinical psychology at the universities are developing in the opposite direction by putting more emphasis on what is going on inside the patient's brain or body. Neurobiology as the mainstream "paradigm" for psychiatry and clinical psychology is today more "popular," and has a higher academic prestige than psychosocial approaches wherein the patient is seen as a person — part of a culture and dependent on the social environment. What goes on inside the body, and especially in the brain, seems to be the point of departure to understand, explain and treat psychiatric disorders among the university-educated treatment professions these days. The consumption of psychopharmaca therefore also increases:

> Total consumption of psychopharmaceuticals in psychiatric hospitals increased by 29% over the period 1991–2000. The use of antidepressants increased by 234%, hypnotics/tranquillisers by 134% and mood stabilisers by 77%, while the use of antipsychotics decreased by 19% and antiparkinsonian drugs by 49%. (Rytter and Håberg, 2003)

Too little emphasis is put on the social, cultural, or even psychological functions in the neurobiological tradition of psychiatry. Therefore, other professions with a three-year university college education, like nurses and social workers, have been popular in the services established outside the hospitals and wards. Their number increases rapidly in the new mental health work, to the detriment of the number of psychiatrists.

Psychosocial Processes in Turning Points and the Recovery Process

An appreciation for the psychosocial variables can be gained from our understanding of the "turning points" in patients' lives and the psychosocial process of recovery.

Turning Points. In a survey of more than 1,000 patients who received mental health services in Norway, the patients were asked if they could tell stories about positive turning points and negative experiences. Three-hundred and eighty (380) people responded to the question about telling a turning-point story (Kogstad, 2002).

What patients describe as a positive turning point seems to be an event that pointed to positive opportunities in their daily living. Three main dimensions was mentioned by the patients: (a) receiving help to function in daily life; (b) practical assistance, caring, and help to master and handle emotions and be able to go back to normal life, and (c) the experience of freedom wherein the person grows in self-acceptance and insight, experiences relief, and gains the ability to explore, develop, and fully utilize one's own personal resources. Three-fourths of the informants reported turning points that belong to these dimensions. Nevertheless, medications and some sort of instrumental-practical help seem to play a modest role in a minority of clients' turning point experiences. For the majority however, turning points are associated with a dimension of meaning, created by the help of supporting environments that facilitate insight, self-acceptance and the working-through process. Additional contributing factors to positive turning points are encouraging, supportive people, long-lasting relationships, and certainly the basic necessities of food, shelter, and clothing. With such support, individuals can gain increased control over their lives, personal power, a sense of self, and meaning or purpose in life, more satisfying relationships, and the ability to contribute in a community (Spaniol et al. 2002). These results are consistent with literature describing recovery as a process of self-discovery, renewal and transformation that involves adjustment of attitudes, feelings, perceptions, beliefs, roles and goals in life (Spaniol, et al. 2002; Davidson and Strauss, 1992; Mead and Copeland 2000). The outcome may not be full recovery, freedom and a new life, but an increased ability to function satisfactorily and to manage life outside the hospital.

The Recovery Process. Experiences from different services illustrate that support, encouragement, confirmation, safety, continuity and reflection upon life events cannot be taken for granted. Nevertheless, in a setting where clients do not expect this obligingness, but still experience kindness, this may serve as a starting point towards recovery, marked by a sense of value and acceptance. To start a recovery process one should focus not only on phases and clients' readiness, but also on environmental factors, and especially those that create a sense of value, safety, acceptance and confirmation.

Borg and Kristiansen (2004) explored helping relationships from the perspective of service recipient experiences. The 15 informants were service users with lived experiences of severe mental illness, the majority diagnosed with schizophrenia. Certain common factors about helpful relationships were identified. Service users valued professionals who conveyed hope, shared power, were available when needed, were open regarding the diversity in what helps, and were willing to stretch the boundaries of what is considered the "professional" role. Recovery-oriented professionals were those who had the courage to deal with the complexities and the individuality of the change process, and were able to use their professional skills and expertise in a collaborative partnership with the service user. A recovery-orientation in professionals also involves the willingness and ability to shape services to the needs and preferences of each individual service user.

It is a challenge to organize services in such a way that they can contribute to recovery and a better life for more people. To obtain this, it seems to be of great importance to include clients' experiences and competence in goal-setting, planning and clinical decisions.

From Medical Psychiatry to Mental Health Work: New Concepts

Since the first half of the nineteenth century the deviant and "mad" subpopulation was taken care of by the medical profession. Calling the asylums *psychiatric hospitals* underscored the dominance of the medical specialty *psychiatry*. During the twentieth century, the terms "psychiatry" and "psychiatric services" designated what today are called the *mental health services*. "Mental health work" is used today as a concept for what was earlier labeled *"psychiatric treatment."* Another reason for this change in terminology is to underline that what is needed is not so much the knowledge of a medical speciality, but a combined and multiprofessional effort to help patients to get work or a meaningful activity, a place to live, and to increase their social network and social relations to get a decent life outside the institutions.

Psychologists as General Practitioners in the Primary Health Care System

The mental health services in Norway are expected to function as a *chain* of continuous care, wherein the different parts cooperate in a smooth manner. Patients can move back and forth along the chain of services depending on their needs for treatment and care at the moment. A chain is no better than its weakest links, and there are still some weak elements in the mental health system in Norway. One of them is the very first professional part, the general practitioners who are medical doctors. Patients often contact their personal GP when they have mental health problems and the GPs frequently become the patient's first contact with the health services. Many patients treated in the specialist mental health services are referred by the GPs. They also prescribe most of the medication for minor psychiatric disorders like anxiety and depression. The GPs therefore have had an important role in the chain of services. They are however, not very well-integrated into the mental health system at the present time, and they are hardly mentioned in the National Mental Health Programme. It is expected that the health authorities will make efforts to improve the coordination between the GPs and the mental health services in the future. Over several decades great investments have been made in building up publicly-supported somatic health facilities at the local level, and the medical doctor has been given responsibility for the primary care. Generally, psychologists have been considered as "second-line" health personnel, to be called upon by "first-line" health personnel when they encounter problems beyond their own level of competence. It sounds reasonable from this point of view to improve the integration of the general physicians into the mental health services.

Another option would be to develop comparable mental health facilities at the local level, due to the massive demand, and accepting that important differences exist between physical and mental disorders. The medical doctors, focusing primarily on illnesses in the body, are not necessarily the most qualified to deal with mental disorders. To increase the number of "general" or municipal psychologists in the local communities and in the primary care could therefore be a better option. One justification for psychologists as a general practitioner for the mental health field is that it is

> . . . generally agreed that most GPs (general medical practitioners) have neither the training nor the time adequately to deal with psychological problems. Their

frequent efforts to do so are expensive both in terms of their own time and the cost to the Health Service.... (McPherson and Feldman, 1977)

Not to have psychological expertise in the first-line of the health and social services is a costly and not a very rational solution, considering the prevalence and new character of the mental health problems today and the extensive demand for help on a low level of intervention. Routh et al. (1983) has formulated the arguments in this way:

> ... psychological consultation in primary care settings may well reduce the inappropriate overutilization of medical services ... when such consultation is available, psychological problems are quickly recognized as such. Many problems can thus be successfully dealt with in brief consultation with the psychologist, avoiding the need for other health care personnel to spend expensive time with patients unnecessarily. In other cases, appropriate referrals can quickly be made.... As far as taxpayers are concerned, the strongest argument for adding psychological services to universal primary health care ... is the likelihood that services will become less expensive. (p. 97)

Christiansen, Iversen, and Stephansen (1983) have taken the argument of cost-effectiveness further. They call attention to a deficiency of the primary health system today, namely that the professional agencies, and especially the General Practitioners (GPs) are not qualified to provide better help than the informal helpers in the local community. They hold onto people instead of offering necessary, appropriate, and qualified treatment. A consequence of this is that emotional problems get somaticized, treated by medication, because the emotional and cognitive dysfunctions are transformed into a modality of expression congruent with the general practitioners' concerns and knowledge. Consequently, by handling pseudo-problems, the GPS to some extent impede more than facilitate proper solutions.

To further improve the quality of the public services for people suffering from mental disorders and distress in Norway it is necessary to give priority to specialized and long-term treatment, care and assistance to people with severe disorders, and also to establish low-threshold services in the communities based on general practitioners with psychological knowledge.

REFERENCES

http://www.ks.no/upload/47468/nasjonal_arsrapport_no_2_003.pdf

http://www.nordictelemed.org/papers/1

http://www.samdata.sintef.no/?p=psykisk_helsevern/sektorrapport_psyk_helse.htm

Alnæs, R. (1996). *Psykoanalysen – mellom psykiatri og psykologi.* Høyskoleforlaget As. Norwegian Academic Press.

Andersen, T. (1978). *Ill Health in Two Contrasting Communities* (Ph.D Thesis.). Tromsø: University of Tromsø.

Ayuso-Mateos, J.L., Vazquez-Barquero, J.L., Dowrick, C., Lehtinen, V., Dalgard, O.S., Casey, P., Wilkinson, C., Lasa, H., Page, H., Dunn, G., Wilkinson, G., & the ODIN Group (2001). Depressive disorders in Europe: Prevalence figures from the ODIN study. *British Journal of Psychiatry 179,* 308–316.

Beck, A.T., Steer, R.A., & Garbin, M.G. (1988). Psychometric properties of the Beck Depression Inventory: Twenty-five years of evaluation. *Clinical Psychology Review 8*(1), 77–100.

Bentsen, B.G. (1970). *Illness and general practice.* Oslo: Universitetsforlaget.

Berg, J.E., & Johnsen, J.E. (2004). Are admission rates to acute psychiatric care higher for immigrants from non-Western countries than for the traditional Norwegian population? *Tidsskr Nor Lægeforen 124,* 634–6.

Bjørngaard, J.H. (2002). *SAMDATA Psykisk helsevern* [SAMDATA Mental health Services]. Report 1/02, Trondheim: SINTEF Unimed.

Borg, M., & Kristiansen, K. (2004). Recovery-oriented professionals: Helping relationships in mental health services. *Journal of Mental Health 13*(5), 493–505.

Christiansen, B., Iversen, B., & Stephansen, M. (1983). Psykologtjenesten i kommunene. Fremvekst, evaluering, fremtidsperspektiver. [Psychological services in the municipalities. Development, evaluation and perspectives for the future]. *Tidsskrift for Norsk Psykologforening.* Monografiserien; Nr. 9.

Dalgard O.S. (1980). *Bomiljø og psykisk helse.* [Housing environment and mental health]. Oslo: Universitetsforlaget.

Dalgard, O.S. (2002). Psykiatrisk epidemiologi i Norge – et historisk tilbakeblikk. [Psychiatric Epidemiology in Norway – A historical retrospect]. *Norsk Epidemiologi 12*(3), 163–172.

Dalgard, O.S., Kringlen, E., & Dahl, A.A. (2002). Psykiatrisk epidemiologi. [Psychiatric Epidemiology]. *Norsk Epidemiologi 12*(3), 161–162.

Davidson, L., & Strauss, J.S. (1992). Sense of self in recovery from severe mental illness. *British Journal of Medical Psychology 65*, 131–145.

Derogatis, L.R., Lipman, R.S., Rickels, K., Uhlenhuth, E.H., & Covi, L. (1974). The Hopkins Symptom Checklist (HSCL): A self-report symptom inventory. *Behavioral Science 19*, 1–15.

Ekeland, T.J. (1999). Evidensbasert behandling; kvalitetssikring eller instrumentalistisk mistak. [Evidencebased treatment; quality assurance or instrumentalistic failure]. *Tidsskrift for Norsk Psykologforening 36*, 1036–1048.

Engedal, K. (2002). Diagnostikk og behandling av demens. [Diagnostic work-up and treatment of dementia]. *Tidsskr Nor Lægeforen 122*, 520-4.

Goffman, E. (1961). *Asylums. Essays on the social situation of mental patients and other inmates.* New York: Doubleday-Anchor.

Hagen, H. (1992). *Pasienter i psykiatriske institusjoner 1. november 1989* [Patients in psychiatric institutions November 1 1989]. Report 6/92. Trondheim: SINTEF/NIS.

Hagen, H. (1997). *Pasienter i psykiatriske institusjoner 1. november 1994* [Patients in psychiatric institutions November 1 1994]. Report 97. Trondheim: SINTEF/NIS.

Hagen, H. (2001). *Pasienter i psykisk helsevern for voksne [Patients in the mental health services for adults]* Report 5/01. Trondheim: SINTEF Unimed Helsetjenesteforskning.

Hagen, H. (Ed.). (2003). *Opptrappingsplanen for Psykisk Helse – Status etter fire år* [The National Mental Health Programme – Status After Four Years]. Report 3/03. Trondheim: SINTEF/Helse.

Hagen, H., & Ruud, T. (2004). *Pasienter i psykisk helsevern for voksne 20. november 2003.* [Patients in the mental health services for adults November 20th 2003]. Rapport 3/04. Trondheim: SINTEF/Helse.

Halsteinli, V. (1998). Nasjonale utviklingstrekk i BUP [Development in BUP]. In H. Hagen (Ed.) *Psykiatritjenesten - på rett veg?* Trondheim: SINTEF/Unimed, pp. 81–99.

Halsteinli, V., Magnussen, J., & Kittelsen, S.A.C. (2001). Scale, efficiency and organization in Norwegian psychiatric outpatient clinics for children. *Journal of Mental Health Policy and Economics 4*(2), 79–90.

Halsteinli, V., Magnussen, J., & Kittelsen, S.A.C. (2003). *Productivity growth in Norwegian psychiatric outpatient clinics. A panel data analysis of the period 1996–2001.* Health Economics, Research Programme at the University of Oslo.

Hartvig, P., & Østberg, B. (2004). Psykisk lidelse og avvik blant norske fengselsinnsatte [Prevalence of psychiatric disorders among inmates in Norwegian prisons: estimates given by different vocational groups]. *Tidsskr Nor Lægeforening 124*, 2091–2093.

Hatling, T., Krogen, T., & Ulleberg, P. (2002). Compulsory admissions to psychiatric hospitals in Norway – International comparisons and regional variations. *Journal of Mental Health 11*(6), 623–34.

Helse- og omsorgsdepartementet, *Statsbudsjettet*, St.prp.1, 2005. Oslo: Author.

Hjort, H. (2000/2003). *Ideer i norsk psykoterapi. Utviklinglinjer og brytninger.* [Ideas in Norwegian psychotherapy]. Oslo: Unipub forlag.

Hordvin, O. (2004). *Narkotikasituasjonen i Norge 2003.* [The narcotics situation in Norway]. Oslo: Statens institutt for rusmiddelforskning.

Hubble, M.A., Duncan, B.I., & Miller, S.D. (1999). *The heart & soul of change.* Washington D.C: American Psychological Association.

Husby, R., Østberg, B., & Hartvig, P. (2003). Får psykiatriske pasienter behandling på riktig omsorgsnivå? [Bed-blockers: A cross sectional study of three psychiatric departments]. *Tidsskr Nor Lægeforen 123*, 1178–1180.

Johannessen, J.O. (2002). Schizophrenia – incidence and significance. *Tidsskr Nor Lægeforen 122*, 2011–2014.

Kogstad, R. (2002). Vendepunkt – byggesteiner i bedrings-presenter (Turning points – components in the recovery process). *Tidsskrift for psykisk helsearbeid 1*(4), 41–49.

Kolstad, A. (1983). *Til diskusjon om sammenhengen mellom sosiale forhold og psykiske strukturer. En epidemiologisk undersøkelse blant barn og unge* [An epidemiological study of children and adolescents]. (Ph.D Thesis). Aalborg: Universitetet i Aalborg.

Kringlen, E., Torgersen, S., & Cramer, V. (2001). A Norwegian psychiatric epidemiological study. *Am J Psychiatry 158*, 1091–1098.

Lambert, M.J. (1992). Implications of Outcome Research for Psychotherapy Integration. In J.C. Norcross & M.R. Goldfried (eds.). *Handbook of psychotherapy intergration.* New York: Basic.

Langeveld, H., & Melhus, H. (2004). Blir psykiske lidelser i fengsel fanget opp av helsetjenesten? [Are psychiatric disorders identified and treated by in-prison health services?]. *Tidsskr Nor Lægeforening 124*, 2094–2097.

Lavigne, J.V., Gibbons, R.D., Christoffel, K.K., et al., (1996). Prevalence rates and correlates of psychiatric disorders among preschool children. *Journal of the American Academy of Child & Adolescent Psychiatry 35*, 204–214.

Lavik, N.J. (1976). *Ungdoms mentale helse.* [Adolescents mental health]. Oslo: Universitetsforlaget.

Lien, L. (2002). Are readmission rates influenced by how psychiatric services are organized? *Nordic Journal of Psychiatry 56*(1), 23–28.

Løchen, Y. (1965). *Idealer og realiteter i et psykiatrisk sykehus.* [Ideals and realities in a psychiatric hospital]. Oslo:Universitetsforlaget.

McPherson, I.G., & Feldman, M.P. (1977). A preliminary investigation of the role of the clinical psychologist in the primary care setting. *Bulletin of British Psychological Society 30*, 242–246.

Mead, S., & Copeland, M.E. (2000). What recovery means to us: Consumers' perspective. *Community Mental Health Journal 36*, 315–328.

Moum, T., Falkum, E., Tambs, K., & Vaglum, P. (1991). Sosiale bakgrunnsfaktorer og psykisk helse. In T. Moum (ed) *Helse i Norge. Sykdom, livsstil og bruk av helsetjenester.* Oslo: Gyldendal, pp. 47–63.

Norwegian Act on Health Enterprises (Lov 2001-06-15-93 om helseforetak m.m. helseforetaksloven) [in Norwegian only]. (http://www.lovdata.no/all/nl-20010615-093.html)

Norwegian Ministry of Health and Care Services (2005). *Mental health services in Norway. Prevention – treatment – care*. Oslo: Author.

Øgar, B. (1981). *Pasienter i psykiatriske institusjoner 1. november 1979* [Patients in psychiatric institutions November 1. 1979]. Report 5/81, Trondheim: SINTEF/NIS.

Øgar, B., Kolstad, A., & Kindseth, O. (1986). *Pasienter i psykiatriske institusjoner 1. november 1984* [Patients in psychiatric institutions November 1. 1984]. Report 5/86, Trondheim: SINTEF/NIS.

Pedersen, P.B. (1999). Theories on the de-institutionalization of psychiatric services: Does politics matter? Paper at the *7th National Conf. in Political Science*, January, 1999, Røros, Norway.

Pollock, D. (2000). Physician Autobiography: Narrative and the Social History of Medicine. In: C. Mattingly & L. Garro (ed.) *Narrative and the cultural construction of illness and healing*. University of California Press.

Rosenvinge, B.H., & Rosenvinge, J.H. (2003). "Prevalence of depression in the elderly: A review of the literature from 1990 to 2001." *Tidsskr Nor Lægeforen 123*, 928–9.

Routh, D.K., et al. (1983). Psychology and primary health care for children. *American Psychologist 38*, 95–98.

Rytter, E., & Håberg, M. (2003). Drug consumption in Norwegian psychiatric hospitals *Tidsskr Nor Lægeforen 123*, 768–71.

Sandanger, I., Nygård, J.F., Ingebrigtsen, G., Sørensen, T., & Dalgard, O.S. (1999). Prevalence, incidence rate and age at onset of psychiatric disorders in Norway. *Soc Psychiatry Psychiatr Epidemiol 34*, 570–579.

Sandanger, I. (2003). Changes in incidence rates of depression during the 1990-2000 period. Paper presented at 27th Nordic Psychiatric Congress. Promoting psychiatric care, 13-16 August, 2003. Abstract in: *The Icelandic Medical Journal, Fylgirit, 48*.

Scheff, T.J. (1966). *Being mentally ill: A sociological theory*. Chicago: Aldine.

Seip, Å.A. (2004). Private Initiative for Public Health – The Emergence of Child Psychiatry in Post-War Norway. In A. Andersen, K.T. Elvebakken & W.H. Hubbard (eds.). *Public health and preventive medicine 1800–2000. Knowledge, co-operation, and conflict*, Rokkansenteret, Report 1, pp. 97–103.

Sosial- og helsedepartementet (1997). *St. Meld. 25 (1996–97): Åpenhet og helhet. Om psykiske lidelser og tjenestetilbudene*. [Openness and comprehensiveness. Psychiatric disorders and the mental health services]. Oslo: Ministry of Health and Social Affairs.

Sosial- og helsedepartementet (1998). *St Prp 63 (1997–98): Om opptrappingsplanen for psykisk helse*. [National Programme for Mental Health]. Oslo: Ministry of Health and Social Affairs.

Spaniol, L., Wewiorski, N., Gagne, C., & Anthony, W.A. (2002). The process of recovery from schizophrenia. *International Review of Psychiatry 14*, 327–336.

Tranøy, J. (1990). *Forfalskningen av lobotomiens historie på Gaustad sykehus* [The falsification of the history of lobotomy at Gaustad Hospital]. Oslo: Institutt for kriminologi og strafferett, Universitetet i Oslo, Stensilserien nr. 64.

Tranøy, J. (1992). *Lobotomi i skandinavisk psykiatri*, [Lobotomy in Scandinavian Psychiatry]. Oslo: Institutt for kriminologi og strafferett, Universitetet i Oslo - KS-serien nr. 1.

Tranøy, J., & Blomberg, W. (2005). Lobotomy in Norwegian psychiatry. *History of Psychiatry 16*(1), 107–10.

Wampold, B.E. (2001). *The great psychotherapy debate. Models, methods, and findings*. New Jersey: Lawrence Erlbaum Associates.

World Health Organization (1992). *International statistical classification of diseases and related health problems, ICD-10, Volume1 (Revision 1996)*. Geneva: WHO.

World Health Organization (1993). *Composite international diagnostic interview (CIDI) Version 1.1*. Geneva: WHO.

World Health Organization (1994). *Schedules for clinical assessment in neuropsychiatry, Version 2.0. Manual*. Geneva: WHO.

Chapter 4

HEALTH AND MENTAL HEALTH IN CANADA

JOHN L. ARNETT

PART ONE: DESCRIPTION OF THE MENTAL HEALTH SYSTEM

Introduction

Geography and Demographics

With a landmass of approximately 10 million square kilometers (km) (3.85 million square miles), Canada is the second largest country in the world, second only to Russia in size. Greatest distance East-West is 5,187km (3,223 miles); North-South is 4,627km (2,875 miles). Including its mainland and islands, Canada's coastline is about 244,000km (151,500 miles). Elevations range from sea level to 5,950 meters (19,520 feet) at Mount Logan (*The World Book Encyclopedia*, 1980, v. 3, p. 87).

Thirty-two million people live in Canada's ten provinces and three territories. This yields an extremely low population density of approximately three individuals per square kilometer. Ninety percent of Canada's total population lives within 100 miles (160 kilometers) of the 4,000 mile-long border with the northern-most U.S. states (*CIA – The World Factbook*, 2004). There are vast areas unpopulated or with very sparse population, separated by great distances in Canada. While Canada is a highly urbanized nation (about 80% of the population live in urban centers of 10,000 people), a substantial number of Canadians live in rural and relatively remote regions of the country. This makes rural health initiatives particularly important in Canada.

Canada is ethnically, culturally, religiously, and linguistically quite diverse. Indeed, Canada fosters respect for diversity and as a matter of public policy attempts to make its health services sensitive and responsive to these differences among Canadians. Canada's rich multicultural heritage is reflected in the fact that people from more than 200 different ethnic origins were identified in the 2001 Canadian census (Statistics Canada, 2001a). Visible minorities constitute over 13 percent of Canada's population with the single largest visible minority group being Chinese. The proportion of visible minorities in the Canadian population has nearly tripled since 1981 when this group constituted only about 4.7 percent of Canada's population.

Historically, most of Canada's immigrants have been of European descent. However, most new immigration to Canada is from Asian countries. This shift over the last 40 years has largely resulted from immigration patterns related to Canada's immigration policies and international events (Statistics Canada, 2001a).

The 2001 Canadian Census (Statistics Canada, 2001b) reported that between 1996–2001 Canada's population growth rate was only four percent and that immigration accounted for more than 50 percent of this population growth. While Canada's population growth rate exceeded that of Italy, Germany, Japan, the United Kingdom, and France, it trailed the population growth rates of the United States, Australia, and Mexico as well as the overall world population growth rate of about seven percent. When Canada's population growth rate is considered in the context of its aging population, the growing importance of immigration becomes apparent.

Like many other countries, Canada's population is aging and at present half the population is over 38 years of age. In 1966, Canada's median age was just over 25 years. In terms of median age, Canadians are older than residents of the United States and Russia but younger than citizens of Japan, Germany, and Italy. In 2001, Canadians aged 45–64 accounted for about 25 percent of Canada's total population and by 2011 this age cohort is expected to increase to approximately 33 percent of Canada's population.

Canada's fertility rate, which is the average number of children that women aged 15–49 will have in their lifetime, was 1.5 in 2002. This compared with a fertility rate 2.0 in the United States, 1.9 in France, 1.6 in the United Kingdom, 1.4 in Germany, 1.3 in Japan, and 1.2 in Italy at the same point in time. In 2002, the number of live births per 1000 population in Canada dropped to 10.5 (328,802 babies born). This was the lowest rate since 1921 when vital statistics began being collected nationally in Canada. Furthermore, the birth rate in Canada has declined more than 25 percent over the last 10 years alone. Thus, indications are that this trend is likely to continue into the future. If Canada's population is to grow more rapidly in the future it will likely have to occur through immigration, which also will impact the nature of the health and mental health services that must be provided.

Language is a very important matter in Canada and immigration has made Canada a very linguistically diverse nation. While Canada is officially a bilingual country (French and English), in 2001 approximately two-thirds of the population was able to converse only in English while about 13 percent spoke only French. About 18 percent were bilingual and able to converse in both English and French while 1.5 percent spoke neither French nor English (Statistics Canada, 2001c). The language used in the workplace in Canada is predominantly English (77%), though 23 percent use French most often at work. While 70 percent of the people in Quebec use French most often at work, in the rest of Canada, English is overwhelmingly used most often at work (Statistics Canada, 2001d). A wide variety of Aboriginal languages were identified in the 2001 Canadian census, and other languages spoken by 225,000 people or more in Canada included Italian, Portuguese, Spanish, Polish, Arabic, Punjabi, Cantonese, Chinese, Hindi, and Tagalog (Filipino) (Statistics Canada, 2001e).

North American Indians, Métis, and Inuit are identified in the *Constitution Act*, 1982 as Canada's Aboriginal peoples. These groups of people form an important part of the multicultural mosaic of Canada. Approximately 1.3 million people reported having at least some Aboriginal ancestry in the 2001 Canadian census (Statistics Canada, 2001f), representing just over four percent of Canada's total population. However, this segment of the population is increasing at a faster rate than the overall Canadian average and hence their relative percentage of the total population will increase in the future. Consequently, culturally appropriate health services must be a significant factor in the development of health and mental health services.

The largest population gain among Aboriginal people was among the Métis who grew by 43 percent between 1996–2001. During this same period, the North American Indian population increased by 15 percent, and the Inuit population by 12 percent. The average age of Canada's Aboriginal population (25 years) is also much younger than the median age of non-Aboriginals (38 years). However, the Aboriginal population over 65 years increased by 40 percent between 1996–2001 while the non-Aboriginal population over age 65 increased by 10 percent during the same period.

The highest concentrations of Aboriginal people are in Canada's North and in the Prairie Provinces. Just under half (47%) of Canada's North American Indian population lived on Indian reserves in 2001. Metropolitan Winnipeg was home to the single largest number of North American Indians living in any metropolitan area in Canada. Nearly 70 percent of Canada's Métis lived in Canada's urban areas in 2001. Just over 7,000 lived on reserves, although the number living on reserves more than doubled in the time period from 1996–2001. Forty-five thousand Inuit, about half the population of this group, lived in Nunavut Territory in 2001. In fact, 85 percent of the population of Nunavut identified themselves as Inuit. At a median age of just under 21 years, the Inuit were the youngest of Canada's three official Aboriginal groups.

Although Canada is quite diverse in terms of religion, the majority of Canadians identify themselves predominately as Christians. Forty-three percent reported that they were Roman Catholic, the single largest religious group. The next single largest group identified themselves as Protestant (29%). However, nearly five million Canadians, 16 percent of Canada's population, reported no religious affiliation. Furthermore, the group reporting no religious affiliation grew significantly by 44 percent from 1991–2001. Muslims constituted about two percent of Canada's population, while the Jewish, Buddhist, Hindu, and Sikh populations each formed about one percent of Canada's population based on self-reported religious affiliation (Statistics Canada, 2001g).

Political System: A Constitutional Monarchy with Parliamentary Rule

Canada is a relatively young country in relation to its entry into the community of nations. Canada was created when Queen Victoria gave royal assent to the British North America Act (BNA) on March 29, 1867 (now renamed the Constitution Act of 1867). That Act came into effect on July 1, 1867 and established Canada as the self-governing Dominion of Canada within the British Empire. The BNA essentially served as Canada's constitution, granting more independence to Canada; however, foreign policy remained under British control and Canada's highest court of appeal remained the Judicial Committee of the British Privy Council. In addition, amendments to Canada's constitution had to be done in Britain. Canada did not become fully independent until 1931 with the passage of the *Statute of Westminster* in Britain. The Canadian constitution was not formally repatriated to Canada until 1982. On March 29, 1982 Queen Elizabeth II gave royal assent to the Canada Act 1982 and it was signed into law in Ottawa on April 17, 1982. With the passage of the Canada Act 1982, the United Kingdom revoked its right to issue further amendments to the Canadian constitution.

As a historical note, the Canada Act 1982 was imposed in spite of the fact that Quebec refused to ratify the Canadian constitution in 1982. The long delay in repatriating the Constitution was due at least in part to the inability of Canada's provinces to agree on a formula for amending the BNA. As part of the Constitution Act 1982, a Charter of Rights and Freedoms was enshrined in the Constitution to define and guarantee the personal rights and fundamental freedoms of Canadians. The delay in repatriating the Constitution is not only of historical interest; it is also important because it reflects the ongoing debates between the federal and provincial and territorial governments about issues of public policy and practice. Nowhere is the debate between levels of government more evident, and at times more acrimonious, than in public policy related to health matters. No doubt the spirited dynamics of the relationship between levels of government regarding health is fueled by the fact that about 40 percent of provincial government spending across Canada is currently consumed by health care costs. In Canada, 16.2 percent of the all government spending for the nation in 2001 was consumed by health care costs (WHO, 2004, Annex Table 5, p. 136).

Canada is governed as a federation in which the powers and responsibilities are divided between the federal government and 10 provincial governments (British Columbia, Alberta, Saskatchewan, Manitoba, Ontario, Quebec, New Brunswick, Prince Edward Island, Nova Scotia, and Newfoundland and Labrador). In contrast to the provinces, the three territorial governments (Northwest Territories, Nunavut, and Yukon Territory) are not sovereign units; their powers are delegated to them by the Parliament of Canada.

Federal Government. In spite of Canada's independence, Queen Elizabeth II remains Canada's official head of state, and she is represented within the federal government by the Governor General. In the provinces, a Lieutenant Governor represents the Queen in each province. Since federal legislation must receive the assent of the Governor General as the Queen's representative, Canada is a constitutional monarchy.

The Parliament of Canada is composed of (a) the House of Commons consisting of 301 members elected by Canadian citizens; (b) the Senate, currently consisting of 98 members who form the Upper House of Parliament, are appointed by the Governor General on the recommendation of the Prime Minister of Canada, and (c) a Governor General, who is effectively appointed by the Prime Minister with the ceremonial approval of Queen Elizabeth II. Elected members of the House of Commons play the leading role in forming and running the federal government of Canada, while the Senate is intended to study and make recommendations on economic and social issues of importance to Canadians. Although Senators are appointed and therefore do not participate in the electoral political process, typically they are aligned with one of the major political parties in Canada. With few exceptions, for federal legislation to become law there must be approval by the House of Commons, the Senate, and the Governor General.

The effective leader of the Government of Canada is the Prime Minister, although the Queen remains the official head of state. However, unlike the United States, in which citizens vote directly for the President as head of state, the leader of the political party that elects a majority of members to the House of Commons becomes the Prime Minister. Thus, Canadians do not vote directly for the Prime Minister. The leader of the political party with the second highest number of elected seats to the House of Commons typically becomes Leader of the Official Opposition. The Prime Minister selects a Cabinet from among the elected members of the majority party in the House of Commons and these members assume responsibility as Ministers of the government for the operation of the various federal government departments, including health.

Provincial and Territorial Governments. In addition to the federal government, Canada has provincial and territorial governments. *Provincial* governments are elected and function in an analogous manner to the federal system although they do not have a Senate. The leader of the provincial governing body is referred to as the Premier of the province. In order to become law, provincial legislation has to be approved by the provincial assembly and then by the Lieutenant Governor of the province as the Queen's provincial representative. *Territorial* governments elect territorial assemblies and function similarly to the federal and provincial governments. The leaders of the territorial assemblies, however, are referred to as Commissioners rather than as Premiers.

There is a noteworthy degree of ambiguity and overlap in relation to the shared responsibilities of the federal and provincial governments in many areas of vital interest to Canadians. However, the Canadian Constitution does specifically confer responsibility to the federal government for matters related to banking, criminal law, national defense, foreign affairs, and the postal system. Provincial governments have constitutional responsibility for civil justice, property, and municipal institutions. Both federal and provincial governments are involved in issues related to agriculture, transportation, communication, immigration, health and health services, social assistance, and the environment. Of particular interest in relation to the division of federal and provincial powers is the fact that in Canada criminal law is the sole responsibility of the federal government. Thus, issues related to competence to stand trial in relation to one's mental health status is under federal jurisdiction rather than provincial or territorial law.

Canada's Economy

Canada is an economically strong and relatively wealthy country. The basic monetary unit is the Canadian dollar (CDN). For 2003, the GDP for Canada had reached 1,199 billion CDN. Based on the 2003 exchange rate of 1.40, the GDP was US$856.6 billion. Per capita GDP was US$27,100 and per capita at current prices and purchasing power was US$30,500 (OECD, 2005). Canada's Gross Domestic Product (GDP) now exceeds one trillion Canadian dollars and its economy is among the world's 10 largest economies. It is a member of the G8, and its trading relationship with the United States produced two-way trade in goods and services that exceeded 441 billion Canadian dollars (US$315) in 2003, making this the largest international trading relationship in the world. In 2003, 20 percent of all U.S. exports went to Canada. In fact, Canada has been the single largest purchaser of U.S. exports since 1946. Canada is also the biggest customer for goods exported by 37 of the 50 U.S. States.

Canada is the single largest supplier of energy to the U.S., providing 88 percent of U.S. natural gas imports, 17 percent of its oil imports and nearly 100 percent of its electricity imports. Canada is the major provider of electricity to the New England states, New York, the upper Midwest, and the Pacific Northwest and California. In 2003, Canada supplied three times more energy to the U.S. than did Saudi Arabia. Total energy sales to the U.S. in 2003 exceeded 41 billion CDN (US$29.3 billion). These statistics reflect the large degree of economic integration between Canadian and U.S. Industries (Canadian Embassy, 2004).

Canada is a highly industrialized country. Following the Second World War, Canada experienced considerable growth in manufacturing, mining and the service sectors. This has transformed the nation from a rural to an industrial and urban economy. Approximately 69 percent of its GDP is derived from the provision of services and approximately 29 percent is composed of industry. Agriculture accounts for approximately two percent of Canada's GDP at the present time. Approximately four percent of the labor force is in service occupations, 15 percent in manufacturing, five percent in construction, and approximately three percent in agriculture and other occupations. Canada is energy independent and exports more oil and gas than it consumes. Canada is a substantial exporter of electricity, much of which is produced from hydroelectric generating plants.

Despite the current strength of Canada's economy, there are human resource issues that may affect both the health of the economy as well as the health of Canadians. The aging of the work force in Canada will likely result in a shortage of workers in a wide range of occupations over the next decade (Statistics Canada, 2001a). This includes not only professionals such as physicians and nurses but also skilled technical service providers such as electricians and plumbers. By 2011, 20 percent of Canadian baby boomers will be at least 61 years of age. Canada will have to rely nearly exclusively on immigration to fill various occupational positions. Consequently, facilitating the credentialing and certification processes for foreign-trained professionals and skilled trades, which now can be cumbersome and problematic, will be increasingly important to Canada's economy and the well-being of its population.

Cultural Values Expressed in Policies and Programs

The federal government sets and administers national principles for health care services. One very important vehicle for doing this is the *Canada Health Act of 1984*. This Act sets forth five basic principles, which express underlying cultural values that guide public policy. The principle of *universality* is intended to ensure that public health care insurance is provided to all Canadians on a uniform basis. The principle of *comprehensiveness* is meant to guarantee that all medically necessary hospital and physician services, including mental health services, as well as dental services that require hospitalization, are covered by public health care insurance. The principle of *accessibility* is meant to ensure that financial barriers (such as user charges) to the provision of publicly-funded medical and surgical-dental services are discouraged so that necessary services are available regardless of income. The principle of *portability* is designed to ensure that Canadians are covered under public health care insurance wherever they may travel within Canada and when they move from one province to another. The principle of *public administration* focuses on the means of ensuring that health care is publicly funded under a single insurer model. Thus, since 1984, societal values embodied in the *Canada Health Act* have endorsed a publicly administered, universal health insurance system, which affords comprehensive, accessible, and portable benefits. These same values undergird the mental health system.

Overview of the Health Care System

Canada's mental health system is an element of the broader health care system, which is described next. In the division of powers between the federal government and the provinces and territories, the provinces and territories are responsible, with some notable exceptions to be outlined below, for the administration and delivery of health care services across Canada. With financial assistance from the federal government, which is contingent on meeting certain conditions set forth in the 1984 *Canada Health Act* (outlined below), provinces and territories plan, finance, organize, evaluate, and assess the need for the wide range of required health services and ensure that the required personnel are in place to meet the needs for health services.

The federal government is responsible for health care services to specific populations of Canadians. Included among these are 735,000 First Nations and Inuit people as well as Canadian military personnel, veterans, the Royal Canadian Mounted Police (RCMP), and inmates of federal prisons in Canada. The federal government notes that when the provinces and territories calculate the federal financial contributions to provincial and territorial governments in support of health services, they tend to ignore or minimize the federal government's own direct fiscal contributions to health services provided to the above populations, many of whom reside within provinces and territorial jurisdictions.

In 1994, the National Forum on Health (Health Canada, 2003) was launched and chaired by the Prime Minister of Canada to seek advice from Canadians and various professionals on innovative ways to improve the nation's health system and the health of the Canadian people. Their report recognized the fact that peoples' views about desired change hinge on what they see and hear around them, individual personal circumstances, and the options they believe are available to them. They also noted that what people say they want when asked is significantly influenced by the messages delivered by articulate special interest groups.

The report by the National Forum on Health made several observations and recommendations. Five are cited here. *First*, if the health care system was to be built from scratch today, it would likely be less reliant on hospitals and physicians, and it would provide a broader range of community-based services by multidisciplinary teams with much greater emphasis on illness prevention. *Second*, the system would also examine the skills of the various health care professionals and remove the barriers that impede the best use of their abilities. The report advocated *thirdly* for a nationwide health information system that would maintain a standardized set of longitudinal information on health status and health system performance in order to advance a population health agenda. *Fourth*, the report recommended that the federal government assume a leadership role in the development of a national vision for the health system and in facilitating partnerships among governments and health stakeholders to attain the vision, without pushing the provinces and territories too fast in an area in which they have primary responsibility. *Fifth*, in addition to providing long-term and adequate levels of funding, the federal government was seen as essential in developing a national research agenda for health. Indeed, the federal government's contribution to health does include funding for health research agencies such as the Canadian Institute of Health Research (CIHR) and the Social Sciences and Humanities Research Council (SSHRC).

The Need for Mental Health Services

A Report on Mental Illnesses in Canada (Health Canada, 2002) was a collaborative effort prepared by numerous partners including academic psychiatry department heads, professional associations related to mental health, self-help groups, various Canadian government agencies, and the Canadian Institute for Health Information (CIHI). This group gathered and summarized information on mood disorders, schizophrenia, anxiety disorders, personality disorders, eating disorders, and suicidal behavior in Canada. The report identified a compelling need for effective mental health services in Canada. Approximately 20 percent of Canadians will experience a mental health disorder in their lifetime. Mental illnesses affect people of all ages, educational levels, walks of life, cultures, and socioeconomic levels. In 1993, the cost of mental illnesses was estimated to be over $7 billion CDN (US$5.4 billion at the 1993 exchange rate of 1.29). By 1998, only five years later, the estimated cost of mental disorders had doubled to over $14 billion CDN (US$9.4 billion at the 1998 exchange rate of 1.48). Thus, the need for cost-effective, comprehensive, patient-focused, accessible, and high quality mental health services is compelling and pressing.

Prevalence Data

The *Report on Mental Illnesses in Canada* (Health Canada, 2002) included estimates of the prevalence of particular mental disorders for adults and separately for children and adolescents to age 19. Adult disorders are discussed first. The report predicted an adult life-time prevalence rate for *major depression* of about eight percent, with most mood disorders usually first occurring during adolescence. And in any given year, four to five percent of the population will suffer a major depression (Canadian Psychiatric Association, 2001). The rate of occurrence of depression in women in Canada is about double the rate in men (Bland, 1997, pp. 367–377). In 1999/2000 the hospitalization rates for women with major depression were significantly higher at virtually all ages compared to men and peaked for women in the 40–44 year age range at about 158 admissions per 100,000. For men, admission rates for depression during the same period peaked in the 85–89 year age range at about 102 admissions per 100,000.

The average length of stay for depression following admission to general hospitals in Canada remained relatively stable between 1987–1999 at 15–19 days. While the Canadian general hospital admission rates for individuals diagnosed with bipolar disorders from 1987–1999 were much lower than they were for depression, for both men and women, the average length of stay for bipolar disorder was higher at between 21–28 days during this time period. The risk of suicide significantly increased with all mood disorders.

The point prevalence rate of *schizophrenia* in Canada is approximately one percent (Hafner & an der Heiden, 1997, pp.139–151). Up to ages 45–49 years, hospitalization for schizophrenia is higher in men. However, after 50 years of age the rate of hospitalization in Canadian general hospitals is higher for women with schizophrenia. The rate of admission for schizophrenia among men between the ages of 20–39 is particularly high at about 180 admissions per 100,000. Furthermore, over half the admissions due to schizophrenia in Canadian general hospitals occur among those aged 25–44 years.

Anxiety disorders are the single most common group of mental disorders affecting Canadians between the ages of 15–64. About 12 percent of Canadians experience anxiety disorders (9% of males and 16% of females) that impair their functioning to at least some extent (Offord, Boyle, Campbell, et al. 1996, pp. 559–563). Specific phobias and social phobia are by far the most common anxiety disorders in Canada with a period prevalence rate of between 6–8 percent for specific phobias and 7 percent for social phobia. Obsessive-compulsive disorder has a one-year prevalence rate of about two percent while generalized anxiety disorder and panic disorder have prevalence rates of approximately one percent and 0.7 percent, respectively. Hospitalization rates for anxiety disorders are relatively low and are more common among women at virtually all ages. Admission rates for anxiety disorders show a tendency to progressively increase for both males and females after the age of 65 years. From 1987 to 1999, the average length of stay in Canadian general hospitals following admission for anxiety disorders has remained relatively stable at about 10 days.

Canadian data on the prevalence of *personality disorders* are very limited. Prevalence estimates of 6–9 percent are based on U.S. data (Samuels, Nestadt, Romanoski et al. 1994, pp. 1055–1062). These estimates vary depending on the specific personality disorder within this cluster of disorders and the diagnostic criteria used. Admission rates to general hospitals in Canada for personality disorders are higher for females at most age ranges and are highest between the ages of 15–54. The rates peak in females between the ages of 35–39 years at a rate of approximately 63 admissions per 100,000. The admission rates for males peak at 20–24 years but remain relatively constant between the ages of 20–39 at about 33 admissions per 100,000. The *Report on Mental Illnesses in Canada* (Health Canada, 2002) cautions that since most individuals with personality disorders are treated in the community and are not hospitalized, the hospitalization data has significant interpretive limitations.

Eating disorders, including anorexia and bulimia, are disorders that predominately affect women in Canada. About three percent of women will suffer an eating disorder in their lifetime (Zhu and Walsh, 2002, pp. 227–234). Steiger and Seguin (cited in Millon, Blaneyu, & Davis, 1999) estimated that 0.5–4 percent of women will develop anorexia while between 1–4 percent will develop bulimia About two percent of the population will develop binge eating disorder (Bruce and Agras,1992, pp. 365–373). However, the rate of binge eating disorder is almost as common in males as in females. It is estimated that 35 percent of those affected by binge eating disorder are male (Spitzer, Yanovsky, Wadden et al. 1993, 137–153). Hospitalization rates for females peak between the ages of 15–19 at approximately 66 admissions per 100,000 and remain noticeably high between the ages of 10–39 years at a hospitalization rate of at least eight admissions per 100,000.

Waddell and Shepherd (2002) estimated the average overall community prevalence rate for mental disorders in *children* and *adolescents* up to 19 years of age. Kirby (2004) reported that the Standing Senate Committee on Social Affairs, Science and Technology used these data to project the prevalence of mental disorders in children and adolescents across Canada by multiplying the prevalence rates found by Waddell and Shepherd (2002). The Committee based its estimates on Statistics Canada's calculation that there were just under eight million individuals aged to 19 years in Canada in July, 2002. This data is presented in Table 4.1. Clearly anxiety disorders were the most common mental disorders in this fairly wide age range. Conduct disorders and ADHD were the second most common disorders identified.

Table 4.1. *Estimated Prevalence of Mental Disorders in Canadian Children and Adolescents to 19 Years of Age.*

Mental Disorder	Prevalence (%)	Number of Cases in Canada
Depressive disorder	2.1	165,990
Bipolar disorder	<1	7,904
Schizophrenia	0.1	7904
Substance abuse	0.8	63,234
Obsessive-Compulsive disorder	0.2	15,809
Anxiety disorder	6.5	513,780
Conduct disorder	3.3	260,842
Eating disorder	0.1	7904
ADHD	3.3	260,842
Any Disorder	15	1,185,645

Note: Source is Waddell and Shepherd (2002).

The *Canadian Community Health Survey (CCHS) – Mental Health and Well-Being* assessed the prevalence during the previous 12 months of a range of mental health and addiction problems among Canadians aged 15 years and older (Statistics Canada, 2002a). Thirty-seven-thousand Canadians from across Canada were interviewed in 2002. The survey used the *World Mental Health-Composite International Diagnostic Interview (WMH-CIDI)* (World Health Organization, 1990) which yields a diagnostic evaluation that is consistent with the definitions used in the *Diagnostic and Statistical Manual of Mental Disorders*, 4th Edition (DSM-IV) (American Psychiatric Association, 1994). Table 4.2 summarizes the information derived from this survey of Canadian adults 15 years of age and older (Statistics Canada, 2002a).

The following discussion is based on more detailed data from the *Canadian Community Health Survey* (CCHS) for the more restricted age group of 15 to 24 years. This group was most likely to suffer from major depression, particularly among women (8.3%), and more likely than other age groups to have experienced suicidal thoughts in the year prior to the survey, especially among females (7.3%) more than males (4.7%). Women were most likely to be at risk for eating disorders (3.8%) while males in this age range were most at risk for alcohol dependence (9.6%). Social phobia occurred most frequently in this age group, particularly among females (6.1%). Substance dependence was much more frequent among 15–24 year-old Canadians of both genders (18.4%)

Table 4.2. *Prevalence of Mental Disorders and Substance Abuse among Canadian Adults Ages 15 Years and Older in the Past 12 Months.*

Disorder	Total Number	Total %	Males Number	Males %	Females Number	Females %
Major Depression	1,195,955	4.8	451,618	3.7	744,337	5.9
Bipolar Disorder	190,000	0.8	90,000	0.7	100,000	0.8
Manic Episode	239,350	1.0	116,757	1.0	122,593	1.0
Any Mood Disorder	1,210,000	4.9	460,000	3.8	750,000	5.9
Alcohol Dependence	640,632	2.6	472,159	3.8	168,473	1.3
Substance Dependence	740,000	3.0	540,000	4.4	200,000	1.6
Panic Disorder	375,973	1.5	125,430	1.0	250,543	2.0
Agoraphobia	183,448	0.7	44,214	0.4	139,234	1.1
Social Phobia	746,103	3.0	313,485	2.6	432,618	3.4
Any Anxiety Disorder	1,180,000	4.7	440,000	3.6	740,000	5.8
Illicit Drug Dependence	193,643	0.8	134,819	1.1	58,824	0.5
Total – Any Disorder or Substance Dependence	2,658,581	10.6	1,215,393	9.9	1,443,187	11.4

Note: Source is the *Canadian Community Health Survey: Mental Health and Well-Being* (Statistics Canada, 2002a).

with females having the highest rate (19.5%). Alcohol dependence was particularly high among males (9.6%) and illicit drug dependence was more frequent among males (3.5%) than in any other age range.

Despite the relatively high prevalence of difficulties in the group aged 15–24 years, just over nine percent reported having had contact with services and/or received support for problems concerning emotions, mental health or the use of alcohol and drugs. Also, males (5.7%) were much less likely to have had contact with caregivers than were females (12.7%). This may in part be due to the fact that this age group self-rated their mental health as "very good or excellent" more frequently than did any other age group, and they were least likely of any age group to self-rate their mental health as "fair or poor." Overall, the 15–24 year age group reported much more frequently that their health care needs with regard to mental health problems went unmet (7.7%). This was particularly true for females (10.2%), but males in this age group were also more likely to report unmet needs with regard to mental health issues (5.3%) than were males in any other age group in the survey.

These data clearly suggest that the health and mental health care systems are not meeting the perceived needs of this age group very well. Lower utilization rates among this age group 15–24 years is consistent with their more frequent reports than other age groups that there were barriers to their access to mental health services based on acceptability and accessibility issues. *Acceptability* issues involve such matters as competing demands on the individual's time, a preference for self-managing one's problems, doubts that seeking assistance would help, fear of asking for help, language issues and attitudes toward illness, health care providers or the health system. *Accessibility* refers to practical issues such as cost (e.g., most psychological services provided by psychologists are not covered by the national health insurance), lack of transportation, lack of knowledge about where to seek help, and issues such as child care or scheduling.

Further analysis of the *Canadian Community Health Survey: Mental Health and Well-Being* (Statistics Canada, 2003a) revealed that 18 percent of Canadians aged 15–24 years reported symptoms consistent with at least one of the five major mental disorders or substance dependencies assessed in the survey. Symptoms were present in 12 percent of those aged 25–44 years, eight percent of those aged 45–64, and three percent of those 65 years of age and older. In addition, nearly eight percent of the 15–24 year age group reported substance dependencies.

Interestingly, less than one-third of Canadians reporting symptoms suggestive of a mental health disorder or substance abuse problem contacted a health professional about these issues. Moreover, in spite of the relatively higher prevalence of mental health problems in those aged 15–24 years, only about 25 percent of them sought help. However, 45 percent of those aged 25–64 and 33 percent of those aged 65 years or older reported they sought assistance with regard to their symptoms. Among those who did consult a health care professional, family physicians were the professional most likely to be consulted. About 26 percent of individuals across all age groups consulted family physicians with regard to their symptoms, while 12 percent consulted a psychiatrist, ten percent saw or discussed their problems with a social worker, and slightly over eight percent consulted a psychologist. Approximately four percent sought consultation from a religious or spiritual advisor. Thus, people who seem to be most in need of assistance were least likely to seek help from the health, social, or religious systems designed to provide assistance. Reasons for not seeking help varied from a preference to manage the problem themselves (31%) to not getting around to, or not bothering to seek help (19%), while 18 percent reported they were afraid to ask for help or were fearful of what others might think if they did so.

Another major study of prevalence of mental disorders is the *Canadian Forces 2002 Canadian Community Health Survey (CCHS) Supplement*. This study was conducted to assess mental health problems present in full-time and reserve members of Canada's armed forces (Statistics Canada, 2002b). This study involved a sample of 5000 Regular and 3000 Reserve members of Canada's military forces and was conducted between May and June, 2002. This was a separate and somewhat different study than the *Canadian Community Health Survey* conducted with Canada's general population. The *Supplement* aimed to capture issues of particular interest to the military. However, it maintained sufficient commonality with the survey of the general Canadian population for comparative purposes.

The *Supplement* measured several mental disorders, including major depression, social phobia, post-traumatic stress disorder, panic disorder, general anxiety and other disorders. Table 4.3 presents a summary of the major findings of this study in comparison to the Canadian General population.

These survey data suggest that the prevalence of depression in Regular Canadian Forces members is

Table 4.3. *Prevalence of Mental Health Problems and Perception of Adjustment and General Health Over the Past 12 Months in Canadian Forces (CF) Regular and Reserve Members Relative to Each Other and to the Standardized Canadian General Population.*

Population Problem	*Canadian Forces* **Regular** *Members* Year Prevalence %	*General Population* **Standardized to Regular** *Members* Year Prevalence %	*Canadian Forces* **Reserve** *Members* Year Prevalence %	*General Population* **Standardized to Reserve** *Members* Year Prevalence %
Ability to handle day-to-day demands rated as fair to poor	3.4	4.5	1.8	4.6
High levels of distress	1.8	2.2	0.7	2.4
Self-rated mental health as fair to poor	9.1	6.4	4.8	6.3
General Anxiety Disorder	1.8	–	1.0	–
Panic Disorder	2.2	1.4	1.4	1.7
PTSD	2.8	–	1.2	–
Social Phobia	3.6	3.2	2.3	3.5
Depression	7.6	4.3	4.1	5.0
Alcohol Dependence	4.2	4.6	6.2	5.7
Dissatisfied with life	5.0	4.9	3.8	4.8
Self-rated general health as fair to poor	6.1	6.5	2.4	6.2

Note: Source is Canadian Forces 2002 CCHS Supplement (Statistics Canada, 2002b).

significantly higher [7.6%], nearly twice the rate as in the Canadian general population [4.3%] and in the Reserve Canadian Forces [4.1%]. In addition, members of the Regular Canadian Forces subjectively rated their *mental* health as fair or poor [9.1%] at almost twice the rate as did Reserve members of the Canadian Forces [4.8%], and about a third more often than did the general Canadian population. Panic disorder, although relatively infrequent, was significantly more common in the Regular Canadian Forces members [2.2%] than in the general Canadian population [1.4%]. However, alcohol dependence did not appear to occur at a higher rate in either Regular or Reserve Canadian Forces relative to the general Canadian population. Overall, the rate of depression in Regular Canadian Forces members was among the most notable findings in the analysis.

A subsequent summary analysis of this data by Statistics Canada (2003a, Sept. 5) indicated that the rate of symptom reporting was higher in the lower ranks of the military and that the symptom reporting rate was higher for women than for men. The analysis suggested also that there may also be a dose-response relationship between the prevalence of Post-Traumatic Stress Disorder (PTSD) and a higher number of military deployments. Among the regular forces that had served three or more deployments, the PTSD symptom rate was 4.7 percent while in those who had served one or two deployments the rate was 2.7 percent and only 1.7 percent in those regular Canadian Forces members who had not served any deployments. About one-quarter of the regular members of the Canadian Forces received help for a mental health disorder or drug or alcohol problem and judged this assistance to be sufficient. However, an additional 27 percent received help but believed that additional or different help was needed for the problem. Twelve percent did not receive help, though they felt that help was needed.

In addition to prevalence data on Canada's general population and military personnel samples, Canada has data from Correctional Service Canada, reported April 2004, regarding the *lifetime* prevalence of mental disorders among inmates of Canada's federal prisons. These data were reported as a brief in The *Report on Mental Health, Mental Illness and Addiction* by the Standing Senate Committee on Social Affairs, Science And Technology (Senate of Canada, 2004 Kirby and Keon, 2004). This report indicated that for the period 1988/1989, 14 percent of males and 33 percent of females experienced major depression, 32 percent of males and 20 percent of females

Table 4.4. *Prevalence of Major Disorders by Gender.*

Disorder	Male (1988)	Female (1989)
Major Depression	13.6	32.9
General Anxiety Disorder	31.9	19.7
Psychosocial Dysfunction	19.6	34.2
Antisocial Personality Disorder	57.2	36.8
Alcohol Use/Dependence	47.4	63.2
Drug Use/Dependence	41.6	50.0

Note: Source is Report 1, Senate Committee (Kirby & Keon, 2004).

experienced general anxiety disorder, 47 percent of males and 63 percent of females were alcohol dependent, 42 percent of males and 50 percent of females were drug dependent, and 57 percent of males and 37 percent of females met criteria for antisocial personality disorder. This is shown in Table 4.4.

To estimate the prevalence of addictive disorders, the *Canadian Addiction Survey* was conducted between December 2003 and April 2004 in order to examine the Canadians' use of alcohol and drugs. This was one of the most comprehensive surveys of the period and lifetime prevalence, incidence, and frequency of alcohol and drug use in the Canadian population. The survey sampled 14,000 Canadians from across Canada, 15 years of age and older, with a minimum of 1,000 interviews in each province (Health Canada, 2004).

For the 12-month period prior to the survey, 79 percent of the Canadians reported consuming alcohol, 44 percent of which reported drinking weekly. The alcohol consumption rate was somewhat higher in males (82%) than in females (77%). Seven percent were heavy-frequent drinkers (5 drinks or more, more than once/week). In general, males, 18–24-year-old males and females, and single men and women were the most likely to be heavier consumers of alcohol. Twenty-three percent of the drinkers exceeded the Low-Risk Drinking Guidelines (weekly alcohol intake exceeding 14 standard drinks for males and nine standard drinks for females). Those most likely to do so were males, men and women between 18–24 years of age, and single individuals. Based on the *Alcohol Use Disorders Identification Test (AUDIT)* (Babor, de la Fuente, Saunders et al. 1992), 17 percent of drinkers (14% of all Canadians) are considered high-risk drinkers. Among male drinkers 25 percent are considered high risk while nine percent of women drinkers are high risk. About 10 percent of consumers of alcohol reported experiencing harm from their drinking, most often due to negative effects on their physical health (5%). However, about 33 percent of drinkers reported having been harmed by the drinking of others, most often as a consequence of having been insulted or humiliated (22%), having been verbally abused (16%), or having been exposed to arguments (16%).

Nearly half (44.5%) of all Canadians reported using cannabis at least once in their lifetime. Males (50%) were more likely to have used the drug than females (39%). Fourteen percent of the survey sample admitted to using cannabis within the year prior to the survey and, again, males were more likely to have used it (18%) than females (10%). Seventy percent of those 18–24 years old have used cannabis. Lifetime cannabis use tended to increase with higher levels of both education and income.

Other than cannabis, hallucinogens were the most commonly used illicit drugs in Canada, with 11 percent of Canadians reporting at least some use during their lifetime. Eleven percent of Canadians reported using cocaine, six percent used speed and four percent used ecstasy. One percent or fewer Canadians used inhalants, heroin, or intravenously administered drugs. The lifetime use of drugs other than cannabis by Canadians was about 17 percent, but one percent or fewer had used these drugs in the year prior to the survey, with the exception of cocaine, which was used by just under two percent of Canadians. The lifetime, including the past year, use of drugs other than cannabis was higher among men (21%) than women (4%) and among 18–24 year old Canadians. About 10 percent of Canadians reported experiencing harm from their own drug use; physical harm was the most common negative effect of drug use reported by 10 percent of drug users.

Although a major new study entitled the Canadian Substance Abuse Cost Study is now underway to update the social and economic costs to Canadian society of alcohol, tobacco and illicit drug use in Canada, Single, Robson, Xie, and Rehm (1996) estimated the 1992 economic costs of alcohol and tobacco use in Canada to be very high. In this study *direct workplace losses* are costs associated with EAP and health promotion programs as well as drug testing costs in the workplace while *productivity losses* consist of losses due to morbidity, mortality, and crime. These costs are outlined in Table 4.5.

Mortality and Disability Estimates

In 1997, suicide was the cause of death for approximately two percent of all deaths in Canada (Statistics

Table 4.5. *1992 Economic Costs of Alcohol and Tobacco Abuse in Canadian Dollars (CDN) and US$*

Expenditure	CDN	US$
Total costs of alcohol abuse	7.5 billion	5.8 billion
Direct health care costs	1.3 billion	1 billion
Direct workplace losses	14 million	10.8 million
Worker's compensation costs	48 million	37.2 million
Social welfare and other costs	3.6 million	2.8 million
Direct costs: prevention and research	141 million	109 million
Law enforcement costs	1.4 billion	1.1 billion
Productivity losses	4.1 billion	3.2 billion
Traffic accidents/ fire damage	518 million	401.6 million
Total illicit drug use costs	1.4 billion	1.1 billion
Total tobacco use costs	9.6 billion	7.4 billion
Direct health care costs of tobacco	2.7 billion	2.1 billion
Lost productivity due to mortality from tobacco use	6.7 billion	5.2 billion

Note: Source is Canadian Centre on Substance Abuse, 1996. Exchange rate used was 1.29 for 1993.

Canada, 1997). The World Health Organization reported that in 1998 the suicide rate in Canada was 19.5 males and 5.1 females per 100,000 (WHO, 2003). Thus, the male suicide rate in Canada is approximately four times the female rate of suicide. The overall suicide rate in Canada of 24.6 per 100,000 is higher than the rate in the United States (21.7/100,000 in 1999) and the United Kingdom (15.1/100,000 in 1999), but lower than in Norway (26.3/100,000 in 1999).

Statistics Canada (2005) reported that in 1997 the highest suicide rate per 100,000 was among males (25.5) in the 45–64 year age group, followed by comparable rates of 25 in the 25–44 year age group, 24.9 in the 20–24 year age group, and 19.9 in the 15–19 year age group. Among females, the highest suicide rate per 100,000 was 7.6 in the 45–64 year age range and 6.6 in the 25–44 year age range (Statistics Canada, 2004). Statistics Canada (2004) reported that the suicide rate among immigrants to Canada was lower than native-born Canadians. The combined male and female immigrant suicide rate per 100,000 in 1996 was 7.9 compared to 13.3 among native-born Canadians. While the male immigrant suicide rate was higher than the female rate, the gender difference in suicide rates was narrower among immigrants to Canada than among native-born Canadians.

Canada's Aboriginal people have not fared as well as other Canadians with regard to suicide rates. In 1995, the *Canadian Royal Commission on Aboriginal Peoples* concluded that conservative estimates of suicide rates across all age groups of aboriginal people were on average approximately three times higher than the nonaboriginal Canadian average (Chenier, 1995). The suicide rate for registered Indians was estimated to be 3.3 times the nonaboriginal Canadian average, while the Inuit rate of suicide was 3.9 times the Canadian average. Moreover, adolescents and young adults were at highest risk. For aboriginal youth aged 10–19 years the suicide rate was five to six times higher than the Canadian average of nonaboriginal youths. However, the suicide rate peaked among First Nations males in the 20–24 year age group at approximately 150 suicides/100,000. The Commission concluded that four groups of major risk factors contributed to the high suicide rates: (a) psychobiological factors (e.g., unresolved grief), (b) situational factors (e.g., disruption of family life, forced attendance at boarding schools, adoption, drugs and alcohol to relieve unhappiness), (c) socioeconomic factors (e.g., poverty, limited education and employment opportunities, inadequate housing, and inadequate sanitation and water quality), and (d) cultural stress factors (loss of confidence in the ways of understanding life and living that their culture had taught them) (Chenier, 1995).

Statistics Canada (2002) contacted individuals across Canada (35,000 adults aged 15 years and older and 8000 children under age 15 years) who had reported a *disability* on the 2001 Census utilizing the *Participation and Activity Limitation Survey (PALS)*, which was based on an earlier survey using the *Health and Activity Limitation Survey (HALS)*. Disability was defined as a health-related condition or problem that limited everyday activities. The overall response rate was 83 percent. Over 15 percent of adults reported activity limitations due to psychological conditions, which were defined as the presence of emotional, psychological, or psychiatric condition such as phobia, depression, schizophrenia, drinking, or drug problems. Thus, about 2.2 percent of the Canadian population reported psychological disabilities of one sort or another.

The Global Business and Economic Roundtable on Addiction and Mental Health reported that depression costs the Canadian and U.S. economies a combined total of $60 billion U.S. dollars a year, with more than half the cost being due to *lost productivity* (Wilson and Joffe, 2000). They also reported that disability from all sources represents from four to 12 percent of payroll costs in Canada, and that since 1994 disability costs to industry as a percentage of payroll have grown dramatically. This group reported more recently that mental disorders are the leading drivers of employee long-term disability costs. Depression was reported as the leading source of worker disability in Canada that, on average, keeps an employee off work for 40 days. Furthermore, the longer an employee is off work, the lower the probability that the employee will ever return to work. Seventy-five percent of employees off work for 12 weeks return to work, whereas only two percent of employees off work for one year ever return to work. In addition, antidepressant medications are the principle prescribed drugs utilized by employees in the 25–44 year age range, based on an analysis of group drug plans of some of Canada's major employers (Wilkerson, 2004).

The impact of work-life conflict and demands on Canada's health care system was examined in a report sponsored by the Public Health Agency of Canada (2004). Over thirty-one thousand Canadian employees working for organizations of 500 or more employees in the public, private, and not-for-profit sectors of the Canadian economy from across Canada were surveyed. Levels of work-life conflict centered around four main areas: *Role overload:* having too much to do in a given time; *Work to family interference:* work demands make it difficult to fulfill family role responsibilities; *Family to work interference:* family demands make it difficult to fulfill work responsibilities; and *Caregiver strain:* physical, financial, or mental stress associated with taking care of an elderly or disabled dependent.

Survey results indicated that combining work and dependent care impacted negatively on perceived health for both genders, and on mental health but not on physical health. While it was associated with visits to mental health professionals, it was not related to utilization of either inpatient or outpatient physician services, nor to utilization of emergency departments.

Employees with high versus low *role overload* were almost three times more likely to rate their health as fair or poor and two and a half times more likely to seek help from a mental health professional. In addition, they were more likely to have (a) received both in-and out patient hospital care, (b) visited a physician significantly more often, (c) spent more than $300 on prescription medication, and (c) to have visited a hospital emergency department. Clearly this significantly impacted costs to the health care system.

Those employees with high levels of *work to family interference* also appeared to be in poorer physical and mental health and made greater use of Canada's health care system. They were more than twice as likely to rate their health as fair or poor relative to those with low work to family interference and their use of the health care system incurred direct costs of $2.8 billion per year.

Family to work interference was not found to be as strongly related to use of the health care system or perceived health in comparison to the other work-life conflicts, but these individuals were more than twice as likely to rate their health as fair or poor in relation to those with low family to work interference. Furthermore, employees with high levels of family to work interference were nearly twice as likely to seek help from mental health professionals compared to those with low family to work interference.

Based on the 2004 exchange rate of 1.30, overall health care-related costs associated with high work-life conflict were approximately $6 billion CDN (US$4.6 billion) per year as a consequence of role overload; $5 billion CDN (US$3.8 billion) per year attributable to high caregiver strain; $2.8 billion CDN (US$2.2 billion) per year related to high work to family interference; and $500 million CDN (US$385 million) per year to family to work interference, for a total of $14 billion CDN (US$395 billion). The problems associated with *role overload* were seen as being significantly related to employee downsizing strategies of the 1980s and 1990s. If true, the downsizing strategy to improve profits and productivity levels within the corporate and public sectors may largely have shifted costs from these sectors to the health care system. In essence, the authors of the survey suggest that, in effect, Canadian taxpayers are subsidizing through their taxes such organizational practices as "doing more with less" by the increasing costs to the publicly funded health care system. They argue that Canada simply cannot afford to ignore the issues of work-life conflict and remain globally competitive economically.

Stephens and Joubert (2001) reported that mental disorders cost Canada a total of US$9.7 billion ($14.4 billion CDN) in 1998, making these the third most costly disorders to treat. The *direct* and *indirect* costs associated with mental health disorders are outlined in Table 4.6. Clearly, this points to the need for cost-effective mental health services in Canada.

Table 4.6. *Estimated Costs of Mental Disorders 1998.*

Item	CDN	US$
Total costs of mental disorders	**14.4 billion**	**9.7 billion**
Estimated total *direct* costs	6.3 billion	4.2 billion
Indirect costs related to medications	642 million	433 million
Physician fees	854 million	575 million
Hospital costs	3.9 billion	2.6 billion
Other health institutional costs	887 million	597 million
Estimated total *indirect* costs	8.1 billion	5.5 billion
Short-term disability	6.0 billion	4.0 billion
Long-term disability	1.7 billion	1.1 billion
Premature deaths	400 million	270 million

Note: Source is Stephens and Joubert (2001). The 1998 exchange rate of 1.48 has been applied.

Policies and Programs

Canada's national mental health policies and programs are addressed in this section under the following headings: The Canada Health Act 1984; the medical necessity standard; national health system standards; federal privacy legislation; mental health legislation; and the national health insurance.

The Canada Health Act, 1984

While over 30 federal laws have relevance to health in Canada, the *Canada Health Act 1984* is Canada's single most important federal health insurance legislation. It states clearly that the primary objective of Canadian health care policy is ". . . to protect, promote, and restore the physical and mental well-being of residents of Canada and to facilitate reasonable access to health services without financial or other barriers." The legislation sets the conditions and criteria with which the provinces and territories must comply in order to receive full federal funding for both insured and extended health care services (e.g., residential and home health care). The intention of the *Canada Health Act* is to ensure that all eligible residents of Canada have reasonable access to medically necessary insured services on a prepaid basis without any direct charges at the point of service delivery. As previously discussed, the guiding ethical principles for this legislation are universality, comprehensiveness, accessibility, portability, and public administration. Also noted earlier, this legislation does not apply to members of the Canadian military, the Royal Canadian Mounted Police (RCMP), and inmates of federal prisons. For these latter groups the federal Government of Canada is the direct funder/provider of health care services.

The Medical Necessity Standard

The *Canada Health Act* defines insured services as "medically necessary hospital, physician and surgical-dental services provided to insured persons." Thus, the legislation does not cover all health services that Canadians may either need or want. It is a common misconception of the Canadian health care system that all health care services are insured services. This is simply not the case. Outpatient mental health services by nonphysicians were excluded in this federal legislation.

"Medically necessary" services are in theory determined by physicians in conjunction with the provincial and territorial health insurance plans. However, what constitutes "medically necessary" and who decides is not always straightforward. A policy paper prepared for the Romanow Commission on the Future of Health Care in Canada presented in September 2002 noted that the *Canada Health Act* neither defines what the term medically necessary means nor does it provide a process for doing so (Romanow, 2002). Furthermore, the term is seen as being too restrictive since it is largely limited to services provided by physicians and hospitals as well as a limited range of surgical dental procedures. It is also true that provinces and territories may decide somewhat arbitrarily that certain services are no longer medically necessary, and consequently not covered as insured services. Thus, the province or territory would no longer pay for these services. Certain surgeries that are regarded as cosmetic might fall into this category. Moreover, "medically necessary care" does not include other elements of health care that may have a beneficial impact on maintaining and/or promoting good health.

Insured services under the *Canada Health Act* include inpatient and outpatient services such as room and meals at a public ward level, or special accommodations if required. Other services covered are nursing care, diagnostic tests and interpretation of them, drugs and other biological preparations when administered in hospitals. The use of operating rooms, anesthetics, medical and surgical equipment and supplies, radiotherapy, and physiotherapy facilities are also covered in addition to the services of hospital staff. Insured physician services include "medically required services rendered by medical practitioners." Insured surgical-dental services are those provided by a dentist in a hospital, that is, when a hospital setting is required to properly perform the dental procedure. "Extended health care services" include certain aspects of long-term residential care and the health aspects of home care and ambulatory care services. However, this should not be misinterpreted to mean that nursing home care is an entirely insured service in Canada.

National Health System Standards

The *Canada Health Act* establishes nine requirements that the provinces and territories must meet in order to receive full federal cash contributions. These performance standards were briefly noted in the introduction of this chapter, where they were discussed as underlying cultural values and guiding principles. They are elaborated here.

Section 8 of the Canada Health Act affirms the *public administration* criterion. This criterion intends to ensure that health care insurance plans are administered and operated in provinces and territories on a nonprofit basis by a public authority that is *accountable* to the government of the province or territory regarding both benefit levels and services, and that the records and accounts of the public authority are publicly audited.

Section 9 of the *Act* expresses the standard of *comprehensiveness*. It requires that the provincial and territorial health care insurance plans "must insure all insured health services provided by hospital, medical practitioners or dentists (i.e., surgical-dental services which require a hospital setting) and, where the law of the province so permits, similar or additional services rendered by other health care practitioners." Mental health services mandated in Section 9 include *inpatient* services provided by both physicians and other mental health professionals, and *outpatient* services provided by physicians only.

Section 10 of the *Act* addresses the criterion of *universality*. It requires that all insured residents in the provinces and territories shall be entitled to the insured health services provided by the health care insurance plans on uniform terms and conditions. It stipulates that new immigrants to Canada as well as

Canadians resuming residence in Canada shall not be subjected to eligibility waiting periods exceeding three months to receive insured health care services.

Section 11 of the *Act* mandates *portability*. This provision of the Act is intended to ensure that residents moving from one province or territory to another must be covered by their "home" provincial or territorial insured health care plan during any waiting period imposed by the new province or territory of residence. Residents who are temporarily absent from their home province or territory, or from Canada, must continue to be covered by their territorial or provincial health insurance plan. It is also the intent of Section 11 of the Act to ensure that Canadians temporarily away on vacation or business are insured to receive necessary emergent services in another province, territory or country. However, not all costs for such services need to be covered by the home plan. This is particularly true when Canadians may require health care services in countries where health care expenses are much higher than they are in Canada (e.g., United States), and when repatriation to the home province requires expensive travel arrangements (e.g., air ambulance transportation).

Section 12 of the *Act* is the standard of *reasonable accessibility*. The intention expressed here is that insured residents of a province or territory have reasonable access to insured hospital, medical and surgical-dental services on uniform terms and conditions, unimpeded, either directly or indirectly, by user fees or extra billing by facilities or health care providers or by other means. It also stipulates that physicians and dentists must be reasonably compensated and that payments to hospitals cover the costs of providing the services. *Reasonable access* follows the "where and as available" rule, which means that residents are entitled to access on uniform terms and conditions to insured services at a setting "where" the services are provided and "as" the services are available in that setting. It does not preclude lengthy waiting lists, although there is an expectation that they will be managed equitably for all residents. In addition, not all services are necessarily provided in close proximity to where a person lives. Nor does it guarantee that all services that a person may need will be available — only that a person has equitable access to the services that are actually provided.

Section 13 of the *Canada Health Act* stipulates that the provincial and territorial governments provide information to the federal Minister of Health as may be reasonably required regarding provincial and territorial insured health care services and extended health care services. It also requires the provincial and territorial governments to appropriately recognize the federal contributions toward insured and extended health care services.

Section 18 of the *Act* is intended to discourage physicians and dentists from extra billing for services they provide in amounts over and above the fees that they receive from the provincial and territorial insured service plans. Prior to the *Canada Health Act* it was a common practice among many physicians to directly bill and/or collect additional fees for services that were insured services under provincial and territorial insured health service plans. Extra billing is seen as a barrier or impediment for people seeking medical care, and it is therefore contrary to the accessibility criterion. Service providers may, however, charge fees for noninsured services such as letters to lawyers and insurance companies and other such services.

Section 19 of the *Act* relates to *user charges*. These are any charges, other than extra billing, which are permitted by a provincial or territorial health care insurance plan and are not payable by the plan. For example, a charge by a hospital to an insured person receiving a service would be regarded as a facility fee and considered a user charge. Facilities may charge reasonable fees for the rental of such supplies as crutches. The Act provides for a reduction of federal government transfer payments to the provinces or territories if either extra billing or user charges are proven.

Privacy Legislation

In addition to the *Canada Health Act*, health policy has been influenced by federal legislation concerning patient rights. Two federal privacy laws have been enacted in Canada in order to protect the privacy of Canadians. The Office of the Privacy Commissioner of Canada outlined the basic provisions of the *Privacy Act* that came into effect in 1983. It imposed obligations on 150 federal government departments and agencies to limit their collection, use, and disclosure of personal information on Canadians. It also permitted Canadians access to personal information about them held by federal government organizations and to correct inaccurate information.

In 2001, the *Personal Information Protection and Electronic Documents Act* (PIPEDA) set rules regarding how organizations in the *private* sector may collect, use, or disclose personal information in the conduct of commercial activities. This *Act* also gave Canadians the right to view information held about them and to request that corrections be made to inaccurate information.

Since the beginning of 2002, this law has applied not only to information held about employees but also to personal information collected about customers, and used or disclosed by a *federally regulated* sector in the course of commercial operations. It also applies to information that is sold across provincial and territorial borders. As of January 2002 the *Act* has been applied to personal health information collected, used or disclosed by private sector organizations. As of January 2004, the Act covered the collection, use, or disclosure of personal information in the course of any commercial activity within a province, including provincially regulated organizations. The federal government has the prerogative to exempt from the requirements of this law any organizations or activities in provinces that have enacted privacy laws that are in large measure similar to federal legislation.

Shields and Tétrault (2001) provided an overview of privacy and personal health information laws in Canada. They noted that the basic concepts underlying personal health information in both federal and provincial legislation are similar. Under both provincial and federal statutes, information related to an individual's physical and mental health is covered with regard to health services that have been provided. Moreover, information about donations of bodily parts or substances, and information obtained from individuals when they register to receive a health service is also covered under the legislation (e.g., health identification number, address, telephone number, etc.). In general, the collection of personal health information is permitted only after an individual has been given sufficient information regarding the purpose for which the information is being collected in order to ensure the individual makes an informed decision and thereafter gives voluntary consent. Even after consent is given, those collecting information from individuals are expected to adopt a *de minimis* approach, namely, to collect the least amount of information that is adequate to achieve the authorized purposes for which the information was collected. Thereafter, the custodians of the information are constrained from using or disclosing the personal health information collected other than as authorized by the individual or as permitted under relevant legislation.

Typically, the specific uses or disclosure of personal health information that may be undertaken *without consent* include (a) providing health services, (b) conducting research, (c) uses authorized by specific regulations or by another specified law, (d) uses intended to address financial mismanagement or professional misconduct, and (e) uses related to internal management purposes, including audit, quality assurance, monitoring, etc. Custodians of personal health information are expected to take substantial precautions to ensure that personal health information is maintained with a high degree of confidentiality and security. While federal and the various provincial legislative initiatives are conceptually similar, they are not identical. Consequently, those working across provincial boundaries have to be familiar with the specific provisions of the legislation in the different jurisdictions of Canada.

In December, 2003, the College of Family Physicians of Canada (CFPC) prepared a critical review of privacy legislation in Canada for family physicians (CFPC, 2003). This work is of sufficient generality to provide a broad understanding of how all health care providers should act to facilitate compliance with privacy legislation in Canada. Privacy legislation is built on two fundamental principles: *consent* and *confidentiality*. However, exceptions to consent, to collect, use, and/or disclose information are also important to ensure appropriate care is provided in a timely fashion. These situations typically include those in which there is a need to provide immediate care (e.g., during an emergency, in the conduct of legal proceedings, in order to prevent serious harm or injury to another person, when contacting the relatives or next of kin of someone seriously ill, and/or when obtaining payment for health care services).

The CFPC review noted that the federal *Personal Information Protection and Electronic Documents Act* (PIPEDA) was crafted to deal with privacy matters associated with "commercial activities" and not with regard to personal health information. However, because no specific federal Act exists with regard to personal health information, PIPEDA may by default become the standard in law for privacy associated with the collection and use of personal health information.

With regard to the issue of consent, the CFAC expressed the view that *implied* consent was acceptable for disclosures between physicians, laboratory technicians, pharmacists and presumably others directly involved in the care of an individual. However, more explicit consent should be obtained for uses or disclosures that a patient might not reasonably expect such as disclosures for research. Canadian Supreme Court decisions have addressed an individual's right to access one's own personal information contained in a health record, hence access should not ordinarily be denied unless it would risk serious harm to the individual or reveal personal information about a third party.

The CFPC review of personal health information identified ten basic principles with regard to managing personal health information within the context of privacy legislation in Canada:

1. *Accountability:* consider designating an individual to be responsible for overseeing and managing the use of personal health information and ensure that all staff are familiar and adhere to the appropriate management of personal health information.
2. *Identifying Purpose:* ensure that both patients and staff are able to identify and understand why they are collecting personal health information at the time or before the information is collected.
3. *Consent:* ensure that patients are aware of the reasons for collecting personal health information and are made aware that they may withdraw their consent at any time and the consequences of doing so. Implied consent appears acceptable in most circumstances except when a patient in not likely to be aware of the purpose for which the information may be used.
4. *Limiting collection:* collect only the personal health information needed to provide care for the person.
5. *Limiting Use, Disclosure and Retention:* obtain oral or written consent for all new uses of personal health information aside from care and treatment and only disclose information consistent with the use for which it was collected. Develop guidelines for the retention and destruction of personal health information contained in records.
6. *Accuracy:* maintain accurate personal health information and allow individuals to correct inaccurate information with appropriate documentation of the time of the modification.
7. *Safeguards:* ensure the safety and security of all personal health information in hard copy or electronic form, and that access to the information for care is only available to authorized personnel.
8. *Openness:* provide information in written form to individuals to reassure them that confidentiality of their personal health information is important.
9. *Individual Access:* individuals should have access to their personal health information and be allowed to correct inaccurate information with a process that tracks changes made to the records.
10. *Challenging Compliance:* develop a process for responding to complaints related to the collection and use of personal health information and correct any perceptions of inappropriate management of personal health information.

Mental Health Legislation

Specific mental health legislation exists in all provinces and territories of Canada. At the present time some provinces are in the process of revising their *Mental Health Acts*. Significant differences exist in the specific provisions contained in the provincial and territorial pieces of legislation, which lead to variations in how people with identical mental health problems are likely to be treated in the various jurisdictions of Canada. Gray and O'Reilly (2001) examined the mental health acts in all Canadian jurisdictions to determine how the clinical management of a routine case might be handled differently in the various jurisdictions. They found that there were clinically significant differences with regard to how cases would be managed in the different Canadian jurisdictions based on differences among the mental health acts in the various provinces and territories. The authors concluded that in some Canadian jurisdictions existing legislation would prevent individuals from receiving what was deemed to be appropriate treatment, whereas in other jurisdictions that treatment would be permitted.

Involuntary admissions. Gray and O'Reilly (2001) paid particular attention to aspects of legislation related to admission criteria in relation to whether or not *involuntary admission* and treatment was permitted under various circumstances. The six factors to be considered were whether the person was (a) suitable for voluntary admission, (b) met the criteria or definition for having a mental disorder, (c) was deemed to be a risk for physically harming themselves or someone else, (d) was judged likely to suffer substantial mental or physical deterioration without admission, (e) was in need of treatment, and (f) was capable of making a treatment decision. They found significant variation from one jurisdiction to another with regard to whether an individual with the same clinical presentation could be involuntarily admitted to hospital. They also examined the review and appeal procedures that exist in all jurisdictions and found that they also vary among jurisdictions. In addition, conditional leave and community treatment orders also vary from one province or territory to another. This leads to individuals having different rights and being treated differently as a function of where they live in Canada.

Fitness to stand trial. The federal Criminal Code of Canada governs all criminal offenses everywhere in Canada, and it plays an important role in mental health, particularly in relation to assessment of fitness to stand trial for offences associated with mental illness. In October, 2004, the Canadian Department of Justice introduced planned reforms to the laws and procedures that apply to individuals who are found unfit to stand trial or deemed not to be criminally responsible due to a mental disorder. Under existing law, if an individual is tried for an offense and found not criminally responsible because of a mental disorder, the person is not considered to have been convicted, acquitted, or sentenced. In this case, a court or Review Board decides on an appropriate course of action that may range from an absolute discharge to committal to a hospital on the basis of rules set forth in the Criminal Code. The proposed amendments include expanding the powers of review boards regarding detention decisions, supervision, and the release of individuals found unfit to stand trial or not criminally responsible due to mental illness (Department of Justice, Canada, 2004).

Attempted and assisted suicide. Until 1972, attempted suicide was considered a criminal act under the Code. In 1972 Minister of Justice Otto Lang removed attempted suicide from the provisions of the Criminal Code of Canada. Minister of Justice Lang explained his decision as follows: "We have removed the offense of attempted suicide, again on the philosophy that this is not a matter which requires a legal remedy; that it has it roots and its solution in sciences outside of the law and that certainly deterrence under the legal system is unnecessary." However, counseling or assisting suicide remains a criminal act in violation of Section 241 of the Criminal Code. The latter provision reads "Everyone who (a) counsels a person to commit suicide, or (b) aids or abets a person to commit suicide, whether suicide occurs or not, is guilty of an indictable offense and liable to imprisonment for a term not exceeding fourteen years" (Health Canada, 1994).

Canada's National Health Insurance Program: Medicare

Medicare has played an extremely important role in Canada for the last half-century and is among the most highly valued public services provided by Canadian governments. Ekos Research Associates has tracked the priorities of Canadians on a range of programs and issues. Health care has topped the list since 1995 and in December, 2003 ninety-three percent of Canadians surveyed rated health care as a high priority for government funding. Moreover, the priority of health care generally increased between 1995 and 2003 (Ekos Research Associates, 2004). Medicare evolved in two distinct phases. In the first phase, hospital and diagnostic service charges were paid for by a government-sponsored insurance plan. In the second phase, physician fees were covered by a government-sponsored health insurance plan. Medicare was first introduced in the province of Saskatchewan and gradually evolved into a national, publicly funded, single-payer health insurance system.

In 1947, the province of Saskatchewan, under the leadership of Premier Tommy Douglas, introduced publicly funded, universal hospital insurance to cover hospital and diagnostic expenses for the citizens of Saskatchewan. Saskatchewan's initiative to cover hospital and diagnostic expenses was implemented by other Canadian provinces and, following the federal government's *Hospital Insurance and Diagnostic Services Act* (1957), all Canadian provinces and territories covered hospital and diagnostic expenses for Canadians by 1961. The federal legislation created a cost sharing arrangement between the federal and provincial governments to pay for expenses related to hospitalization and diagnostic services. In 1962, under then Premier W.S. Lloyd, Saskatchewan implemented universal public health insurance to pay for medical care and physician fees provided *outside* of hospitals. This legislation was a logical extension of the public insurance that paid for hospitalization costs. Covering physician fees along with hospital and diagnostic service costs significantly limited the financial exposure of citizens to potentially financially crippling costs associated with illness.

In 1962, the former Premier of Saskatchewan Province, Tommy Douglas explained the two-fold rationale for implementing government-funded medicare. *First*, he argued that existing *private* health plans levied the same premiums regardless of family income level, and thus did not take into consideration a family's ability to pay. Less affluent families were at a significant financial disadvantage under such a system. Only a government plan, in the context of a progressive taxation system, could take into consideration a family's ability to pay. *Second*, he noted that to remain solvent, private plans had to eliminate coverage for certain groups of people who most needed health insurance coverage in the first place. These were people with chronic conditions and congenital illnesses as well as those with existing medical illness and older people who were more likely to be high users of services. Only a government plan that spread the financial liability for health care across all citizens could address this issue. Following lengthy negotiations between the federal and provincial governments regarding cost-sharing arrangements, the Saskatchewan model of public health insurance was adopted nationally and universal medicare became a reality across Canada by 1972.

Physicians in Saskatchewan did not like their fees being paid from government coffers and they waged a withdrawal of services. They also enlisted the public to protest against the government legislation on the basis that it was an infringement of the individual rights of both the doctors and the public. The doctors argued that the legislation also created a government monopoly on health care matters, and they feared that a government-funded program would lead to the government dictating to them how to go about their business. However, while drawing some support from the public, the public response was less than they had hoped for, and after three weeks they ended their strike. The dye was thus cast for Medicare in Canada to become a federally funded, national health insurance program.

In 1979, Canadian Supreme Court Justice Emmett Hall was asked by the federal government to review the strengths and weaknesses of the Canadian health care system. Two major concerns that prompted this review related to (a) hospitals implementing user charges and (b) physicians billing patients' directly additional fees over and above the tariffs provided to them by the provincial and territorial health care plans. Justice Hall also noted in his report that Canadians were running into difficulty receiving health care services when traveling to another province outside their home province, contrary to the principle of portability, which was affirmed later in the 1984 *Canada Health Act*. Justice Hall also commented on the lack of accessibility that existed because some individuals were not sure whether or not they were covered in light of health care premiums being charged by some provinces. He recommended against both user fees charged by hospitals and extra billing by physicians. At the same time, Justice Hall recognized the right of physicians to be compensated adequately for their services and acknowledged that provincial governments did not have the right to essentially conscript physicians and pay them whatever they pleased. He recommended that physician fees be established through negotiation and, if necessary, through binding arbitration. It is clearly evident that Justice Hall's report profoundly influenced the basic principles later articulated in the federal *Canada Health Act* (1984).

Romanow and Marchildon (2003) pointed out that the manner in which Medicare developed in Canada has "historically privileged" both hospital and physician services. It has also tended to focus health services more on physical ailments than on the provision of mental health services. Under Medicare the existing fee-for-service billing arrangement for physicians was maintained, but the government became the single payer of health care costs rather than individual citizens or private insurers. Although there have been persistent demands over the years by the provinces for more money from the federal government to pay for health care costs, and with some merit to their demands, the fundamental aspects of Canadian Medicare have not changed a great deal in the last half century (Romanow and Marchildon, 2003, pp. 283–295).

There is evidence that hospitals in some jurisdictions are now increasingly being micromanaged directly by provincial governments and that the days of hospitals being provided with global budgets to manage as they see fit are becoming a thing of the past. In some jurisdictions, health ministries are mandating that specific programs be instituted in hospitals and recommending, if not requiring, that specific personnel be hired to meet program priorities that have been established by the governments. With the high costs of health care, one has to wonder about the degree to which economics and politics influence the personnel recommendations of governments. While governments no doubt have the health interests of people at heart, and they have been given a mandate through public elections to govern and make choices about important programs in public institutions, it is undoubtedly difficult for political leaders to avoid confounding political pressures with long-term health priorities.

Canada's Mental Health Delivery System

The Canadian system for delivering mental health services is discussed first in the primary care sector, then in specialized mental services. Typical mental health services are illustrated from the province of Manitoba.

Mental Health Services in Primary Care

Canada's approximately 32,000 family physicians, constituting just under half of Canada's physician population, are the single largest providers of mental health services in Canada (College of Family Physicians of Canada, 2004) This is the case because of (a) the fairly large number of family physicians relative to other publicly funded service providers, (b) their high regard by the public, and (c) their relative accessibility in the country. The fact that mental health services provided by physicians are covered as insured services under provincial and territorial health plans also contributes to these physician services being more readily available to Canadians of all financial means.

Pharmacotherapy is often the first line of treatment by physicians with regard to mental health problems. Unfortunately, the support that family physicians often receive from other medical and nonmedical colleagues in helping them to assist individuals with mental health problems is quite inadequate. Eighty percent of psychological services in Canada, for example, are not funded by any government program and are thus not equally available to Canadians at all financial levels. Psychological consultations are also not readily available to family physicians to assist them in dealing with patients' mental health problems. This compromises the health care provided to Canadians and renders it less comprehensive than it should be and more likely, with respect to mental health issues, to be more biologically focused than is often appropriate.

Specialized Mental Health Services

Psychiatric health services had been *excluded* from the statutory definition of hospital services in the *Hospital Insurance and Diagnostic Services Act (1957)*, and the federal government did not provide funding to the provinces for general hospital expenditures related to psychiatric services, with the exception of some emergency mental health services. This created a clear distinction between physical and mental illnesses and encouraged the prevailing inclination to separate mental health facilities from the "regular" health system facilities (Romanow and Marchildon, 2003). This legislation encouraged the continued development of independent psychiatric hospitals in Canada, separate from general-medical hospitals in the primary health care sector.

Although funding for nonphysician services provided in hospitals within the context of Medicare has expanded over time in Canada to cover a range of other services (e.g., psychology, social work, occupational therapy), these funded services are generally not available as publicly funded services outside of hospitals and some community clinics. In addition, staffing for these nonmedical services in hospitals is limited and variable across jurisdictions in Canada. Thus, for Canadians to access nonphysician clinical services (e.g., psychology services), Canadians often have to enter and navigate a complex hospital system that even their family physicians may not completely understand very well. While hospitals and various clinical services have attempted to make the system more user-friendly, accessibility remains a challenge for many people.

Mental health services are organized in most provinces within the context of *Regional Health Authorities*, which are responsible for all health services in both the institutional and community sectors. Ontario is at this time one major exception to this administrative arrangement, although the province is moving toward a form of regionalization in which the regions are identified as *Local Health Integration Networks (LHINs)*. Mental health programs have been the subject of countless reviews in the provinces and territories over the last decade. While there have been changes in programs and advances made, many of the recommendations have never been implemented in spite of kind words said about them by policymakers.

In 1997, a discussion paper entitled *Best Practices in Mental Health Reform*, (Clarke Institute of Psychiatry, 1997) was funded by the Federal/Provincial/Territorial Advisory Network on Mental Health (ANMH). The objective of the review was to identify the best practices in mental health reform and strategies for their implementation, with an emphasis on the two percent of the population with chronic and severe mental illness. They reported that *Assertive Community Treatment (ACT)* had a strong body of research supporting its superiority in improving the clinical status of individuals and in reducing hospitalization. The report advocated the need for a range of housing options in the community and noted the need for staffed residential housing options for those individuals with special needs. Long-stay patients in psychiatric hospitals were reported to do best if moved into the community, with a strong link with both family physicians and mental health professionals. The report appeared to be supportive of self-help and other consumer initiatives, but it noted that there was variability in the quality of research underlying this area. More research on family self-help was recommended and there was support for refocusing traditional vocational services to support employment. The report strongly advocated the creation of a separate funding envelope that combined the multiple funding streams involved in the delivery of mental health services. It also advocated establishing distinct mental health authorities at regional and local levels to plan, organize, monitor services, control human resources, and to administer the funding. This funding and governance model would thus create a separate and distinct mental health system within a region, separating mental health from the rest of health care services.

While a number of the initiatives recommended in the 1997 *Discussion Paper* have been implemented in various jurisdictions, to date no such completely autonomous funding and governance model has been fully implemented in any jurisdiction in Canada. While the discussion paper argued that the desirability for such a funding and administrative arrangement would improve patient outcomes, it also acknowledged the widely-held belief that mental health programs often do not fare well when they compete for resources with physical health programs. Thus, there is often a desire for separation and autonomy in one form or another. Unfortunately, this recommendation would also lead to the separation of mental health services from other medical services, which appears contrary to the intent of primary health care reform that advocates greater integration of mental and physical health care systems.

Canada's provinces and territories provide a wide range of mental health services. As might be expected from decentralized administration, there are both commonalities as well as differences in the services that are provided in the various jurisdictions of Canada. A general outline of the range and type of services is provided here, although no attempt is made to provide detailed descriptions of the various programs. The guide to the mental health system in Manitoba serves as an example of the types of mental health services that are available in Canada (Manitoba Health, 2004).

Typical Mental Health Services: The Example of Manitoba

Acute care treatment facilities provide psychiatric care and treatment in inpatient psychiatric units in general hospitals and community health centres.

Assertive community treatment focuses on individuals with severe and persistent mental illness who experience great difficulty in meeting their basic daily needs in the community. They are at high risk for requiring hospitalization and/or homelessness and frequently have co-occuring disorders.

Child and adolescent centres provide services to children and adolescents requiring mental health services ranging from brief interventions to intensive long-term treatment, including inpatient services.

Community mental health services provide comprehensive assessment, case management, rehabilitation/treatment, supportive counseling and crisis intervention, community consultation and education. The objective is to help individuals with mental health problems develop coping and living skills necessary to meet their living needs and individual goals. The staff includes community mental health workers capable of working with children and adolescents, adults, and elderly individuals.

Crisis lines offer telephone-based crisis intervention and suicide prevention services that can also provide referral to other available mental health services.

Crisis stabilization units are short-term community-based facilities for individuals in crisis who do not require hospitalization. Patient stays in these facilities usually do not exceed two weeks.

Safe houses are short-term residential housing for those who require assistance to manage a mental health crisis. These are not appropriate for individuals who require medical management.

Critical incident stress debriefing provides immediate and short-term support to individuals who have experienced a traumatic event (e.g., suicides, murders, major accidents). They provide post-traumatic debriefing, education and, when necessary, referral to other resources.

Forensic community services focus on treatment and rehabilitation services to individuals monitored by the Criminal Code Review Board. Coordinates work with mental health agencies and other health care providers to address the daily living and safety needs of the clients and their families as well as those of the community.

Forensic inpatient services provide inpatient mental health services to individuals referred by the courts subsequent to a breach of the Criminal Code of Canada.

Help lines provide information to individuals with emotional or mental health crises and make referrals to crisis lines and other mental health services.

Housing and community living assist people in finding and maintaining housing in the community, which may range from residential care facilities to supportive housing options.

Intensive case management programs focus on intensive psychosocial rehabilitation with individuals who have reasonably well-identified goals with regard to work, school, etc. Individuals in these programs are believed to be strongly motivated to make changes in their lives that may be facilitated with support and assistance.

Mobile crisis units provide crisis intervention and suicide prevention in the community, typically in the home of the individual experiencing a mental health crisis. Services include screening and mental health assessment, crisis intervention, short-term follow-up, and referral to other resources.

Outpatient services are provided at hospitals and health centres that include assessment, treatment and case management for individuals with mental health disorders.

Psychiatric hospitals offer long-term treatment for forensic patients and for individuals with severe and persistent mental health disorders whose needs cannot be met by other mental health resources.

Psychosis early intervention services are programs oriented toward intervening in psychotic conditions early in the course of these conditions.

Self-help groups offer support that is typically provided by those affected by mental health problems or by their families. The activities provided include mutual support, public education, advocacy and consumer-oriented services.

Social and recreational programs provide support and skills development for individuals with mental health problems who are interested in becoming involved in social and leisure activities.

Specialty clinics are units designed to assess and intervene in particular disorders (e.g., anxiety, mood, obsessive-compulsive, etc.).

Vocational and employment supports provide assistance to those pursuing employment. Services may include career guidance, education and training, referral and assistance finding employment.

Direct Service Personnel

One of the major objectives of primary care renewal in Canada is the enhancement of interprofessional collaboration in order to facilitate the development of patient-centered, multidisciplinary care. In order to fully achieve meaningful and noncompetitive collaboration, the various health care professions need to be placed on a more equal legislative and remunerative footing. This does not necessarily mean a leveling of incomes among the various professions, but it does mean that the system must facilitate greater equality of financial opportunity, security, and professional status across the professions. At present, physicians are virtually guaranteed independent incomes through Medicare no matter where they choose to practice in Canada, whereas all other health care professionals are subjected to the uncertainty of seemingly arbitrary budget cuts that occur in cycles. Furthermore, legislation and regulations confer specific privileges and responsibilities on physicians, many of which could be equally well, if not better exercised by other health care professionals in a more cost-effective manner. These suggestions are not meant to be critical of physicians or to diminish their responsibilities or authority. However, the present system is not one that creates ideal conditions for collaboration and interprofessional cooperation, and therefore changes need to be made. After all, little has changed in the remunerative system in Medicare in Canada in the last 50 years and it is time for a review of the system in order to make it work better for all Canadians.

Report 3 from the Senate Committee on mental health, mental illness and addiction (Kirby and Keon, 2004) noted that no national data base currently exists to provide even a crude assessment of Canada's human resource base in mental health and addiction. There are data reporting the numbers of professionals in a range of regulated health professions in Canada, but the information does not provide a specific estimate of the numbers of practitioners working in mental health or the time that they devote to these activities. While it appears reasonable to assume that most psychiatrists and registered psychiatric nurses primarily provide of mental health services, it is more difficult to estimate the proportion of time or the number of practitioners specifically devoted to mental health services by social work, occupational therapy, psychology, etc. Clearly, these professionals provide at least some mental health services and the level of services is likely to be substantial with 16,000 psychologists, 9,600 occupational therapists, and 47,000 social workers in Canada. However, since these professions provide services throughout the health care system, it is not possible to precisely estimate the amount of overall service that is specifically allocated to mental health and addiction. With a total population of 32 million people, Canada's 16,000 psychologists yield a ratio of approximately 50 psychologists per 100,000 citizens or 1:2000 inhabitants. However, estimating that about one-third of the total number of psychologists in Canada are actively involved in providing direct clinical services at any point in time yields a ratio of approximately 17 clinical service provider psychologists per 100,000 population, or 1:5,882 population.

It is even more problematic to estimate the number of professionals working in mental health from the large number of so-called *unregulated* health professions in Canada. This includes health professionals such as marriage and family therapists, counselling personnel, addiction counsellors, etc. However, like the regulated health professions, the amount of service provided by unregulated health professionals is generally thought to be quite significant.

In general, the most comprehensive information available with regard to the regulated health professions is gathered with respect to medicine and nursing. This is not surprising since there are now over 60,000 physicians in Canada and medicine was among the first of the regulated health professions. Based on the National Physician Database, published by the Canadian Institute of Health Information in 2004, in 2002–2003 there were approximately 4,000 psychiatrists and neuropsychiatrists in Canada with a full-time equivalent of just over 3,500 physicians. Nursing as a profession is increasingly assuming more diverse roles and, with approximately 240,000 Registered Nurses in Canada, it is currently the single largest of all the regulated health professions. In western Canada (British Columbia, Alberta, Saskatchewan, and Manitoba), there are an *additional* 5,000 Registered Psychiatric Nurses who add to the overall nursing resource pool. These nurses are particularly important to the mental health system. However, the Registered Psychiatric Nursing profession has been diminishing in numbers over the last decade.

Regulation of Specialized Mental Health Professions

The regulation of health professions is well-developed in Canada as a means of protecting the public from harm and attempting to ensure high quality services. The regulated professions are typically governed by a professional body or regulatory authority that is empowered to establish entry requirements, set standards of practice, assess whether applicants possess the appropriate credentials for safe and effective practice, and discipline registrants or licensees as necessary in order to protect the public. While there are many specialty certification bodies that are national in scope in Canada, such as the Canadian Register of Health Service Providers in Psychology and the Royal College of Physicians and Surgeons, the professional regulation of practitioners is a constitutionally guaranteed provincial responsibility. As might be expected, there is considerable variability with regard to regulation, including which specific health professions are regulated in the various provinces and territories across the country. For example, while the province of Alberta regulates acupuncturists, hearing aid practitioners, naturopaths, paramedics, and social workers as health professionals under the *Health Professions Act*, the province of Ontario does not regulate any of these as health professions under its *Regulated Health Professions Act*. However, there clearly are commonalities across provinces with regard to which professions are regulated as health professions such as medicine, nursing, dentistry, psychology, etc.

Some health professions believe that the provinces' failure to properly recognize their contributions and capabilities by refusing to regulate them under health profession legislation (e.g., Marriage and Family Therapists in Ontario) is unfair. They feel that the failure to do so is largely arbitrary and has the effect of lumping together, in an unregulated professions category, professions whose standards are as strict as other professions that are regulated under legislation. Moreover, they argue that failure to regulate them as health professionals conveys an inaccurate impression that these professions are less legitimate than other professions that are regulated.

The *self-regulation* of professional groups under legislative authority, although clearly not infallible in protecting the public, is nevertheless an important element in the maintenance of quality services across the regulated health professions. On a national level, the Canadian Council on Health Services Accreditation (CCHSA) is an accrediting body in Canada that focuses attention on health care organizations in an effort to maintain high quality services and appropriate standards. The Board of Directors of CCHSA itself has consumer representatives as well as members of organizations that provide health care. CCHSA is extremely important in assisting health care organizations to be more accountable to the public through an accreditation process provided by an independent, nonprofit, nongovernmental agency. The accreditation process is predicated on the belief that by undergoing an objective, peer-review assessment of the quality of services measured against a recognized and valid set of national standards, health care organizations will be provided with a guide that will assist them in making improvements in care and services that will benefit the public.

The process begins with an extensive self-evaluation conducted internally by the organization or system undergoing evaluation. Each accreditation evaluation includes feedback from clients, families, community partners as well as front-line health care staff who provide the services that the public receives. The standards adopted by CCHSA are derived through consultation with health experts from across

Canada. Evaluation using these standards proceeds with on-site survey visits by senior health professionals who examine all aspects of the visited organization including governance and management, environmental management, human resources, and information management. In addition, client services are evaluated across a wide range of health sectors.

Administrative Personnel

Health service executives assume important leadership, management, and administrative roles in the Canadian health care and mental health care and addiction systems. However, in spite of the important and responsible roles that they assume, over the last decade their numbers have been steadily decreasing as governments often specifically target administrative roles in cost-saving initiatives. In 2002, there were approximately 2,300 members of the Canadian College of Health Service Executives (CCHSE) while in 1994 there were nearly 3,000 members. An accurate measure of the amount of administration in the mental health care and addiction systems that is provided by health care administrators and others is very difficult to obtain. Furthermore, front-line health care workers do a considerable amount of administrative work although it is not always counted as such. For example, it is not uncommon to observe nursing staff on Canadian hospital wards filling in an ever-increasing number of forms, often related to accountability measures. The absence of expenditure data for administrative personnel and services makes it difficult to estimate the efficiency of the Canadian mental health system. The most recent estimate by the Canadian Institute for Health Information (CIHI) is that about four percent of total health expenditures in 2005 went to pay for administration costs (CIHI, 2005).

Financing Strategies

Public Sector Financing Strategies

Federal Allocations to Provinces. The major vehicles by which the federal government provides funding to the provinces and territories are: (a) by transferring cash through the Canada Health Transfer (CHT), (b) by providing tax transfers to the provinces by which the federal government agrees to reduce its taxation by the exact amount it allows the provinces and territories to raise their taxes, and (c) by the federal government providing funding through equalization payments. *Equalization funding* is based on a complex formula that essentially redistributes wealth from financially better off provinces to provinces that are less economically advantaged. The aim of equalization is to ensure that the provinces and territories have the financial means to provide a reasonably comparable level of services while maintaining similar taxation levels. In order for the provinces and territories to receive federal funding they must agree to adhere to the principles outlined in the *Canada Health Act.* These fiscal measures constitute important levers by which the federal government influences health policy in the provinces and territories.

Veldhuis and Clemens (2003) examined the Government of Canada's contribution to Medicare with the goal of clarifying the relative contributions of the federal, provincial, and territorial governments to Medicare. At the beginning of universal health insurance in Canada in 1972, the federal government split the costs of hospital and physicians' billings with the provinces on a 50–50 percent basis. This led to the mistaken notion that *all* Medicare or health care costs were to be shared equally between the federal and provincial governments. In fact, from the very beginning only hospital and physician billings were to be split equally between the federal and provincial governments. Moreover, these costs were always only a portion of the total amount of funding required for health care in the provinces. Thus, the federal government never covered 50 percent of the costs of health care funding in Canada. This notion of 50–50 sharing of costs appears to have contributed to setting the stage for the now virtually continuous debates between the federal and provincial governments in Canada regarding funding for health care. The discussions have also become increasingly acrimonious as health care funding requirements increased and consumed, on average, about 40 percent of provincial governments overall budgets.

In 1977, Established Programs Funding (EPF) was introduced as a means by which the federal government provided cash and tax transfers to the provinces in support of health care and postsecondary education. This program represented a significant shift from a 50–50 federal-provincial cost sharing of hospital and physician costs to providing funding on a *block grant* basis. This program change was motivated by different objectives on the parts of the federal and provincial governments. The federal government was increasingly concerned about escalating costs and wanted to limit its open-ended financial liability that occurred in the previous cost-sharing program. The provinces wanted more flexibility in using federal funding in support of social programs.

In 1996, EPF was replaced by the Canada Health and Social Transfer (CHST) and the Canadian Assistance Plan (CAP), which gave the provinces still greater flexibility with regard to their spending priorities. The CHST was the largest federal funding transfer to the provinces to help support health care, postsecondary education, social assistance, and social services. In April, 2004, the CHST was replaced by two new programs with the intent of enhancing the transparency and accountability of federal funding. A Canada Health Transfer (CHT) was created in order to provide federal support to the provinces and territories for health. A Canada Social Transfer (CST) was created to support the provinces and territories with respect to postsecondary education, social assistance, and social services as well as early childhood development. The existing CHST cash and tax transfers were apportioned between the CHT and CST.

Federal-provincial/territorial disputes related to the relative proportions that each government jurisdiction contributes to health care depend in significant measure on what is counted. However, there is little doubt that the federal government at present contributes a lower proportion of funding relative to the provincial/territorial contributions in support of health care than it did in the past. The provinces argue that the federal government's off-loading of expenses related to health care onto them is one factor that has permitted the federal government to post large budget surpluses over the last several years. However, the federal government announced in September, 2004 that 41 billion CDN (US$31.5 billion at the 2004 exchange rate of 1.30) in additional federal funding would be provided to the provinces and territories over the next ten years through the Canada Health Transfer (CHT). This additional funding will change the balance of federal-provincial funding allocated to health care. Most observers expect, however, that the federal-provincial/territorial discussions and debates related to health care funding will continue in the foreseeable future.

It is difficult to determine precisely what Canada spends on mental health specifically because Canada lacks a standardized data collection system for tracking mental health expenditures across the country. Consequently, determining mental health expenditures across jurisdictions is both complex and requires assumptions and estimates that impede accuracy. At present, some jurisdictions collect and/or make publicly available information that other jurisdictions either do not collect at all or collect but do not make publicly available. In other instances the manner in which the funding for the various aspects of mental health services are accounted for vary widely. Given this situation it is difficult to determine the absolute level or proportion of public funding allocated specifically to mental health and even more difficult to determine how much private money individuals spend on mental health services.

The Canadian Mental Health Association (CMHA), Ontario Division, conducted a careful and sophisticated analysis to examine the Province of Ontario's mental health expenditures (Canadian Mental Health Association, 1999). In this review of funding CMHA also sought to determine how well the Province of Ontario was doing with regard to a 1993 commitment by the Ontario Ministry of Health to reallocate funding from the institutions to community care as part of mental health reform. Despite gaps in the available financial data from Ontario, after searching for mental health expenditures in various government budget locations, the CMHA concluded that in 1997/1998 the Province of Ontario spent 8.8 percent of its total health care budget on mental health services. This was an increase in the proportion of health care funding spent on mental health from 1994/1995 when the province spent 7.3 percent of its total health care budget on mental health. Relative to prevalence estimates of 20 percent of the population experiencing mental disorders, the 8.8 percent of total health care budget in Ontario appears to be disproportionately low.

With regard to spending on institutional versus community-based mental health services, in 1994/1995 expenditures for hospital-based mental health services exceeded community-based service funding by a ratio of 4.5:1. At the 1994 exchange rate of 1.37, 644 million CDN (US$471 million) was spent on hospital-based services and 144 million CDN (US$105 billion) were spent on community services. In 1998/1999 the ratio of hospital-based mental health service expenditures to community-based service funding had narrowed to 3.5:1 with 856 million CDN (US$577 million) spent on hospital-based services and 243 million CDN (US$164 million) spent on community-based services and. Thus, in 1998/1999 for every dollar spent on community-based mental health services, three and a half dollars were spent by the Province of Ontario on hospital-based mental health services. Consequently, while more money is now spent on community mental health services than was the case in the past, hospital spending continues to dominate mental health spending in Canada.

Sealy and Whitehead (2004) summarized data showing the impact of deinstitutionalization on both psychiatric hospitals and general hospitals in Canada. From 1965 to 1981 there was a 71 percent decrease in the number of beds in Canada's psychiatric hospitals. In 1965, there were 69,128 beds in Canada's psychiatric hospitals while in 1980/1981 there were 20,302 beds, a net decrease of 48,827 beds over this time period. There was, however, a significant increase in the number of psychiatric beds in Canada's general hospitals from 844 psychiatric beds in 1960 to 5,836 beds in 1976, an increase of 4,992 beds (or 591%). There was also significant variation in the rate at which deinstitutionalization occurred among the provinces in Canada. Sealy and Whitehead (2004) noted that there has been a steady decline in the total operating expenditures for both Canada's psychiatric hospitals and psychiatric units in general hospitals since the 1980s (317 million CDN or US$254 million at an exchange rate of 1.25) through the mid-1990s ($221 million CDN or US$177 million). However, there has been a significant increase (about fifteenfold) in funding for community-based psychiatric services over the same period of time, from $8 million CDN (US$6.4 million) in the late 1980s to $82 million CDN (US$60 million at the 1994 exchange rate of 1.37) in 1994/1995, to $113 million CDN (US$76 million at the 1998 exchange rate of 1.48) in 1998/1999.

Canada's overall health care expenditures are much clearer than are the expenditures related specifically to mental health. This is in part due to the National Health Expenditure Database of the Canadian Institute for Health Information (CIHI). Canada spent a total of 130 billion CDN (US$100 billion at the 2004 exchange rate of 1.30) for health care in 2004. This represented a 5.9 percent increase in spending over 2003, although the rate of growth in health care spending from 2003 to 2004 was the smallest since 1997. Overall per capita health care spending by Canada is currently over 4,000 CDN (US$3,077) per Canadian per year. There has been a relatively steady increase in health care spending in Canada since the mid-1970s. This is illustrated in Figures 4.1 and 4.2 with data from CIHI in Canadian dollars.

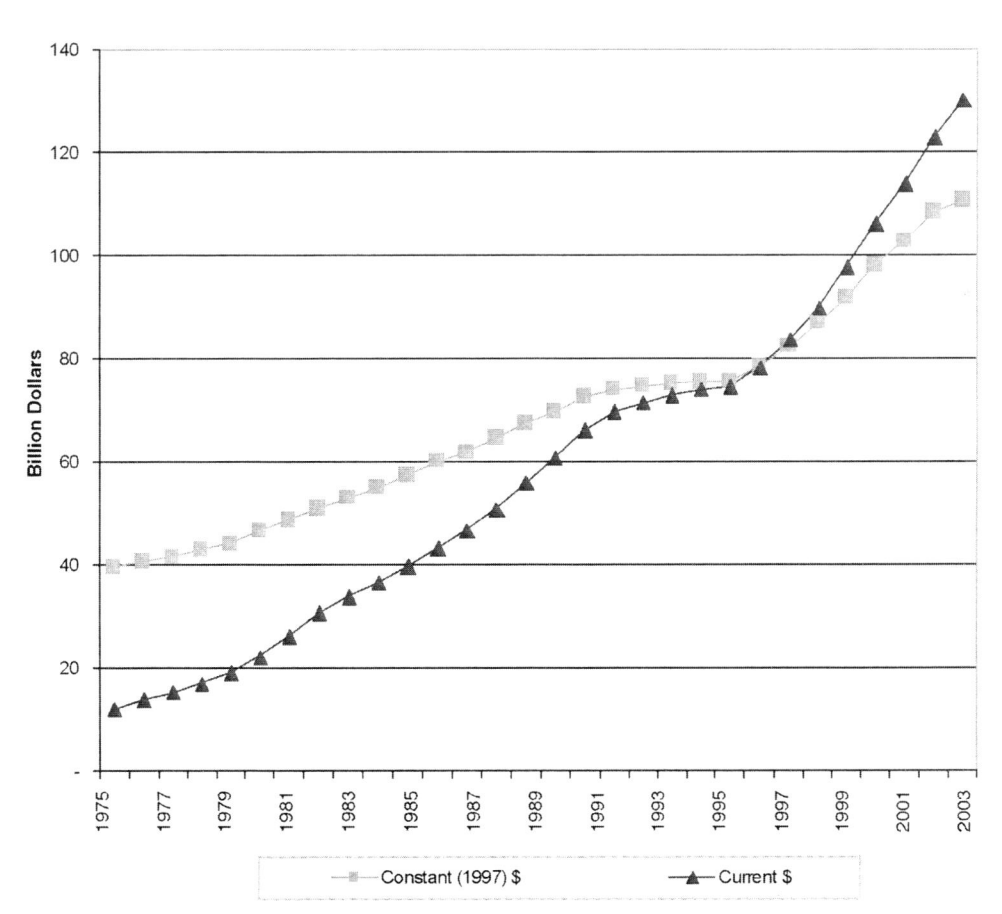

Figure 4.1. Canadian Health Care Expenditures in Current and Constant (1997) Dollars, 1975–2004. *Note:* Soure is Canadian Institute for Health Information (CIHI).

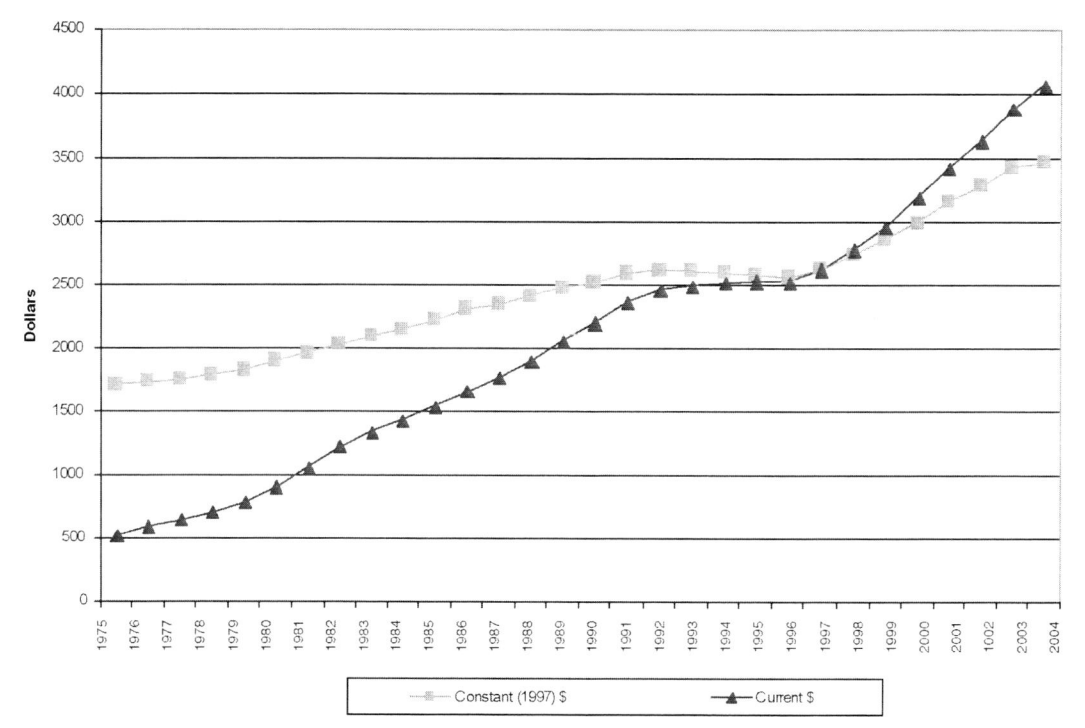

Figure 4.2. Canadian Per Capita Total Health Expenditures in Current and Constant (1997) Dollars. *Note:* Source is Canadian Institute for Health Information (CIHI).

Canadian health care spending as a percentage of Canada's Gross Domestic Product (GDP) has also shown a general trend upward since the mid-1970s, although there have been periods when health care spending has decreased in relation to the economic growth of the country. At the present time Canada spends just over ten percent of GDP on health care. Thus, Canada spends less of its GDP on health in comparison to the United States (approximately 15% of its GDP). The Canadian patterns of health care spending in relation to GDP are shown in Figure 4.3.

Private Sector Financing Strategies

It is perhaps less well-known that Canadians pay a substantial amount of money each year on health care out of their own pockets or through private or corporate insurance plans. In 2004, private sector expenditures by Canadians for health care totaled approximately $32 billion US ($42 billion CDN) while public (government) expenditures were approximately $72 billion US ($94 billion CDN). The rise in both government and private health care expenditures has been fairly steady since the mid-1970s, although the rate of growth of government expenditures appears to have been somewhat greater than private expenditures.

Figure 4.5 shows the relative proportions of various health care expenditures that are funded by government and through private health care spending.

In 2002, physician fees (98.3%) were covered almost entirely by government funding. This is not surprising since covering this cost has always been one of the main objectives of the Canadian Medicare system. The small proportion of physician costs not covered by public funding might include, for example, costs for insurance medical examinations, opinions in legal proceedings, and the like. By contrast, nearly 91 percent of the services by nonphysician health care professionals (with certain exceptions such as nurses and other professionals working in hospitals) are paid for through private funding. This situation creates a significant disparity in the average Canadian's access to the broad range of health care services provided by nonphysicians (e.g., psychologists), both because of affordability and also because public funding for physicians provides assured capital funding for expansion of their services and development of new initiatives. Nearly all hospital costs are publicly funded, which was the other major historical objective of Canadian Medicare. Thus, public funding of both physician costs and the hospital institutions that are integral to the conduct of many of their

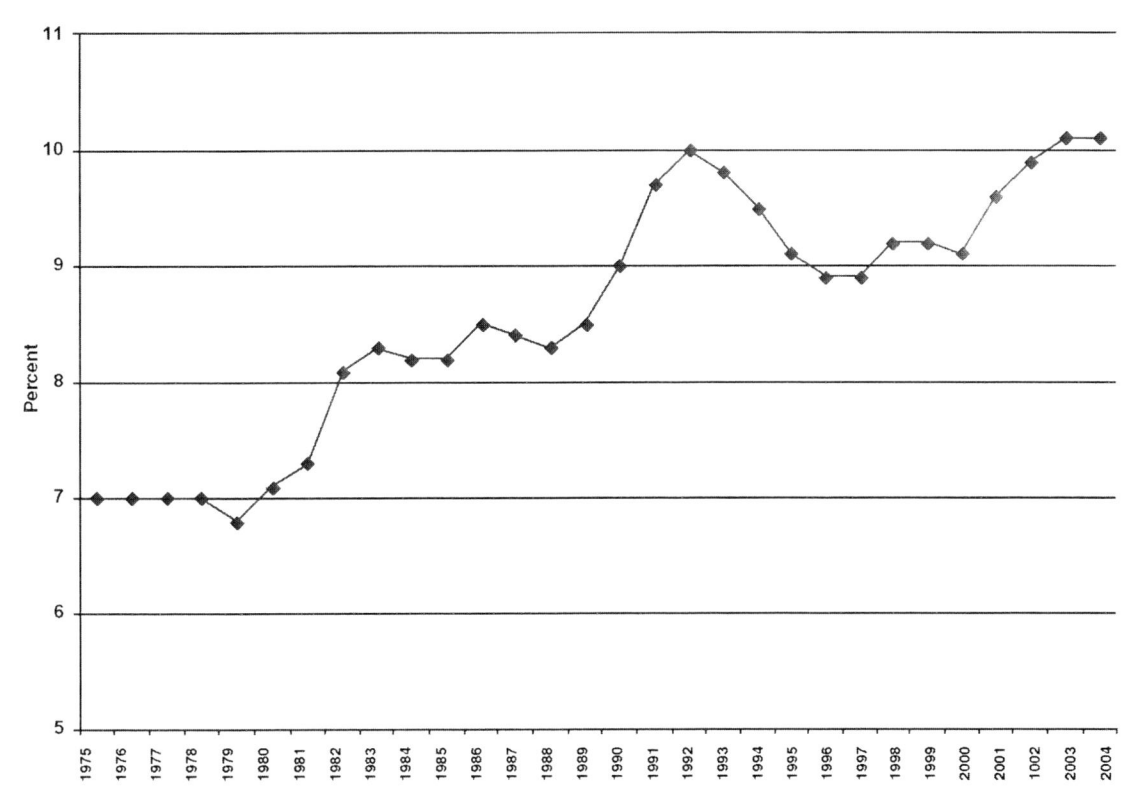

Figure 4.3. Total Health Expenditures as a Percentage of Gross Domestic Product: Canada 1975–2004. *Note:* Source is Canadian Institute for Health Information (CIHI).

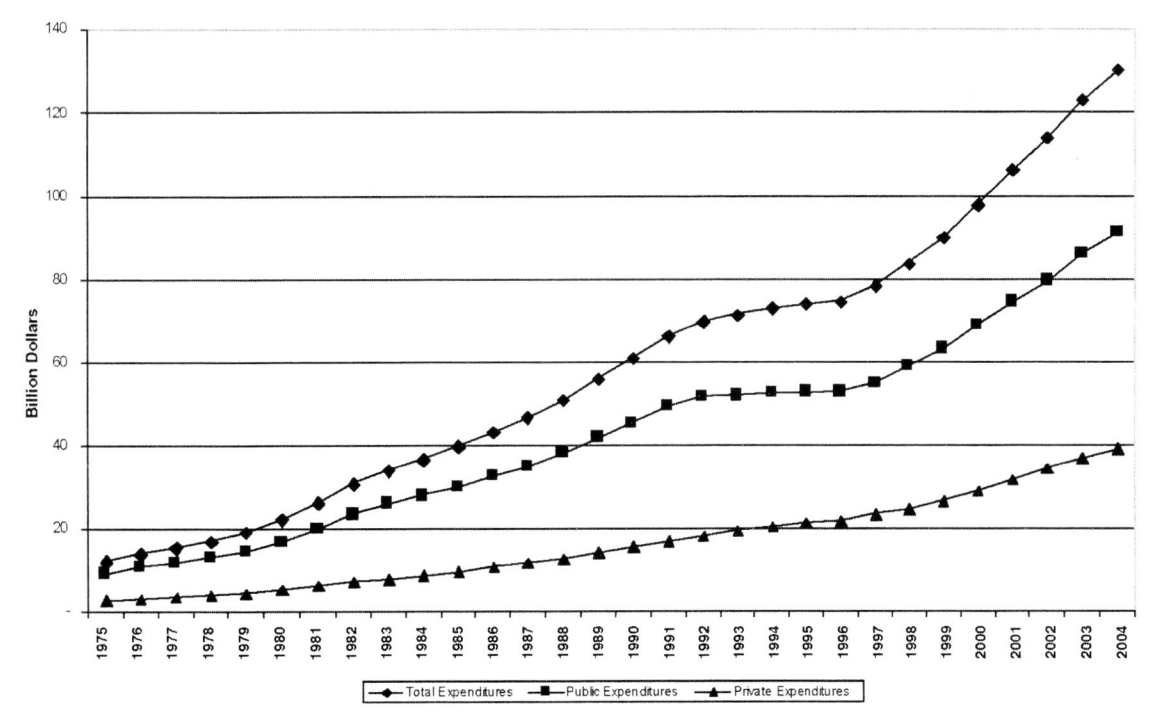

Figure 4.4. Canadian Health Expenditures by Source of Finance, 1975–2004. *Note:* Source is Canadian Institute for Health Information (CIHI).

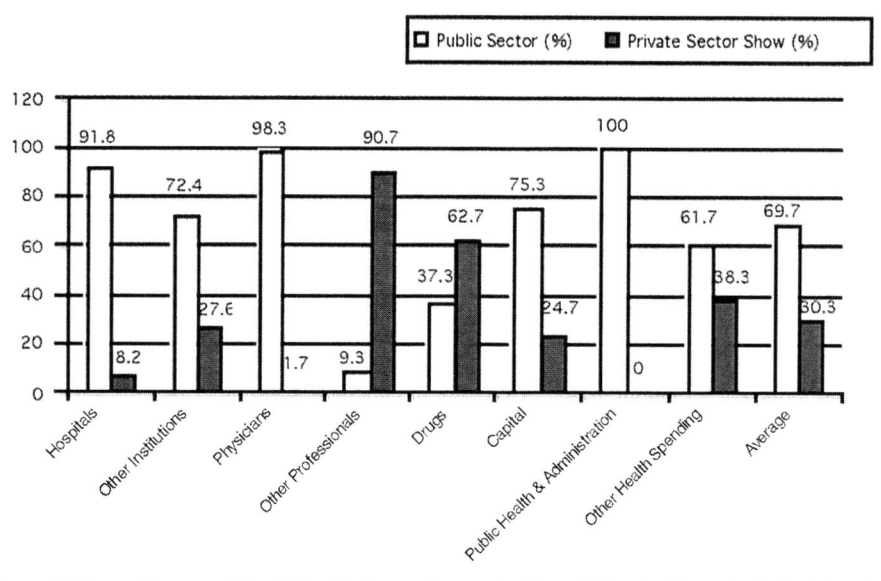

Figure 4.5. Public and Private Shares of Total Health Expenditures by Use of Funds, Canada 2002. *Note:* Source is Canadian Institute for Health Information (CIHI).

activities are provided at public expense while neither the fees, nor capital investments, nor operating costs of most other health care professionals are covered by public expenditures. It is no wonder therefore that Romanow and Marchildon (2003) recognized physicians as "privileged" providers of health care services from the beginning of Medicare in Canada. The present Medicare arrangement not only creates an uneven playing field among health care professionals; it also tends to maintain the status quo and reduces constructive competition that often leads to improved services. In addition, it encourages many general practice physicians to provide services (e.g., psychotherapy) for which other professionals may be better trained.

Table 4.7 shows the relative categorical distribution of Canada's total public and private health care spending for the years 2002, 2003, and 2004.

It is clear from these Figures that hospitals consume the single largest proportion of Canadian health care spending (approximately 30%) that has basically remained steady at about 30 percent, even though this proportion has been decreasing slightly over the last few years. Prescribed and nonprescribed drugs and other health care products (e.g., diabetic test strips) are the next largest category of expenditures at 16–17 percent of total costs and this category is increasing in the relative proportion of health care dollars it consumes. Physician fees are now the third

Table 4.7. *Total Public and Private Canadian Health Expenditures and Percent of Total Expenditures by Category ($ billions CDN).*

Category	2002 $	2002 %	2003 $	2003 %	2004 $	2004 %
Hospitals	34.4	30.1	36.4	30.0	38.9	29.9
Other Institutions	10.8	9.4	11.6	9.5	12.5	9.6
Drugs	18.4	16.1	19.6	16.2	21.8	16.7
Physicians	15.1	13.2	15.6	12.9	16.8	12.9
Other Professionals	13.1	11.5	14.5	11.9	14.6	11.2
Other Health Spending	9.9	8.7	10.2	8.4	11.2	8.6
Public Health & Administration	7.5	6.6	7.9	6.5	8.7	6.7
Capital	4.9	4.3	5.6	4.6	5.9	4.5

Note: Source is Canadian Institute for Health Information (CIHI).

largest proportional category of health care expenditures, holding at about 13 percent of total expenditures for 2004. Other professionals costs, most of which are *privately* funded, constitute approximately 11.2 percent of total health care expenditures and this category has shown noteworthy growth since 2002. Administration costs have remained relatively stable at about 6.5 percent of total health care expenditures.

An Organization of Economic Cooperation and Development (OECD) analysis of public and out-of-pocket spending by citizens on health care in 22 OECD countries in 2000 revealed that the Canadian governments finance 71 percent of health care costs. At this level of public spending, Canada provides less than the median level of public funding to finance health care (75%) across the 22 countries in the survey. In addition, Canadians incurred out-of-pocket health care expenses of 16 percent. This level is precisely at the OECD median level for out-of-pocket expenses for health care incurred by citizens of the 22 countries in the survey. In the United States, only 44 percent of health care expenditures were covered through government support while in Norway 85 percent of health care costs were assumed by government spending (Directorater Employment, Labour, and Social Affairs, 2003).

Cost Containment Strategies

One major way that cost containment is achieved in Canada's mental health system is by limiting the volume of services. There was a net saving to the system as mental hospitals were closed and more limited mental health services and beds were placed in Canada's general hospitals. Although there were strong reasons aside from cost containment to close Canada's mental hospitals, cost saving was undoubtedly one factor that was important to government. A significant approach to cost containment has been to reduce inpatient psychiatric beds. Community-based services and supports that were intended to facilitate deinstitutionalization were never put in place to the extent necessary to ensure that individuals discharged from Canada's mental hospitals could be appropriately assisted in the community. This has contributed to the "revolving-door" phenomenon in which severely and chronically mentally ill individuals are frequently admitted and discharged repeatedly to Canada's general hospital inpatient mental health units. Psychotropic medications, historically comparatively inexpensive, are now very costly and as a consequence are more difficult to add to the formulary.

The range of mental health services in Canada's mental health system, although variable across facilities and provinces, is becoming increasingly limited, particularly in some provinces. This encourages individuals to seek services in the private sector and saves the public system money. The clinical services provided by nonmedical personnel working in hospitals are frequently the targets of cost containment initiatives, in spite of the fact that this often further narrows the range of services available in the public system.

PART TWO: EVALUATION

Prior to addressing the evaluation criteria selected for comparisons among countries, this section introduces the recent, comprehensive evaluation conducted by a Canadian Senate Committee. The report provides an historical perspective and addresses deinstitutionalization, community mental health programs, and recommended treatment for addictions, dual disorders, and children and adolescents. Another recent report by the Romanow Commission (2002) is cited, which noted the fragmentation of services and proposed a more integrated "shared care" model. The dominant biomedical model is then discussed, and the lack of health promotion and prevention programs is noted. This introduction ends with the call for a national policy framework. Thereafter, the Canadian mental health system is evaluated according to the standard criteria of access and equity, quality and efficacy, cost and efficiency, financing and fairness, protection and participation, and population relevance. Recommendations in these latter areas are offered in Part Three.

Senate Evaluation Report, 2004

In late November, 2004, the Canadian Senate Standing Committee on Social Affairs, Science, and Technology released the first comprehensive report on mental health, mental illness and addiction in Canada (Kirby and Keon, 2004). This report provided an overview of the policies and programs that exist in Canada. It also provided a commentary on various aspects of mental health and addiction services in Canada. Not only did the Committee report survey the relevant literatures on mental health and addiction; it also received testimony and was able to question in Senate hearings a wide range of experts in mental health from across Canada. This provided the Committee with a unique perspective on mental health, mental illness and addiction services. This section relies significantly on the Senate report.

The Committee concluded that neither the mental health nor addiction services in Canada have garnered sufficient public support or adequate government funding to provide Canadians with mental health services equal in quality to the clinical services they receive when they suffer from a physical illness. Implicit within this conclusion are deficiencies in financing, quality, and equity.

Historical Development of Canada's Mental Health System

The Committee reviewed the evolution of Canada's mental health system, noting that it has evolved in a series of relatively distinct stages. From 1900–1960 large mental hospitals emerged across Canada, often in remote geographic locations, with some individuals being admitted involuntarily. Treatments common during this period included hydrotherapy, insulin coma, psychosurgery/lobotomy, and electroconvulsive therapy without anesthesia or muscle relaxants, the latter often causing complications including prolonged seizures, elevated blood pressure, abnormal heart rhythms, and compression fractures of the spine. The lack of effective treatments during this period, if not the relative brutality of the treatments, contributed to the low esteem in which psychiatry was held during this period. By 1950, the approximately 66,000 patients in psychiatric hospitals exceeded the number of patients in nonpsychiatric hospitals and most psychiatric hospitals functioned at 100 percent capacity. Understaffing, overcrowding, and ineffective treatments led to a custodial rather than therapeutic environment. The mental health services were not accessible, equitable, efficient, or effective.

Deinstitutionalization: 1960s to the Present

Deinstitutionalization began in 1960 and continues to the present day. This occurred as a result of a variety of factors including (a) inefficiencies associated with overcrowding and understaffing at Canada's mental hospitals, (b) enhanced recognition of the negative effects on people of long-term institutionalization, (c) the development of neuroleptic medications that were effective in controlling at least some of the major symptoms of mental illness, and (d) federal and provincial funding was made available to develop psychiatric units in general hospitals.

In 1964, the Royal Commission on Health Services, chaired by the distinguished Justice Emmett Hall, advocated that mental health services should be integrated with services related to physical health and that "any distinction in the care of physically and mentally ill individuals should be eschewed as unscientific for all time" (Canada, 1964). The degree of integration of care is considered as one of the criteria for judging the quality of mental health services.

The Senate Committee identified three phases of deinstitutionalization: *first*, the venue of care changed from mental hospitals to psychiatric units in general hospitals; *second*, mental health services in the community and away from institutions was envisioned; and *third*, the focus became the integration of mental health services in the community and improving their effectiveness.

The Committee noted that both psychiatric and general hospitals resisted these changes. The general hospitals did not want psychiatric patients and the psychiatric hospitals did not like the significant reduction in their budgets. In fact, the shift in patients from mental hospitals to general hospitals was not accompanied by a commensurate shift in resources from the mental hospitals to the general hospitals. In addition, adequate funding was not provided to communities in order for them to provide the necessary support for individuals discharged from hospitals. As a result, there was a high frequency of relapse among patients with severe mental illnesses and high re-admission rates to hospitals (revolving door syndrome), increased homelessness, and increased criminal behavior and incarceration. Consequently, in too many instances jails and the streets, instead of the hospitals, have become the new residences for those with severe and persistent mental illnesses. The problem has not been with deinstitutionalization per se, but rather with inadequate resources and inefficient organization of the mental health system to make the transition to community-based care.

The Senate Committee pointed out that for community programs to be effective there needs to be an array of supports in place. Nine are mentioned here: (a) appropriate housing, (b) vocational rehabilitation programs, (c) employment opportunities, (d) income support, and (e) effective case management to facilitate the coordination of services in the community delivery system. In addition, there is a recognized need for (f) more frequent home visits, (g) outreach services, (h) enhanced working relationships with self-help groups, and (i) mobile crisis teams to assist with acute situations that arise.

Treatment of Addictions

With regard to addictions, the Senate Committee identified five distinct phases of evolution in Canada. *First*, in the 1940s little attention was paid to treatment and the prevailing view of those with addiction problems was that they lacked appropriate will power and/or had personality deficits. In the *second* phase, there was a degree of enlightenment as most provinces added services and established administrative institutions to coordinate and/or provide addiction treatment services. Although the initial focus was on problems associated with the excessive use of alcohol, over time there was an expansion of focus that included other drugs as well. *Third*, beginning in the mid-1960s addiction services rapidly expanded, with the most rapid expansion in Canada occurring between the early and mid-1970s. *Fourth*, in the 1980s there was diversification and specialization of alcohol and drug treatment services with the development of specialized services for women, adolescents, and Aboriginal peoples. In addition to medical treatments, psychologically-based treatment strategies were made available including, for example, cognitive behavior therapy. By the early 1990s, the *fifth* phase of evolution identified by the Committee was implemented. In this final phase addiction services were integrated into the community and social services delivery systems, better integrating alcohol and drug services, and adopting a more holistic and population health perspective that recognizes the impact of multiple dimensions such as social, economic, cultural, etc. as important factors in health and well-being.

Fragmented Services for Dual Disorders

The Senate Committee identified a number of common problems with the provincial and territorial frameworks that are primarily responsible for providing mental health and addiction services. After much analysis, the Committee concluded that the mental health and addiction system is, in fact, not truly a system at all; rather, it is a complex array of services that are delivered through federal, provincial, territorial, and municipal jurisdictions, by private providers and self-help services initiated by individuals with mental illness and addiction themselves. The system . . .

> is a mix of acute care services in general hospitals, specialized services for specific disorders or populations, outpatient community clinics, community-based services providing psychosocial supports (housing, employment, education, and crisis intervention) and private counseling, all of varying capacity and quality, often operating in silos, and all-too-frequently disconnected from the health care system. (Kirby and Keon, 2004)

The Senate Committee described the system as lacking integration and being highly *fragmented*, with services being delivered by many different agencies with many different access points and with data systems that are not adequately linked. These deficiencies make it virtually impossible to monitor the quantity, distribution, quality, and cost-effectiveness of mental health and addiction services other than those provided in hospitals or in primary health care settings. The Committee also observed that current mental health services are largely *institutionally focused* rather than patient-centered and community-based. Also, the mental health services system is not *comprehensive* in terms of providing a continuum of services and supports. Thus, individuals requiring mental health or addiction services do not have equal *access* to the services that they need when and where they need them.

The Senate Committee noted further that mental health services in Canada are underfunded. The inadequate financial support is particularly problematic for those individuals with severe and persistent mental health disorders, which is an issue of equity of services. They felt that the mental health sector had significant human resource shortages and that it lacked appropriate measures of accountability to ensure quality and cost-effectiveness. The lack of coordination was compounded by the absence of clear lines of authority.

Concerns about fragmented mental health services were expressed not only by the Senate Committee, but also by the Canadian Royal Commission on the Future of Health Care in Canada in a recent publication entitled, *Building on Values: The Future of Health Care in Canada* (Romanow, 2002). The Romanow Commission noted that mental health has been described as the "orphan child" of health care (page xxxi). The Commission observed that "mental health care remains one of the least integrated aspects of health care" (p.178). The Commission also cited the following comments by the Canadian Mental Health Association:

> For many former (mental) hospital residents, the new (deinstitutionalized) system meant either (a) abandonment, demonstrated by the increasing numbers of homeless mentally ill people; (b) "transinstitutionalization": living in grim institution-like conditions such as those found in the large psychiatric boarding homes; or (c) a return to family, who suddenly had to cope with an

enormous burden of care with very little support. In addition, fears and prejudices about mental illness, in part responsible for the long history of segregation in institutions, compounded the problems in the community. These attitudes increase the barriers to access to community life in such areas as employment, education, and housing. (Romanow, 2002, p.178)

Child and Adolescent Services

The prevalence of mental health disorders in children and adolescents reported in Table 4.1 is believed to greatly exceed the capacity of the system, which limits access to needed services. This often leads to significant waiting times for services. Furthermore, mental health policies and programs have largely been oriented to the treatment of adults, and services for children and adults have developed relatively slowly. Child and adolescent mental health services are inadequately funded and there has been relatively little emphasis placed on prevention and early intervention. The Senate Committee (2004) concluded that many effective treatments are not as widely available to children and adolescents as should be the case, while ineffective interventions that are both more costly and restrictive continue to be used. Clear goals and objectives are often not set, and indicators of outcome relevant to children and adolescents are not regularly reported, thus making it difficult to assess the performance and effectiveness of child and adolescent mental health services. In short, the Senate report found the mental health services for children and adolescents were deficient on the criteria of access, financing, and efficacy.

The mental health and addiction services for children and adolescents (as well as adults) are often perceived to function in parallel rather than in an integrative fashion. As a result, an individual who suffers from both an addiction and mental health problem may be excluded from both systems. Once again, *fragmentation* is seen as a major concern with regard to the delivery of high *quality* services. Moreover, the impact of fear and stigma associated with both mental illness and addiction may discourage an individual from seeking treatment and increase the risk of self-treatment (often with alcohol or other drugs).

In terms of both criteria of access and equity, the *distribution* of mental health and addiction services is uneven in Canada and especially in rural areas that often lack an appropriate level of services. This is also true for many Aboriginal communities that are often located in relatively remote areas of the country. This inefficient distribution of mental health and addiction services forces many people to leave their communities in order to receive appropriate assessment and treatment. While telehealth initiatives have improved this situation, they have not eliminated it, particularly with regard to treatment.

Integrating Primary and Specialist Services: A Shared Care Model

The first professional most often contacted by an individual with a mental health or addiction problem is a family physician functioning within the primary health care system. However, the Senate Committee often heard testimony that many family physicians lack sufficient knowledge, training, and skills to screen and manage individuals with mental illness and addiction. Nevertheless, family physicians provide mental health services to over 50 percent of those individuals with mental health problems who seek and receive care (College of Family Physicians of Canada, 2002). Thus, there is a need for family physicians and psychiatrists to position themselves to better provide for the needs of individuals with mental illness.

Psychiatrists and family physicians both recognized the need to strengthen the role of the family physician and also to enhance the consultative role of psychiatry in improving the quality of care that patients with mental health problems receive. The intent of shared mental health care has been to increase collaboration between psychiatrists and family physicians in order to improve the *quality* of mental health care for patients, improve *access* to psychiatric consultation as necessary, and to improve patient access to psychiatric services as required. For the providers of services, the intent was (a) to increase the competence and confidence of family physicians in managing mental health problems, (b) to enhance the effectiveness of psychiatrists as consultants and supports to family physicians, and (c) to increase mutual support among psychiatrists and family physicians in managing complex mental health problems. The *shared care model* of mental health care was seen as one important vehicle to achieve these objectives.

Three key principles and objectives guiding this more integrative approach are (a) to improve communication between psychiatrists and family physicians, (b) to build new linkages between family physicians and psychiatrists and psychiatric services, and (c) to integrate psychiatrists and psychiatric services within primary care settings. These were seen as the fundamental principles to enhance collaborative care. This approach was also seen as one component that held promise to facilitate more *efficient* use of resources, to reduce fragmentation, and to improve integration of mental health care within the general health care system.

In practice, it would appear that the success of the model has been disappointing. In the *2001 National Family Physician Workforce Survey* that was released in December, 2002 (Table 8, page 14), only 26 percent of the family physicians rated their perceived access to the services of psychiatrists as good (16.1%), very good (6.9%), or excellent (3.2%), whereas 73.7 percent rated their access as fair (29.2%) or poor (44.5%) (College of Family Physicians of Canada, 2002). Thus, approximately five years after the shared care model agreement was affirmed by the respective professional organizations of Canadian psychiatry and Family Medicine, almost half of the family physicians reported their access to psychiatrists was poor.

As noted earlier, only one-third of Canadians suffering from mental health problems and/or addictions seek professional help for these difficulties. In addition, those aged 15–24 years, who on average experience proportionally more difficulty, are least likely to seek assistance. While stigma remains a potent deterrent to seeking professional help, this relatively *low utilization rate* also raises serious questions about the perceived relevance and/or value of many existing professional mental health and addiction services for the majority of Canadians. We have to continue to challenge ourselves to examine whether our services are truly patient-focused or whether they remain largely focused around the interests of the professional providers of mental health and addiction services. Population relevance is an important criterion for evaluating a mental health system, in addition to criteria of access, quality, cost, equity, and fair financing.

The Dominant Biomedical Model

Although there is a range of providers of mental health and addiction services in Canada and a variety of program initiatives, the mental health system remains largely controlled by physicians and consequently, dominated by the biomedical model. The Standing Senate Committee on Social Affairs, Science and Technology (2004) stated this by noting that the current services that governments have chosen to finance are "narrowly defined biomedical services" (p.163). As was the case 50 years ago, the national health insurance program (Medicare) continues to be largely oriented to covering the costs associated with physician services and hospital care, rather than a broader range of providers and a broader range of community-based services. While community-based mental health and addiction services have increased in recent years, the majority of funding remains captured by the hospital care system. This likely reflects the clear notion among many influential policymakers that mental health and addiction problems are fundamentally diseases that should be approached largely from a biomedical perspective.

The mental health services model that is adopted is extremely important not only because it reflects beliefs about the etiology of mental health disorders, but also because it profoundly affects which services are offered, where they are provided, and who is primarily responsible as well as the degree to which the therapeutic approaches are integrated or not with other factors that affect mental health (e.g., housing, work, etc), the type of research that is supported, and the focus and degree to which illness prevention and health promotion is pursued. Clearly, the model matters a great deal in terms of the specific services that ultimately are made available, as well as the organization and delivery of those services.

For some time now there has been an increasing tendency to medicalize, and perhaps overly medicalize, a wide range of social problems. It appears as though people have become so conditioned and accustomed to think of both personal and interpersonal problems in terms of the biomedical model, that this model is often uncritically and reflexively adopted in explanatory terms for an increasingly wide range of problems. For example, when people hear of a heinous crime directed against other people it is not uncommon for them to reflexively think of the perpetrator as "sick" or mentally ill, in spite of the fact that mental illness does not underlie the vast majority of serious crimes committed by individuals. Moreover, the illness model often leads to the stigmatization of those with mental illness and to etiological hypotheses focused primarily on biological factors. Despite society's fascination with images of the brain and other biological systems provided by sophisticated imaging machines and technology, there has not been a significant reduction in mental illness associated with the use of these biomedical technologies. Furthermore, in the treatment of mental health problems, nonbiological approaches to treatment work just as well, and in some cases better, than biological approaches (Antonuccio, D.O., Danton, W.G.

and DeNelsky, G.Y.,1995; Barlow, D.H., Gorman, J.M., Shear, M.K. and Woods, S.W. ,2000; DeRubeis, R.J., Gelfand, L.A., Tang, T.Z. and Simons, A.D., 1999; Gould, R.A., Otto, M.W., and Pollack, M.H., 1996; Jarrett, R.B., Schaffer, M., McIntire, D., Witt-Browder, A., Kraft, D. and Risser, R. C., 1999; Keller, M.B., McCullough, J.P., Klein, D.N., Arnow, B., Dunner, D.L., Gelenberg, A.J., Markowitz, J.C., Nemeroff, C.B., Russell, J.M., Thase, M.E., Trivedi, M.H., and Zajecka, J., 2000).

While biology is clearly important in mental health and health in general, the biomedical model appears to be too narrow to fully conceptualize and plan optimal interventions for the wide range of mental health problems that exist. The Senate Report 1 on mental health, mental illness and addiction (Kirby and Keon, 2004) outlined the importance of a population health approach to mental health. The Senate Committee noted that mental health, mental illness and addiction are strongly influenced by a wide range of factors including biology and genetics, income and educational achievement, employment, social environment, and more. This fact points clearly to the need to address mental health, mental illness and addiction from a population health approach, a broad perspective extending well beyond health care *per se* (Kirby and Keon, 2004, p. 209).

Clearly, the biomedical model has led to an increasing emphasis on pharmacological treatments for mental health problems and rapidly growing costs associated with the increasing use of psychotropic medications across the age span, including children. With governments overwhelmed by the ever-growing costs associated with health care, it is not surprising that they do not often seek to diversify services and add new providers under provincial and territorial health plans. Although not perfect, Engle's (1977) biopsychosocial model provides a broader and more comprehensive way of conceptualizing the nature, etiology, and treatment of mental health disorders than does the biomedical model. The biopsychosocial model undergirds and guides the practice of clinical and counseling psychology.

Promotion/Prevention Is Lacking

One might expect that the large costs associated with the provision of health care services would prompt Canadian policymakers to seek to prevent problems in the health and mental health areas, in addition to diagnosing and treating them. In fact, the efforts by governments at all levels in Canada have been nothing short of anemic in terms of health promotion and illness prevention strategies, in spite of the fact that most, if not all, appear to be philosophically in tune with this approach. Had they chosen to seriously follow this approach they would have had access to an excellent conceptual model that was provided by the Government of Canada in 1974. Unfortunately, this work has largely gathered dust in the more than 30 years that have passed since this work was presented in the Canadian House of Commons. In 1974 Marc LaLonde, as the federal government's Minister of Health and Welfare, released a green paper entitled, *A New Perspective of the Health of Canadians*, which clearly articulated the fundamental principles of the population health perspective and highlighted the importance of health promotion and illness prevention as public health strategies.

The working group on Striking a Balance (2003) was given the mandate by the National Forum on Health to make recommendations on how to best allocate Canada's resources to protect, restore, and promote the health of Canadians. They recommended against pitting the resources associated with caring for the ill against those required for health promotion, suggesting that illness will always take precedence over prevention. They suggested that promoting health required a reconfiguration of resources throughout the economy. Thus, all sectors of the economy and government would have to consider changes in policy in relation to their impact on health, not merely the health care system. This would be a far-reaching approach that would extend considerably beyond the health sector of the economy. The reader is referred to previous discussion in this chapter on the effects of work-related stress as an example.

The positive relationship between good health and higher income is very clear and robust, and it is cited repeatedly in the population health literature. Few would argue against the wisdom of working toward enhancing the well-being of children, not only as an intrinsic good, but also because of its potential value to later reduce costs associated with health and mental health problems as children become adults. In Canada, 18.4 percent of the children currently live in poverty. This is actually a slightly higher rate than 10 years ago when about 18.2 percent of children lived in low-income families. This example is meant to demonstrate that improvements in health do not necessarily involve the health care system directly. The problem of child poverty is clearly a matter that requires resolution by Canadians and the governments of Canada.

The Need for a National Policy Framework

The Senate Standing Committee on Social Affairs, Science and Technology (2004) noted that Canada's mental health, mental illness, and addiction systems are plagued "by a serious lack of leadership" (p. 204). The Committee also noted that Canada lacks a national action plan on mental health, mental illness, and addiction, and that Canada, unlike similar G-8 countries, lacks a national mental health policy that reaches across jurisdictional boundaries in the country. Furthermore, the Committee noted that there is little indication that a coordinated strategy is being developed within the federal government relating to services that it provides or populations of people for which it is responsible. The Committee strongly advocated that, in spite of federal-provincial jurisdictional issues, better links between the federal and provincial and territorial governments and among the various overlapping government departments (e.g., health, justice, family services, etc.) are needed to facilitate the health and mental health of Canadians. Clearly, the absence of a national framework impedes needed developments in the areas of child and adolescent mental health, aboriginal mental health, suicide prevention (which is particularly high in Quebec and among some Aboriginal populations), the various adult mental health problems, as well as the difficulties encountered by specific populations (e.g., military, inmates of correctional institutions).

A national system for gathering data on mental health expenditures needs to be developed to permit comparisons across jurisdictions. This would not only facilitate financial comparisons; it would also serve as a means of monitoring accountability and quality. Given the existence of a national database to track all health care expenditures across Canada, there would not appear to be any significant jurisdictional issues that would prevent the development of such a system. The lack of development to date seems to be largely a function of the overall lack of leadership in mental health and addictions in Canada.

Canada's health and mental health care systems are far from perfect. However, it is also true that they are among the best in the world in terms of quality, equity, and access to care irrespective of an individual's financial status and/or ability to pay. The critical comments in this chapter are intended to make the systems better. The comments that follow address more specifically the evaluation criteria selected for this comparative analysis among four countries.

Access and Equity

The Canadian Medicare system does not provide comprehensive coverage for all types of mental disorders, nor does it provide an adequate level of services to meet in a timely fashion the needs and demands that exist in areas it does seek to cover. In fact, the system does not purport to provide comprehensive services; rather it aims to ensure equal access among citizens to the services that are available and deemed to be "medically necessary." The Canadian Mental Health Association observed in its brief to the Canadian Senate Standing Committee on Social Affairs, Science and Technology (Canadian Senate Mental Health, Mental Illness and Addiction, Report 1) that in order to obtain services "about half of the adult population who need (mental health) services must wait for eight weeks or more" (CMHA Brief, November 2004, p.161). The Senate Committee itself noted that "many low and middle-income individuals, together with people who are unemployed and/or do not have private health care insurance cannot afford to pay for private psychological services which are not covered under publicly funded provincial health care insurance" (Senate Report 1, p.161). In reality, even those fortunate enough to have private, supplementary health insurance to cover nonmedical mental health services are not greatly advantaged due to the typically inadequate level of coverage provided under the terms of most supplementary insurance plans.

Access to the mental health system is limited not only by income levels, but by an insufficient number and uneven distribution of mental health providers. The Senate Committee report commented, "long waiting lists and significant delays in diagnosis, treatment and support are direct by-products of a mental health system that lacks the human resources to deliver care effectively" (Senate Report 1, p.161). When people do access the publicly-funded mental health system it will often be in hospitals. There they will encounter a system that is primarily focused on biomedical approaches to mental health disorders with a strong emphasis on pharmacotherapy. This partly reflects the fact that the single largest group of publicly-funded providers is physicians, many of whom retain a strong biomedical orientation from their medical education.

The strong biomedical orientation and reliance on physicians to provide mental health services are a consequence of the way in which medicare was first established and has been maintained over the last half century in Canada. This point was emphasized by Roy Romanow, a former Premier of Saskatchewan and

Commissioner of the most recent Royal Commission on the Future of Health Care in Canada, when he wrote "although the CHA *(Canada Health Act)* has never blocked the (Canadian) provinces from providing a broader range of services under their respective health plans, it has meant that both hospital services and primary care physician services are historically privileged" (Romanow and Marchildon, 2003, p.4). It is also largely the case that hospitals tend to see nonmedical approaches to mental health problems and other health problems as expendable. For example, the Senate report (2004) on mental health, mental illness and addiction noted that "as general hospitals face budgetary constraints their departments of psychology are frequently reduced or eliminated" (p. 161).

Overall, the proportion of funding allocated to mental health services, although difficult to calculate with precision, is relatively low given the 20 percent prevalence of mental health disorders in Canadian society. In its submission to the Canadian Senate Standing Committee on Social Affairs, Science and Technology, the Canadian Alliance on Mental Illness and Mental Health observed that governments tend to favor physical medicine over mental health in the allocation of resources to the health care system. The Alliance commented "governments choose to make their health investments in narrowly defined biomedical services at the expense of services for the mentally ill and those with psychological complications in physical illness and disability" (Kirby and Keon, 2004, Senate Report 1, p. 164).

The *Canadian Senate Report on Mental Health, Mental Illness and Addiction* noted significant weaknesses in the child and adolescent mental health service system in terms of both the level of services available and their quality. The report indicated that many effective interventions were not widely available and that many ineffective approaches continue to be utilized in spite of being more expensive and restrictive than available alternatives. The report noted a lack of adequate funding for child and adolescent services as well as inadequate emphasis on prevention and early intervention. Indeed the Senate report followed the Romanow Commission Report and noted comments from several witnesses who referred to child and adolescent mental health services in Canada as the "orphan's orphan" of the health care system (Senate Report 1, p.155). Clearly, this reflects a conclusion that adult mental health services constitute the original "orphan" of the Canadian health care system.

Services to Canada's aboriginal populations and people living in remote and northern areas are clearly inadequate at the present time. The Senate Report 1 on mental health, mental illness and addiction reflected the testimony that it heard related to the paucity of mental health services in rural and remote areas of Canada by characterizing the available services as "Greyhound Therapy" (Kirby and Keon, 2004, p.158). This term was used to reflect the reality that for those individuals living in rural and remote areas of the country, including most Aboriginal communities, it was necessary to travel long distances from their homes in order to receive the mental health services that they required.

The vast majority of funding for nonmedical approaches to mental disorders is derived from private funding sources including out-of-pocket spending by citizens themselves and various private insurance programs derived through employment benefit plans. Consequently, nonmedical mental health services are largely available to more affluent individuals in Canada at present. This reflects poorly on the 1984 *Canada Health Act* principle of comprehensiveness, in spite of the narrow framework of medical necessity in which that term is used. The primary objective of the Canadian health care policy is "to protect, promote, and restore the physical and mental well-being of residents of Canada and to facilitate reasonable access to health services without financial or other barriers."

To the extent that utilization of mental health services represents one measure of access, the *Canadian Community Health Survey* suggests that Canadians aged 15–24 years largely avoid the current mental health system in spite of the fairly high prevalence of mental health problems among people in this age group (Canadian Community Health Survey: Mental health and well-being, Statistics Canada, 2003). The work of Tommy Douglas in initiating and providing the model for Canadian Medicare has increased access to health care services and spared many Canadians from financial ruin related to the cost of illness. Unfortunately, the lack of innovation and fundamental change in Canadian Medicare over the last 50 years has spawned a mental health care system that is (a) primarily focused on acute care services based in hospitals, (b) functions largely on the basis of a biomedical model of illness with a strong emphasis on pharmacotherapy, and (c) directs minimal effort toward health promotion and illness prevention initiatives.

The seemingly insatiable appetite of this system for funding has left relatively little residual money available for activities aimed at some of the root causes of mental illness identified through population health studies or facilitated more extensive initiatives directed toward illness prevention and health promotion. It has also impeded greater development and involvement of nonmedical mental health providers in the publicly-funded mental health system that in turn has limited the availability of a wider range of mental health services for Canadians, in spite of their desire for such services when given a choice (Dwight-Johnson, et al. 2000; Walker et al. 2001).

There are clear signs that governments recognize some of the problems with the current health and mental health care systems in Canada. The Government of Canada recently created the Public Health Agency of Canada not only to deal with potential pandemics and other major threats to public health, but also to stimulate increasing movement toward health promotion that is long overdue in health and mental health. Nevertheless, governments in Canada tread very carefully on issues related to health because Canadians have become accustomed to the current system and are prone to perceive major change that occurs too quickly as an indication that government is withdrawing services or inadequately supporting them. Either perception can be fatal for a government at election time. Indeed, The Filmon provincial government in Manitoba was defeated in 1999, in part because it was successfully painted by the opposition and perceived by the electorate as providing inadequate support to the health care system.

The National Forum on Health Values Working Group Synthesis Report (*Canada Health Action: Building on the Legacy – Volume II*, National Forum on Health, 1997) found when studying the responses of focus groups of Canadians that many individuals viewed "health reform" as a code for the withdrawal of health services. This was particularly troubling to participants since the majority of them saw Medicare as an essential part of their national identity as Canadians and a major distinguishing feature between Canada and the United States. Influential health professional associations, although often critical of the current health care system, as well as powerful commercial interests in the pharmaceutical and medical equipment manufacturing industries, have a vested interest in maintaining and expanding the current system.

The National Forum on Health final report *(Canada Health Action: Building on the Legacy – Volume I, 1997)* noted that people's responses to opinion polls, when asked what needs to change in health care, are significantly influenced by what they see and hear around them, by their immediate personal circumstances, and by the choices offered to them. They also noted that public opinion may be swayed significantly "by articulate (special) interests." Thus, changing the current mental health care system, even if it is not ideally meeting people's needs, will not be easy given (a) the fears that people have that change likely entails loss, and (b) the range of special interest groups that will view change to open the system more broadly as contrary to their self-interests. Nevertheless, there is evidence that change is in the wind. The recently formed Health Council of Canada (HCC) recommended in its January, 2005 report that, in order to facilitate greater emphasis on health care teams and to permit more flexibility in the way team members work, legislative barriers that artificially and unnecessarily restrict the scopes of practice of various health professionals should be removed.

Quality and Efficacy

In spite of the concerns and problems outlined above, there does not appear to be wholesale dissatisfaction with the mental health system in Canada by the majority of Canadians. Based on the *Canadian Community Health Survey: Mental Health and Well-Being* (Statistics Canada, 2002a), approximately 21 percent of individuals who reported experiencing any of the surveyed mental disorders or substance dependencies expressed the opinion that they did not receive the help that they needed during the year prior to the survey interview. Furthermore, over 82 percent of individuals reporting symptoms of the mental disorders or substance dependencies that were surveyed indicated that they were either satisfied or very satisfied with the services that they received from the professional provider whom they consulted. Nevertheless, the 21 percent who did not seek help for the problems that they acknowledged represents a significant number of people that felt that the system did not entirely meet their needs. While approximately 50 percent of these individuals reported that they either preferred to manage their problems themselves or did not get around to seeking help, another 18 percent were afraid to seek help or feared what others would think if they did so. Thus, at least four percent of the Canadian population appears to be so concerned with stigma that they fail to seek help when they recognize that they need it. It is also likely that a significant proportion of those who did not seek help because of an expressed preference to manage their own problems, or because they didn't get around to it, were likely also impacted by some degree of stigma. Thus stigma would appear to constitute a significant problem associated with the current mental health system. It does not appear to be a large inferential leap to postulate that the illness model that currently prevails in much of the Canadian mental health system acts to discuourage significant numbers of people from seeking assistance.

The Senate report on *Mental Health, Mental Illness and Addiction. Report 1* (Kirby and Keon, 2004) noted significant fragmentation within the mental health system and a lack of community services resulting in (a) a high frequency of relapse and increased hospital readmission rates, (b) increased homelessness, and (c) increased criminal behavior and incarceration. Thus, to some extent the criminal justice system appears to be serving some of the same functions once served by the Canada's former mental hospitals. In addition, there appears to be less than optimal coordination between the various components of the mental health system including, for example, housing, income support, employment assistance, hospital-based mental health services and community mental health services, etc. Moreover, the "institutionally-driven philosophy of care" was found to prevail to a great extent by the Senate committee studying mental health, mental illness, and addictions (Senate Report 1, p.154). Also, the mental health system appears to lack appropriate leadership and, according to the Senate report, "nobody appears to be in charge" (Senate Report 1, p.156).

Moreover, the Senate committee found the coordination between mental health reform and primary health care reform to be virtually nonexistentent with each proceeding independently of the other. This cannot be helpful to the quality of mental health services in Canada. The absence of a national policy on mental health in Canada and the lack of a national data base permitting the collection of comparable data on the mental health systems across Canada inevitably impede management and the quality of the system across the country. The different legislative and regulatory provisions across Canada with regard to the involuntary treatment of individuals affected with severe and persistent mental illness likely results in variations in quality and individual rights across Canada. Finally, the limited focus on the early detection and intervention with regard to most mental health problems as well as a significant lack of emphasis on preventon of mental disorders impedes optimal quality services from developing.

Cost and Efficiency

To facilitate comparisons among the four countries discussed in this book, data from the World Health Organization (2005) are reported here on several national health accounts indicators related to levels of expenditure of health in general. These data are reported to the WHO by member countries. To facilitate discussion of any trends, data are presented for 1998 and the most recent year reported (2002). Comments on these data follow presentation of Table 4.8.

Table 4.8. shows that health care expenditures are consuming an increasing proportion of Canada's economy in terms of health expenditures in relation to Canada's GDP. In addition, overall government spending on health is also increasing. With an aging population, this trend is likely to continue in the future. This table also shows that private insurance plans are

Table 4.8. *WHO National Health Account Indicators: 1998 and 2002.*

Indicator	1998	2002
Total expenditure on health as a % of GDP	9.2	9.6
General government expenditure on health as a % of total health expenditure	70.6	69.9
Private expenditure on health as a % of total expenditure on health	29.4	30.1
General government expenditure on health as a % of total government expenditure	14.3	15.9
External resources for health as a % of total expenditure on health	0	0
Social security expenditure on health as a % of general govt. expenditure on health	1.8	2.1
Out-of-pocket expenditure as a % of private expenditure on health	55.2	50.3
Private prepaid plans as a % of private expenditure on health	38.1	42.1

Note: Source is the World Health Organization (2005). Annex Table 5, pp. 192–199.
Note: See Tables 1.2 and 1.3 for comparisons for the year 2002, and Table 6.9 for the year 2003.

Table 4.9. *Total and Government Per Capita Expenditures on Health, 1998 and 2002.*

Indicator	1998	2002
Per capita total expenditure on health	$1,842	$2,222
Per capita government expenditure on health	$1,300	$1,552
Government percent of total health expenditure	70.6%	69.8%

Note: Source is WHO (2005). Annex Table 6. Figures are in US$ at average exchange rates.

increasing which probably reflects a belief by Canadians that the publicly-funded health care system is not likely to fully meet their health care needs in the future, thus necessitating the need for private insurance.

Per capita expenditures on health for 1998 and 2002 are presented in Table 4.9 in U.S. dollars at the average annual exchange rates.

Table 4.9 indicates that for the five-year period 1998–2002, per capita *total* expenditures on health increased by $380 (20.6%) and per capita *government* health expenditures on health increased $252 (19.4%).

Subtracting the government expenditures from the total expenditures yields an estimate of *private sector* expenditures in Canada for the same years. For 1998 and 2002 respectively, those private sector per capita amounts were $542 (29.4%) and $670 (30.2%). The estimated amount and percent increase in private sector per capita health expenditures from 1998 to 2002 are $128 (23.6%). Private sector per capita expenditures increased 4.2 percent more than government per capita expenditures over the same time period (23.6% private versus 19.4% government).

Canada spent approximately $130 billion CDN (US$100 billion) on health care in 2004 (2004 exchange rate was 1.30). This represents just over ten percent of Canada's GDP with the per capita health care cost in 2004 being just under $4,100 CDN (US$ 3,154) for every Canadian.

Accurate estimates of total *mental health* expenditures are very difficult to obtain. This is because of (a) the large number and diversity of providers (many of whom operate mainly in the private sector), (b) the absence of a national data base of mental health expenditures or even an approach that is comparable across provinces and territories and within the federal government, (c) accounting systems that not infrequently make it difficult to identify and determine precisely how government money for health is spent,

(d) differences among jurisdictions in what health expenditures are reported and how they are reported, (e) coding practices in physician billing schedules that may not always clearly identify the precise nature of the problem associated with the billing, etc.

The Canadian Mental Health Association estimated that 8.8 percent of total health expenditures in the province of Ontario in 1998–1999 were spent on mental health. If 8.8 percent of Canada's 2004 total health expenditures on health ($130 billion CDN; US$100 billion at the 2004 exchange rate of 1.30) had been spent on mental health, then the total Canadian national expenditure on mental health would have been estimated at $11.4 billion CDN (US$8.8 billion). However, this would likely underestimate total expenditures significantly since it would not, for example, capture money spent on private sector services. Furthermore, all provinces and territories do not necessarily allocate similar proportions of their budgets to mental health. We know that Canadians spent approximately $39 billion CDN (US$30 billion) of their own money or supplementary insurance coverage on health care in 2004, but it is not clear precisely what proportion of these expenditures were spent on mental health services. Disability costs associated with mental health disorders, particularly depression, are now among the major cost drivers of disability insurance. Administration costs are reported to be approximately 6.5–7 percent of total health care expenditures in Canada. However, this figure may underestimate administration expenses as the increasing emphasis on accountability requires line staff to spend increasing amounts of time completing forms and responding to requests for information. This time is not always captured in its entirety in estimates of administration time and costs.

Stephens and Joubert (2001) provided an estimate of the economic burden of mental health problems in Canada in 1998 using data from Statistics Canada's *National Population Health Survey (NPHS)*, 1996/1997. Recognizing that failure to account for mental health problems treated outside the medical system would miss substantial mental health services provided, they attempted to calculate the cost of psychologist and social worker visits by Canadians who sought services independent of the publicly-funded health care system. They calculated that Canadians, aged 12 years and older, made three million visits in 1998 to psychologists and social workers for assistance with depression and distress at a cost of $278 million CDN (US$187 million at the 1998 exchange rate of 1.48). They recognized that the two problems assessed in the NPHS (depression and distress) did not constitute an exhaustive list of the mental health problems experienced by Canadians. However, their study was the first attempt to estimate at least some of the costs incurred by Canadians when seeing nonmedical mental health providers outside the health care system.

As an estimate of costs related to mental health problems in Canada, Stephens and Joubert's (2001) calculated costs for depression and distress in 1998. Calculated here based on the 1998 exchange rate of 1.48, the costs were $3.9 billion CDN (US$2.6 billion) for hospitalization, $887 million CDN (US$598 billion) for other institutional costs, $854 million CDN (US$576 million) for physician fees, $642 million CDN (US$433 million) for prescribed medications, and $278 million CDN (US$187 million) for psychologist and social worker costs. They acknowledged that they were unable to tabulate costs for over-the-counter medications that may have been used by people in an effort to assist with mental health problems (e.g., nonprescription sleeping pills).

Overall, Stephens and Joubert (2001) estimated that *direct* treatment costs for mental health problems in 1998 amounted to $6.3 billion CDN (US$ 4.3 billion). The *indirect* costs for mental health problems (including short and long term disability and early death) amounted to even more at a total of $8.1 billion CDN (US$5.5 billion) in 1998. This led to a combined estimated cost for mental health problems in Canada for 1998 identified from the NPHS data at approximately $14.4 billion CDN (US$9.7 billion). Even this very large cost likely represents an underestimate of the true cost of all mental health problems in Canada.

These data provided the basis for concluding that mental health problems constitute one of the most costly health problems facing Canada today, and projections that these costs will likely increase in relation to other health problems in the future. The data underscores the need to greatly enhance efforts directed at illness prevention and health promotion in mental health. Adding more and more services aimed primarily at treatment alone will not stem the tide and will eventually lead to greater service limitations and an even narrower range of available services.

Overall, given the high cost associated with mental health problems and the frequently long waiting times for services leads to one inescapable conclusion: Including (a) patient transfers from the mental hospitals to the general hospitals, (b) the near exclusive focus on the biomedical model of illness, (c) the retention of the basic illness philosophy that was embodied in the mental hospitals, and (d) minimal effort at illness prevention and health promotion, the manner in which mental health problems have been dealt with to date is both inefficient and unsustainable in the long term.

Financing and Fairness

The mental health system in Canada is largely paid for by public tax dollars that originate with the provincial and territorial governments, as well as funding provided by federal government transfers of money and tax points to the provinces. As mentioned, the federal government directly funds and/or provides health services for specified populations, including the military, Royal Canadian Mounted Police (RCMP), inmates of federal prisons, etc. In most provinces funding is transferred from the provinces to *Regional Health Authorities* and, in some instance, to health care facilities directly. In theory, all Canadians have equal access to the available publicly-funded health services, including mental health services. In brief, Canada has a publicly financed, single-payer system for insured health services.

In functional terms, the publicly-funded services are often underfunded and underresourced which leads to waiting lists and delays for people when accessing services. While emergencies are usually dealt with promptly and without major delay, most problems do not meet the criteria established for true emergencies and people are forced to wait. In this situation, individuals who are able to either afford to pay out-of-pocket for mental health services or who have supplementary private insurance to pay for such services usually are in a position to access a wider range of mental health services faster than those who must rely on the publicly-funded health care system. Frequently, the publicly-funded health care system chooses to fund mental health personnel who are seen as essential to, or who facilitate medical personnel in carrying out their tasks, rather than professionals whose services are valued in their own right.

Protection and Participation

Individuals usually have the right to refuse mental health treatment. However, the legislation and regulations regarding involuntary admission and care, as mentioned earlier in this chapter, vary significantly among jurisdictions in Canada. In some provinces, individuals deemed to be incompetent may be treated involuntarily while in other provinces that same individual would not be allowed to be treated. In all jurisdictions there are safeguards built into legislation and regulations that are intended to balance and maintain the rights of individuals in relation to the province or territory, but they vary from place to place.

Professional practice in the various mental health disciplines, although not necessarily all providers of mental health services, is regulated by the provinces and territories in Canada. Various regulatory bodies attempt to ensure the professional competence of practitioners, to remove or rehabilitate incompetent practitioners, and to discipline professionals who use their positions of trust for unethical purposes.

Most mental health professionals attempt to work collaboratively with their clients in planning the assessment and treatment strategy, although strong philosophical differences may emerge between professionals and individuals seeking treatment. When individuals are being treated on an involuntary basis, particularly when they feel that they are being forced to take medicine or undergo procedures to which they object, considerable conflict and dissatisfaction may result. Overall, however, there appears to be a satisfactory level of protection for and participation of individuals in their mental health care in Canada.

Population Relevance

Presently, the mental health system in Canada does not comprehensively meet the mental health service needs of Canadians. There is good evidence that the system is underresourced in urban areas and even less accessible in the more remote and northern areas of Canada, particularly for Canada's Aboriginal populations. The mental health system is largely institutionally based and there are inadequate community services. These limitations have not changed much over the years in spite of provincial government promises. Mental health services are poorly coordinated and there is little linkage between primary care, mental health services, housing, income support, etc. In general, there is a significant absence of strong leadership. The underlying philosophy that guides the development of clinical services, particularly in health care institutions, is typically based on a biomedical and illness model of mental health problems for which pharmacotherapy is the mainstay of treatment.

Although there does not appear to be a major public revolt aimed against the current mental health system in Canada, the system is used by only about one-third of those experiencing mental health problems. This suggests that most people tend to avoid the system. In fact, those aged 15–24, a group that appears at particular risk for mental health problems based on the Canadian Community Health Survey, use the mental health system least of all Canadians. Many people of financial means seek private mental health services. Overall, and in spite of years of reform, the fundamental components of the institutionally-based mental health system appear to be similar to the way they were prior to reform, except smaller. The fundamental biomedical model has remained intact and may, in fact, have strengthened.

PART THREE: RECOMMENDATIONS

Recommendations concerning Canada's mental health system are addressed in this section according to the same evaluation criteria, and in the same order.

Access and Equity

It is clear that mental health services in Canada are not equally accessible to all Canadians. This is partly due to an inadequate level of resources that are provided by governments in Canada's publicly funded, single payer health care system. However, a major contributing factor underlying both the inadequate level and range of mental health services relates to the principal model upon which Canada's publicly-funded mental health system is substantially based, the biomedical model. This model tends to focus clinical mental health services in and around expensive health care institutions and also significantly restricts the range of providers who are funded to provide services. The biomedical model, which works well in acute care medicine, does not work particularly well in most areas of mental health and leads to limitations in the range and extent of services that are funded and made available to Canadians.

A second major problem, which is related to the biomedical model, is the "medically necessary" principle that applies broadly in Canadian Medicare. Since the concept of medical necessity is often not defined precisely in law or in regulations, it may be used to limit the scope of available mental health services.

Not only does the conceptual primacy of the biomedical model and the principle of medical necessity limit available mental health services, but also these concepts significantly impact on the scope of a variety of other important elements within the mental health system. The biomedical model and medical necessity tend to substantially influence where mental health services are provided and the range of providers, the administration of the mental health system, the research agenda, the relative balance between institutional and community care, the degree of coordination or lack thereof between the various elements of the mental health system, and the focus of health promotion and illness prevention objectives in mental health. Moreover, they tend to maintain the status quo of the mental health system and make it highly resistant to change.

In many ways the fundamental thinking and structures present in today's inpatient mental health units in general-medical hospitals resemble those of Canada's former mental hospitals. In short, patients are seen to have a biomedical disorder that is most often treated with medications and other procedures. Most non-medical interventions are viewed as secondary to the primary importance of medical treatments.

While senior policymakers have succeeded in making the footprint of inpatient mental health services smaller through downsizing, they have had less success in changing the underlying conceptual model that drives existing services. Adopting a population-based, public health approach in both principle and function, as outlined by the Senate Committee (Report 1) on mental health, mental illness and addiction (Kirby and Keon, 2004), would go a long way toward both diversifying the available mental health services and modifying the mental health system to improve access and equity for Canadians.

Quality and Efficacy

There is no doubt that competent and high quality mental health services are available in Canada. Also, widespread citizen criticism of Canada's mental health system was not found in the most recent *Canadian Community Health Survey: Mental Health and Well-Being* (Statistics Canada, 2002a) However, the fact that the majority of Canadians experiencing mental health problems do not use the publicly-funded mental health system, particularly in the 15–24 year old age group that experiences the single highest incidence of mental health difficulties, speaks volumes about the perceived quality and/or acceptability of the current mental health system in Canada.

The Senate Committee (Report 1) on mental health, mental illness and addiction in Canada (Kirby and Keon, 2004) went so far as to suggest that the high degree of fragmentation in Canada's mental health and addiction system implied that it is not, in fact, a system at all. Rather, it consists of a conglomeration of services with multiple entry points, poor coordination among the component parts, and a serious lack of leadership and accountability. The Senate Committee noted that Canada's mental health and addiction system lacks comprehensiveness in providing the continuum of services and supports that characterize a good mental health service system.

Weakness was particularly evident in mental health services for children and adolescents, with costly and often ineffective services remaining in place while available and more effective services are not implemented. Child poverty in Canada also contributes to child and adolescent mental health difficulties, and child poverty has actually increased slightly over the last decade. Deficiencies in mental health services also exist and need to be addressed with regard to Canada's senior citizen population and with Aboriginal and other Canadian residents who live in rural areas of Canada.

Illness prevention and early intervention services need to be substantially beefed-up and emphasized much more than they are today in Canada's mental health system. Shortages of trained human resources also need to be addressed in the system.

The poor coordination between the mental health and primary care systems contributes to less than optimal care and compromises continuity of care. These systems need to be much better coordinated as they undergo reform than is the case presently. While self-help initiatives are important components of a comprehensive mental health system, government must not regard them as economical alternatives to comprehensive professional mental health services. Furthermore, care must be taken to ensure that the necessary broadening of the scope of clinical services is not accomplished at the expense of maintaining appropriate professional standards and practitioner qualifications.

The absence of both a federal and national mental health policy arching across jurisdictions in Canada is a serious problem that needs to be addressed by all levels of government, including funding of research on mental health services and outcomes. High quality services are typically supported by a thriving and broadly-based research enterprise. Canada currently spends less on mental health research than is appropriate. The argument advanced to justify this under expenditure is that the existing scientific base in Canada is limited, hence spending more money would not result in more high quality science. This argument is unconvincing. The Canadian Institute of Health Research (CIHR) appears to have a bias in favor of supporting biologically-based mental health research at present. While CIHR's supposition that there are not enough researchers to support more biomedical research may have merit, many social scientists who could contribute significantly to mental health research go unfunded at present despite meritorious and highly-regarded research proposals.

Overall, in order to enhance the quality, efficacy, and range of available mental health services, a population health approach to mental health service delivery should be established within which the biomedical approach to mental health disorders is a major and important component part.

Cost and Efficiency

Canada now spends nearly $4100 CDN (US $3,154 at the 2004 exchange rate of 1.30) per citizen per year on health care, which makes the country one of the top six spenders on health care among OECD countries. However, the country lacks and very much needs a mental health care financial data base that would permit an accurate tracking of mental health expenditures across jurisdictions in Canada. The absence of such information makes it difficult to assess the efficiency of the mental health system. The study of mental health funding by the Canadian Mental Health Association using data from Ontario clearly suggests that mental health is significantly underfunded in Ontario and, by extension, in Canada. This is consistent with Report 1 by the Senate Committee studying mental health, mental illness and addiction (Kirby and Keon, 2004), which also concluded that mental health and addiction is significantly underfunded in Canada. However, the lack of comprehensive data on the current level of mental health and addiction funding and the multiplicity of dimensions that might be considered in evaluating how much funding is sufficient render the appropriate level of funding question unclear at this point. For example, should the appropriate level of funding be tied to the prevalence of mental health disorders, the economic burden they account for, mortality associated with mental illness, and/or other factors, etc?

The efficiency of the mental health system is called into question by the observation that published research often takes years to find its way into clinical service delivery systems. In addition, less effective or ineffective treatment approaches frequently remain in place for long periods of time in spite of significant questions about their clinical efficacy. This points to the critical need for the incorporation of valid evaluation measures to assess clinical outcomes with respect to patient care activities.

Financing and Fairness

It is clear that the range of nonmedical mental health services within the public system is inadequate and tends to worsen with financial crises that arise periodically within the health care system. Nonmedical clinical services are among the first clinical services to be cut during financially difficult times. To a significant degree, this is due to Medicare being presently structured only for services that are "medically necessary" and insured. This results in very limited nonmedical clinical services being available within the publicly-funded mental health system. This impact is particularly negative on the less affluent members of Canadian society who often do not have the financial means to purchase these services within the private system. Clearly, a reformed mental health system must address this significant unfairness in the public mental health system.

Protection and Participation

The federal government needs to develop specific federal law that guards personal health information since no specific federal act now exists in this regard. Existing federal legislation was developed largely to deal with commercial activities and corporate transactions. Given the emergence of electronic health records, federal legislative action is essential to deal with the regulation of health information, particularly across the various jurisdictions in Canada.

In order to enhance the availability of a broader range of clinical mental health services within the publicly-funded mental health, the *Canada Health Act* and Medicare legislation should be revised to remove or broaden the "medically necessary" construct and to extend the list of insured providers beyond physicians and dentists since this significantly limits mental health services at the present time.

Population Relevance

The mental health system in Canada needs to address the inadequacy of the available level of services, particularly with respect to children and adolescents, Canada's Aboriginal populations, the growing senior citizen population, and the residents of remote and rural areas of Canada. Also, a national suicide prevention strategy must be developed and implemented along with a national mental health strategy. Patient safety within the health care system and mental health care systems requires urgent attention and, in fact, significant system efforts are now underway. There needs to be increased effort in this regard directed at developing enhanced psychologically-based services for mental health disorders, particularly including anxiety and depression, as a means of reducing the rising tide of work disability problems related to these conditions. Also, the public tends to prefer psychologically-based treatments to medications when given the choice. A shift to a biopsychosocial model of mental disorders will provide both the impetus and vision for more comprehensive services relevant to the Canadian population.

REFERENCES

Agras, S. (1992). Binge eating in females: A population-based investigation. *International Journal of Eating Disorders, 12,* 365–73.

American Psychiatric Association.(1994) *Diagnostic and statistical manual of mental disorders,* 4th ed. Washington, DC: American Psychiatric Association.

Antonuccio, D.O., Danton, W.G. & DeNelsky, G.Y. (1995). Psychotherapy versus medication for depression: Challenging the conventional wisdom with data. *Professional Psychology: Research and Practice, 26*(6), 574–585.

Babor, T.F., de la Fuente, J.R., Saunders, J., Grant, M. (1992). *The Alcohol Use Disorders Identification Test. Guidelines for use in primary health care.* Geneva, Switzerland: World Health Organization.

Barlow, D.H., Gorman, J.M., Shear, M.K., & Woods, S.W. (2000). Cognitive-behavioral therapy, imipramine, or their combination for panic disorder: A randomized controlled trial. *Journal of the American Medical Association, 283*(19), 2529–2536.

Bland, R.C. (1997). Epidemiology of affective disorders: A review. *Canadian Journal of Psychiatry, 42,* 367–77.

Canada (1964). *Royal Commission on Health Services Report # 2.* Ottawa, ON: Hall EM.

Canadian Centre on Substance Abuse (1996). *The Costs of Substance Abuse in Canada: Highlights of a Major Study of the Health, Social and Economic Costs Associated with the Use of Alcohol, Tobacco and Illicit Drugs.* Retrieved March 8, 2005 from http://www.ccsa.ca/pdf/ccsa-006277-1996.pdf

Canadian Department of Justice (2004, Oct 8). *Newsroom: Government Moves to Modernize Mental Disorder Provisions in the Criminal Code.* Retrieved January 2, 2005 from http://canada.justice.gc.ca/en/news/nr/2004/doc_31250.html

Canadian Embassy (2004). *United States – Canada: The World's Largest Trading Relationship.* Retrieved December 21, 2004 from http://www.canadian embassy.org /trade/wltr2004-en.asp

Canadian Institute for Health Information (2005). *Total health expenditures, by use of funds, Canada, 1975–2005-current dollars.* Retrieved December 20, 2005 from http://secure.cihi.ca/cihiweb/en/media_07dec2005_tab_c11_e.html

Canadian Mental Health Association. (1999). *Trends in Mental Health Expenditures: Evaluating the Ministry of Health's Commitment to Mental Health Services and Supports.* Canadian Mental Health Division – Ontario Division, May 27.

Canadian Psychiatric Association (2001). Canadian clinical practice guidelines for the treatment of depressive disorders. *Canadian Journal of Psychiatry, 46,* Supplement 1.

Chenier, N.M. (1995). *Suicide Among Aboriginal People: Royal Commission Report.* Library of Parliament, MR-131.

CIA – *World Fact Book – Canada.* Retrieved November 17, 2004, from http://www.cia.gov/cia/publications/factbook/geos/ca.html

Clarke Institute of Psychiatry (1997). *Best Practices in Mental Health Reform.* Health Systems Research Unit – Clarke Institute of Psychiatry.

College of Family Physicians of Canada, Canadian Medical Association, & Royal College of Physicians and Surgeons of Canada. (2004, November). *Initial Data Release of the 2004 National Physician Survey.*

College of Family Physicians of Canada (2003, December). *Privacy Legislation: A Critical Review for Family Physicians.*

College of Family Physicians of Canada (2002, December). *Profile of Family Physicians/General Practitioners (FPs) in Canada: Perceived Access to Health Care Services in their community.*

Commission on the Future of Health Care in Canada (2002). *Medically necessary: What is it and who decides?* University of Manitoba, Winnipeg, MB: September 17, 2002.

DeRubeis, R.J., Gelfand, L.A., Tang, T.F.Z., & Simons, A.D. (1999). Medications versus cognitive therapy for severely depressed outpatients: Mega-analysis of four randomized comparisons. *The American Journal of Psychiatry, 156,* 1007–1013.

Directorate for Employment, Labour, and Social Affairs (2003). *OECD Health Data 2003,* 2nd edition. Paris, France: OECD.

Dwight-Johnson, M., Sherbourne, C.D., Liao, D., Wells, K.B. (2000). Treatment preferences among depressed primary care patients. *Journal of General Internal Medicine, 15,* 527–534.

Ekos Research Associates (2004, January). *Tracking Public Priorities.* Retrieved March 8, 2005 from http://www.ekos.com/admin/articles/publicpriorities04jan2004.pdf

Engel, GL. (1977). The need for a new medical model: A challenge for biomedicine. *Science, new series, 196,* 4286, Apr 8, 1977,129–36.

Gould, R.A., Otto, M.W., & Pollack, M.H. (1996). A meta-analysis of treatment outcome for panic disorder. *Clinical Psychology Review, 15*(8), 819–844.

Gray, J. E, & O'Reilly, R. L. (2001). Clinically significant differences among Canadian mental health acts. *Canadian Journal of Psychiatry, 46,* 315–321.

Hafner, H., & an der Heiden, W. (1997). Epidemiology of schizophrenia. *Canadian Journal of Psychiatry, 42,* 139–151.

Health Canada (2002). *A Report on Mental Illnesses in Canada.* Ottawa, Canada.

Health Canada (2003). *Canada health action: Building on the legacy – volume I – The final report.* Ottawa, Canada.

Health Canada (1994). *Update of the report of the task force on suicide in Canada.* Mental Health Division – Health Canada.

Health Canada (2004). *Canadian Addiction Survey (CAS).*

Jarrett, R.B., Schaffer, M., McIntire, D., Witt-Browder, A., Kraft, D., & Risser, R. C. (1999). Treatment of atypical depression with cognitive therapy or phenelzine: A double-blind, placebo-controlled trial. *Archives of General Psychiatry, 56,* 431–437.

Keller, M.B., McCullough, J.P., Klein, D.N., Arnow, B., Dunner, D.L., Gelenberg, A.J., Markowitz, J.C., Nemeroff, C.B., Russell, J.M., Thase, M.E., Trivedi, M.H., & Zajecka, J. (2000). A comparison of nefazodone, the cognitive behavioral-analysis system of psychotherapy, and their combination for the treatment of chronic depression. *The New England Journal of Medicine, 342*(20), 1462–1470.

Kirby, J.L., & Keon, W.J. (2004). *Mental Health, Mental Illness and Addiction: Overviews of Policies and Programs in Canada (1).* The Standing Senate Committee on Social Affairs, Science and Technology.

Manitoba Health. (2004). *Mental Health – Guide to the Mental Health System in Manitoba.* Retrieved November 8, 2004 from http://www.gov.mb.ca/health/mh/system.html

Millon T, Blaneyu, P.H., David, R, (Eds.) (1999). *Textbook of psychopathology.* New York: Oxford University Press.

Offord, D.R., Boyle, M.H., Campbell, D, Goering, P., Lin, E., Wong, M., et al. (1996). One-year prevalence of psychiatric disorder in Ontarioans 15–64 years. *Canadian Journal of Psychiatry, 41,* 559–563.

Organization for Economic Development and Cooperation (OECD) (2005). *Fact book 2005. National accounts of OECD Countries. Vol. 1. Gross domestic product per capita for OECD countries.* Retrieved July 19, 2005 from http://www.oecd.org/dataoecd/4815/34244925.xls

Public Health Agency of Canada (2001). *The economic burden of mental health problems in Canada.* Retrieved January 5, 2004 from http://www.phac-aspc.gc.ca/publicat/cdic-mcc/22-1/d_e.html

Public Health Agency of Canada. (2004, March). *Exploring the link between work-life conflict and demands on Canada's health care system.*

Romanow, RJ, & Marchildon, GP. (2003). Psychological services and the future of health care in Canada. *Canadian Psychology, 44*(4), 283–95.

Romanow, R.J.(2002, November). *Building on values: The future of health care in Canada.* Commission on the Future of Health Care in Canada.

Samuels, J.F., Nestadt, G., Romanoski, A.J., Folstein, M.F., McHugh, P.R. (1994). DSM-III personality disorders in the community. *American Journal of Psychiatry, 151,* 1055–62.

Sealy, P., & Whitehead, P.C. (2004). Forty years of deinstitutionalization of psychiatric services in Canada: an emperical assessment. *Canadian Journal of Psychiatry, 49*(4), April.

Shields, R., Tetrault, M. (2001). *Privacy and personal health information in Canada: An Overview.* Ottawa, ON: Riley Information Services Conference, September 29, 2001.

Single, E., Robson, L., Xie, X., Rehm, J. (1996). *The costs of substance abuse in Canada.* Canadian Centre on Substance Abuse.

Spitzer, R.L., Yanovsky, S., Wadden, T., Wing, R., Marcus, M.D., Stunkard, A., et al. (1993). Binge eating disorder: Its further validation in a multi-site study. *International Journal of Eating Disorders, 13*(2), 137–153.

Statistics Canada (1997a). *Selected leading causes of death by sex – suicide.* Retrieved January 28, 2005 from http://www.statcan.ca/English/pgdb/health36.htm

Statistics Canada (1997b). *Suicides and suicide rate, by sex and age group.* Retrieved November 5, 2004 from http://www.statcan.ca/English/pgdb/health01.htm

Statistics Canada (2001a). *Canada's etthnocultural portrait:The changing mosaic.* Retrieved January 27, 2005 from: http//www12.statcan.ca/english/census01/products/analytic/companion/etoimm/canada.cfm. (Information had been modified by Stats Canada on January 21, 2003.)

Statistics Canada (2001b). *Canada's 2001 population: Growth rates and trends.* Retrieved December 12, 2005 from http://geodepot.statcan.ca/diss/highlights/page2/page2_e.cfm

Statistics Canada (2001c). *Knowledge of official languages, Canada.* Retrieved December 22, 2004 from http://www12.statcan.ca/english/census01/products/standard/themes/RetrieveProductTable.cfm?Temporal=2001&PID=55537&APATH=3&GID=431515&METH=1&PTYPE=55440&THEME=41&FOCUS=0&AID=0&PLACENAME=0&PROVINCE=0&SEARCH=0&GC=99&GK=NA&VID=0&FL=0&RL=0&FREE=0

Statistics Canada (2001d). *Frequency of language of work by provinces and territories – Quebec, Census 2001.* Retrieved December 22, 2004 from http://www40.statcan.ca/l01/cst01/demo44a.htm

Statistics Canada (2001e). *Language spoken at home, Census 2001.* Retrieved December 22, 2004 from http://www12.statcan.ca/english/census01/products/standard/themes/RetrieveProductTable.cfm?Temporal=2001&PID=55536&APATH=3&GID=431515&METH=1&PTYPE=55440&THEME=41&FOCUS=0&AID=0&PLACENAME=0&PROVINCE=0&SEARCH=0&GC=99&GK=NA&VID=0&FL=0&RL=0&FREE=0\

Statistics Canada (2001f). *Aboriginal peoples of Canada, Census 2001*. Retrieved January 27, 2005 from http//www12.statcan.ca/english/census01/products/analytic /companion/abor/canada.cfm

Statistics Canada (2001g). *Religions in Canada*. Retrieved December 20, 2005 from http://www12.statcan.ca/english/census01/products/analytic/companion/rel/canada.cfm

Statistics Canada (2001h). *Census 2001: Age and sex profile: Canada*. Retrieved December 22, 2004 from http://www.12.statcan/english.census01/products/analytic/companion/age/canada.cfm

Statistics Canada (2003). Canada's 2001 population: growth rates and trends. Retrieved January 27, 2005 from http://geodepot.statcan.ca/diss/highlights/page2/page2_e.cfm

Statistics Canada (2002a). *Canadian community health survey: Mental health and well-being*. Retrieved August 12, 2004 from: http://www.statcan.ca/Daily/English/030903.htm

Statistics Canada (2002b). *Canadian forces mental health survey*. Retrieved December 24, 2004 from http//www.forces.gc.ca/health/information/op_health/stats_can/en-graph /MH_Survey_e.asp

Statistics Canada (2002c). *Participation and activity limitation survey*. Retrieved January 5, 2004 from http://www.statcan.ca/English/sdds/3251.htm

Statistics Canada (2003a, February 11). *The Daily*. Retrieved January 27, 2005 from http//www.statcan.ca/daily/english/030211/d030211a.htm

Statistics Canada (2003b, September 3). *The Daily*. Retrieved January 28, 2005 from http//www.statcan.ca/daily/english/030903/d030903a.htm

Statistics Canada (2003c, September 5). *The Daily*. Retrieved January 28, 2005 from http://www.statcan.ca/Daily/English/030905/d030905b.htm

Statistics Canada (2004, March 29). *The Daily*. Retrieved December 30, 2004 from http://www.statcan.ca/Daily/English/040329/d040329a.htm

Statistics Canada (2005). *Suicides, and suicide rate, by sex and by age group*. Retrieved December 20, 2005 from http://www40.statcan.ca/101/cst01/health01.htm?sdi–suicide%20rates

Stephens, T., & Joubert, N. (2001). *The Economic Burden of Mental Health Problems in Canada. Chronic Diseases in Canada 22*(1). Retrieved March14, 2005 from http://www.phac-aspc.gc.ca/publicat/cdic-mcc/22-1d_e.html

The World Book Encyclopedia (1980). Volume 3.

Veldhuis, N, Clemens, J. (2003). Clarifying the Federal Government's Contribution to Health Care. *Fraser Forum, February 2003:* 3–5.

Waddell, C., & Shepherd, C. (2002). Prevalence of Mental Disorders in Children and Youth. *British Columbia Ministry of Children and Family Development*.

Walker. J.R., Ediger, J., Joyce, B., Furer, P., Vincent, N., & Kjernisted, K. (2001). Poster presentation. *Anxiety Disorders Association of America, 21st National Conference*, Atlanta, Georgia: March, 2001.

Wilkerson, B. (2004, November). *Mental health, the economy, and work in Canada and Ontario*. Toronto, ON: Global Business and Economic Roundtable on Addiction and Mental Health.

Wilson, M, Joffe, RT. (2000). *Global business and economic roundtable on addiction and mental health*. Toronto, ON, Centre for Addiction and Mental Health.

World Health Organization. (2003). *Suicide Rates (per 100,000), by Country, Year, and Gender*. Retrieved December 30, 2004 from http://www.who.int/mental_health/prevention /suicide/suiciderates/en/print.html

World Health Organization. (1990). *Composite International Diagnostic Interview*. Geneva, Switzerland: World Health Organization.

Zhu, A.J., & Walsh, B.T. (2002). Pharmacologic treatment of eating disorders. *Canadian Journal of Psychiatry, 47*(3), 227–34.

Chapter 5

MENTAL HEALTH CARE IN THE UNITED STATES

DANNY WEDDING, PATRICK H. DELEON, AND R. PAUL OLSON

PART ONE: DESCRIPTION OF THE MENTAL HEALTH SYSTEM

Introduction

Mental health care in the United States is a patchwork of segmented systems, lacking both coherence and good evidence of effective outcomes. The limitations in providing mental health care reflect the larger problem of a failure of the government of the United States to effect systematic and meaningful health care reform measures. In fact, the Institute of Medicine (IOM, 2002) has expressed the view that:

> The American health care system is confronting a crisis. The cost of private health insurance is now increasing at an annual rate in excess of 12 percent, while at the same time individuals are paying more out of pocket and receiving fewer benefits.... One in seven Americans is uninsured, and the number of uninsured is on the rise.... The health care delivery system is incapable of meeting the present, let alone the future needs of the American public.... (p. 1).

The IOM was established in 1970 by the National Academy of Sciences in order to secure the services of eminent members of appropriate professions in the examination of policy matters pertaining to the health of the public. It acts under the responsibility given to the National Academy of Sciences by its congressional charter to be an adviser to the federal government and, upon its own initiative, to identify and study issues of medical care, research, and education. One of the IOM's most thought-provoking conclusions has been that: "The lag between the discovery of more efficacious forms of treatment and their incorporation into routine patient care is unnecessarily long, in the range of 15 to 20 years. Even then, adherence of clinical practice to the evidence is highly uneven" (IOM, 2001, p. 155).

As individuals who have spent many years of our professional lives being intimately involved in both the mental health field and the public policy process at both the state and national level, it is our observation that it is very important to appreciate that historically there simply has not been sufficient appreciation of the importance of mental health care (or psychological care) to one's overall *health* status by our nation's health care policy experts, or over the years within the various Administrations (regardless of party affiliation) or by the legislative branches of government. It is true that high level Administration personnel have *talked about* the importance of quality mental health care, but we have yet to see the national commitment which we genuinely feel is required. Moreover, along the lines that the IOM has suggested, in our judgment, society has yet to truly understand the importance of the psychosocial-economic-cultural gradient of health care, including the value of mental or psychological care. Accordingly, one needs to appreciate the context in which the mental health delivery system operates, including its geography, demographics, its political and economic systems, and dominant cultural values.

Geography

The United States is the fourth largest country in the world, both in area and in population. It covers the full width of the North American continent from the Atlantic to the Pacific Oceans, and extends north to Alaska and south to Hawaii. The total area is about 3.6 million square miles, which includes about 78,250 square miles of inland waters and about 14,000 square miles of coastal waters. Including both Alaska and Hawaii, the greatest distance east to west is 2,807 miles; north-south is 1,598 miles; with a total coastline of about 12,380 miles. According to the *World Book Encyclopedia* (1980, v. 20), the land of the United States is as varied as it is vast.

> It ranges from the warm beaches of Florida to the frozen northlands of Alaska, and from the level Midwest prairies to the snow-capped Rocky Mountains. The United States is the land of the spectacular Grand Canyon, the mighty Mississippi River, and thundering Niagara Falls. (p. 42)

Elevations range from 282 feet below sea level in Death Valley in California to 20,320 feet above sea level at Mt. McKinley in Alaska. Temperatures range significantly from –30 degrees Fahrenheit in northerly winters to 110 degrees in the Southwest summers.

Demographics

Initially a wilderness occupied by indigenous Native American tribes, the United States became a melting pot of emigrants from Europe, Africa, and Asia, each wave bringing unique cultural traditions and a common quest for freedom, opportunity, and greater equality.

As of July, 2004, the United States has an estimated population of 293,027,571. The aging of a large cohort of "baby boomers" (those individuals born in the years immediately after WWII) has resulted in a rapidly growing number of seniors, and it is difficult to overestimate the importance of this demographic shift. At the beginning of the twentieth century, life expectancy in the United States was 42 years, but today it is 77 years; most people once died at home, but now most die in hospitals; most medical expenses were paid by families, while today most expenses for the approximately 36 million elderly are covered by Medicare; in 1900 there was usually little disability before death, now the average person will be disabled for two years before dying (Field and Cassel, 1997). Those individuals over 80 years of age represent the fastest growing segment of the U.S. population, and there are over 70,000 centenarians in the United States. In terms of mental health, the aging of the U.S. population portends increasing numbers of citizens with Alzheimer's disease and other dementias, as well as other chronic, debilitating and disabling illness (Suthers, Kim, and Crimmins, 2003).

The population of the United States is predominately white (77.1%). Other racial groups reported in the U.S. 2000 census include African Americans (12.9%), Asians (4.2%), Amerindians and Alaska natives (1.5%), native Hawaiians and other Pacific islanders (0.3%), and others (4%). However, these demographics are also shifting, with profound implications for the United States (Aponte and Crouch, 2000). Especially significant changes include dramatic increases in the numbers of racial and ethnic minorities in the United States population, a decreasing proportion of non-Hispanic Whites, a growing foreign-born population and a larger number of Americans who speak a language other than English at home (2000 census). These changes will have a profound impact on the need and demand for mental health providers in the United States (Wilk et al. 2004).

The American Political System

In the late eighteenth century, the Americans ended their status as a British colony through the Revolutionary War and became an independent, democratic Republic characterized by a federation of states, separation between church and state, freedom of religion, speech, and the press, and protection of other civil liberties affirmed in its written Constitution and Bill of Rights.

The United States is a federation of states governed in principle as a constitutional democracy. The federal government consists of three branches of government: Executive, legislative and judicial. Three independent branches were established to provide checks and balances on concentrations of power. The legislative branch is made up of a bicameral Congress comprised of a Senate (100 seats; two members are elected from every state) and House of Representatives (435 seats allocated in direct proportion to population). Elections of both the President and Congress are through national and state elections.

Presidential elections are held every four years in a national election based on an electoral college system that gives the candidate with the most votes in a state all of the number allocated to the stated based upon population size. A candidate can become president with less than a majority of the popular vote as occurred in the 2000 presidential election. The President is limited to two terms of four years each.

As a federation of states, the United States has multiple levels of government: Federal, state, county, and local governments. All citizens have the constitutional rights to vote and to petition their government.

The United States is a country founded on a set of documents known as the Declaration of Independence (1776), Articles of Confederation ratified in 1781, the Constitution and Bill of Rights ratified in

1788, and a total of about 25 Amendments. The first three articles of the Constitution define the powers, restraints and duties of the Legislative, Executive, and Judicial branches of the federal government. The remaining Articles address the relationship of the states to each other and to the federal government (Article IV), the method of amending the Constitution (V), the preempting authority of federal Constitution and law (VI), and methods for ratifying the Constitution (VII). These Articles and subsequent Amendments constitute the framework for the American federal system and express some of the fundamental values upon which it is founded. Together with the Declaration of Independence they affirm basic human rights and entitlements of American citizenship, including "liberty and justice for all" expressed in the Pledge of Allegiance taken by citizens.

Economy

The United States is a largely urbanized, industrialized nation with a mixed economy of semi-regulated capitalism. Major sectors of the economy include manufacturing, construction, and mining, a growing service sector (hospitality, financial services), agriculture and fishing, transportation and communications, the health and insurance industries, education and entertainment.

The United States is presently one of the major economies in the world with a total Gross Domestic Product (GDP) of about $12 trillion ($37,800 per capita). About 20 percent of the GDP is accounted for by the total federal budget with projected outlays of $2.6 trillion in 2006 (Budget Summary, 2006, Table S-1). Despite the country's wealth and substantial public expenditures, "long-term problems include inadequate investment in economic infrastructure, rapidly rising medical and pension costs of an aging population, sizable trade and budget deficits, and stagnation of family income in the lower economic groups" (CIA World Factbook, 2005).

The uneven distribution of the U.S. population, including health care professionals, both across the country and in urban versus rural areas, presents a challenge for the delivery of health care services to all American citizens. Embedded within a predominantly competitive and capitalist economy, the health care system has both significant strengths and serious weaknesses.

Cultural Values

The original purposes for creating an independent, constitutional democracy were "to establish justice, promote the general welfare, and secure the blessings of liberty to ourselves and our posterity." Justice, liberty, and the common good are defining aspirations in the American culture. The people of the United States also value individualism and opportunity, equality and progress, work and family. However, the values of individualism and liberty may limit the willingness of the American people to support mental health parity, and the commitment to equality has heretofore been insufficient to support an egalitarian health care system with universal access to high quality, affordable health care.

Overview of the U.S. Mental Health System

Nearly three decades ago, President Carter's Commission on Mental Health released their landmark report.

> In assessing mental health care in 1978 we have been struck by the inconsistencies that exist between what we know should be done and what we do. We know that services should be tailored to the needs of people in different communities and circumstances, but we do not provide the choices that make this possible. We know that people should seek care when they need it, but we do little to change the public attitudes that often keep people from seeking help. We know that people are usually better off when care is provided in settings that are near families, friends, and supportive social networks, yet we still channel the bulk of our mental health dollars to nursing homes and State mental hospitals. (p. 12)

Under President Clinton in 1999, we witnessed the first White House Conference on Mental Health and the first Secretarial Initiative on Mental Health prepared under the aegis of the Department of Health and Human Services. In his Surgeon General's *Report on Mental Health*, David Satcher proclaimed:

> Previous Surgeons General reports have saluted our gains while continuing to set ever higher benchmarks for the public health. Through much of this era of great challenge and greater achievement, however, concerns regarding mental illness and mental health too often were relegated to the rear of our national consciousness. Tragic and devastating disorders . . . affect nearly one in five Americans in any year, yet continue too frequently to be spoken of in whispers and shame. Fortunately, leaders in the mental health field – fiercely dedicated advocates, scientists, government officials, and consumers – have been insistent that mental health flow in the mainstream of health. I agree and issue this report in that spirit. . . . We know more today about how to treat mental illness effectively and appropriately than we know with certainty about how to prevent mental illness

and promote mental health. Common sense and respect for our fellow humans tells us that a focus on the positive aspects of mental health demands our immediate attention. Even more than other areas of health and medicine, the mental health field is plagued by disparities in the availability of and access to its services. These disparities are viewed readily through the lenses of racial and cultural diversity, age, and gender. A key disparity often hinges on a person's financial status.... We have allowed stigma and a now unwarranted sense of hopelessness about the opportunities for recovery from mental illness to erect these barriers. It is time to take them down. Promoting mental health for all Americans will require scientific know-how but, even more importantly, a societal resolve that we will make the needed investment. The investment does not call for massive budgets; rather, it calls for the willingness of each of us to educate ourselves and others about mental health and mental illness, and thus to confront the attitudes, fear, and misunderstanding that remain as barriers before us. It is my intent that this report will usher in a healthy era of mind and body for the Nation. (U. S. Department of Health and Human Services, 1999, p. 7)

President G.W. Bush convened The President's New Freedom Commission on Mental Health, which submitted their report on July 22, 2003. The Commission wrote:

Dear Mr. President: On April 29, 2002, you announced the creation of the New Freedom Commission on Mental Health, and declared, "Our country must make a commitment. Americans with mental illness deserve our understanding and they deserve excellent care." You charged the Commission to study the mental health service delivery system, and to make recommendations that would enable adults with serious mental illnesses and children with serious emotional disturbance to live, work, learn, and participate fully in their communities. We have completed the task. Today, we submit our final report, *Achieving the Promise: Transforming Mental Health Care in America.*

After a year of study, and after reviewing research and testimony, the Commission finds that recovery from mental illness is now a real possibility. The promise of the New Freedom Initiative – a life in the community for everyone – can be realized. Yet, for too many Americans with mental illnesses, the mental health services and supports they need remain fragmented, disconnected and often inadequate, frustrating the opportunity for recovery. Today's mental health care system is a patchwork relic – the result of disjointed reforms and policies. Instead of ready access to quality care, the system presents barriers that all too often add to the burden of mental illnesses for individuals, their families, and our communities.

The time has long passed for yet another piecemeal approach to mental health reform. Instead, the Commission recommends a fundamental transformation of the Nation's approach to mental health care. This transformation must ensure that mental health services and supports actively facilitate recovery, and build resilience to face life's challenges. Too often, today's system simply manages symptoms and accepts long-term disability. Building on the principles of the New Freedom Initiative, the recommendations we propose can improve the lives of millions of our fellow citizens now living with mental illnesses. The benefits will be felt across America in families, communities, schools, and workplaces. (p. 1)

And yet, we must not forget that back in 1974, Marc Lalonde the Minister of National Health and Welfare for Canada reported:

Good health is the bedrock on which social progress is built. A nation of healthy people can do those things that make life worthwhile, and as the level of health increases so does the potential for happiness. The Governments of the Provinces and of Canada have long recognized that good physical and mental health are necessary for the quality of life to which everyone aspires. Accordingly, they have developed a health care system which, though short of perfection, is the equal of any in the world.... At the same time as improvements have been made in health care, in the general standard of living, in public health protection and in medical science, ominous counter forces have been at work to undo progress in raising the health status of Canadians.... For these environmental and behavioural threats to health, the organized health care system can do little more than serve as a catchment net for the victims. Physicians, surgeons, nurses and hospitals together spend much of their time in treating ills caused by adverse environmental factors and behavioural risks. It is evident now that further improvements in the environment, reductions in self-imposed risks, and a greater knowledge of human biology are necessary if more Canadians are to live a full, happy, long and illness-free life....

The Government of Canada now intends to give to human biology, the environment and lifestyle as much attention as it has to the financing of the health care organization so that all four avenues to improved health are pursued with equal vigour. Its goal will continue to be not only to add years to our life but life to our years.... Past improvement has been due mainly to modification of behaviour and changes in the environment and it is to these same influences that we must look particularly for further advances.... More concretely: It is estimated that about half the burden of illness is psychological in origin and this proportion is growing.... And yet mental health, as opposed to physical health, has been a neglected area for years; unfortunately there is still a social stigma attached to mental illness. (Lalonde, 1974, p. 5)

We strongly suggest that a major and underlying reason for this unfortunate situation has been the lack of systematic interest in, and appreciation for, the nuances of the public policy process within professional psychology and the mental health community. We are, however, making significant progress. For example, Ron Levant, 2005 President of the American Psychological Association, wrote:

> The historical separation of physical from mental throughout our healthcare system is precisely the problem that my "Health Care for the Whole Person" Presidential initiative was designed to solve. By collaborating with a broad range of health care organizations on a public statement on the role of psychology in health care, I hope to promote the integration of physical and psychological health care in a reformed health care system in which health care professionals team up to treat the whole person. I have been ... talking with leaders of key health care groups, including physicians groups, other provider groups, consumer groups, and health policy groups. We have found a tremendous degree of enthusiasm for, and consensus on, the importance of integrating behavioral sciences into the very heart of health care, and of delivering health care through multidisciplinary teams using the biopsychosocial model. So far, the following groups have become partners with APA in the Health Care for the Whole Person Presidential initiative: the American College of Nurse Practitioners, American Nurses Association, American Public Health Association, Association of Academic Health Centers, Center for the Advancement of Health, Consumers Union, Families USA, National Association of County and City Health Officials, and the Society for Behavioral Medicine. (Ron Levant, personal communication, April 2005)

Recall that under former American Psychological Association President Norine Johnson, the membership voted overwhelmingly in 2002 to expressly include "health" in the association's underlying mission statement. Definite progress for psychology and the behavioral sciences is evident; and yet, the underlying extraordinarily critical issue remains, namely, the absence of a national health vision and commitment to access to quality, affordable health care for all Americans.

The mental health care system is embodied in a complex matrix of payor systems that include private financing from out-of-pocket payment by patients and families, private insurance, employer paid health insurance, and public financing of federal insurance and health programs (Medicare, Medicaid, State Children's Health Insurance Program, the Federal Employees Health Benefits Program, the Department of Defense and Veterans Administration health care system and Indian Health Service). The system is clearly inequitable, and as many as 44 million American citizens have no health insurance, while millions of other Americans have inadequate coverage (Mills and Bhandari, 2003). As of August, 2005, the U.S. Census Bureau reported the number of uninsured had increased to 45.8 million equal to 15.6 percent of the total population. The number of Americans without health insurance is approximately equal to the number of Americans covered by the federal insurance program for the elderly and disabled called Medicare (Mundinger, Thomas, Smolowitz and Honig, 2004).

Starfield (2000) has noted that the belief that rising health care costs in the United States are associated with enhanced health or extended life is an illusion. Various international comparisons using indices such as life expectancy, low-birth-weight and infant mortality typically place the United States low in the bottom half of industrialized nations. Starfield compares the United States to Japan (generally ranked as the healthiest of nations) and highlights the problems associated with access to health care in the United States. She argues that the inadequacy of the U. S. health care system is actually the third leading cause of death in the United States.

There is little evidence to suggest that the United States is in any way superior to other industrialized nations in the provision of mental health services (as the other chapters in this volume document). This failure to provide adequate mental health services continues across generations. As a National Council on Disability (2002) report notes:

> Children and youth who experience dysfunction at the hands of mental health and educational systems are much more likely to become dependent on failing systems that are supposed to serve adults. In parallel fashion, adults whose mental health service and support needs are not fulfilled are very likely to become seniors who are dependent on failing public systems of care. In this fashion, hundreds of thousands of children, youth, adults and seniors experience poor services and poor life outcomes, literally from cradle to grave. (p. 1)

Summarizing the pervasive problems in the U. S. mental health system, Bell and Shern (2002) note:

- Although millions of Americans rely on public mental health services, thousands of people in need do not have access to these services. Children and older adults are particularly underserved.
- Stigma, discrimination, and the lack of insurance coverage for mental illnesses continue to inhibit access to care for many Americans.
- A lack of community mental health care has led to widespread, inappropriate use of hospital emergency departments, crisis stabilization units, and institutional

and residential care, including jails, prisons, and juvenile justice facilities.
- Our nation's prisons have become, in effect, our largest mental hospitals. In many states, a greater number of individuals with severe mental illness are incarcerated than are hospitalized in state psychiatric facilities.
- Desperately needed support and rehabilitation services (housing, transportation, employment, disability benefits, health care, etc.) are often not available, especially for persons with severe mental illness. The lack of support services results in an exacerbation of symptoms and leads to higher costs than would have occurred had adequate support services been available.
- Billions of dollars are spent on public mental health across multiple sectors, but funds are often disproportionately allocated to deep end, intensive services. At the same time, many critical prevention and early intervention programs are underfunded. (p. 1–2)

The Need for Mental Health Services in the United States

In addition to three major epidemiological studies discussed subsequently, the need for mental health services in the United States is clearly documented in two seminal publications: *Healthy People 2010* (U.S. Department of Health and Human Services, 2000; Chapter 18) and *Mental Health: A Report of the Surgeon General* (U.S. Department of Health and Human Services, 1999). For example, *Healthy People 2010* notes:

> Mental disorders generate an immense public health burden of disability. The World Health Organization, in collaboration with the World Bank and Harvard University, has determined the "burden of disability" associated with the whole range of diseases and health conditions suffered by peoples throughout the world. A striking finding of the landmark *Global Burden of Disease* study is that the impact of mental illness on overall health and productivity in the United States and throughout the world often is profoundly underrecognized. In established market economies such as the United States, mental illness is on a par with heart disease and cancer as a cause of disability. Suicide – a major public health problem in the United States – occurs most frequently as a consequence of a mental disorder.

The *Global Burden of Disease* report alluded to in *Healthy People 2010* was a collaborative research study between the World Health Organization, the World Bank and Harvard University. This study estimates that mental illness accounts for over 15 percent of the burden of disease in established market economies such as the United States; it is striking to note that this is more than the burden of disease attributed to all cancers (National Institute of Mental Health, 2001).

The relative rankings for the various disorders are displayed in Table 5.1.

The second federal government estimate of need is the Surgeon General's *Report on Mental Health*, which takes a public health approach in documenting the need for mental health services, and estimates that about 20 percent of the U. S. population is affected by mental disorders during any given year (U.S. Department of Health and Human Services, 1999, Chapter 2). The estimate is the same for adults and for children and adolescents; however, the report notes that the epidemiology of mental illness is well-documented only for adults. The latter studies estimate higher rates of prevalence.

Three Epidemiological Studies of Prevalence

The current generation of mental health epidemiology in the United States began in the 1980s with the development of the Diagnostic Interview Schedule (DIS) at Washington University by Lee Robins and her colleagues for use in the *Epidemiological Catchment Area* (ECA) study (Kessler, Koretz, Merikangas, and Wang, 2004). The DIS was closely linked to the diagnostic labels included in the third edition of the Diagnostic and Statistical Manual of the American Psychiatric Association (DSM-III).

Funded largely by the National Institute of Mental Health, the *Epidemiologic Catchment Area Survey* investigated the prevalence and incidence of mental disorders, as well as the use of mental health services. There were five study sites, and five of the country's major research universities collected data: New Haven, Connecticut (Yale); Baltimore, Maryland (Johns Hopkins); St. Louis, Missouri (Washington University); Durham, North Carolina (Duke); and Los Angeles, California (UCLA). The ECA study involved interviews with over 8,000 people and indicated that approximately 28 percent of American adults are affected annually by mental and addictive disorders, but only one in three of these individuals will seek help for their problems (Reiger, Narrow, Manderscheid, Locke and Goodwin, 1993).

About a decade after the ECA study, the most comprehensive epidemiological study of mental illness in the United States was the *National Comorbidity Survey* (NCS) funded by the National Institute of Mental Health (NIMH). This study involves a nationally representative sample taken from hundreds of different communities in 48 states during the period 1990–1992. Linked to the revised edition of the

Table 5.1. *Leading Sources of Disease Burden, 1990.*

The Leading Sources of Disease Burden in Established Market Economies, 1990	Total (millions)	Percent of Total
All Causes	98.7	
1. Ischemic heart disease	8.9	9.0
2. *Unipolar major depression*	6.7	6.8
3. Cardiovascular disease	5.0	5.0
4. Alcohol use	4.7	4.7
5. Road traffic accidents	4.3	4.4
6. Lung & UR cancers	3.0	3.0
7. Dementia & degenerative CNS	2.9	2.9
8. Osteoarthritis	2.7	2.7
9. Diabetes	2.4	2.4
10. COPD	2.3	2.3
Mental Illness as a Source of Disease Burden in Established Market Economies, 1990	**Total (millions)***	**Percent of Total**
All Causes	98.7	
Unipolar major depression	6.7	6.8
Schizophrenia	2.3	2.3
Bipolar disorder	1.7	1.7
Obsessive-compulsive disorder	1.5	1.5
Panic disorder	0.7	0.7
Post-traumatic stress disorder	0.3	0.3
Self-inflicted injuries (suicide)	2.2	2.2
All mental disorders	15.3	15.4
Disease Burden by Selected Illness Categories in Established Market Economies, 1990		**Percent of Total**
All mental illness including suicide		15.4
All malignant disease (cancer)		15.0
All respiratory conditions		4.8
All alcohol use		4.7
All infectious and parasitic disease		2.8
All drug use		1.5

Note: Measured in DALYs (lost years of healthy life regardless of whether the years were lost to premature death or disability).

DSM-III, this national survey found that approximately 30 percent of the respondents reported having experienced symptoms consistent with a diagnosis of mental illness within the previous year, and almost half of the sample (48%) reported experiencing mental illness at some point in their life. The lifetime prevalence is considerably higher than those reported in the ECA study. Kessler et al. (1994) were struck with the extent to which comorbidity was present, and noted:

> The most common disorders were major depressive episode, alcohol dependence, social phobia, and simple phobia. More than half of all lifetime disorders occurred in the 14 percent of the population who had a history of three or more comorbid disorders. These highly comorbid people also included the vast majority of people

with severe disorders. Less than 40 percent of those with a lifetime disorder had ever received professional treatment, and less than 20 percent of those with a recent disorder had been in treatment during the past 12 months. Consistent with previous risk factor research, it was found that women had elevated rates of affective disorders and anxiety disorders, that men had elevated rates of substance use disorders and antisocial personality disorder, and that most disorders declined with age and with higher socioeconomic status. (p. 8)

The NCS data are consistent with the ECA data in suggesting that men are more likely to develop addictive disorders and antisocial personality disorders, while women are more likely to develop mood disorders (with the exception of mania) and anxiety disorders (Kessler et al. 2004).

The third national epidemiological study of the American population was the *National Comorbidity Survey-Replication* (NCS-R), conducted in 2001–2002 with a stratified sample of 9,090 cases from 48 states. This replication expanded the original NCS study (e.g., it included assessment of intermittent explosive disorder and pathological gambling, neither of which had been assessed in the NCS). The study also applied the DSM-IV revision for defining and classifying mental disorders and included estimates of severity, age of onset, co-morbidity, and service utilization rates.

In general, the NCS-R data on annual 12-month prevalence (26%) showed a small decrease from previous estimates (ECA – 28%, NCS – 30%), and there was a slight decrease in the estimated number of people who have met the criteria for lifetime presence of a mental disorder (46.4% in NCS-R versus 48% in NCS) (Kessler et al. 2004). "About half of Americans will meet the criteria for a DSM-IV disorder sometime in their life, with the first onset usually in childhood or adolescense" (Kessler, et al. 2005a, p. 593).

Collectively, these epidemiological studies (ECA, NCS and NCS-R) document that there are pervasive mental health problems in the United States. At an average annual prevalence of 28 percent based on the three studies cited, and a current population of about 293 million, the estimated number of people with mental disorders is a staggering 82 million Americans. The NCS-R study estimated that about 60 percent (49 million) manifest moderate or serious impairment; however, the study also noted that even "... disorders that were classified as mild were associated with levels of impairment equivalent to those caused by clinically significant chronic physical disorders" (Kessler, et al.,

Table 5.2. *Best Estimate 1-Year Prevalence Rates Based on ECA and NCS, Ages 18–54.*

	ECA Prevalence (%)	NCS Prevalence (%)	Best Estimate (%)
Any Anxiety Disorder	13.1	18.7	16.4
Simple Phobia	8.3	8.6	8.3
Social Phobia	2.0	7.4	2.0
Agoraphobia	4.9	3.7	4.9
GAD	(1.5)	3.4	3.4
Panic Disorder	1.6	2.2	1.6
OCD	2.4	(0.9)	2.4
PTSD	(1.9)	3.6	3.6
Any Mood Disorder	7.1	11.1	7.1
MD Episode	6.5	10.1	6.5
Unipolar MD	5.3	8.9	5.3
Dysthymia	1.6	2.5	1.6
Bipolar I	1.1	1.3	1.1
Bipolar II	0.6	0.2	0.6
Schizophrenia	1.3	–	1.3
Nonaffective Psychosis	–	0.2	0.2
Somatization	0.2	–	0.2
ASP	2.1	–	2.1
Anorexia Nervosa	0.1	–	0.1
Severe Cognitive Impairment	1.2	–	1.2
Any Disorder	19.5	23.4	21.0

Table 5.3. *Children and Adolescents Ages 9 to 17 with Mental or Addictive Disorders, Combined MECA Samples.*

Type of Disorder	Prevalence (%)
Anxiety disorders	13.0
Mood disorders	6.2
Disruptive disorders	10.3
Substance use disorders	2.0
Any disorder	20.9

2005a, p. 600). Compared with other countries that participated in the WHO-WMH Survey Initiative, the NCS-R prevalence estimates are consistently higher than in these other countries (Kessler, et al. 2005b, p. 624). Unfortunately, the NCS-R study also revealed that 60 percent of those with a mental disorder receive no treatment in the health care system, and only 32.7 percent reported mental health services that met criteria for minimally adequate mental health care.

The NCS study in particular documented the extent to which mental illnesses tend to be co-morbid. As Kessler et al. (2004) note, "the major burden of psychiatric disorder in this sector of our society [persons aged 15–54] is concentrated in a group of highly comorbid people who constitute about one-sixth of the population" (p. 162).

The Surgeon General's *Report on Mental Health* (U.S. Department of Health and Human Services, 1999) drew on the first two epidemiological studies previously described (ECA, NCS) to produce the "best estimate of 12 month prevalence rates . . . ages 18–54" presented in Table 5.2. Table 5.3 presents prevalence rates for children and adolescents ages 9 to 17.

The Surgeon General's Report also looked at mental disorders among older adults (ages 55 years and older), noting:

> estimates generated from the ECA survey indicate that 19.8 percent of the older adult population has a diagnosable mental disorder during a 1-year period. . . . Almost 4 percent of older adults have SMI, and just under 1 percent has SPMI . . . these figures do not include individuals with severe cognitive impairments such as Alzheimer's disease. (p. 48)

The best estimates of prevalence rates of mental illness in older adults (age 55+) from the ECA study (excluding substance abuse) are presented in Table 5.4.

These estimates of mental disorders for older adults ranging from 19.8 percent to 21.0 percent of mental disorders are lower than the prevalence rates for all adults reported by the three epidemiological studies (ECA -28%; NCS -30%; NCS-R – 26.2%). The average of the latter three studies (28%) seems to be a more comprehensive estimate because it includes substance abuse disorders.

Need Estimated from Medication Expenditures

A somewhat different approach to estimating the prevalence of mental health disorders involves looking at the expenditures in the United States for psychotropic medications. In 1987, spending for the top five conditions totaled $13.7 billion (in 2001 dollars), and mental health conditions were not included in the top five categories of expenditures, as seen in Table 5.5.

In contrast, by 2001, total expenditures for the top five conditions had climbed to $55.9 billion (in 2001 dollars), and mental health disorders had climbed to second place on the list (Table 5.6). *Note that the total spending for mental health conditions alone in 2001 exceeded the total for the top five conditions in 1987.* Total annual prescription medicine expenditures for mental health conditions for the U. S. civilian noninstitutionalized population increased more than tenfold from $1.3 billion in 1987 to $14.3 billion in 2001 (using inflation adjusted 2001 dollars; Stagnitti and Pancholi, 2004).

Table 5.4. *Best Estimate Prevalence Rates Based on Epidemiological Catchment Area, Age 55+.*

	Prevalence (%)
Any Anxiety Disorder	11.4
Simple Phobia	7.3
Social Phobia	1.0
Agoraphobia	4.1
Panic Disorder	0.5
Obsessive-Compulsive Disorder	1.5
Any Mood Disorder	4.4
Major Depressive Episode	3.8
Unipolar Major Depression	3.7
Dysthymia	1.6
Bipolar I	0.2
Bipolar II	0.1
Schizophrenia	0.6
Somatization	0.3
Antisocial Personality Disorder	0.0
Anorexia Nervosa	0.0
Severe Cognitive Impairment	6.6
Any Disorder	19.8

Table 5.5. *Medication Expenditures, 1987.*

1987 Top Five Household-Reported Conditions Related to a Prescribed Drug Purchase	Total Annual Expenditures
1. High blood pressure	$5.5 billion
2. Heart disease	$3.5 billion
3. Arthritis	$1.9 billion
4. Diabetes	$1.5 billion
5. Asthma	$1.3 billion
Total of Top Five Conditions	$13.7 billion

Note: Expenditures are in 2001 dollars.

These data partially reflect the development of new and more efficacious psychotropic medications; however, they also reflect pressure from managed care companies to treat mental health conditions with medication rather than psychotherapy, as well as the effectiveness of aggressive media campaigns and direct to consumer marketing plans.

Health insurance companies have increasingly turned to preferred drug lists (PDLs) to cope with the escalating costs of prescription medications, requiring prior authorization before patients can use their insurance benefits to purchase drugs that are not included on the PDL. In addition, insurers advocate for the use of generic (cheaper) drugs whenever they can be substituted for more expensive medications. In 2005, a limited prescription drug benefit was added to Medicare, and the same year drug companies banded together as the Partnership for Prescription Assistance (PPA) to provide free medication to those individuals unable to afford to fill their prescriptions. It is too early to tell is either initiative will have a significant impact on health care cost or quality.

Table 5.6. *Medication Expenditures, 2001.*

2001 Top Five Household-Reported Conditions Related to a Prescribed Drug Purchase	Total Annual Expenditures
1. High blood pressure	$15.1 billion
2. Mental health disorders	$14.3 billion
3. Diabetes	$9.5 billion
4. Asthma	$9.0 billion
5. High cholesterol	$8.0 billion
Total of Top Five Conditions	$55.9 billion

Note: Expenditures are in 2001 dollars.

Although more epidemiological and drug expenditure research is needed to fully document the need for mental health services in the United States, the data we do have indicates that there are significant – and unmet – needs for mental health services, and that there is an increasing tendency to use medication to treat behavioral problems.

Policies and Programs

There is some ambiguity in the concept of "mental health services," and it is not always clear whether these include treatment for addictions and social services such as housing, financial assistance or job training (Fellin, 1996). We include substance abuse treatment under the general rubric of mental health services, but not related social services, (e.g., subsidized housing, vocational rehabilitation, social security disability), realizing the interdependence of various services provided for needy individuals. In addition, we acknowledge the complexity of the health care crisis we face in the United States, and fully understand that health care policy is affected by a number of interrelated geographic, demographic, and social factors including the growing federal debt and deficit, increases in the proportion of retirees per each working individual, increases in life expectancy, advances in medical technology, a growing number of uninsured individuals and an ever growing number of children being raised in poverty.

Two of the major federal and state health insurance programs are Medicare and Medicaid. Respectively, these programs cover about 42 million elderly and disabled and about 50 million lower income individuals and families. The policies governing these programs are significant, not only because of the number of people affected, but also because these public programs serve as benchmarks for private insurance plans.

In 1990, the General Accounting Office (GAO), a nonpartisan, federal agency, released a report exploring the availability of information on mental health services. The report focused on Medicaid, the program financed jointly by the federal and state governments, but administered by the states. The report underscores the lack of a comprehensive and standardized national plan:

> The availability of mental health services under Medicaid has been a concern to many health experts. In an earlier report, we summarized changes that state Medicaid and mental health officials believe could improve the delivery of such services.... Medicaid, authorized

under title XIX of the Social Security Act, is a federally aided, state-administered medical assistance program for low-income people.... The Health Care Financing Administration (HCFA) [now Centers for Medicare and Medicaid Services (CMS)], within the Department of Health and Human Services (HHS), is the federal agency responsible for developing program policies, setting standards, and ensuring compliance with Medicaid legislation and regulations. Each state has considerable flexibility concerning its Medicaid program. Within broad federal guidelines, states determine who will be eligible, what services will be provided, and what limits will be placed on the services. As a result, between the states over the years, wide variations have developed in Medicaid services in general and mental health services in particular. Mental health services are provided to treat a variety of mental conditions including developmental, behavioral, and emotional problems, as well as substance abuse, schizophrenia, and depression. At a minimum, Medicaid mental health services cover long-term institutional care, outpatient hospital care, and consultations with a physician, as well as clinic and laboratory services. Drug therapy might also be provided. Medicaid specifically excludes federal reimbursement for the care of the mentally ill aged 22 through 64 in institutions for mental diseases. These are defined in Medicaid regulations as institutions primarily engaged in providing diagnosis, treatment, or care (which includes medical attention, nursing care, and related services) for people with mental diseases. States are not required, but have the option to provide institutional care for the mentally ill who are under 21 years of age and 65 years or age or older. If the states exercise this option, the federal government will pay its share of the cost of such institutional care. Each state is allowed to set use and dollar limitations on the duration, scope, and dollar amount of Medicaid coverage. Each state also has the option of covering or not covering certain mental health services. As a result, there is considerable variation across states in the nature and extent of mental health services available to Medicaid recipients. (pp. 1–2)

A decade later, another GAO report (General Accounting Office, 2000) highlighted the continuing necessity for state and federal health policy dialogue and collaboration, this time focusing upon the pressing needs of individuals with serious mental illness (SMI).

Mental disorders take an enormous toll on the nation's families and finances. The indirect costs of mental illness, such as for lost productivity, were estimated at $78.6 billion in 1990. In 1997, $73 billion was spent on mental health services. The Surgeon General has estimated that about 20 percent of the U.S. population is affected by a mental disorder in a given year. About 5 percent of the population are considered to have a serious mental illness (SMI). SMI, which includes, among other diseases, schizophrenia, bipolar disorder, and major depression, is a chronic condition that can substantially limit a person's ability to function in many areas of life such as employment, self-care, and interpersonal relationships. Effective treatment can reduce the severity of these problems for the majority of people with SMI. Much of this treatment can now be provided in the community rather than in institutions....

Between 1987 and 1997, the growth in mental health spending in the United States roughly paralleled the growth in overall health care spending. After adjusting for overall inflation, spending on mental health services grew by 4 percent a year, on average, compared with 5 percent a year for spending on all health care. However, federal mental health spending grew at more than twice the rate of state and local spending. This led to the federal government's share surpassing that of state and local governments, while the share attributable to private sources declined slightly. Increasing Medicaid and Medicare expenditures accounted for the larger federal share, with combined federal and state Medicaid expenditures accounting for 20 percent of all mental health spending in 1997. The focus of care for adults with SMI has continued to shift from providing services in psychiatric hospitals to providing services in the community....

HCFA has also supported states' use of Medicaid managed care waivers to provide a wider array of community-based mental health services. However, incentives associated with capitated payment can lead to reduced service utilization. Recognizing the risks for people with specific health care needs, such as serious mental illness, the Congress required HCFA to take steps to ensure that beneficiaries enrolled in managed care receive appropriate care.... Effective oversight to ensure that adequate safeguards are implemented will be essential to provide meaningful protection to this vulnerable population. SAMHSA and HCFA commented on a draft of this report and generally agreed with our findings. (pp. 3–5)

Concluding Observations – As people with SMI increasingly receive their care in the community, it is important that they have access to the variety of mental health and other services they need. Because of the nature of SMI, people with this condition are often poor and must rely on the public mental health system for their care. Recently, states have stepped up their efforts to provide community-based services that give ongoing support to adults with SMI. These services are especially critical for people making the transition from institutions to the community, to help prevent their becoming homeless or returning to institutions.... The use of managed mental health care by some state Medicaid programs has resulted in the flexibility to provide a wider array of services. However, given the potential for managed care providers reducing access to needed services, it is important for HCFA and state Medicaid programs to ensure that beneficiaries enrolled in managed care receive appropriate care. (pp. 3–5, 19)

The United States has few clearly articulated and integrated health care policies; the policies that exist address segmented populations, yet they tend to overlap (e.g., Department of Defense and Veterans Health Administration), and/or the policies leave significant gaps in coverage; the policies often reflect state rather than federal law; and there is wide variation across states in both mental health policy and law. In addition, regulatory guidelines as well as law establish health policy, and these guidelines are shaped and influenced by administrators, executives, and a wide variety of deeply invested stakeholders. In general, health policies address different aspects of access, cost containment and quality for segregated categories of people. Some of the key factors influencing the positions of policymakers on health care policy legislation include philosophy (e.g., belief in health care as a universal right), attitudes about the role of government vs. private sector financing and service delivery and the role of employers in providing health insurance, and the willingness to learn from the experience and mistakes of health policies enacted in other countries. Federal policies established by Congress are also influenced by campaign contributions and lobbying by various constituencies.

Federal health policy formulation involves both the executive and legislative branches of government. The executive branch sets health policy, based on the advice and counsel of political, health policy, economic and budget advisors. Decisions made by the President and his staff affect Medicare and Medicaid payment policies, the Federal Employees Health Benefits Plan, and the health care priorities of the Veterans Administration, Indian Health Service and the Department of Defense health services. Federal law establishes health care *entitlements*; these are important features of the health care landscape because they are funded automatically and do not require specific appropriations. Entitlements include Social Security, Medicare, Medicaid, Food Stamps and Temporary Assistance to Needy Families (TANF). Designated as mandatory expenditures, entitlements do not receive the congressional scrutiny applied to other spending bills, and they are often indexed to cost of living increases. With an aging American population, projected to more than double from about 36 million in 2005 to 77 million Americans by 2011, the growth of entitlement spending (especially Medicare) is an important part of the current escalation in health care costs and our looming health care crisis. Total mandatory obligations projected in the federal budget for FY 2006 amount to $1.4 trillion, equal to about 53 percent of the projected total federal expenditures of $2.6 trillion (Budget Summary 2006, Tables S-1 & S-10).

Health care is routinely included on the list of the most important issues for voters, and the availability of health insurance, Medicare and the cost of prescription drugs were important health care policy issues debated in the 2004 Presidential election. Another key issue in the election was the safety and availability of imported drugs from Canada; in the final Presidential debate in 2004, President Bush appeared to open the door for importation, remarking, "If [foreign drugs] are safe, they're coming." This policy decision is important to the mental health community because many of the newer psychotropic medications are too expensive for mental health consumers who don't qualify for entitlement programs. Unfortunately, importation of medications has not been authorized by federal legislation or regulation to date, and the Bush Administration has actually discouraged it as unsafe.

The U.S. Congress influences health care policy by enacting legislation relevant to health care delivery and financing. Senate and House committee staff conduct most of the work in the health care area. Key health-related committees in the Senate include the Finance Committee (and its Subcommittee on Health Care); Health, Education, Labor and Pensions; Appropriations; and the Budget Committee. Key committees in the House of Representatives include Ways and Means (and its Subcommittee on Health); Appropriations (and its Subcommittee on Labor, HHS and Legislation); Energy and Commerce (and its Subcommittee on Health) and the Budget Committee.

Members of Congress often become quite knowledgeable about health care policy issues. For example, in the (current) 109th Congress, Representatives Dennis Hastert (R-Illinois) and John Dingell (D-Michigan) are widely acknowledged as experts on health care policy; likewise, in the Senate, Bill Frist (a cardiologist; R-Tennessee) and Ted Kennedy (D-Massachusetts) are both respected health policy experts. Important health policy issues that must be addressed by the 109th Congress include oversight of health care fraud, maintaining public confidence in the safety of drugs, medical malpractice reform, and the establishment of effective policies to reduce runaway health care spending (a perennial issue).

Two of the sea changes in health care policy in the United States occurred in 1996 with the enactments of the *Health Insurance Portability and Accountability Act* (HIPAA) and the *Mental Health Parity Act*. Since both federal laws relate to improvements in patient protection, they are discussed later in Part Two of this chapter.

Medicare and Medicaid are the two largest health insurance programs created by federal health policy in the United States. President Lyndon Johnson signed both into law on July 30, 1965. The signing occurred in Independence, Missouri at the Truman Library; this had considerable symbolic significance insofar as President Harry Truman had proposed a program for national health insurance as early as 1945. When the Medicare program was fully implemented in 1966, there were approximately 19 million individuals enrolled; today Medicare funds health care services for approximately 40 million Americans. Both Medicare and Medicaid programs were administered formerly by the Health Care Financing Administration (HCFA), which in 2001 was renamed the Centers for Medicare and Medicaid Services (CMS).

The Federal Medicare Health Insurance Program

Significant modifications to Medicare occurred in 2004 with the signing of the Medicare Modernization Act (MMA), including the addition of a limited outpatient prescription drug benefit, one of the more controversial changes. Under the MMA, participant co-payment was adjusted as a function of beneficiary income for the first time in Medicare history.

In general, Medicare benefits are available to all citizens when they reach age 65, some people with disabilities and anyone with end-stage renal disease (ESRD). The program is available to anyone over the age of 65 without regard to economic need. For this segment of the population, Medicare functions as a publicly financed, single payer, national health insurance system.

The Medicare program is divided into two parts: Medicare Part A is designed to pay for the costs associated with medical and psychiatric hospitalization. Medicare Part B pays for outpatient care and associated costs such as psychotherapy, diagnostic tests and laboratory tests (Norris, Molinari and Rosowsky, 1998).

Medicare's Prospective Payment System (PPS) went into effect in 1983. The PPS model involves fixed payment for any given diagnosis; payment is set in advance of treatment, based on Diagnostically Related Groups (DRGs). Providers working with prospective payment systems must budget their resources judiciously to ensure that costs do not exceed capitated rates; to the extent that costs are contained below the capitated amount, the provider makes money. To the extent that costs exceed capitation, the provider loses money. It is obvious that such a system shifts risk from the payor to the provider of services, and from an incentive for overtreatment to an incentive for undertreatment.

Most mental health hospitals and programs were exempt from DRGs because of the difficulty of using diagnosis to predict resource use. This change in policy suddenly made the care of psychiatric patients desirable for hospitals that could now use their beds to attract a small pool of cost-based reimbursement (Mechanic, 1999).

With legislative authorization expressed in the Medicare Modernization Act of 2003 (PL108-173), total funding for Medicare is projected at $340 billion for FY 2006 (Budget MMS 2006). According to Thomas R. Saving, senior fellow with the National Center for Policy Analysis and a public trustee of Social Security and Medicare, Medicare is today America's second largest federal entitlement program, behind Social Security, which is projected at $540 billion for FY 2006. In 2004, Medicare accounted for about 13 percent of the federal budget. By the year 2076, Saving projects that Medicare will consume nearly all of the government's revenue from income taxes (Minnesota Senior News, July 2005, p. 14). Revenue from individual income taxes for FY 2006 is projected at $967 billion and another $220 billion from corporate income taxes (Budget Summary 2006, Table S-8).

The Federal/State Medicaid Program

Medicaid is a complex federal program that has been set up to assist States to pay for health care for individuals and families with very low incomes. Medicaid is jointly funded by the federal government and state governments. Total funding for Medicaid in FY 2006 is projected to be $338 billion, about $193 billion of which is paid by the federal government and the remainder by the States (Budget MMS 2006).

There are certain categorical groups that qualify for Medicaid; these include children, pregnant women, adults in families with dependent children, individuals with disabilities and individuals age 65 and over. Within these broad guidelines, each state establishes its own eligibility criteria, determines what services will be covered by Medicaid, sets payment rates, and administers the program.

Medicaid covers more people than Medicare, and the Medicaid program pays for over half of all HIV/AIDS care and nursing home care. It often fills in the gaps in Medicare coverage for the elderly and disabled. However, Medicaid costs have been increasing dramatically in recent years, with the bulk of the increases attributable to the escalating costs of prescription drugs. The higher costs for prescription drugs under the Medicaid program reflect increased utilization, the development of new medications, high costs for existing medications, and pharmacy-driven increases in capitation rates for managed care organizations. Attempts by states to control Medicaid spending have involved putting controls on the availability and cost of prescription drugs, reducing or freezing provider payment rates, restricting eligibility, reducing benefits, or increasing co-payment levels.

Though funded with both federal and state revenues, Medicaid programs are administered by the individual states within parameters set by federal regulations. There is marked variance across states in the quality and scope of Medicaid coverage, and state government has considerable latitude in setting Medicaid standards. For example, within hours of taking office, Matt Blunt, the new Republican governor of Missouri, set the maximum income level for Medicaid at 30 percent of the federal poverty level, reducing it from 75 percent of poverty. This single decision eliminated more than 89,000 people from Missouri's Medicaid roles. Under the Blunt standards, a family of three is disqualified from Medicaid if they earn more than $4,700 per year; under the previous administration, families with incomes below $11,752 qualified for Medicaid services. Likewise, the Governor proposed shutting down the First Steps program, which served 8,100 toddlers with Down's syndrome, cerebral palsy, spina bifida and other developmental disabilities. These draconian core budget cuts and program closings will save the state of Missouri more than $700 million per year – in part by eliminating services for 89,000 Medicaid recipients and cutting back services for another 370,000 (*Columbia Daily Tribune*, 2000). This supply-side strategy for containing costs is a blatantly inequitable reduction in the volume and accessibility of health care services for the poor.

Medicaid pays for most community-based mental health services, and it is the only program that finances the full range of rehabilitative services required by people with mental health needs. In addition, Medicaid pays for the medical and surgical care that may be needed by people with mental disorders. It is ironic that in a country that purports to value families, many families, with incomes too high to qualify for Medicaid but too low to pay for private health insurance, have given up their children to the state to make them eligible for the services they need (General Accounting Office, 2003).

People diagnosed with mental illness currently represent slightly over 10 percent of Medicaid enrollees, but account for almost 44 percent of Medicaid payments. These data reflect the severe, ongoing and chronic needs of individuals with serious mental illnesses (Koyanagi, Mathis and Semanskky, 2003). In a Bazelon Center for Mental Health Law policy paper that examines options for Medicaid reform (e.g., replacing the Medicaid entitlement with block grants), Koyanagi et al. note:

- Medicaid is increasingly the only financing source of community services for people with serious mental disorders.
- Medicaid is the single most important source of revenue for state mental health systems. From 1987 to 1997, a national study shows Medicaid's share (federal funds and state match) of state and locally administered mental health program costs increased by 50 percent, rising from slightly more than one-third to one-half of state and local spending.
- Medicaid contributes half of all revenue for community services and thereby supports state initiatives to integrate people with psychiatric disabilities in the community.

Although Medicaid does cover many mental health services, payment rates are frequently dramatically lower than those in the private sector, and Medicaid enrollees often find it difficult to locate a provider willing to accept Medicaid payment rates. Those providers who accept Medicaid patients frequently respond to the low payment levels by setting up a "mill" approach that maximizes the number of patients who can be seen on any given day.

In addition to the major federal programs of Medicaid and Medicare, there are a number of other federal government programs with legislative authority insuring and/or providing health care for selected segments of the population. Among these publicly financed programs are the State Children's Health Insurance Program (SCHIP); federal, state, and county employee benefit plans; Department of Defense health services and insurance (TRICARE); the Veterans Health Administration; and Indian Health Service. These programs are discussed here with the exception of the VHA, which is described subsequently in this chapter to illustrate federal health care delivery systems.

State Children's Health Insurance Program (SCHIP)

In 1997, the U.S. Congress enacted title XXI as part of the Balanced Budget Act. This legislation created the State Children's Health Insurance program (SCHIP). It offered State governors flexible funding to create or expand subsidized coverage for some of the nation's eleven million uninsured children. It was the largest single federal investment in health insurance since Medicare and Medicaid in the 1960s. Since 1998, SCHIP contributed about $40 billion over ten years for States to administer, and enrolled about five million children by 2003. Although Medicaid is expected to serve more than 46 million Americans in 2006, SCHIP provides States with more flexibility than Medicaid, allowing States to cover their own selected populations, incorporate private sector insurance options, provide appropriate benefit packages, and maximize public dollars.

Compared with the Medicaid program, SCHIP relies more heavily on federal funding, but leaves the State governments with greater freedom to design and administer the allocations. The program retains a broad base of political support at both federal and state levels for several reasons: "it reaches beyond the poorest population, is not an entitlement, has been marketed along the lines of a private insurance plan, and has thrown off some of the shackles of the Medicaid bureaucracy" (Weil, 2001, p. 77).

Of particular relevance to mental health services, a state's SCHIP plan must include mental health coverage that is equivalent to 75 percent of the actuarial value of one of three federal benchmark health insurance plans: (a) the Federal Employees Health Benefits Program (FEHBP) Blue Cross standard option plan; (b) the state's own employee health benefit plan, or (c) the health maintenance organization (HMO) with the largest number of commercially insured members in the state (Howell, Buck, and Teich, 2000).

Based on SCHIP data gathered from several states, Howell, Buck, and Teich (2000) concluded that mental health coverage is considerably less extensive in SCHIP plans than in Medicaid expansion plans. "While both types of plans cover traditional inpatient and outpatient [mental health] care, Medicaid expansion plans are much more likely to cover residential, partial hospitalization, case management, and school health services" (p.291). Moreover, SCHIP plans are allowed to charge co-payments for mental health services and medications (not allowed under Medicaid expansion plans), and SCHIP plans are more likely to limit the number of inpatient days and outpatient visits. Despite these limitations, evaluations of the SCHIP policy initiative have been favorable with respect to increasing health insurance coverage, hence access to the health care delivery system, for nearly four million children (Kenney and Chang, 2004).

The Congressional authorization for SCHIP expires at the end of 2007. The 2006 Budget proposes to reauthorize it early due to its success in enrolling millions of previously uninsured children (Budget HHS 2006). Projected federal expenditures for SCHIP in 2006 are about $6 billion (Budget Summary 2006, Table S-10), which combined with Medicaid allotments, yields a total of $199 billion paid by the federal government and largely financed by individual income taxes.

The Federal Employees Health Benefit Program (FEHBP)

Other forms of publicly funded health insurance coverage for a selected segment of the population include the plans provided to employees of federal, state, and country governments. The federal plan will be discussed by way of illustration since it has the widest enrollment.

Functioning like a publicly financed, single payer, national health insurance plan for all federal employees and their dependents, the FEHBP is administered by a federal agency called the Office of Personnel Management (OPM). For FY 2006, OPM projects expenditures of $33 billion in health benefits for about eight million enrollees and their dependents. Adding expenditures for both human services and health yields a projected total of $68.9 billion (Budget OPM 2006, Tables S-1 & S-3). Both the enrollment and level of expenditures make the FEHBP the largest employer-based health insurance program of its kind in the country, and the federal government the largest, single employer funding employee health benefits in the entire public and private employment-based health insurance sector. Total personnel costs (compensation plus benefits) in all branches of the federal government and its agencies, including the active military, was about $338 billion in 2004, and projected at $345 billion in the Budget for 2006. (Budget FEC 2006, Table 24–4).

Department of Defense and TRICARE

The federal Department of Defense (DoD) provides health care services for active duty military personnel and their families, and a health insurance benefit (TRICARE) for health care is provided for them in the civilian sector. Of its total $426 billion budget request for 2006, the DoD projects $19.8 billion expenditures to provide service men and women and their families with comprehensive and quality health care.

In addition, the DoD has expanded access to medical care for reservists and their family members before, during, and after mobilization for the current military operations in Afghanistan and Iraq. For those reservists, retirees, and families not using DoD's own medical care system, the DoD provides TRICARE. The latter program reimburses both civilian physicians and allied health care providers (Budget DoD 2006, p. 91). The Ronald W. Reagan National Defense Authorization Act for 2005 (P.L. 108-375) provided permanent, indefinite appropriations to finance the cost of TRICARE benefits accrued by all uniformed service members. The total permanent, indefinite amount for FY 2006 is estimated at $10.7 billion (Budget DoD 2006, pp. 1–3).

The Indian Health Service

The Indian Health Service (IHS) is another federal program targeted to address the needs of a segment of American society, in this case, the indigenous population of Native Americans. The IHS was created by the Act of August 5, 1958 (68 Stat. 674); it was expanded subsequently by the Indian Self-Determination Act, the Indian Health Care Improvement Act, and Titles II & III of the Public Health Service Act (p.1). As of 1988, this federal program was administered by an agency of the Public Health Service of the Federal Department of Health and Human Services. Appointed by the President, the Director of the Indian Health Service reports to the Assistant Secretary of the Department of Health and Human Services.

Functioning like a publicly financed, single payer system for Native Americans, the IHS account provides funding for medical care, public health services, and health professions training opportunities for American Indians and Alaska Natives. Counting all clinical services, preventive health, urban Indian health, and Indian health professions funding, a total of about $2.4 billion is allocated for health care in FY 2006 (Budget HIS 2006, pp. 1, 2, & 4). These amounts exclude capital expenditures and costs to administer this federal program. Expenditures for mental health and substance abuse services were not listed as separate budget categories, though a national plan for mental health prevention and treatment services was given budgetary authorization in the U.S. Code Title 25 – Indians; Chapter 18 – Indian Health Care; Subchapter II-Health Services; Section 1621h – Mental health prevention and treatment services) and by Title 25/Chapter 18/Subchapter V-A – Substance Abuse Programs.

This brief review of federally funded health insurance and health care services reveals (a) substantial investment of public funds in the American health care system, (b) which are appropriated and administered publicly through multiple, separate programs to selected segments of the population, and moreover, (c) the patchwork of federally funded programs suggests a "system" of several national, single payer health insurance plans for segmented populations. The multiple federal programs are complex and confusing; adding the thousands of health insurance companies and health plans operating in the private sector highlights the inordinate complexity of the American health care system, and helps to account for the lack of standardization of benefits and eligibility requirements, unequal access to health care services, and marked inefficiencies due to substantial duplication in the administration and delivery of health insurance services. The mixture of public and private programs is, nevertheless, what one would expect in a health care system embedded in a mixed economy characterized as semi-regulated capitalism.

Delivery Systems

Multiple provider groups deliver mental health care in the United States in numerous and diverse settings in both fee-for-service and prepaid insurance programs. Many of these public and private settings operate relatively independently and make up the *de facto* mental health system. This system involves four primary sectors: (a) *specialty mental health care*, with services provided by mental health professionals with specialized training (psychologists, psychiatrists, psychiatric nurses, and social workers); (b) *general medical/primary care*, with services provided by professionals with generic health and medical training (family physicians, internists, nurse practitioners, pediatricians, etc.); (c) *human services*, with care provided by professionals and paraprofessionals with relevant skills other than health training (e.g., probation officers, religious leaders, teachers, and similar helping professions); and (d) *voluntary support networks*, which include groups like Alcoholics Anonymous that focus on education and support (Wedding and Mengel, 2004).

According to *Mental Health: A Report of the Surgeon General* (U.S. Department of Health and Human Serivces, 1999), about 15 percent of all adults and 21 percent of U. S. children and adolescents use services in the *de facto* mental health system each year. Altogether, slightly less than six percent of the adult population and about eight percent of children and adolescents (ages 9 to 17) use *specialty* mental health services in a year. In contrast, more than six percent of the adult U.S. population use the *general medical sector* for mental health care, with an average of about four visits per year – far lower than the average of 14 visits per year found in the specialty mental health sector. About five percent of adults use the *human services sector*, but a much larger percent of children receive services in the human services sector, primarily through school mental health services (U.S. Department of Health and Human Services, 1999). The mental health usage data from the Surgeon General's report are provided in more detail in Tables 5.7 and 5.8.

In the discussion that follows, mental health services are described first in primary care settings, including publicly funded Health Centers, and subsequently in specialist mental health care settings such as Community Mental Health Centers, Veterans Health Administration, State and County Mental Hospitals, Private Psychiatric Hospitals, Psychiatric Units in General Hospitals, and Residential Treatment Centers.

Mental Health Services in Primary Care Settings

Because psychological disorders often result in physical symptoms (e.g., the malaise and fatigue associated with depression; the insomnia associated with manic episodes), individuals with mental illness frequently bring their concerns first to their primary care providers. Therefore, it is not surprising that much if not most mental health care is delivered in primary care settings (Regier, Narrow, Rae, Manderscheid, Locke and Goodwin, 1993), often by physicians

Table 5.7. *Proportion of Adult Population Using Mental/Addictive Disorder Services in One Year.*

Total Health Sector	11%
Specialty Mental Health	6%
General Medical	6%
Human Services Professionals	5%
Voluntary Support Network	3%
Any of Above Services	15%

Table 5.8. *Proportion of Child/Adolescent Populations (Ages 9–17) Using Mental/Addictive Disorder Services in One Year.*

Total Health Sector	9%
Specialty Mental Health	8%
General Medical	3%
Human Services Professionals	17%
School Services	16%
Other Human Services	3%
Any of Above Services	21%

Note: Totals of all sectors and services add to more than the final category of "any of the above services" because an individual may request services from more than one sector.

and nurses with only rudimentary training in the diagnosis and treatment of mental illness.

A number of compelling studies have documented the extent to which mental health concerns present in the offices of primary care providers. Over 40 years ago, Cummings and colleagues initiated a seminal series of studies that documented that 60 percent of physician visits were by patients who had no physical illness or whose psychological problems were exacerbating their physical illness (Cummings and Follette, 1968; Cummings, Kahn, and Sparkman, 1962; Follette and Cummings, 1967). Likewise, Kroenke and Mangelsdorff (1989) found that 40 percent of outpatient visits could be attributed to one of ten core symptoms (chest pain, fatigue, dizziness, headache, swelling, back pain, shortness of breath, insomnia, abdominal pain, and numbness); however, a biological cause could be identified for the symptoms in only 26 percent of primary care visits.

Druss, Rohrbaugh, Levinson and Rosenheck (2001) conducted a randomized clinical trial to test an integrated model of primary medical care for a cohort of patients with serious mental disorders. Those patients in the integrated care condition received "on-site primary care and case management that emphasized preventive medical care, patient education, and close collaboration with mental health providers to improve access to and continuity of care" (p. 861). This study demonstrated that on-site, integrated primary care for patients with mental disorders resulted in both improved quality of care and improved outcomes. Likewise, Unutzer et al. (2001) documented that a quality improvement program aimed at fostering collaboration between mental health care specialists and primary care doctors could significantly enhance the quality of care provided for depressed patients.

Several models of integrated care have been developed in which psychologists and other mental health providers work closely with primary care providers, often in the same building. This practice is sometimes referred to as "integrated behavioral health care;" it is defined by co-location, joint training, and shared continuing education of primary care providers and mental health specialists. The idea is surprisingly simple, but it has proved difficult to implement fully for a variety of reasons, including the sociology of professions, our history of training health care providers in disparate settings, and fears of loss of power and autonomy by high-status providers, most often physicians. However, when the model has been implemented and tested, it has been found effective and satisfying for both patients and those providers working in the integrated system (McDaniel, 1995; Wedding and Mengel, 2004).

Healthy People 2010 set an explicit goal (18-6) of increasing the number of people seen in primary health care who receive mental health screening and assessment; integrated care is the most cost-effective and expeditious way to meet this goal. In a book targeting psychologists, DeLeon, Rossomando and Smedley (2004) argued that "the future is primary care."

Federally Funded Health Centers

In an effort to extend primary health care to the poor by making health care services more accessible, the federal government initiated the Neighborhood Health Centers Program. Started in 1965, it was administered through the federal Office of Economic Opportunity. At the time, this demonstration program was a highly visible component of President Lyndon Johnson's War on Poverty, and today it is truly the "safety net" for our nation's uninsured and underinsured citizens. In 1975, Congress provided explicit federal legislative authority for the health center program for the first time by enacting the Special Health Revenue Sharing Act of 1974 (P.L. 94–63). To do so, they overrode the veto of this bill by then President Gerald Ford. Nearly 40 years later, the number of public Health Centers has increased substantially.

Health Centers deliver high-quality, affordable, primary and preventive health care to nearly 14 million patients, regardless of ability to pay, at 3,740 sites across the United States annually. In 2006, Health Centers are predicted to serve an estimated 16 percent of the nation's population at or below 200 percent of federal poverty line. The poverty line in 2004 was $18,850 for a family of four; 200 percent of that equals a family income of about $37,000. These figures are increased another 25 percent for immigrants (HHS, 2004).

Another 1,200 new or expanded Health Center sites to serve an additional 6.1 million people have been proposed for 2006. Almost 2.4 million additional individuals will receive health care in 2006 through over 570 new or expanded sites in rural areas and underserved urban neighborhoods. The federal budget for 2006 includes $26 million to fund 40 new Health Center sites in high-poverty counties. Faith-based and community programs will be encouraged to compete for these grants (Budget HHS 2006, p. 136).

The Health Centers are faced with the challenge of embedding culturally- and community-appropriate mental health services into their primary care programs – a task that requires significant innovation and financial resources. Federal health centers regulations require that all "new start" centers in 2006 and those centers that receive federal expansion funds include mental health and substance abuse services in their array of primary care services. Accordingly, in our judgment, not only is the door open to psychologists, but health centers have an urgent need for psychologists to help them comply with these new service mandates. Our personal discussions with health center personnel consistently reinforce the notion that behavioral health is one of their top priorities, especially the prevention and treatment of depression and family violence (DeLeon, Giesting and Kinkel, 2003).

Community Mental Health Centers

That same legislation authorizing Health Centers to provide primary health care contained standards and implementation guidelines for Community Mental Health Centers, establishing from the very beginning parallel and separate systems for providing physical health care and mental health care. Many individuals almost automatically think of community mental health centers (CMHCs) when they reflect on the delivery of mental health services, and, from a public health perspective, these centers "represent the 'safety net' for a significant and steadily growing proportion of our citizenry – the uninsured and others who, according to research, face significant health status disparities as a result of ethnic and geographical considerations" (DeLeon, Giesting and Kenkel, 2004, p. 598).

The community mental health center movement began when President Kennedy signed the Mental Retardation Facilities and Community Mental Health Centers Construction Act of 1963 into law. Missouri was awarded the first federal CMHC construction grant for the Mid-Missouri Community Mental Health Center in Columbia, Missouri (Ahr, 2003). These centers were viewed as attractive and humane alternatives to the "warehousing" of psychiatric patients that occurred in massive state hospitals, and the development of CMHCs provided a foundation for the deinstitutionalization of millions of patients. This deinstitutionalization was one of the sea changes that occurred in mental health during the twentieth century.

The CMHCs were federally mandated to provide specific and carefully defined services: inpatient care, outpatient care, 24-hour emergency services, partial hospitalization, and consultation and education (Callicutt, 1997). In addition, they replaced institutional care with community care; provided service to the entire community, with a focus on prevention; planned for services for the mental health of the community; and provided continuity of care with an emphasis on providing the least restrictive care possible (Fellin, 1996). The bulk of funding for community mental health centers has traditionally come from the mental health block grant.

CMHCs serve catchment areas of 75,000 – 200,000 individuals; the low end of this range is large enough to be cost-effective, while the high end is small enough to be manageable. They make it possible to treat people with mental illness in their home communities, provide a continuum of care, make it possible for multidisciplinary teams to work with individual patients, and allow for linkage with other community organizations and agencies (Ahr, 2004). CMHCs have been demonstrated to be cost-effective venues for training mental health professionals (Greenberg, Cradock, Godbole, and Temkina, 1998).

Veterans Health Administration

The Veterans Health Administration (VHA) is the nation's largest health care delivery system, and it employs and trains a large portion of the nation's mental health work force. For example, the VHA hires and retains more psychologists than any other agency (approximately 1,350 are involved in patient care); these psychologists work in over one hundred health care systems and in 1,134 VA facilities in 50 states plus the District of Columbia, Guam, the Philippines, Puerto Rico and the Virgin Islands (Cannon et al. 2001; Department of Veterans Affairs, 2005).

President Herbert Hoover established the Veterans Administration in 1930; its motto, "to care for him who shall have borne the battle, and for his widow and his orphan," comes from Lincoln's second inaugural address. The health care arm of the Veterans Administration initially focused on treating wounded veterans, but over time, the Veterans Health Administration has evolved to the point where it is a mainstay of the health care system in the United States. For example, in 2004 the VHA served approximately 4.9 million patients. One-hundred and seven Veterans Administration Medical Centers (VAMCs) are affiliated with medical schools in the United States, and approximately 60 percent of all U.S. health professionals receive at least part of their training in these sites; the patients treated in these facilities tend to be male, older (49% are over age 65), sicker and poorer than other patients being treated in the U. S. health care system (Yevich, 2005).

In recognition of the sacrifices made by military personnel, United States veterans, their children, and survivors can receive multiple financial benefits; these benefits include disability compensation, educational, vocational, and rehabilitation benefits, employment benefits, insurance (life, disability, mortgage), pension and burial benefits, and guaranteed housing loans. The VHA both insures and provides medical and mental health services.

Spending for mental health services in the VHA shifted substantially during the period 1995–2001, when there was a 21 percent decrease in overall spending on mental health services. These changes in part reflect a dramatic shift from inpatient care to outpatient mental health services. The VHA managed to achieve these cost savings despite a significant increase in outpatient medication costs during this same period (Chen, Smith, Wagner and Barnett, 2003). Rosenheck and Stolar (1998) used census data to evaluate the use of Veterans Administration mental health services in each U. S. county and found that 2.0 percent of U.S. veterans used mental health services.

Budgeted expenditures for all VHA medical services for FY2006 are projected at about $19.8 billion. Of that amount, VHA psychiatric services for FY 2006 total about $1.6 billion, including psychiatric care ($1 billion), medical administration ($232 million), and psychiatric facilities ($389 million) (Budget MP 2006, pp. 3, 15, & 19).

The VHA has been a leader in the development of both clinical guidelines and performance measures. As examples of the latter, the VHA reported that health care services were rated as very good or excellent by the majority of surveyed patients (inpatient – 73% and outpatient – 74%). Moreover, 93 percent and 94 percent, respectively, reported that primary and specialist care appointments were scheduled within 30 days of the desired date. There was also a 77 percent utilization of clinical practice guidelines (Budget MP 2006, pp. 8 & 9).

The VHA has grown increasingly sensitive to the need for treating veterans experiencing post-traumatic stress disorder (PTSD), a condition noticed in previous wars but then labeled as combat neurosis or battle fatigue. This is a problem that is not limited to veterans of Vietnam; in fact, it is estimated that 15 percent of service members serving in Iraq and Afghanistan will experience post-traumatic stress disorder (PTSD) (General Accounting Office, 2004).

The Iraq-Afghanistan conflict has brought home to the nation the importance of the psychological sequelae of war. Reviews of the fiscal year 2006 appropriations and authorization committee recommendations include new and improved resources, as well as hiring incentives for mental health personal. For example, "The Committee directs the Department of Veterans Affairs and Department of Defense to jointly study mental health care, the onset and nature of PTSD, panic disorder, and bipolar disorder. Also to improve mental health testing, tracking of returning combat duty servicemen, to include the Reserve Component for a period of not less than 10 years. In addition, the Departments of Defense and Veterans Affairs are encouraged to establish a classification for psychiatric nurses, and increase hires of individuals with those capabilities." Further, "The Committee notes that more than 20 years ago, the Congress established a Department of Veterans Affairs Special Committee on Post-Traumatic Stress Disorder to determine the Department's capacity to provide assessment and treatment for PTSD and to guide the Department's educational, research, and benefits activities with regard to PTSD. The Special Committee has provided the Department of Veterans Affairs and the Congress with annual reports that contain recommendations for improving PTSD programs and some progress has been made. But it is also clear from the most recent report, dated October, 2004, that much more needs to be done so that this issue is given its proper attention." And, "In the opinion of most experts in the field, mental health issues will be the most pressing problem for the Department of Veterans Affairs in the coming years. . . ." (Military quality of life, pp. 15, 58). The APA Education Directorate was successful in having a new item included, proposing $4 million in the House legislation for psychology's relevant training efforts.

State and County Mental Hospitals

Until the 1950s, most mental health care was provided in large institutions that were supported with state funding. These institutions, often little more than human warehouses, offered custodial care for thousands of patients who received minimal treatment (Talbott, 1978). However, with the development and adoption of genuinely effective psychotropic medications (e.g., Thorazine) in the mid-fifties, coupled with a need to shift the cost of care for mental patients from the states to the federal government, a massive transfer of patients from state hospitals to alternative (outpatient) settings began. This sea change in the treatment of people with mental illness is generally referred to as deinstitutionalization. It is a change that continues today because of managed care (Mechanic, 1998).

Public mental hospitals in the United States had a total population of about 560,000 resident patients at their peak in 1955; in contrast, there are fewer than 60,000 public mental hospital patients today, despite considerable growth in the general population (Mechanic, 2002). Although hundreds of thousands of patients were ostensibly being discharged "to the community," this was often a euphemism for simply returning patients to their families. "[A]s parents died, or families broke under the stress of caring for untreated patients, or the mentally ill restlessly wandered off, rooming houses, single-room occupancy hotels (SROs), streets, and jails increasingly supplemented the family as alternatives to mental hospitals" (Isaac and Armat, 1990).

Deinstitutionalization continued throughout the late sixties as states took advantage of the opportunity to divest themselves of responsibility for the treatment of people with mental illness, all the while purporting to do so in the name of client rights, empowerment, individual liberty and a commitment to providing less restrictive care. The patients who were discharged were often poorly prepared to cope with the demands of life outside an institution, and the communities to which they were discharged were hardly prepared to assume responsibility for their care. In addition, with the passage of Medicaid in 1965, it became economically viable for residential care facilities and small group homes to support patients who could only have received care previously in state hospitals and similar asylums.

It is widely acknowledged that the plan to transfer patients *en masse* from state hospitals to community mental health centers was a failure. Writing in *Madness in the Streets: How Psychiatry and the Law Abandoned the Mentally Ill*, Isaac and Armat (1990) note:

A vacuum of aftercare followed the collapse of the mental hospital as a place offering asylum for the severely and chronically mentally ill. President Kennedy had promised to replace 'the cold mercy of custodial isolation' with the 'open warmth of community concern and capability.' But this rhetoric reflected . . . 'remarkably romantic ideas about the nature of 'the community.' In fact, 'the community' was neither warm, concerned nor capable, when it came to the mentally ill. (p. 287)

State mental hospitals today deal with the poorest, sickest, most disabled, and most difficult of patients. They are less likely than private hospitals to provide meaningful therapeutic activities for patients (New York Commission, 1996). They are more likely to use seclusion and restraint. In 1999, Senator Joseph Lieberman testified before a Senate Subcommittee to protest the abuse of restraint in psychiatric settings, citing a story in a Hartford newspaper that described 142 deaths that had resulted from the use of restraint and seclusion in mental health facilities (Lieberman, 1999).

Despite being smaller and treating only a fraction of all patients with mental illness, these state and county mental hospitals "continue to consume from one-half to two-thirds of state mental health budgets. . . . [despite the fact that] [t]heir share of all treated episodes continues to decline relative to private psychiatric hospitals, and particularly general hospitals, which have become a major provider of psychiatric acute inpatient care" (Mechanic, 1999, p. 16).

Private Psychiatric Hospitals

Two key features define the private psychiatric hospital: it focuses primarily on treating individuals with mental illness or addictions, or both, and the majority of funding comes from private insurance rather than from federal, state or local resources (entitlement programs, block grants, mil taxes, etc.) McLean Hospital in Belmont, Massachusetts is the quintessential example of a private psychiatric facility; it is the facility portrayed in Susan Kaysen's autobiography *Girl Interrupted* and in the film of the same name.

In 1993, the National Association of Private Psychiatric Hospitals changed its name to the National Association of Psychiatric Health Systems (NAPHS) in response to trends sweeping through the health care system: the evolution from hospitals to systems of care; the change from independent organizations to integrated delivery systems; and the change from treating illness in individuals to maintaining healthy communities (Sharfstein, Stoline and Szpak, 2001). Another change in the private hospital *Zeitgeist* is the emergence of specialty services or wards dedicated to treating particular problems such as eating disorders or adolescent depression.

The number of private psychiatric hospitals increased dramatically after the implementation of Medicare and Medicaid legislation in 1965. For example, during the period between 1970 and 1992, the number of private psychiatric hospitals increased tenfold, while the number of residential treatment beds for emotionally disturbed children doubled (Mechanic, 1999). There are few more striking examples of the influence of payment policy on hospital practice.

In general, private psychiatric hospitals offer high quality care to patients with private insurance and to a growing number of children and elderly who have access to Medicaid and Medicare (under federal guidelines, private hospitals can only bill Medicaid for services provided to individuals under age 21 or over age 64). Patients in private hospitals generally participate in more therapeutic programs and activities, have more visits with psychiatrists and other mental health providers, experience fewer episodes of restraint and seclusion, and have better follow-up after discharge (New York Commission, 1996). With private hospitals increasingly accepting Medicaid and Medicare patients, the lines between the private and public sectors are becoming increasingly blurred.

Managed care has seriously eroded the income potential of private psychiatric facilities, and these hospitals have been forced to turn to providing services to the elderly and indigent mentally ill covered by Medicare and Medicaid. Between 1989 and 1993, managed care reduced length of stay in New York psychiatric hospitals by 18 days (New York Commission, 1996). Likewise, the average length of stay in private psychiatric hospitals throughout the United States decreased from over 30 days in 1987 to only 10 days in 1999 (Sharfstein, Stoline and Szpak, 2001). Unfortunately, shortening the time available for treatment in mental health settings may be counterproductive; for example, Appleby et al. (1993) documented a greater likelihood that brief-stay patients will be rehospitalized within 30 days after discharge than patients treated for longer periods.

Rosenau and Linder (2003) reviewed studies comparing the performance of for-profit and nonprofit psychiatric inpatient care providers in the United States. Sixteen of the 17 studies (96%) reviewed by these investigators found that the performance of the nonprofit psychiatric inpatient care providers was better than or equal to that of their for-profit counterparts across all performance criteria. The nonprofit care providers were found to have performed best in 70 percent of the comparisons. Twenty-six percent of the comparisons indicated no difference between the for-profit and nonprofit providers.

Many private psychiatric hospitals will offer treatment for both substance abuse and mental health problems, recognizing the co-morbidity that is present in these two populations. The recent national epidemiological study (NCS-R) noted the presence of co-morbidity in about 45 percent of people with mental disorders (Kessler, et al. 2005b, p. 617). Inpatient treatment utilizing multiple treatment approaches often offers the best hope for treating the patient with a dual (mental illness and substance abuse) diagnosis (Drake, Muesner, Brunette, and McHugo, 2004; Goldsmith and Garlapatia, 2004). These combined services are sometimes offered under the rubric of behavioral health services.

A significant limitation in access to mental health services available through private psychiatric hospitals is presented by insurers who limit the risk of "adverse selection" by discouraging enrollment in insurance programs by individuals with a history of mental illness or substance abuse. Typically, this history is defined as a pre-existing condition, and individuals with such a history are denied insurance or forced to accept policies with significant restrictions in mental health benefits (Druss and Rosenheck, 1998).

Psychiatric Units in General Medical Hospitals

Kiesler, Simpkins and Morton (1991) examined medical records for patients being discharged from general medical-surgical hospitals to determine the frequency of mental and substance abuse disorders. They found that 12 percent of all cases treated in these facilities had dual diagnoses: 5.5 percent had a primary diagnosis of an alcohol or drug disorder, and almost 20 percent of all cases had two or more mental or substance abuse disorders. Interestingly, those patients with coexisting disorders had shorter mean hospital stays than those with mental disorders only.

In a related study, Kiesler and Simpkins (1992) examined a large national discharge database and found that total episodes of psychiatric care decreased between 1980 and 1985, but there was more focused concentration on the treatment of schizophrenia and affective disorders. During this same period, specialty hospitals decreased treatment of mental disorders but increased their treatment of chemical dependency. Kiesler and Simpkins attribute at least part of the changes observed to Medicare's prospective payment policies.

Residential Treatment Centers

Residential treatment centers (RTCs) provide 24-hour care for small groups of patients with either mental disorders or substance abuse problems. The goal of the RTCs is to help these patients function at the highest possible level, and, in the case of addicts, to stay clean and sober.

A 1999 Supreme Court decision (*Olmstead* v. *L. C.*) had important implications for residential treatment centers. This case involved two women who had been held in a Georgia psychiatric hospital far beyond the time that the hospital staff considered them ready for community care. They were detained because of a shortage of space in community settings. The Supreme Court ruled that "unjustified isolation . . . is properly regarded as discrimination based on disability" (Petrila and Levin, 2004, p. 49). The Olmstead decision supported the rights of people with mental and other disabilities to live in community settings, and found that unnecessary institutionalization of people constituted discrimination under the Americans with Disabilities Act. The requirement for enforcing Olmstead falls primarily on the states (Arons et al. 2004).

Direct Services Personnel

The best available data on the kinds and numbers of personnel working in the mental health field are found in *Mental Health, United States*, 2002 (Manderscheid and Henderson, 2004). This volume is updated on a biennial basis with input and assistance from major professional organizations within the mental health field (e.g., the Office of Research of the American Psychological Association). Chapter 21 addresses mental health practitioners and trainees.

It is notoriously difficult to define the mental health work force with any precision, and the problem is compounded by the facts that many therapists work part-time and a given individual may identify with more than one mental health profession at the same time (e.g., a therapist may be both a social worker *and* a marriage and family therapist). However, we know that in 2002 there were 40,867 clinically active psychiatrists practicing in the United States; this reflects a 41 percent increase in the number of psychiatrists since 1982. In contrast, there were about 88,500 licensed psychologists in 2002 and almost 100,000 clinically trained social workers. Social work represents the largest professional group of mental health and therapy service providers (Duffy et al. 2004).

These numbers stand in marked contrast to a far smaller number of psychiatric nurses: only 8,519 clinical nurse specialists were providing psychiatric-mental health nursing in 2002 (Duffy et al. 2004). There were approximately 50,000 marriage and family therapists providing clinical services in the United States in 2002, but this number is growing rapidly, and an increasing number of these providers hold doctorates. In 2002, there were 111,931 credentialed professional counselors practicing in the United States, and almost all states now license or certify the practice of counseling. A variety of counseling and mental health services may also be provided by professionals who identify themselves as rehabilitation counselors, guidance counselors, pastoral counselors, school psychologists, or clinical sociologists (Wedding, 2005). The latter are not generally considered among the "core mental health professions." Excluding the latter groups, the estimated total number of mental health specialists is nearly 400,000. For a population of 293 million Americans, the ratio of providers to population, is 1:733 the highest of the four countries included in this study.

A fascinating development which we see evolving within each of the current systems is the collective interest of a wide range of nonphysician health care providers in systematically expanding their historical scope of clinical practice to include prescribing medications, which for those with mental health training would primarily involve psychotropic medications. This movement began with U.S. Senator Daniel K. Inouye's address at the Hawaii Psychological Association annual convention in November, 1984 in which he urged psychologists to seek prescriptive authority in order to improve the availability of comprehensive, quality mental health care. In June, 1994 then-APA President Bob Resnick attended the graduation ceremonies for the first two Department of Defense (DoD) psychopharmacology fellows, Navy Commander John Sexton and Lt. Commander Morgan Sammons. Ten military colleagues would ultimately graduate from this DoD program. The following year, at the New York City annual convention meeting of the APA Council of Representatives, obtaining prescriptive authority for appropriately trained psychologists became formal APA policy, and model legislation and a model training curriculum were adopted. In March, 2002, New Mexico enacted their prescriptive authority law and in May, 2004, Louisiana followed with APA Council Representative Glenn Ally reporting:

"On February 18, 2005, the first prescription was written by a civilian 'medical psychologist' in Baton Rouge, Louisiana under the new RxP law signed by Governor Blanco. Dr. John Bolter wrote the first prescription – a prescription for Remeron (for the trivia folks). This was an historic moment for the Louisiana Academy of Medical Psychology, for the citizens of Louisiana, and for psychology as a profession" (Glenn Ally, personal communication, February 22, 2005). Indiana and Guam also have enacted appropriate prescriptive authority laws for psychologists that are currently in the implementation process. As Russ Newman of the APA Practice Directorate and the DoD graduates have clearly described, the psychological approach to the use of psychotropic medications is qualitatively different than that historically utilized by medicine. In our judgment, this development possesses the potential to truly revolutionize the delivery of quality mental health care throughout the nation, and particularly within the public sector.

In recent years, psychologists and social workers have come closer to achieving the status of medical therapists, especially in the areas of insurance reimbursement, participation in federal health programs, and admission to psychoanalytic training. Psychologists also have gained hospital admitting privileges in many states, and now psychologists who have received advanced training in psychopharmacology can prescribe medications for their patients in Louisiana, New Mexico and Guam. Other groups that practice counseling or psychotherapy are making rapid strides toward achieving some of the privileges now available to psychologists and social workers (Wedding, 2005).

One perennial challenge facing the U.S. mental health system is overcoming the uneven distribution of mental health professionals across the country, and especially the gap between rural and urban areas. As an example of this disparity, in 2005 there were only two or three full-time psychologists in private practice in Fremont County in Wyoming, a jurisdiction one-and-a-half times the size of the State of Connecticut, but with a population of only 37,000 (Thomas, 2005). Another illustration is the uneven distribution of mental health professionals by setting. The U.S. federal prison system has 114 facilities, 183,000 inmates, and about 500 doctoral psychologists' positions, many of which remain unfilled. The former regional administrator for psychological services within the Federal Bureau of Prisons, Thomas W. White, noted: "There are not enough qualified mental health professionals in the prison system to care and provide treatment for the sheer number of inmates coming into the system that are mentally ill" (Gill, 2005, p. 19).

Administrative Personnel

There are no available data on the numbers of administrative personnel who support the mental health delivery system in the United States or the cost of this system to the nation. However, an article in the *New England Journal of Medicine* (Woolhandler and Himmelstein, 1997) estimated overall administrative costs of 26 percent of total hospital costs; administrative costs of 34 percent of total costs in for-profit hospitals, 24.5 percent at private not-for-profit hospitals, and 22.9 percent for public hospitals. These findings are consistent, albeit slightly higher, than a previous study using the same methodology (Woolhandler and Himmelstein, 1991).

The mental health care system in the United States is at least as complex as the general health care system, and there is no compelling reason to believe that the administrative burden would be less significant for the mental health sector.

Information Technology

In reviewing our nation's overall health care system, the IOM noted that:

> Health care delivery has been relatively untouched by the revolution in information technology that has been transforming nearly every other aspect of society.... Although growth in clinical knowledge and technology has been profound, many health care settings lack basic computer systems to provide clinical information or support clinical decision making. The development and application of more sophisticated information systems is essential to enhance quality and improve efficiency.... The Committee believes information technology must play a central role in the redesign of the health care system if a substantial improvement in quality is to be achieved over the coming decade. (Institute of Medicine, pp. 15–16)

Similarly, President G.W. Bush has concluded:

> The way I like to kind of try to describe health care is, on the research side, we're the best. We're coming up with more innovative ways to save lives and to treat patients. Except when you think about the provider's side, we're kind of still in the buggy era. And the health care industry is missing an opportunity.... It's like IT, information technology, hasn't yet shown up in health care yet. (Bush, April, 2004, p. 699) Nevertheless, within the public sector, mental health is consistently one of, if not the, top utilizers of telehealth technology.

Financing Strategies

A patchwork of financing strategies characterizes health care in the United States, and the situation is even more chaotic in the case of mental health care. Funding for health care can come from the federal government or the states; it can be linked to voluntary, employer-based insurance, the public sector (Medicare and Medicaid, SCHIP, Federal Employees Health Insurance program, Indian Health Services, Department of Defense and the Veterans Health Administration) or community hospitals (charity care). In an ever-increasing number of cases, financing is out of pocket for the individual receiving care through premiums, deductibles, and co-payments at the point of service. Mental health financing frequently requires combining financing strategies (e.g., mixing state and federal dollars through the Medicaid "match," or using private insurance to pay for part of outpatient services while paying the remaining costs with personal funds).

It is impossible to separate the discussion of the economics of mental health care in the United States from the broader question of financing health care in general. Health care in the United States is more expensive than health care provided in any other country (by at least 40%), and there is little evidence that U.S. citizens are getting a good return on the prodigious investments in health care they make each year. (See Tables 5.9, 5.10, and 6.3 for comparison with the other three countries included in our study.)

While health care expenditures rise with per capita income,

> ... the United States is a notable outlier, spending 56% more per capita than would be predicted by our average income.... Despite spending the most per capita on health care, the United States ranks generally in the bottom half of industrialized countries in relation to life expectancy and infant mortality, and the relative ranking is worsening. (Mehrotra, Dudley and Luft, 2003, p. 386)

There are multiple reasons for the rapidly escalating cost of health care in the United States, and some of the reasons proffered for these costs include the aging population, the exorbitant costs of end of life care, the costs associated with new technology, excessive incomes for health care providers, the rapidly escalating costs of prescription drugs, managed care and the underfunding of public health (Mehrotra, Dudley and Luft, 2003).

While all of these factors no doubt contribute to the rise in health care spending, there is widespread agreement that the cost of health care in the United States is excessive at least in part because of the administrative costs associated with for-profit care. For-profit hospitals have been shown to be 3–11 percent more expensive than not-for-profit hospitals, and these hospitals spend far more on administration than not-for-profit hospitals (Woolhandler and Himmelstein, 1997, 1999). In a more recent article, Woolhandler and Himmelstein (2004) note:

> How does investor ownership increase hospital costs? Successful executives at for-profit hospitals reap princely rewards, and these rewards raise their personal stake in "gaming" the payment system. When the chief executive officer of Columbia/HCA, the industry leader, resigned in the face of federal fraud investigations, he left with a $10 million severance package and $269 million in company stock. Incentive bonuses averaged 41.5 percent of administrators' pay at for-profit hospitals, as compared with 19.7 percent at not-for-profit hospitals. In 1995, 25 percent of Columbia/HCA's administrators received profit-related bonuses that amounted to at least 80 percent of their salaries; many who did not were forced out of the company. (p. 1814)

Woolhandler and Himmelstein conclude this article by noting, "Behind false claims of efficiency lies a much uglier truth. Investor-owned care embodies a new value system that severs the community roots and Samaritan traditions of hospitals, makes physicians and nurses into instruments of investors, and views patients as commodities. Investor ownership marks the triumph of greed" (p. 1815).

While Woolhandler and Himmelstein estimate that the approximately $209 billion is spent annually on medical administration in the United States, Henry Aaron (2003), using a different methodology, estimates annual administrative spending of $159 billion, suggesting that Woolhandler and Himmelstein overestimate the administrative burden of the U. S. health care system by $50 billion. However, while challenging the methodology and the amount, Aaron does not question the reality of administrative waste in the U. S. system, noting:

> like many other observers, I look at the U.S. health care system and see an administrative monstrosity, a truly bizarre mélange of thousands of payers with payment systems that differ for no socially beneficial reason, as well as staggeringly complex public systems with mind-boggling administered prices and other rules expressing distinctions that can only be regarded as weird. (p. 801)

Private insurance policies frequently "carve out" mental health benefits, and it was estimated a decade ago that at least one-half of all Americans with insurance (including public plans) were enrolled in some type of "carved-out" managed behavioral health care plan (Frank, McGuire and Newhouse, 1995). Some of the reasons for the rapid development of managed behavioral health care plans include dissatisfaction with the quality of existing mental health services, improved technology to treat mental illness (e.g., SSRIs and atypical antipsychotics; assertive community treatment; case management), expanded consumerism and enhanced involvement of families, and growing concerns about the cost of mental health as a percentage of overall health care costs (Mowbray, Grazier and Holter, 2002). However, a naturalistic experiment that occurred in 1996 when TennCare (Tennessee's Medicaid program) carved out mental health benefits suggests that the practice is not without risks; as a consequence of the change, medication adherence in high-risk patients being treated for psychosis declined dramatically after the change, and there was a substantial loss of continuity of outpatient care (Ray, Daugherty and Meador, 2003).

There are also compelling data to document that financial incentives offered to health care providers under managed care contracts influence the decisions that providers make about patient care. For example, Rosenthal (1999) demonstrated that when a managed behavioral health organizations (MBHOs) changed provider incentives by moving from a fee-for-service plan to a fixed per patient case rate, irrespective of services provided, mental health visits decreased by 25 percent. Under the case rate scenario, patients were far more likely to receive medication and be referred to self-help programs and/or the community mental health center. As an example, despite evidence like this, the Minnesota Department of Health approved a case rate of about $325 for providers of outpatient mental health services to enrollees of one of the three large HMOs in the state (Health Partners). About that time, their enrollees were being informed that their benefit included up to 20 outpatient sessions. As of August, 2005, this capitated mode of payment to individual providers remained in effect, but the number of sessions it was to cover was judged as privileged information by the health plan, and not available through the Minnesota Department of Health, Managed Care Systems Section.

Mental health parity legislation at the state level increasingly requires insurance companies selling insurance in the states in question to offer mental health services (and sometimes substance abuse services) at the same level as physical health benefits. President Bush has publicly indicated the support of his administration for full mental health parity (Hogan, 2003); however, he has not pressured Congress to pass parity legislation, and several bills that would support federal parity have not received the support necessary to enact them into law.

Historically, mental health services have been provided at the state level, and the states have assumed responsibility for financing the care of the most disabled citizens with the greatest need. Up until the mid-1950s, mental health services were provided in large institutions ("state hospitals") that were often relatively self-contained communities. However, in part due to the widespread adoption of effective antipsychotic medications, these hospitals began to downsize and state financed mental health services became increasingly delivered in outpatient settings, often in the community mental health centers described above. These centers were often not sufficiently staffed to manage the increased workloads that resulted from deinstitutionalization, and many individuals who had lived in state hospitals for many years found themselves homeless and without access to even minimal mental health services.

In a somewhat desperate effort to control escalating health care costs, states have turned to managed care models that include management information systems, incentive contracts and fee negotiations. Beginning in the 1960s, with the advent of Medicare and Medicaid, states began to use a mix of state funds and federal funds to pay for services, often partnering with community mental health centers. By the late 1970s, the state mental health authorities were contracting for many of the mental health services needed by their citizens, and increasingly the state mental health authorities became managers of the financing of a complex array of services that included inpatient residential care, contracts for outpatient services and collections from third-party payers, including the federal government. Some of the managed care tools used by the states included prior authorization, utilization review, concurrent review of claims, analysis of computerized claims data, the use of networks of providers and negotiated rates (Essock and Goldman, 1995).

EVALUATION OF THE MENTAL HEALTH SYSTEM

Access and Equity

There are multiple barriers to access to health care in the United States, and not even the staunchest advocates of the *status quo* would argue that the U.S. health care system is equitable. This overall systemic problem is only compounded when one examines access to mental health services.

The Uninsured

U.S. citizens who have mental or emotional problems often find they are denied insurance coverage because their psychological difficulties are identified as preexisting conditions; as a result, there exists an underground service economy in which payments for treatment of mental illness (e.g., depression) or substance abuse are made in cash so there is no formal (insurance) record of the treatment, virtually guaranteeing that one's history of treatment will not be used against an individual in the future. Of course, this practice contributes to the stigma associated with treatment for mental or emotional problems.

Even for people with health insurance, access to mental heath care may be unavailable because of limited benefits, a "carve out" for mental health, provider panels with few or inexperienced mental health providers, or the existence of primary-care gatekeepers who receive financial inducements for limiting the number of patients who are referred to specialists (e.g., mental health) providers. Druss and Rosenheck (1998) examined a database of over 77,000 interviews and concluded:

> [P]eople with mental disorders may face substantial barriers to obtaining and maintaining both health insurance and necessary health care . . . they were more likely to have had difficulty in procuring their insurance (as represented by denial for preexisting conditions) and had more concerns about losing their insurance (reflected in staying in their jobs because of fear of losing health benefits) . . . [and] they were about twice as likely to have delayed seeking care or to have been unable to obtain needed medical care. (p. 1766)

Minority Access

Access to health care in the United States is also limited by race and socioeconomic status. Weitzman, Byrd and Auinger (1999), for example, examined black and white middle class children with private health insurance, and found that black children experienced substantially increased rates of asthma, low birth weight and school difficulties. The authors note that "middle class black children, even in the presence of private health insurance, have markedly different sources and patterns of use of medical services"

(p. 151). Likewise, Weinick, Zuvekas and Cohen (2000) report:

> [B]lack Americans have higher death rates from coronary disease, breast cancer, and diabetes than do white Americans, and infant mortality rates are higher among both African American and American Indian/Alaska Native populations. In addition, the data show that there is a higher rate of uncontrolled hypertension among Mexican Americans than among white Americans and that Asian/Pacific Islander, African American, and Hispanic populations all have an elevated incidence of tuberculosis. (p. 37)

These disparities were also noted for mental health care, and black and Hispanic children were shown to receive fewer mental health services and were less likely to be given a prescription for medication.

William Vega and his colleagues have documented serious gaps in service utilization by Mexican Americans with mental health problems, documenting that only about one-fourth of the Mexican Americans with mental health diagnoses in their study had received services over the past 12 months. In addition, Vega et al. documented that Mexican immigrants had a utilization rate that was only two-fifths of that of Mexican Americans born in the United States (Vega, Kolody, Aguilar-Gaxiola and Catalano, 1999, p. 928). These lower rates of utilization for Hispanic individuals may result from cultural differences including the use of native healers (*curanderos* and *curanderas*) and a greater tendency to rely on family support rather than medical services in addressing mental health problems. However, "the transformation of public health care policy and the health care industry poses special and unprecedented challenges for the Mexican American population because of their low insurance coverage and the persistence of cultural-linguistic barriers" (p. 929).

Wang, Berglund and Kessler (2000) conducted a cross-sectional survey using the Midlife Development in the United States (MIDUS) database to examine the quality of care provided for people with mental disorders. They found that only 53.8 percent of respondents with a mental disorder had received care in the preceding year; however, even more alarming was the fact that "only 14.3 percent received care that could be considered consistent with evidence-based treatment recommendations" (p. 284). Predictors of receiving evidence-based care included being white, female, and severely ill and having mental health coverage. Wang et al. conclude that an "epidemic of untreated and poorly treated mental disorders exists in the United States, especially among vulnerable groups such as African Americans and the uninsured. Cost-effective interventions are needed to improve both access to and quality of treatment" (p. 284).

The Medical Expenditure Panel Survey (MEPS) documented significant disparities in perceived mental health as a function of race, with 6.0 percent of white women rating their mental health as "fair or poor" while 10.2 percent of black women selected this category. Age was also a predictor, with older women rating their mental health significantly lower than younger women. However, one of the most dramatic findings appeared to be related to education. Only 3.8 percent of women with more than 12 years of education rated their mental health as "fair or poor" while this category was selected by 14.9 percent of those women with less than a high school education. Interestingly, women who were single without children had the poorest self-reported mental health, while those women with children under age five had the best mental health, at least according to this survey (Altman and Taylor, 2001).

Part of the solution to providing better access to health care for minority groups in the United States may be found in current efforts to train more Hispanic and African American physicians and other health care providers. When Moy and Bartman (1995) examined the relationship between physician race and the care of racial and ethnic minority patients, they found that minority patients were more than four times more likely to receive care from nonwhite physicians than were non-Hispanic white patients. However, they also noted:

> Low-income, Medicaid, and uninsured patients were also more likely to receive care from nonwhite physicians. Individuals who receive care from nonwhite physicians were more likely to report worse health, visit an emergency department, and be hospitalized. Individuals who receive care from nonwhite physicians reported more acute complaints, chronic conditions, functional limitations, and psychological symptoms as well as longer visits.... Nonwhite physicians are more likely to care for minority, medically indigent, and sicker patients. Caring for less affluent and sicker patients may financially penalize nonwhite physicians and make them particularly vulnerable to capitation arrangements. (p. 1515)

Access for Children

As a contemporary federal initiative, the SCHIP legislation of 1997 increased insurance coverage and access to health care services, including mental health services, for nearly four million children in the United States (Kenney and Chang, 2004), though others have observed in one state that the program has not covered the "hard-to-reach" population (Kempe et al. 2003). One proposal for expanding access under SCHIP is to provide more mental health services in the public schools (Nabors and Mettrick, 2001). Another approach is to integrate mental health services into the growing number of publicly funded Health Centers.

Quality and Efficacy

Despite the problems with access and equity alluded to in the previous section, the quality of health and mental health services provided are generally good in the United States vis-à-vis other countries of the world, though not rated the best among the four countries in this study. For example, on the overall level of health attained by the populations serviced, the 1997 WHO comparison ranked Canada 12th, Great Britain 14th, Norway 15th, and the United States 24th of the 191 member countries of the World Health Organization (WHO, 2000, Annex Table 1, pp. 152–155. Cf. Table 6.1 of this volume). There is considerable variability in quality across the states and territories, and considerable variation across urban and rural areas within states.

Some studies have suggested that many people in the United States *do not* receive appropriate care. For example, in one of the few national samples to address the provision of mental health services in the United States, Alexander Young and his colleagues (Young, Klap, Sherbourne, and Wells, 2001) surveyed 1,636 adults with a probable depressive or anxiety disorder as determined by a brief diagnostic interview. The researchers used established treatment guidelines to assess whether or not effective treatment had occurred. They found that 83 percent of their sample of adults with depression or anxiety actually saw a health care provider, usually a primary care provider. Only 30 percent of this group were believed to have received appropriate treatment. However, it is striking in this study that appropriate care was provided for only 19 percent of the patients treated by *primary care providers*, while 90 percent of the patients seen by mental health *specialists* received appropriate care. Men and clients who were black, less educated, younger than 30 or older then 59 years were less likely to receive appropriate care.

Many mental health providers feel that managed care limitations have significantly eroded the quality of care provided in the United States. For example, Wells et al. (2000) used a controlled clinical trial to evaluate the impact of a quality improvement program in enhancing quality in the treatment of depression for patients in managed primary care settings. These researchers assessed the use of antidepressant medication, mental health specialty counseling visits, medical visits for mental health problems, and the total number of medical visits. They found that "when these managed primary care practices implemented QI (Quality Improvement) programs that improve opportunities for depression treatment without mandating it, quality of care, mental health outcomes, and retention of employment of depressed patients improved over a year, while medical visits did not increase overall" (p. 3204).

One consequence of managed care is that patients who might once have been referred to a mental health provider and treated with psychotherapy for depression are now far more likely to be treated by a primary care physician with antidepressants. Stagnitti (2005) examined Medical Expenditure Panel Survey (MEPS) data and found that in 2002, 8.5 percent of the U.S. civilian noninstitutionalized population purchased at least one antidepressant. Higher percentages were observed for the elderly (13.2%), and white non-Hispanics (10.6%). The number of women taking antidepressant medication was more than twice as high as the number of men; likewise, people with insurance were far more likely to have antidepressants prescribed than those citizens with no insurance.

Although mental health providers historically haven't been held to the same quality standards as other providers, this has changed quickly and dramatically over the past two decades as mental health care has moved from being a service to being a business. One manifestation of this change is the proliferation of practice guidelines in mental health. The Agency for Healthcare Research and Quality (AHRQ; formerly the Agency for Health Care Policy and Research) has taken the lead in the United States in promoting practice guidelines, including those relevant to mental health. Almost 1,600 individual practice guidelines can be reviewed by going to the National Guideline Clearinghouse at www.guidelines.gov. A search for guidelines on "depression" yields 319 guidelines, while a search for "anxiety" produces 251 guidelines. While not all of the guidelines will be directly relevant to mental health, many will be and perusing them can be a valuable experience for the mental health provider.

Still another parameter of the growing interest in the United States in the cost and efficiency of mental health services is the growing debate over evidence-based treatments (EBT), also known and discussed in various settings as empirically validated treatment (EVT), empirically supported interventions (ESI) or evidence informed practice (EIP). Nathan and Gorman (1998) wrote one of the seminal publications in this area, *Treatments That Work*. This issue is almost as contentious as prescriptive authority for psychologists, resulting in a marked chasm between those practitioners who view psychotherapy as an art and those who regard it as a science. In the American Psychological Association, the frequently acrimonious debate has often been between members of Psychologists in Independent Practice (Division 42, representing the art of psychotherapy) and the Society of Clinical Psychology (Division 12, and especially Section III, the Society for a Science of Clinical Psychology, representing practitioners and educators committed to science). Corrigan et al. (2001) have described two major barriers to the adoption of evidence-based practices in staff who treat people with serious mental illness: (1) service providers often lack the knowledge and skills required to assimilate evidence-based practices into their ingrained daily practice patterns, and (2) many evidence-based practices require multidisciplinary teams and solo practitioners are not well-positioned to implement new treatment strategies.

Other countries might benefit from the development of more than 27 clinical practice guidelines by the American Department of Defense and the National Clinical Practice Guideline Council of the Veterans Health Administration (Cassidy and Nilan, 2005, June), and by additional guidelines specific to disorders developed by the American Psychiatric Association and the American Psychological Association.

A voluntary quality improvement strategy has been less than successful addressing the U.S. mental health needs and quality of care. Quality assessments of managed behavioral health organizations (MBHOs) such as those by the National Committee for Quality Assurance or URAC accreditation, or use of the Health Plan Employer Data and Information Set (HEDIS) data have had only marginal impact upon employers' decisions about selecting health plans. A recent study by Gabel, et al. (2003) indicated that

> when employers seek new plans, however, their understanding of quality of care is limited. Advocates of new approaches to improve quality and expand consumer choice agree that quality measures are important, but the majority of small and large U.S. employers are unfamiliar with organizations that measure health plan quality. (p. 122)

The survey indicated that a very small percentage of both small and large firms were familiar with quality measures such as HEDIS and other quality monitoring groups such as the Leapfrog Group, or voluntary accreditation of managed behavioral health organizations by the National Committee for Quality Assurance (NCQA) or URAC accreditation.

Program evaluation of mental health services has relied upon structural, process, and outcome measures. Some of these measures have been questionable psychometrically. As an example, a *process measure* was developed by the National Committee for Quality Assurance (NCQR, 1997). The NCQR consists of voluntary members of private managed care organizations, including those that specialize in managed behavioral health care (for mental health and substance abuse disorders). Called the *Health Plan Employer Data and Information Set (HEDIS)*, this standardized survey was created to assist *employers* in selecting health plans based upon their quality ratings. Elements of the HEDIS data set have been adopted by some state departments charged with regulating the operations of managed care organizations (MCOs) in their jurisdiction, even though the HEDIS format was judged unreliable by *Consumer Reports* (1996, August). Several limitations of this format led the Minnesota Health Data Institute (1997, October, p. 66) to reject it in favor of another survey method (CAPHS).

Program evaluations based on actual treatment outcomes remains one of the major areas of development for all four of the countries included in this volume. As an example, when Olson (1999) conducted an evaluation of mental health services provided through managed care organizations operating in Minnesota, none of the health plans had conducted any studies that utilized outcome measures of clinically significant, sustained improvement following treatment. Only one study had been initiated by the Minnesota Health Department, Managed Care Systems Section, and that was a retrospective review of record-keeping of patients treated for depression, without addressing whether the patients improved, to what degree, for how long, at what cost.

Cost and Efficiency

To facilitate comparisons among the four countries discussed in this book, data from the World Health Organization (2005) are reported here for the United States on several national health accounts indicators related to levels of expenditure on health in general. These data are reported to the WHO by member

Table 5.9. *WHO National Health Account Indicators: 1998, 2002.*

Indicator	1998	2002
Total expenditures on health as a % of GDP	13	14.6
General government. expenditure as a % of total health expediture	44.5	44.9
Private expenditure on health as a % of total expenditure expenditure on health	55.5	55.1
General government expenditure on health as a % of total government expenditure	18.5	23.1
External resources for health as a % of total expenditure on health	0	0
Social security expenditure on health as a % of general government. expenditure on health	33.4	30.8
Out-of-pocket expenditure as a % of private expenditure on health	28.0	25.4
Private prepaid plans as a % of private expenditure on health	61.1	65.7

Note: World Health Organization (WHO). 2005. Annex Table 5, pp.1192-199.
Note: See Tables 1.2 and 1.3 for comparisons for the year 2002, and Table 6.9 for 2003.

countries. Data are presented for 1998 and the most recent reported year (2002) to help evaluate trends. Comments on these data follow presentation of Table 5.9.

Table 5.9 shows that from 1998 to 2002, health care expenditures are consuming an increasing proportion of the United States' economy as measured by health expenditures in relation to GDP (13% in 1998 versus 14.6% in 2002). An even larger increase in percent of total *government* expenditures are spent on health care (from 18.5% in 1998 to 23.1% in 2002). Social Security expenditures on health care decreased somewhat from 33.4 percent in 1998 to 30.8 percent in 2002. Of the total health expenditures in the private sector, prepaid health plans account for the largest increase (from 61.1% to 65.7%) relative to out-of-pocket expenditures, which actually decreased from 28.0 percent in 1998 to 25.4 percent in 2002.

Per capita expenditures for health in the United States are provided in Table 5.10 for the years 1998 and 2002.

Table 5.10 indicates that in the five-year period from 1998 to 2002, per capita *total* expenditure on health increased by $1,178 (28.8%) and per capita *government* expenditure on health increased by $545 (29.9%). The average annual rate of increase in both is roughly six percent.

Subtracting the per capita government expenditure from the total per capita expenditure yields an estimate of *private* sector per capita expenditures in the United States for the same years. For 1998 and 2002 respectively those per capita private expenditures are $2,273 (55.5% of the total per capita expenditure) and $2,906 (55.1% of the total per capita expenditure). The estimated amount and percent increase in private sector per capita health expenditures from 1998 to 2002 is $633 (27.8%). Private sector expenditures increased per capita slightly less than government per capita expenditures over the same time period (27.8% private versus 29.9% government).

Third-party payers, insurance companies, employers and clients all have a need to know if particular mental health services are efficacious, cost-effective and efficient. However, these questions are deceptively simple insofar as it is sometimes difficult to quantify the outcomes of psychological interventions or put a dollar value on the benefits that are attained. For example, if a depressed individual starts treatment with a 60 percent likelihood of committing suicide and this risk is cut in half, how much are the psychological

Table 5.10. *Per Capita Expenditures on Health, 1998, 2002.*

Indicator	1998	2002
Per capita total expenditure on health at average exchange rate (US$)	4,096	5,274
Per capita government expenditure on health at average exchange rate (US$)	1,823	2,368

Note: World Health Organization (WHO). 2005. Annex Table 6, p. 203.

services worth? What is the dollar value by reducing the suicide risk still more? How can this risk reduction be measured?

All four countries included in this volume are challenged by rising costs. As indicated by per capita health expenditures, the United States has had greatest difficulty in achieving cost containment, despite its experiment with managed care. Though managed care strategies include reducing both volume of services and provider fees, there is entrenched resistance to price controls by the government due to expectations and demands that private insurance companies and health plans earn a profit for their shareholders and provide extraordinary compensation for their top executives. The successful lobbying by these corporations with the U.S. Congress sustains their privileged positions. A recent example of that is the new Medicare prescription drug benefit (Part D), which prevents Medicare from negotiating the price of prescription drugs with private, for-profit pharmaceutical companies.

In lieu of price controls, the major cost-containment strategy adopted in the American health care system and mental health system has been control of the volume of services. Drastic reductions in inpatient psychiatric hospitalizations and inpatient days have occurred along with severe limits on the number of outpatient mental health visits under managed behavioral health care organizations (MBHCOs), which were estimated to enroll about 164 million Americans in 2002, an increase from 70 million in 1993. Depending on various definitions of managed care, estimates of covered workers in firms carving out mental health benefits to specialized MBCHOs range from 36 percent in HMOs, PPOs, and POS plans, to 66 percent when stand-alone utilization review and case management services are included (Barry, et al. 2003, pp. 132–133).

Reforms to contain costs in the American system have ranged from proposals that address either the supply or demand for mental health services. In general, the United States has favored control of the demand by shifting costs of both privately and publicly insured health care services to the users of these services in the form of increased shares of the constantly rising health insurance premiums, co-insurance, co-payments, and higher deductibles. Despite national legislation such as the Mental Health Parity Act (P.L. 104–204) passed by the U. S. Congress in 1996, and parity regulations passed by 34 states, serious gaps in coverage for mental health persist (Barry, et al. 2003, p. 129).

Employer mandated health insurance coverage was an element of the 1993 reform proposed by the Clinton Administration, which was defeated. The United States continues with a largely voluntary, employment-based health insurance system in the private sector. Job-based health insurance is estimated to cover about 175 million Americans, including 160 million active workers and their dependents, three million early retirees, and twelve million Medicare eligible retirees. But this voluntary system has gaping holes. Of the estimated 59 percent of the nation's firms that have three to nine workers, just over half offer health insurance coverage (Gabel, et al. 2003, pp. 117, 123). This is one explanation for the finding that among the uninsured in America (about 46 million in 2005), approximately 80 percent are from families whose head of the household is employed.

All U.S. workers pay a mandatory Medicare payroll tax, but they cannot benefit from that national single payer system until they are 65 or disabled, though they could buy into the system at an earlier age if they could afford the higher premiums. With the aging population and increased availability of advanced, but costly medical technologies, and a shrinking work force relative to the number of anticipated retirees, the viability of Medicare has been questioned. Medicaid, which is insurance for about 50 million Americans, has served as an important source of mental health coverage for vulnerable, low-income Americans, but reductions in both the federal and states' funding of Medicaid are likely to hamper the program's future success (Rowland, Garfield, and Ellias, 2003, p. 73).

Financing and Fairness

The Reverend Martin Luther King, Jr., once wrote: "Of all forms of inequality, injustice in health care is the most shocking and inhumane." The U.S. health care system is, by any measure, shocking in its inequality, permitting widespread disparities based on race, gender, ethnicity and poverty. The Census Bureau (August, 2005) reported that the number of uninsured Americans reached a new high in 2005 – 45.8 million citizens, representing 15.8 percent of the U.S. population. Nine million American children have no access to regular medical care. While the rates of heart disease and stroke have plummeted in the United States, these benefits are disproportionately enjoyed by the affluent, and wide disparities in health care continue to plague the nation (IOM, 2003).

Budget cuts in Medicaid at both the state and Federal level exacerbate the problem of health care inequity. As recently as May, 2005, Health and Human Services Secretary Michael Levitt established a commission to recommend ways to reduce Medicaid spending by $10 billion over the next five years. Medicaid is the largest source of financing mental health care in the United States and enables about 46 million individuals and families to access critically needed mental health services, especially the poor, unemployed or marginally employed, and uninsured (Gill, 2005, p. 1). Even without further funding cuts, under federal Medicaid law, states have the option of covering or refusing to cover mental health services as part of their own Medicaid program. The result is marked unfairness in public funding for mental health services for the poor.

Mental health benefits may be limited even for those citizens fortunate to have health insurance. Historically, private insurers have been reluctant to provide mental health benefits, fearing high costs associated with long-term treatment. While some insurers simply refused to offer mental health benefits, others limited payment to acute care services or imposed lower annual or lifetime limits to care and/or higher deductibles and copayments. Finally, many private insurers believed that coverage for serious mental illness was a state responsibility, and not one that should be borne by private insurance providers. Mental health parity laws have addressed some of these problems, but these changes are occurring on a state-by-state basis, and the United States still does not have comprehensive national parity legislation. In addition, there is some evidence that employers have resisted parity legislation by requiring more rigorous utilization review for mental health claims than for other health claims, resulting in a $10 billion decrease over the past decade in the percentage of total health spending that is devoted to mental health (Carnahan, 2001).

The issue of fairness in financing the mental health system is part of the broader issue of how all federal government programs are financed. Of the total receipts projected in the federal budget for FY 2006 ($2.178 trillion), $967 billion is from individual income taxes and $220 billion is from corporation income taxes. The substantially lower taxes paid by corporations has led many to characterize the American economy as a system of corporate welfare. Moreover, although the individual income tax system is somewhat progressive, with the percentage of income taxed increasing as income increases (up to a point), the larger proportion of out-of-pocket family income spent on health care by lower income families makes the financing of health care highly regressive.

An illustration will be helpful here. The median annual income for American households in 2005 was about $43,000 (Kiplinger, 2005, p. 130). A 65-year-old man who worked 45 years at an average salary of $40,000 would have earned $1,800,000 in his/her preretirement years. As an employee, she/he would have paid 1.45 percent of $1,800,000, which equals $26,100 as a financial contribution to help fund the Medicare insurance program, or an average of $580/year for 45 years. His employer would have matched that contribution with another $26,100, for a total of $52,200 (or $1,160/year) in Medicare insurance "premiums" charged as mandatory payroll taxes. Thus, funding of Medicare is basically a mandated, employment-based system of financing, and that is why a shrinking work force will create a significant financial crisis for Medicare in the future as the number of workers per retiree declines as the population grows older.

Although one needs to work only ten years to qualify for Medicare at age 65, at the time of retirement the individual will continue to pay premiums, deductibles, and co-payments or co-insurance costs for Medicare health insurance. In 2005, for hospital, medical, and prescription drug benefits (Parts A, B, & D respectively), plus the least expensive privately sold Basic Supplemental Insurance to cover what Medicare does not cover, an individual's costs would be about $2,250 in annual premiums plus another $430 annual deductibles, plus variable co-insurance payments ranging from zero to 50 percent of the total health costs. (The one time deductible for Part A of $912 is excluded here). Excluding all additional co-insurance and co-payments, the premiums plus deductibles alone amount to an estimated cost of about $2,700/person/year for the duration of one's retirement (without factoring in any increases in either premiums or deductibles). There are no premiums for Part A and basically no hospital charges at the time of utilization. Part B (medical expenses) qualify as tax deductible expenses, which reduce gross adjusted income on which income tax is paid (called taxable income). Were a retiree to live 20 years (to age 85), and his/her premiums and deductibles remained constant at $2,700/year (unlikely due to inflation), excluding co-insurance and co-payments, the extra costs would amount to another $54,000 for Medicare insurance. When this cost incurred *after* retirement is added to the preretirement contributions of $26,100 by an employee with an average income of $40,000, the total cost to a former employee/now retiree is about $80,100. The employer's contribution would add another $26,100. With payments like that, it is no wonder Americans have come to view Medicare as an "entitlement." It is clearly not free. With few exceptions, everyone must contribute to help fund Medicare while they are working and throughout their retirement, though in a different manner and rate.

Protection and Participation

Protection

Abuse of people with mental illness was commonplace in the 17th and 18th centuries (Grob, 1994), and even today people with mental illness make up an especially vulnerable population at high risk for abuse and exploitation. All states have licensing boards (e.g., the State Committee on Psychology, in Missouri) that have the power to revoke the licenses of any professionals found to be guilty of abusing patients. Although professionals sit on these boards, they are charged with oversight of the profession and their mandate is to protect the public. Sexual exploitation of mental health consumers continues to be an especially vexing problem for the mental health professions (Wedding, 2005).

Participation

There has been a growing realization that consumers can help one another, and consumers (often known as Consumers/Survivors/Ex-Patients or CSX) have banded together to lobby for the rights of people with mental illness. The efficacy of peer support programs has recently been evaluated by the Substance Abuse and Mental Health Services Administration (SAMHSA) in a multimillion dollar study referred to as the Consumer Operated Services Program (COSP) project. These programs are described in a recent book titled *On Our Own Together: Peer Programs for People with Mental Illness* (Clay, 2005).

Groups such as the Mental Health Association (MHA), the National Association for the Mentally Ill (NAMI), and the National Coalition of Mental Health Professionals and Consumers (NCMHPC) are involved in efforts to empower people with mental illness and their families, providing them with important advocacy and self-help skills. For example, NCMHPC provides an on-line "Guide to Solving Problems with Insurance and Managed Care" (http://www.thenationalcoalition.org/consum.html) that provides tips on how to work effectively to ensure that one gets the care to which one is entitled. They also provide "Eight Incorrect Rationales for Denying Treatment" that include the following stratagems used by insurance companies to deny benefits to clients with mental health problems, along with strategies and arguments to confront the rationalizations: (a) You should have read your policy and manual more carefully to see the reasons that treatment can be denied; (b) treatment is time limited because people get better faster when they know how many sessions they have; (c) most of the possible change occurs in the first few sessions and, therefore, extended therapy is not helpful; (d) patients who are motivated will get over their problems in just a few sessions; (e) if a patient cannot prove steady progress, treatment should be stopped; (f) if a patient cannot be cured, therapy does not make sense; (g) the purpose of therapy is to restore a person to the usual level functioning; and (h) the treatment was not supported by scientifically-based guidelines.

In addition to the efforts by patient and family advocacy groups, progress in protecting the human rights of the mentally ill and in fostering their participation has been made in the United States at various levels through federal and state legislation, by professional organizations, and by judicial decisions. Examples of federal legislation relevant to consumer rights include a variety of bills in Congress to improve access and quality of care, the right to appeal denials of coverage by health plans, the right to sue a health maintenance organization for negligence or malpractice, and parity legislation between medical and mental health coverage. Illustrative federal and state laws include the Americans with Disabilities Act, the Mental Health Parity Act, Mental Health Bills of Rights, the Health Insurance Portability and Accountability Act, state mandated reporting of neglect and abuse, and civil commitment procedures and rights to treatment for persons judged incompetent due to their mental illness.

Americans with Disabilities Act (ADA)

The *Americans with Disabilities Act (ADA)* became federal law July 26, 1990. The law extended the Civil Rights Act of 1964 to include protection of people with physical and mental disabilities from discrimination in employment, public accommodations, and federally funded programs (O'Keefe, 1993). The ADA includes a statutory definition of disability as "a physical or mental impairment that substantially limits one or more of the major life activities; a record of such impairment; or being regarded as having such an impairment" (42 United States Code, Section 12102). This federal law formally recognized the disabling results of mental illness.

Reasonable accommodations in employment must be provided for individuals with psychiatric disabilities (Carling, 1993). Examples of reasonable accommodations include flexible scheduling, providing extra unpaid leave for short-term medical or psychiatric treatment, a private workspace, restructured job duties, and job coaching.

Goodman-Delahunty (2000) informed psychological practitioners about five types of discrimination claims involving mentally impaired individuals and some of the pitfalls in psychological assessments pertinent to such claims. Foote (2000) provided a model for psychological consultation in cases involving ADA claims, and Carling (1993) and Houlihan and Reynolds (2001) outlined strategies and procedures for psychological assessments and consultations with employers. It is pertinent to know that the Equal Employment Opportunity Commission (EEOC) is a federal agency that can sue employers for discrimination of disabled employees, even when individuals have signed agreements to submit to arbitration (*Star Tribune*, Jan. 16, 2000).

Mental Health Parity Act, 1996

Another recent and significant change in federal health policy was expressed in the Mental Health Parity Act of 1996 (42 United States Code, Section 201), which amended both (a) the Employee Retirement Income Security Act of 1994 (ERISA) (29 United States Code Section 10001) and (b) the Public Health Service Act (42 United Stated Code, Section 290). This legislation required health insurance to be portable, private and simple. Moreover, health plans provided by employers with more than 50 employees are required to provide annual and lifetime dollar benefits for selected mental disorders (Erdman, 2001).

Subsequent bills to expand the 1996 Parity Act such as the Paul Wellstone Mental Health Equitable Treatment Act (2001) have languished in Congress. As drafted, the Wellstone bill calls for requiring insurance companies to extend coverage equal to that given medical conditions to the more than 200 mental disorders recognized in the DSM-IV (Bradshaw, 2004).

Mental Health Bills of Rights and Patient Protection Rulings

In addition to federal legislation, several states have written legislation advancing the rights of mental health patients. An illustration is the Mental Health Client Bill of Rights (Minnesota Statutes, Chapter 148B, Section 148B.71) and the State's Patient Protection Act (62J.695-62J.76).

In addition to both federal and state legislation, mental health professionals have articulated statements to protect patient rights. Several national mental health professional organizations made a joint initiative to create a document, entitled *Your Mental Health Rights*, to assist consumers/patients in their dealings with insurance companies and managed care plans with respect to their mental health and substance abuse treatment services.

Managed care has become the dominant model for delivering health care in the United States. DeLeon, VandenBos, and Bulatao (1991) provided a history of the federal policy initiatives leading to the enactment of the Health Maintenance Organization (HMO) Act of 1973. Subsequent to the HMO Act, several federal and state laws and regulations have been passed to protect patients' rights in these and other forms of managed care organizations, including federal Medicare consumer protection rules announced in 2002 (Howatt, 2002). Patients' rights to sue their HMO were supported by a U.S Court of Appeals for the Second Circuit in New York in 2003, but legislation enacted by ten states to allow patients to sue their HMO for *damages* from negligence or malpractice in state courts was overruled by the United States Supreme Court (*The National Psychologist*, July/Aug, 2004).

The latter rulings by the Court reflect the role of the judicial branch of the federal government in either bringing about or blocking reforms in health and mental health services. Additional judicial action could involve antitrust law (Hass-Wilson, 2003) or breach of fiduciary duty lawsuits against managed care organizations (Rosoff, 2001).

Health Insurance Portability and Accountability Act

The most significant recent legislation protecting the privacy of both medical and mental health patients is the Health Insurance Portability and Accountability Act of 1996 (HIPAA). The bill was designed to protect Americans who were previously ill from losing their health insurance when they changed jobs or residences; however, provisions of the Act concerning electronic records and filing claims electronically also had significant implications for the security and privacy of patient health information.

HIPPA limits access to protected health information (i.e., any information that can be linked to specific individuals), provides minimum safeguards to prevent unauthorized access to health information, and achieves administrative simplification through the use of a standard format for exchanging electronic health information. Covered entities under HIPPA include almost all health plans and health care providers.

"Protected health information," such as psychotherapy notes, has become more secure as a result of HIPAA. Nevertheless, despite this mandated protection, a subsequent survey by Lorence (2004) of mental health delivery settings revealed significant variability in levels of protection of confidentiality in both paper and computerized records.

Mandated Reporting of Neglect and Abuse

Although some mental health professionals want to maintain absolute confidentiality of their work with clients, most states impose limits in the form of mandated reporting to legal authorities of abuse and neglect of children and vulnerable adults, and justify breaches of confidentiality when clients are a danger to themselves or to others. However, a study from New Zealand indicates that not all practitioners consistently conform to such mandates. Agar and Read (2002) reviewed the files of 200 users of a community mental health service and found that 46 percent of the files contained documentation of sexual or physical abuse as children or adults, but only 36 percent of summary formulations and 33 percent of treatment plans for the abused clients mentioned the abuse. Only 22 percent of the abused clients received abuse-focused therapy. Response rates were lower for clients who were male and had a schizophrenic spectrum diagnosis, and if the clinician was male or a psychiatrist. The most dramatic finding was that *none* of the alleged crimes (past, recent or ongoing) was reported to legal authorities. The authors of this chapter are not aware of a comparable study conducted in the United States, hence the level of compliance with mandatory reporting statutes is unknown, but based on the New Zealand study, it seems reasonable to hypothesize that compliance will vary depending upon state laws, clinic policies, the gender of clients and clinicians, the client's mental disorder, and the clinician's mental health profession.

Civil Commitment and the Right to Treatment

Another important area of patient rights pertains to the denial of their liberty in cases of involuntary commitments and treatments. Involuntary treatment of mental health patients involves judgments by the courts in civil commitment proceedings, and forced interventions of hospitalized mental patients. Parry (1994) identified seven distinct types of civil commitment that have been and continue to be applied in the United States: Informal, voluntary, third-party, short-term, extended, and outpatient commitments, and recommitment. Most of these legal proceedings result in patients being hospitalized without their consent.

The existence and application of these types of civil commitment proceedings depend partly upon the relative dominance of perspectives and policies influenced by mental health professionals, family members, patients, patient advocates, and the courts. In general, mental health patients and their advocates tend to argue for deinstitutionalization or for a less restrictive alternative. In all models, the state is permitted to serve as the sovereign and guardian for individuals who are legally incapable (incompetent) to care for themselves, or who are a danger to themselves or others (Dallaire, McCubbin, Morin, and Cohen, 2000). Actual proceedings for involuntary civil commitment of mentally ill persons have varied in the United States, both by time and place (Loue, 2002) and by forensic examiner training (Edens, Poythress, Nicholson, and Otto, 1999). The American Psychological Association has published guidelines for participation of forensic psychologists in civil commitment proceedings.

In the United States, involuntary commitment triggers a constitutional right to receive treatment, but also protection of the patient's right to accept or refuse medication, and procedural guidelines concerning the use of restraints and seclusion (Wynaden et al. 2002). The right to accept or refuse medication has been tied to the Fourth Amendment constitutional rights of privacy and due process, and to state constitutions and common law (Loue, 2002). These statutory protections seem consistent with the principles for the protection of persons with mental illness and for the improvement of mental health care (MI Principles) adopted by the United Nations General Assembly in 1991 (Resolution 46/119) to curb the political abuses of psychiatry found in several regions of the world. Maingay et al. (2002) provide a summary of these MI Principles and implementation strategies.

Psychiatric Advance Directives (PADs) are an emerging method for adults with serious and persistent mental illness to document treatment preferences in advance of periods of incapacity. Clinical, administrative, legal, and training issues associated with application of these directives have been discussed by Srebnik and Brodoff (2003), who address some of the concerns that have been raised about PADs by Miller (1998).

Population Relevance

The health care system in the United States fails to meet the overall health care needs of all citizens, and this problem is even more acute when mental health care needs are specifically addressed. There is a dramatic gap between the identified need for mental health services and the availability of those services, and substantial barriers prevent people with mental illness from acquiring the services they need. Druss and Rosenheck (1998) have documented these barriers and the fact that access to general medical providers is not adequate to meet the special needs of this population. They note:

> People with mental disorders may face particular difficulties in obtaining needed medical care. Mental disorders may represent pre-existing conditions that make purchasing new health insurance difficult or make people fearful of losing existing benefits. Restricted provider panels, with or without accompanying utilization review, may prevent people from obtaining needed specialty care even when they have health insurance and a primary care provider. (p. 1775)

Recommendations for Improvement in the Overall Performance of the Mental Health System

Numerous incremental approaches to improving mental health services in the United States are possible, and incremental approaches are more politically viable in the short run than the total revamping of the U. S. health care system that we believe is necessary to effect long-term and substantive health care reform. For example, two of the authors of this chapter have been enthusiastic proponents of prescriptive authority for psychologists (e.g., DeLeon, Dunivin and Newman, 2002; Wallis and Wedding, 2004). Because psychologists are better distributed and more likely to serve rural America, mental health care will be enhanced as psychopharmacology is added to the armamentarium of psychologists. We believe there is a particularly powerful synergy between primary care providers (e.g., family physicians and advanced practice nurses) and psychologists, and this combination of providers may hold the best hope for providing comprehensive mental health care for U. S. citizens (Wedding and Mengel, 2004).

Another serious problem with mental health care in the United States is the established lag between science and practice. The magnitude of this problem has been dramatically underscored by the Institute of Medicine (2001): "Health care today harms too frequently and routinely fails to deliver its potential benefits. . . . Between the health care we have and the care we could have lies not just a gap, but a chasm" (p. 1). However, there is compelling evidence that traditional models of information dissemination (e.g., continuing education lectures and seminars) are *not* effective tools for influencing practice, and "education alone has little impact on practitioner behavior" (Torrey, Finnerty, Evan and Wyzik, 2003, p 883). The mental health field desperately needs to identify ways to meaningfully influence the practice patterns of providers, encouraging them to implement the findings that come out of university and medical school research settings. For example, there is compelling evidence that cognitive behavior therapy (CBT) is an empirically validated therapy that is the treatment of choice for anxiety disorders, but it was used less frequently than dynamic psychotherapy for treating generalized anxiety disorder, panic disorder and social phobia in the United States between 1991 and 1996 (Goisman, Warshaw, and Keller, 1999). Other examples of treatments with known efficacy not being widely adopted include family psychoeducation and behavioral interventions for children with attention deficit hyperactivity disorder. Speaking before the President's New Freedom Commission on Mental Health on behalf of the American Psychological Association, Diane Marsh (July 19, 2002) noted:

> For a variety of social and systemic reasons, our knowledge of what works with these patients and with these disorders is not always translated into clinical practice. A case in point is family psychoeducation, which has documented clinical, social, family, and economic benefits for a range of disorders, including schizophrenia. . . . Yet fewer than 10 percent of families of patients with schizophrenia receive even minimal educational and supportive services in the United States. . . . Another case in point is the treatment of ADHD. Although behavioral interventions are well-validated and highly effective treatments for reducing behavior problems and functional impairment . . . too often these young patients receive only stimulant medication.

The mental health care system in the United States is also likely to benefit from the inclusion of consumers as full participants in their own care, and a growing body of literature documents that mental health consumers do not have to be passive recipients of treatment but in fact can actively facilitate their own recovery. The efficacy of a variety of peer-run programs for people with mental illness has been demonstrated by the SAMHSA funded Consumer Operated Support Program (COSP) (Clay, 2005). These programs include mutual support groups, mentoring services, peer-run multiservice agencies, peer-run drop-in programs, specialized supportive services and peer-run education/advocacy programs (Campbell, 2005).

We believe the future also will see an increasing appreciation for the role of psychologists as primary behavioral care providers, along with the increasing co-location of primary care and behavioral health care services. The practice of co-location allows for convenient "hallway handoffs," dramatically increasing the likelihood that a patient referred for mental health services by a primary care provider will actually follow-up and get the services recommended. Wedding and Mengel (2004) describe the importance of co-located mental health and primary care services as follows:

> Despite the ubiquity of behavioral health problems in primary care settings, up to two-thirds of patients meeting diagnostic criteria for mental illness have these problems go undetected by primary care clinicians (deGruy, 1996; Spitzer et al. 1994), underscoring the importance of a collaborative approach to the delivery of health care services for this population. According to Stoeckle (1995), "Patients bring [to the medical visit] not only the bodily complaints, but also the circumstances of their every day lives – who they are and who they hope to be."... We believe most mental health and behavioral health problems can – and should – be treated in a primary care setting; however, if adequate treatment is to occur, it will require genuine integration of services and close collaboration between primary care providers and providers with specific training in the identification of behavioral health problems and the delivery of meaningful, evidence-based treatments. (pp. 48–49)

Although the implementation of any of the suggestions offered above would enhance the quality of mental health services available in the United States, the authors of this chapter do not believe substantive change in the mental health system will occur without meaningful reform of the total U. S. health care system. We also believe that a publicly financed, single payer health care system is the best possible way for the United States to achieve access to at least a modicum of health care for all of her citizens. This goal has been achieved by each of the other countries discussed in this book, and we fully believe it is a goal that can be attained by the United States.

Most Americans believe health care is a basic human right. This idea is neither novel nor new; for example, Harry Truman almost passed a national health insurance plan in 1945; at that time, he had the support of 75 percent of the American public (Quadagno, 2005), but he was foiled by Southern politicians (who feared national health insurance would lead to racially integrated hospitals) and the American Medical Association (Krugman, 2005).

Somewhat later, in 1981, the Catholic Bishops of the United States wrote:

> Following on these principles and on our belief in health care as a basic human right, we call for the development of a national health insurance program. It is the responsibility of the federal government to establish a comprehensive health care system that will ensure a basic level of health care for all Americans. The federal government should also ensure adequate funding for this basic level of care through a national health insurance program. (p. 17–18)

Article 25 of the *Universal Declaration of Human Rights* states that every person has a right to medical care. It is also striking that the American Medical Student Association has endorsed a single-payer health care system.

Although Dennis Kucinich was the only major Democratic candidate to actively support a single payer health care system in the Democratic primaries for the 2004 Presidential race, there is growing support for a single-payer system; increasingly this takes the form of "Medicare for all." An example of this approach of building upon what is already known to work is provided here to illustrate one American version of a publicly financed, national health insurance program.

A bill was introduced in the 108th Congress in 2003 by Representatives John Conyers (D-Michigan) and Jim McDermott (D-Washington) entitled, *The United States National Health Insurance Act* (HR676). This USNHI bill proposes "expanded and improved Medicare for all." It builds on a successful, well-known program (Medicare) that has been in place for 40 years for a very large, and growing segment of the population, namely those 65 years and older (as well as the disabled and some kidney dialysis patients). It is a uniquely American form of a national health insurance program. Among health care professionals, the bill is supported by a national advocacy group called Physicians for a National Health Program (PNHP), numbering about 12,000 members.

This program would provide (a) universal access to (b) comprehensive coverage, (c) in a publicly financed health insurance program, (c) administered as a nonprofit system, and would be (d) both portable and free at the point of service. According to an executive summary, this landmark bill proposes essentially a national health insurance program to ensure universal access of all U.S. residents to all medically necessary services. *Comprehensive coverage* would include primary care and specialist care, such as mental health services and substance abuse treatment; inpatient, outpatient and emergency services; prescription drugs; durable medical equipment; long term care; dentistry, eye care, and chiropractic care. The bill would preserve patients' choice of providers, hospitals, and clinics, ensure portability, and require no deductibles or co-payments at the point of service.

This bill would convert the entire U.S health care system to a not-for-profit system that is *publicly financed* primarily from payroll taxes. It would actually reduce employers' costs for health care from an average of 8.5 percent of payroll by substituting a payroll tax on all employers of 3.3 percent in addition to maintaining the employer and employee Medicare payroll tax of 1.45 percent each. Some mechanisms would be employed to establish a progressive financing system such as a health income tax on the wealthiest five percent of Americans and closing corporate tax shelters.

The payroll tax revenues would be pooled nationally and allocated through an entitlement outlay set by the U.S. Congress annually. It would be federally administered under the auspices of the Department of Health and Human Services, and incorporate all current Medicare, Medicaid, and SCHIP insurance programs. Oversight of the program would be provided by a National USNHI Advisory Board comprised primarily of health care professionals and representatives of health advocacy groups.

Three methods of provider payments would be applied to include all health care and mental health care providers (not just physicians or psychiatrists): (a) fee-for-service payments to private practitioners based on a negotiated schedule of discounted fees; (b) capitation payments for large group practices and clinics; (c) global budgets for hospital-based health plans to pay salaries for the majority of physicians who now work at least part-time as employees.

Projected savings the first year of $150 billion on paperwork and another $50 billion from using rational bulk purchasing of medications will be more than enough to cover all the nearly 46 million uninsured, improve coverage for everyone else, and include medication coverage and long-term care.

Major opponents to this nationalization of health care are likely to include private sector organizations (health insurance companies, health plans, managed care organizations, pharmaceutical companies), private practitioners resistant to controlled fees, and both for-profit and nonprofit hospitals resistant to operating under budgetary limits set by the government. Current for-profit companies would receive no compensation for their loss of business profits, but only for real estate, buildings, and equipment. Private health insurers would be prohibited under this act from selling coverage that duplicates the benefits of the USNHI program, though they could sell any additional benefits not covered by this Act (e.g., cosmetic surgery and other medically unnecessary treatments). Some state departments of health and human services may be threatened by a federal usurpation of state prerogatives in financing and administering Medicaid and SCHIP programs. A public cynical about big government beholden to special interests will resist this bill. Critical support will be needed from the primary payers in the private sector, namely, employers. If federal and state employee benefits were to be replaced by this bill, their unions can be expected to resist this major reform, especially if benefits are reduced.

A recent communication with Joel Segal in Representative John Conyers office, August 23, 2005, indicated this bill has 51 cosigners in the House of Representatives, but there was no companion bill in the Senate. Endorsements have come from some major unions, but not yet from organizations representing mental health specialists.

Knowing Americans' reflex reaction to federal interventions, perhaps we can learn from Canada. The national health insurance program of Canada began in one province. If one state in America were to serve as a demonstration project, the American version of universal health insurance could be tested, evaluated, and revised before launching a federal system. A similar proposal was defeated recently in Oregon, but related proposals have been offered in Minnesota and California.

Massive lobbying by opposing private health insurance organizations and health plans make these reforms a protracted struggle. There appears to be no constituency with sufficient influence to overcome the present opposition and apathy about the 46 million uninsured and the additional millions of underinsured Americans. Perhaps for a national health insurance program will be able to tap the frustration and anger of enough citizens to pressure Congress for reform. Mere endorsements by various stakeholders – payers, providers, and patients – will not be sufficient to create a movement for major health care reform. Most likely it will take a grass roots organization of citizens as it did in Canada to rebalance power in favor of the public good.

The popularity of Medicare with Americans, who have come to view it as an entitlement, is a reason to be optimistic about health care reform based on expansion of that federally funded health insurance program. Medicare remains popular with Americans even as it has evolved over the years into a more complex and varied set of health insurance options. Administrative costs have been consistently under three to five percent, which are only a fraction of those of private insurers, so it appears to be an efficient system. Moreover, the idea of extending an existing program seems more acceptable to many Americans than imitating another country's health care system (e.g., the Canadian system). Finally, extending coverage under Medicare is not perceived as dramatic or as radical as creating a new and complex health care delivery system as proposed by the Clinton Administration in the Health Security Act in 1993.

In its present form, Medicare can be construed as a publicly financed, single payer, national health insurance program for a large and growing portion of the American population (Kiplinger, 2005). Expansion of this program will be necessitated by the aging of baby boomers from about 36 million elderly Americans in 2005 to an estimated 77 million by 2011. Expanding this program into a universal health insurance program might gain the support of businesses desperate to do something about rising health care costs, workers who have routinely seen their wages rolled back at the bargaining table because of health care costs, and hospitals that have heretofore borne the costs of uncompensated care (a challenge which became even more acute with the cutbacks in Medicaid funding that occurred during the G. W. Bush administration). Both providers and hospital administrators will be attracted by the administrative simplification provided by a single payer system. Under a universal Medicare program, patients would still be able to choose their own doctor and their own hospital. Finally, millions of Americans will be spared the ignominy of living in a country that fails to provide basic access to health care to a growing segment of 45.8 million (15.8%) of the population whose access to health care and mental health care is diminished.

We cannot countenance this glaring injustice in access to the American health care system. This is a significant moral failure in a country that pledges its allegiance to "liberty and justice for all," and proclaims equal rights to "life, liberty, and the pursuit of happiness."

REFERENCES

Aaron, H. J. (2003). The costs of health care administration in the United States and Canada – Questionable answers to a questionable question. *New England Journal of Medicine, 349*, 801–803.

Agar, K., & Read, J. (2002). What happens when people disclose sexual or physical abuse to staff at a community mental health centre? *International Journal of Mental Health Nursing, 11*, 70–79.

Ahr, P. R. (2003). *Made in Missouri: The community mental health movement and community mental health centers, 1963-2003*. Saint Louis: Causeway.

Altman, B. M., & Taylor, A. K. (2001). *Women in the health care system: Health status, insurance, and access to care*. Rockville, MD: Agency for Healthcare Research and Quality. MEPS Research Findings No.17, AHRQ Pub. No. 02-0004.

Andrews, G., Sanderson, K., Corry, J., Issakidis, C., & Lapsley, H. (2003). Cost-effectiveness of current and optimal treatment for schizophrenia. *British Journal of Psychiatry, 183*, 427–435.

Aponte, J. F., & Crouch, R. T. (2000). The changing ethnic profile of the United States in the twenty-first century. In J. E. Aponte and J. Wohl (Eds.). *Psychological intervention and cultural diversity* (2nd ed.) (pp. 1–17). Needham Heights, MA: Allyn & Bacon.

Appleby, L., et al. (1993). Length of stay and recidivism in schizophrenia: A study of public psychiatric hospital patients. *American Journal of Psychiatry, 150*(1), 72–76.

Arons, B., et al. (2004). SAMHSA's Center for Mental Health Services: A decade of achievement, 1992–2002. In R. W. Manderscheid & M. J. Henderson, *Mental Health, United States, 2002* (pp. 1–8). Rockville, MD: Substance Abuse and Mental Health Services Administration.

Bartels, S. J. (2003). Improving the System of Care for Older Adults With Mental Illness in the United States. *American Journal of Geriatric Psychiatry, 11*, 486–497.

Bell, N. N., & Shern, D. L. (2002). State Mental Health Commissions: Recommendations for Change and Future Directions. [Report]. Alexandria, VA: National Technical Assistance Center for State Mental Health Planning, National Association of State Mental Health Program Directors.

Benjamin, L. T. Jr. (2003). Why can't psychology get a stamp? *Journal of Applied Psychoanalytic Studies, 5*, 443–454.

Bickman, L. (1996). A continuum of care: More is not always better. *American Psychologist, 51*(7), 689–701.

Bradshaw, J. (2004). Daschle contends parity could still be enacted this year. *The National Psychologist*, May/June, 14.

Budget of the United States Government, Fiscal Year 2006. Summary Tables. Table S-10: Budget Summary by Category. Retrieved July 13, 2005 from http://www.gpoaccess.gov/usbudget/fy06/browse.html. In-text citation (Budget Summary 2006).

Budget of the United States Government, Fiscal Year 2006. Medicare and Medicaid Services. Retrieved July 7, 2005 from http://www.gpoaccess.gov/usbudget/fy06/browse.html. In-text citation (Budget MMS 2006).

Budget of the United States Government, Fiscal Year 2006. Department of Health and Human Services. Retrieved July 7, 2005 from http://www.gpoaccess.gov/usbudget/fy06/browse.html. In-text citation (Budget HHS 2006).

Budget of the United States Government: Browse Fiscal Year 2006. Other Agencies/Office of Personnel Management. Retrieved on July 7, 2005 from http://www.gpoaccess.gov/usbudget/fy06/browse.html. In-text citation (Budget OPM 2006).

Budget of the United States Government: Fiscal Year 2006, Federal Employment and Compensation. Table 24-4: Personnel Compensation and Benefits. Retrieved July 7, 2005 from http://www.gpoaccess.gov/usbudget/fy06/empl.html. In-text citation (Budget PCB 2006).

Budget of the United States Government: Fiscal Year 2006, Medical Programs. Retrieved July 8, 2005 from http://www.gpoaccess.gov/usbudget/fy06/browse.html. In-text citation (Budget MP 2006).

Budget of the United States Government: Fiscal Year 2006, Department of Defense. Retrieved July 8, 2005 from http://www.gpoaccess.gov/usbudget/fy06/browse.html. In-text citation (Budget DOD 2006).

Budget of the United States Government: Fiscal Year 2006, Indian Health Service. Retrieved July 8, 2005 from http://www.gpoaccess.gov/usbudget/fy06/browse.html. In-text citation (Budget IHS 2006).

Bush, G.W. (2004). Remarks in a discussion on the benefits of health care information technology in Baltimore, Maryland. (April 27, 2004). *Weekly Compilation of Presidential Documents, 40*(18), 697–702.

Callicutt, J. W. (1997). Overview of the field of mental health. In T. R. Watkins & J. W. Callicutt (Eds.). *Mental health policy and practice today*. Thousand Oaks, CA: Sage.

Campbell, J. (2005). The historical and philosophical development of peer-run support programs. In S. Clay (Ed.), *On our own together: Peer programs for people with mental illness* (pp. 17–64). Nashville: Vanderbilt University Press.

Cannon, D. S. et al. (2001). The impact of the Veterans Health Administration (VHA) reorganization on psychology programs: A survey of VHA psychology leaders. *Professional Psychology: Research and Practice, 4,* 373–379.

Carling, P. (1993). Reasonable accommodations in the workplace for individuals with psychiatric disabilities. *Consulting Psychology Journal, 45*(2), 46–66.

Carnahan, I. (2002, January 21). Asylum for the insane. *Forbes,* 33–34.

Cartwright, W. S. (1999). Costs of drug abuse to society. *Journal of Mental Health Policy and Economics, 2,* 133–134.

Cavanaugh, D. A., & Muck, R. D. (2004). Editors' Introduction: Using Research to Improve Treatment for Adolescents: Findings from Two CSAT Demonstrations. *Journal of Psychoactive Drugs, 36,* 1–3.

Chavkin, W., & Breitbart, V. (1997). Substance abuse and maternity: The United States as a case study. *Addiction, 92,* 1201–1205.

Chen, S., Smith, M. W., Wagner, T. H., & Barnett, P. G. (2003). Spending for specialized mental health treatment in the VA: 1995-2001. *Health Affairs, 22,* 256–263.

CIA World Factbook (2005). United States. Retrieved January 30, 2005 from http://www.cia.gov/cia/publications/factbook/geos/us.html.

Clay, S. (Ed.) (2005). *On our own together: Peer programs for people with mental illness.* Nashville: Vanderbilt University Press.

Columbia Daily Tribune (January 28, 2005). Medicaid plan sparks worry: Blunt's cuts would disqualify 89,000.

Crowther, R. E., Marshall, M., Bond, G. R., & Huxley, P. (2001). Helping people with severe mental illness to obtain work: Systematic review. *British Medical Journal, 322,* 204–208.

Corrigan, P., Steiner, L., McCracken, S.G., Blasedr, B. & Barr, M. (2001). Strategies for disseminating evidence-based practices to staff who treat people with serious illness. *Psychiatric Services, 52*(12), 1598–1606.

Dallaire, B., McCubbin, M., Morin, P., & Cohen, D. (2000). Civil commitment due to mental illness and dangerousness: The union of law and psychiatry within a treatment control system. *Sociology of Health and Illness, 22*(5), 679–700. Retrieved February 10, 2004 from http://web5.epnet.com.

Davis, K. (1997). Managed care, mental illness and African Americans: A prospective analysis of managed care policy in the United States. *Smith College Studies in Social Work, 67,* 623–641.

deGruy, F. (1996). Mental health care in the primary care setting. In M. S. Donaldson, K. D. Yordy, K. N. Lohr, & N. A. Vanselow (Eds.), *Primary care: America's health in a new era* (pp. 285–311). Washington, DC: National Academy Press.

DeLeon, P. H. (2003). Foreword – Reflections on prescriptive authority and the evolution of psychology in the 21st century. In M. T. Sammons, R. U. Paige, & R. F. Levant (Eds.), *Prescriptive authority for psychologists: A history and guide* (pp. xi–xxiv). Washington, DC: American Psychological Association.

DeLeon, P. H., Biesting, B., & Kenkel, M. B. (2003). Community health centers: Exciting opportunities for the 21st century. *Professional Psychology: Research and Practice, 34,* 579–585.

DeLeon, P. H., Rossomando, N. P., & Smedley, B. D. (2004). The future is primary care. In R. G. Frank, S. H. McDaniel, J. H. Bray, & M. Heldring, *Primary care psychology* (pp. 317–325). Washington, DC: American Psychological Association.

DeLeon, P. H., Dunivin, D. L., & Newman, R. (2002). The tide rises. *Clinical Psychology: Science and Practice, 9*, 249-255.

DeLeon, P. H., VandenBos, G. R., & Bulatao, E. (1991). Managed mental health care: A history of the federal policy initiative. *Professional Psychology: Research and Practice, 22*(1), 15-25.

Department of Veterans Affairs (2005). Facility locator and directory. Retrieved February 5 from http://www1.va.gov/directory/guide/allstate.asp.

Donohue, J. M., & Frank, R. G. (2000). Medicaid behavioral health carve-outs: A new generation of privatization decisions. *Harvard Review of Psychiatry, 8*, 231-241.

Dougherty, D. (1988). Children's mental health problems and services: Current federal efforts and policy implications. *American Psychologist, 43*(10), 808-812.

Drake, R. E., Mueser, K. T., Brunette, M. F., & McHugo, G. J. (2004). A review of treatments for people with severe mental illnesses and co-occurring substance use disorders. *Psychiatric Rehabilitation Journal, 27*, 360-374.

Druss, B. G., & Rosenheck, R. A. (1998). Mental disorders and access to medical care in the United States. *American Journal of Psychiatry, 155*, 1775-1777.

Druss, B. G., Rohrbaugh, R. M., Levinson, C. M., & Rosenheck, R. A. (2001). Integrated medical care for patients with serious psychiatric illness: A randomized trial. *Archives of General Psychiatry, 58*, 861-868.

Duffy, F. F., et al. (2004). Mental health practitioners and trainees. In R. W. Manderscheid & M. J. Henderson (Eds.), *Mental health, United States, 2000.* Retrieved February 5, 2005 from the National Mental Health Information Center: http://mentalhealth.samhsa.gov/publications/allpubs/SMA01-3537/default.asp.

Edens, J. F., Poythress, N. G., Nicholson, R. A., & Otto, R. K. (1999). Effects of state organizational structure and forensic examiner training on pretrial competence assessments. *Journal of Behavioral Health Services and Research, 26*(2), 140-150. Retrieved April 26, 2005 from http://web34.epnet.com.

Ellis, B. J., Bates, J. E., Dodge, K. A., Fergusson, D. M., Horwood, L. J., Pettit, G. S., & Woodward, L. (2003). Does father absence place daughters at special risk for early sexual activity and teenage pregnancy? *Child Development, 74*, 801-821.

Erb, M., Hodgins, S., Freese, R., Müller-Isberner, R., & Jöckel, D. (2001). Homicide and schizophrenia: Maybe treatment does have a preventive effect. *Criminal Behaviour and Mental Health, 11*, 6-26.

Erdman, C. (2001). The medicolegal dangers of telephone triage in mental health care. *The Journal of Legal Medicine, 22*, 553-579.

Essock, S. M., & Goldman, H. H. (1995). States' embrace of managed mental health care. *Health Affairs, 14*, 34-44.

Feldman, S., Bachman, J., & Bayer, J. (2002). Mental health parity: A review of research and a bibliography. *Administration and Policy in Mental Health, 29*, 215-228.

Fellin, P. (1996). *Mental health and mental illness: Policies, programs, and services.* Itasca, IL: F. E. Peacock.

Field, M. J., & Cassel, C. K. (Eds.) (1997). *Approaching death: Improving care at the end of life.* Washington, DC: National Academy Press.

First, M. B., & Pincus, H. A. (2002). The DSM-IV Text Revision: Rationale and potential impact on clinical practice. *Psychiatric Services, 53*, 288-292.

Foote, W. (2000). A model for psychological consultation in cases involving the Americans with disabilities act. *Professional Psychology: Research and Practice, 31*(2), 190-196.

Frank, R. G., Blevins, N. C., & Dimoulas, E. (2004). Policy and financing of the professional psychology workforce. *Journal of Clinical Psychology in Medical Settings, 11*, 119-125.

Frank, R. G., McGuire, T. G., & Newhouse, J. P. (1995). Risk contracts in managed mental health care. *Health Affairs, 14*, 50-64.

General Accounting Office (December, 2000). *Community-based care increases for people with serious mental illness.* Washington, DC: U.S. General Accounting Office (GAO-01/224).

General Accounting Office (April, 2003). *Child welfare and juvenile justice: Federal agencies could play a stronger role in helping states reduce the number of children placed solely to obtain mental health services.* Washington, DC: U.S. General Accounting Office (GAO-03/397).

General Accounting Office (September, 2004). *More information needed to determine if VA can meet an increase in demand for post-traumatic stress disorder services.* Washington, DC: U.S. General Accounting Office (GAO-04-1069).

Gill, R. E. (2005a). Prisons understaffed for mental health needs. *The National Psychologist, 14*(4), July/Aug.

Gill, R. E. (2005b). Mental health care for needy to plummet if Medicaid is cut. *The National Psychologist, 14*(4), July/Aug, p.1.

Goisman, R. M., Warshaw, M. G., & Keller, M. B. (1999). Psychosocial treatment prescriptions for generalized anxiety disorder, panic disorder, and social phobia, 1991-1996. *American Journal of Psychiatry, 156*, 1819-1821.

Goldsmith, R. J., & Garlapati, V. (2004). Behavioral interventions for dual-diagnosis patients. *Psychiatric Clinics of North America, 27*, 709-725.

Goodman-Delahunty, J. (2000). Psychological impairment under the Americans with Disabilities Act: Legal guidelines. *Professional Psychology: Research and Practice, 31*(2), 197-205.

Goodwin, R. D., Hoven, C. W., Lyons, J. S., & Stein, M. B. (2002). Mental health service utilization in the United States: The role of personality factors. *Social Psychiatry and Psychiatric Epidemiology, 37*, 561-566.

Greenberg, D. J., Cradock, C., Godbole, A., & Temkin, T. (1998). Cost effectiveness of clinical training in a community mental health center. *Professional Psychology: Research and Practice, 29*, 604-608.

Grob, G. N. (1994). *The mad among us: A history of the care of America's mentally ill.* New York: The Free Press.

Harman, J. S., Scholle, S. H., & Edlund, M. J. (2004). Emergency department visits for depression in the United States. *Psychiatric Services, 55,* 937–939.

Hass-Wilson, D. (2003). Managed care and monopoly power: The antitrust challenge. Cambridge, Mass: Harvard University Press. Reviewed by Robert I. Field in *Journal of Legal Medicine, 25,* 369–376.

Henderson, C., Liu, X., Diez Roux, A. V., Link, B. G. & Hasin, D. (2004). The effects of U.S. state income inequality and alcohol policies on symptoms of depression and alcohol dependence. *Social Science and Medicine, 58,* 565–575.

HHS (2004). *Health and Human Services Updates Poverty Guidelines for 2004.* Retrieved July 13, 2005 from http://www.immigrationlinks.com/new/news1898.html. In-text citation (HHS 2004).

HMOs win Supreme court challenge. *National Psychologist* (2004). July/Aug.13(4).

Hogan, M. F. (2003). New Freedom Commission Report: The President's New Freedom Commission: Recommendations to Transform Mental Health Care in America. *Psychiatric Services, 54,* 1467–1474.

Houlihan, J. P., & Reynolds, M. D. (2001). Assessment of employees with mental health disabilities for workplace accommodations: Case reports. *Professional Psychology: Research and Practice, 32*(4), 380–385.

Howatt, G. (2002). Proposed Medicare patient protections echo state laws. Retired 1/20/03 from http://www.startribune.com/stories/535/21286.html.

Howell, E. M., Buck, J. A., & Teich, J. L. (2000). Mental health benefits under SCHIP. *Health Affairs, 19*(6), 291–297.

Isaac, R.J., & Armat, V. C. (1990). *Madness in the streets: How psychiatry and the law abandoned the mentally ill.* New York: Free Press.

Institute of Medicine (IOM). (2001). *Crossing the quality chasm: A new health system for the 21st century.* Washington, DC: National Academy Press.

Institute of Medicine (IOM). (2002). *Fostering rapid advances in health care: Learning from system demonstrations.* Washington, DC: National Academies Press.

Institute of Medicine (IOM). (2003). *The future of the public's health in the 21st century.* Washington, DC: National Academies Press.

International Labor Organization. (n.d.). Disability and Work. Retrieved June 19, 2005 from http://www.ilo.org/public/english/employment/skills/disability/papers/execsummaries20.htm.

Kapp, M. B. (2001). Legal interventions for persons with dementia in the USA: Ethical, policy, and practical aspects. *Aging and Mental Health, 5,* 312–315.

Karlin, B. E., & Duffy, M. (2004). Geriatric mental health policy: Impact on service delivery and directions for effecting change. *Professional Psychology: Research and Practice, 35*(5), 509–519.

Kempe, A., Renfrew, B., Barrow, J., Cherry, D., Levinson, A., & Steiner, J. F. (2003). The first 2 years of a state child health insurance plan: Whom are we reaching. *Health Affairs, 111*(4), 735–740.

Kenkel, M. B., DeLeon, P. H., Mantell, E. O., & Steep, A. (in press). Divided no more: Psychology's role in integrated healthcare. *Canadian Psychology/Psychologie Canadienne.*

Kenney, G., & Chang, D. I. (2004). The State Children's Health Insurance Program: Successes, shortcomings, and challenges. *Health Affairs, 23*(5), 51–62.

Kessler, R. C., Demler, O., Jin, R., Walters, E. E., Berglund, P. Koretz, D., et al. (2003). Treatment of Depression by mental health specialists and primary care physicians: Reply. *JAMA: Journal of the American Medical Association, 290,* 1992.

Kessler, R. C., & Frank, R. G. (1997). The impact of psychiatric disorders on work loss days. *Psychological Medicine, 27*(4), 861–873.

Kessler, R. C., Koretz, D., Merikangas, K. R., & Wang, P. S. (2004). The epidemiology of adult mental disorders. In B. L. Levin, J. Petrila, and K. D. Hennessy (Eds.), *Mental health services: A public health perspective* (pp. 157–176). New York: Oxford.

Kessler, R. C., Berglund, P., Demler, O., Jin, R., Koretz, D., Merikangas, K. R.; et al. (2003). The epidemiology of major depressive disorder: Results from the National Comorbidity Survey Replication (NCS-R). *JAMA: Journal of the American Medical Association, 289,* 3095–3105.

Kessler, R. C., Mickelson, K. D., & Williams, D. R. (1999). The prevalence, distribution, and mental health correlates of perceived discrimination in the United States. *Journal of Health and Social Behavior, 40,* 208–230.

Kiesler, C. A. (1992). U. S. mental health policy: Doomed to fail. *American Psychologist, 47*(9), 1077–1082.

Kiesler, C. A. (2000). National mental health issues. In C. R. Snyder & R. E. Ingram (Eds.). *Handbook of psychological change: Psychotherapy processes and practices for the 21st century* (pp. 681–688). New York: Wiley.

Kiesler, C. A., & Simpkins, C. (1991). The de facto national system of psychiatric inpatient care: Piecing together the national puzzle. *American Psychologist, 46,* 579–584.

Kiesler, C. A., Simpkins, C., & Morton, T. L. (1991). Prevalence of dual diagnoses of mental and substance abuse disorders in general hospitals. *Hospital and Community Psychiatry, 42,* 400–403.

Kimmel, D. C. (1988). Ageism, psychology, and public policy. *American Psychologist, 43,* 175–178.

King, L. J. (2003). Health care reform: Historical and current perspectives. *Annals of Clinical Psychiatry, 15,* 163–170.

Knapp, M., Mangalore, R., & Simon, J. (2004). The global costs of schizophrenia. *Schizophrenia Bulletin, 30,* 279–293.

Koyanagi, C., Mathis, J., & Semansky, R. (2003). *Making the Right Choices: Reforming Medicaid to Improve Outcomes for People Who Need Mental Health Care.* Washington, DC: Judge David L. Bazelon Center for Mental Health Law.

Krugman, P. (2005). One nation, uninsured. New York Times Op-Ed published June 13, 2005. Retrieved June 19 from http://www.nytimes.com/2005/06/13/opinion/13 krugman.html?hp&oref=login.

Lalonde, M. (1974). *A new perspective on the health care of Canadians: A working document.* Ottawa: Government of Canada.

Lichtenberg, F. R. (2003). The economic and human impact of new drugs. *Journal of Clinical Psychiatry, 64,* 15-18.

Lieberman, J. (1999). Testimony of Senator Joseph I. Lieberman on Deaths and Injuries to Mental Health Patients. Senate Appropriations Committee Subcommittee on Labor, Health and Human Services, and Education.

Lorence, D. P. (2004). Confidentialitiy measures in mental health delivery settings: Report of U.S. Health Information managers. *Journal of Behavioral Health Services and Research, 31*(2), 199-207.

Loue, S. (2002). The involuntary civil commitment of mentally ill persons in the United States and Romania. *The Journal of Legal Medicine, 23,* 211-250.

Luchins, D. J. (2004). Pharmacoeconomics: The new dismal science. *Administration and Policy in Mental Health, 31,* 425-427.

Maingay, S., Thormcroft, G., Huxley, P., Jenkins, R., & Szmukler, G. (2002). Mental health and human rights: The MI Principles – turning rhetoric into action. *International Review of Psychiatry, 14,* 19-25.

Manderscheid, R. W., Henderson, M. J. (2004). Mental Health, United States, 2002 Executive Summary. *Administration and Policy in Mental Health, 32,* 49-55.

Mann, R. E., Smart, R. G., & Govoni, R. (2003). The Epidemiology of Alcoholic Liver Disease. *Alcohol Research and Health, 27,* 209-219.

Marsh, D. (2002, July 19). Testimony before the President's New Freedom Commission on Mental Health. Retrieved July 2, 2005, from http://www.apa.org/practice/pcmh-testimony.html.

Mays, W. (2002). Elder abuse and mental health. *Journal of Elder Abuse and Neglect, 14,* 21-29.

McDaniel, S. (1995). Collaboration between psychologists and family physicians: Implementing the biopsychosocial model. *Professional Psychology: Research and Practice, 26,* 117-122.

Mechanic, D. (1998). Emerging trends in mental health policy and practice. *Health Affairs, 17*(6), 82-98.

Mechanic, D. (1999). *Mental health and social policy: The emergence of managed care* (4th Ed.). Boston: Allyn & Bacon.

Mechanic, D. (2002). Mental health policy at the millennium: Challenges and opportunities. In R. W. Manderscheid & M. J. Henderson (Eds.), *Mental health, United States, 2000.* Retrieved February 5, 2005 from the National Mental Health Information Center: http://mentalhealth.samhsa.gov/publications/allpubs/SMA01-3537/default.asp.

Mehrotra, A., Dudley, R. A., & Luft, H. S. (2003). What's behind the health expenditure trends? *Annual Review of Public Health, 24,* 385-412.

Mental Health Bill of Rights Project: A Joint Initiative of Mental Health Professional Organizations. Retrieved 12/18/98 from http://www.psych.org'psych'htdocs'public_info/bill_rights.html.

Meyers, E. (2004). Guest editorial: Part A Medicare coverage for the cognitively impaired resident. *American Journal of Alzheimer's Disease and Other Dementias, 19,* 149-152.

Miller, R. D. (1998). Advance directives for psychiatric treatment: A view from the trenches. *Psychology, Public Policy, and Law, 4*(3), 728-745.

Military quality of life and veterans affairs, and related agencies appropriations bill, 2006 (H.R. 2528). H. Rpt. 109-95. 109th Congress, 1st Session. (May 23, 2005).

Minnesota Senior News, 28(7), July, 2005.

Mills, R. J., & Bhandari, S. (2003). Health insurance coverage in the United States: 2002. Washington, DC: U.S. Department of Commerce, Economics and Statistics Administration, Bureau of the Census.

Morris, S. M., Steadman, H. J., & Veysey, B. M. (1997). Mental health services in United States jails: A survey of innovative practices. *Criminal Justice and Behavior, 24,* 3-19.

Mowbray, C. T., Grazier, K. L., & Holter, M. (2002). Managed behavioral health care in the public sector: Will it become the third shame of the states? *Psychiatric Services, 53,* 157-170.

Mundinger, M. O., Thomas, E., Smoloqitz, J., & Honig, J. (2004). Essential health care: Affordable for all? *Nursing Economics Journal, 22*(5), 1-9. Retrieved January 30, 2005 from http://cpmcnet.columbia.edu/dept/nursing/pdf/nEconJnl.pdf.

Murray, C.J.L., & Lopez, A.D. (1996). *The global burden of disease.* Cambridge, MA: Harvard University Press.

Nabors, L. A., & Mettrick, J.E. (2001). Incorporating expanded school mental health programs in state children's health insurance program plans. *Journal of School Health, 71*(2), Feb., 73-76.

Nathan, P. E., & Gorman, J. (Eds.) (1998). *Treatments that work.* New York: Oxford University Press.

National Council on Disability (2002). *The well being of our nation: An inter-generational vision of effective mental health services and supports.* Washington, DC: Author.

National Institute of Mental Health (2001). The impact of mental illness on society. Fact Sheet. NIH Publication No. 01-4586.

National Mental Health Association (2005). Depression in the workplace. Retrieved June 19, 2005 from http://www.nmha.org/infoctr/factsheets/depressionworkplace.cfm.

New York Commission on Quality of Care for the Mentally Disabled (1996). *Breaking with the past: How New York's private psychiatric hospitals have managed since managed care.* New York: Author.

Newcomer, R. J., Fox, P. J., & Harrington, C. A. (2001). Health and long-term care for people with Alzheimer's disease and related dementias: Policy research issues. *Aging and Mental Health, 5,* 124-137.

Nickelson, D. W. (1996). Behavioral telehealth: Emerging practice, research, and policy opportunities. *Behavioral Sciences and the Law, 14,* 443-457.

Norris, M. P., Molinari, V., & Rosowsky, E. (1998). Providing mental health care to older adults: Unraveling the maze of Medicare and managed care. *Psychotherapy: Theory, Research, Practice, and Training, 35*, 490–497.

Nystuen, P., Hagen, K. B., & Herrin, J. (2001). Mental health problems as a cause of long-term sick leave in the Norwegian workforce. *Scandinavian Journal of Public Health, 29*, 175–182.

O'Keefe, J. (1993). Disability, discrimination, and the Americans with Disabilities Act. *Consulting Psychology Journal, 45*(2), 3–9.

Owen, G. (2004). Living outside mental illness: Qualitative studies of recovery in schizophrenia. *Journal of Mental Health (UK), 13*, 522–522.

Pankratz, M., Hallfors, D., & Cho, H. (2002). Measuring perceptions of innovation adoption: The diffusion of a federal drug prevention policy. *Health Education Research, 17*, 315–326.

Parry, J. (1994). *Involuntary civil commitment in the 90s: A constitutional perspective*, 18 Mental & Physical Disability L. Rep. 320. Cited by S. Loue (2002). The involuntary civil commitment of mentally ill persons in the United Status and Romania. *The Journal of Legal Medicine, 23*, 211–250.

Petrila, J., & Levin, B. L. (2004). Mental disability law, policy, and service delivery. In B. L. Levin, J. Petrila, & K. D. Hennessy, *Mental health services: A public health perspective* (2nd Ed., pp. 42–71). New York: Oxford University Press.

Physicians for a National health Plan (2003). Executive summary of the United States National Health Insurance Act (HR676). "Expanded and Improved Medicare for all bill." Retrieved June 8, 2005 from http://www.pnhp.org/nhibill/nhi_execsumm.html.

Psychiatric Times (2004). Mental illness: Global challenges, global responses. Retrieved June 19, 2005 from http://www.psychiatrictimes.com/ptg031003.html.

Quadango, J. (2005). *One nation uninsured: Why the U. S. has no national health insurance*. New York: Oxford.

Ray, W., Daugherty, J., & Meador, K. G. (2003). Effect of a Mental Health "Carve-Out" Program on the Continuity of Antipsychotic Therapy. *New England Journal of Medicine, 348*, 1885–1894.

Reed, C., Burr, R., & Melcer, T. (2004). Navy Telemedicine: A Review of Current and Emerging Research Models. *Telemedicine Journal and e-Health, 10*, 343–356.

Regier, D. A., Narrow, W. E., Rae, D. S., Manderscheid, R. W., Locke, B. Z., & Goodwin, F. K. (1993). The de facto US mental and addictive disorders service system. Epidemiologic Catchment Area prospective 1-year prevalence rates of disorders and services. *Archives of General Psychiatry, 50*, 85–94.

Ripple, C. H., & Zigler, E. (2003). Research, policy, and the federal role in prevention initiatives for children. *American Psychologist. 58*(6–7), 482–490.

Rosenau, P. V., & Linder, S. H. (2003). A comparison of the performance of for-profit and nonprofit U.S. psychiatric inpatient care providers since 1980. *Psychiatric Services, 54*, 183–187.

Rosenheck, R., & Stolar, M. (1998). Access to public mental health services: determinants of population coverage. *Medical Care, 36*, 503–512.

Rosenthal, M. B. (1999). Risk sharing in managed behavioral health care. *Health Affairs, 18*, 204–213.

Rosoff, A. (2001). Breach of fiduciary duty lawsuits against MCOs: What's left after Pegram v. Herdrich? *The Journal of Legal Medicine, 22*, 55–75.

Sandars, J., & Esmail, A. (2003). The frequency and nature of medical error in primary care: Understanding the diversity across studies. *Family Practice, 20*, 231–236.

Sederer, L. I., & Bennett, M. J. (1996). Managed mental health care in the United States: A status report. *Administration and Policy in Mental Health, 23*, 289–306.

Sharfstein, S. S., Stoline, A, & Szpak, C. (2001). Private psychiatric hospitals. In J. A. Talbott & R. Hales (Eds.), *Textbook of administrative psychiatry: New concepts for a changing behavioral health system* (2nd ed.) (pp. 227–237). Washington, DC, US: American Psychiatric Association.

Spitzer, R., Williams, J., Kroenke, K., Linzer, M., deGruy, F., Hahn, S., Brody, D., & Johnson, J. (1994). Utility of a new procedure for diagnosing mental disorders in primary care: The PRIME-MD 1000 Study. *Journal of the American Medical Association, 272*, 1749–1756.

Srebnik, D., & Brodoff, L. (2003). Implementing psychiatric advance directives: Service provider issues and answers. *Journal of Behavioral Health Services and Research, 30*(3), 253–268.

Stagnitti, M. N. (2005). *Antidepressant Use in the U.S. Civilian Noninstitutionalized Population, 2002*. Statistical Brief #77. Rockville, MD: Agency for Healthcare Research and Quality. Retrieved July 2, 2005, from http://www.meps.ahrq.gov/papers/st77/stat77.pdf.

Stagnitti, M., & Pancholi, M. (2004). *Outpatient Prescription Medicines: A Comparison of Expenditures by Household-Reported Condition, 1987 and 2001*. Statistical Brief #43. Rockville, MD: Agency for Healthcare Research and Quality. Retrieved July 2, 2005, from http://www.meps.ahrq.gov/papers/st43/stat43.htm.

Starfield, B. (2000). Is U.S. health really the best in the world? *Journal of the American Medical Association, 284*(4), 483–485.

Stoeckle, J. D. (1995). Patients and their lives: Psychosocial and behavioral aspects. In M. Lipkin, S. M. Putnam, & A. Lazare (Eds.), *The medical interview: Clinical care, education, and research frontiers of primary care* (pp. 147–152). New York: Springer-Verlag.

Sue, D. W., Parham, T. A., & Santiago, G. B. (1998). The changing face of work in the United States: Implications for individual, institutional, and societal survival. *Cultural Diversity and Mental Health, 4*, 153–164.

Suthers, K., Kim, J. K., & Crimmins, E. (2003). Life expectancy with cognitive impairment in the older population of the United States. *Psychological Sciences and Social Sciences, 58*, S179–S186.

Talbott, J. A. (1978). *The death of the asylum: A critical study of state hospital management, services, and care*. New York: Grune & Stratton.

Thomas, J. (2005). Wyoming psychologist thrives on fabric of his community. *The National Psychologist, 14*(4), July/Aug.

Thornicroft, G., & Maingay, S. (2002). The global response to mental illness: An enormous health burden is increasingly being recognised. *BMJ: British Medical Journal, 325,* 608–609.

Torrey. W.C., Finnerty, M., Evan, A., & Wyzik, P. (2003). Strategies for leading the Implementation of evidence based practice. *Psychiatric Clinics of North America, 26,* 883–897.

Unutzer, J. L., Rubenstein, L., Katon, W.J., et al. (2001). Two-year effects of quality improvement programs on medication management for depression. *Archives of General Psychiatry, 58,* 935–942.

US Catholic Conference (November 19, 1981). *Health and health care: A pastoral letter of the American bishops.* (Washington, DC: Part V, 17–18).

U.S. Department of Health and Human Services (1999). *Mental health: A report of the surgeon general.* Rockville, MD: U.S. Department of Health and Human Services, Substance Abuse and Mental Health Services Administration, Center for Mental Health Services, National Institutes of Health, National Institute of Mental Health.

U.S. Department of Health and Human Services (2000). *Healthy people 2010: Understanding and improving health* (2nd ed.). Washington, DC: U.S. Government Printing Office.

Von Korff, M., & Goldberg, D. (2001). Improving outcomes in depression. *BMJ, 23,* 948–949.

Van Tosh, L., Ralph, R. O., & Campbell, J. (2000). The rise of consumerism. *Psychiatric Rehabilitation Skills, 4,* 383–409.

VandenBos, G. R. (1993). U.S. mental health policy: Proactive evolution in the midst of health care reform. *American Psychologist, 48*(3), 283–290

Vega, W. A., Kolody, B., Aguilar-Gaxiola, S., & Catalano, R. (1999). Gaps in service utilization by Mexican Americans with mental health problems. *American Journal of Psychiatry, 156,* 928–934.

Wallis, N., & Wedding, D. (2004). The battle for the use of drugs for therapeutic purposes in optometry: Lessons for clinical psychology. *Professional Psychology: Research and Practice, 35,* 323–328.

Wang, P. S., Berglund, P., & Kessler, R. C. (2000). Recent care of common mental disorders in the United States. Prevalence and conformance with evidence-based recommendations. *Journal of General Internal Medicine, 15,* 284–292.

Wang, P. S., Demler, O., & Kessler, R. C. (2002). Adequacy of treatment for serious mental illness in the United States. *American Journal of Public Health, 92,* 92–98.

Wasserman, G. A., Jensen, P. S., Ko, S. J., Cocozza, J., Trupin, E., Angold, A. et al. (2003). Mental health assessments in juvenile justice: Report on the Consensus Conference. *Journal of the American Academy of Child and Adolescent Psychiatry, 42,* 751–761.

Wedding, D. (2004). Learning From Our Neighbors. *PsycCRITIQUES,* [np].

Wedding, D. (2005). Contemporary issues in psychotherapy. In R. Corsini & D. Wedding (Eds.), *Current psychotherapies* (pp. 475–492). Belmont, CA: Thompson Brooks/Cole.

Wedding, D., & Mengel, M. (2004). Models of integrated care in primary care settings. In L. Haas (Ed.), *Handbook of psychology in primary care* (pp. 47–62). Oxford University Press.

Weinick, R. M., Zuvekas, S. H., & Cohen, J. W. (2000). Racial and ethnic differences in access to and use of health care services, 1977 to 1996. *Medical Care Research and Review, 57* (Sup 1), 36–54.

Wells, K. B., Sherbourne, C., Duan, M., Meredith, L., Unutzer, J., Miranda, J., et al. (2000). Long-term effectiveness of disseminating quality improvement for depression in primary care. *Archives of General Psychiatry, 58,* 696–703.

Weil, A. (2001). Increments toward what? *Health Affairs, 20*(1), 68–82.

Weitzman, M., Byrd, R. S., & Auinger, P. (1999). Black and white middle class children who have private health insurance in the United States. *Pediatrics, 104,* 151–157.

Wilk, J., Duffy, F. F., West, J. C., Narrow, W. E., Hales, D., Thompson, J., Reiger, D. A., et al. (2004). Looking back, looking forward. In R. W. Manderscheid & M. J. Henderson (Eds.), *Mental health, United States, 2004* (pp. 17–42). Washington, DC: Center for Mental Health Services.

Williams, D. R., & Williams-Morris, R. (2000). Racism and mental health: The African American experience. *Ethnicity and Health, 5,* 243–268.

Wilson, M., Joffe, R., & Wilkerson, B. (2002). The unheralded business crisis in Canada: Depression at work. An information paper for business, incorporating 12 steps to a business plan to defeat depression. Toronto: Global Business and Economic Roundtable on Addiction and Mental Health. Retrieved June 19, 2005 from http://www.mentalhealthroundtable.ca/aug_round_pdfs/Roundtable%20report_Jul20.pdf.

Woolhandler, S., & Himmelstein, D. U. (1991). The deteriorating administrative efficiency of the U.S. health care system. *New England Journal of Medicine, 324,* 1253–1258.

Woolhandler, S., & Himmelstein, D. U. (1997). Costs of care and administration at for-profit and other hospitals in the United States. *New England Journal of Medicine, 336,* 769–774.

Woolhandler, S., & Himmelstein, D. U. (1999). When money is the mission - the high costs of investor-owned care. *New England Journal of Medicine, 341,* 444–446.

World Book-Childcraft International, Inc. (1980). *The World Book Encyclopedia,* volume 20. Chicago: Author.

World Health Organization (2001). *World health report 2001: Mental health – new understanding, new hope.* Geneva: World Health Organization. Retrieved June 19, 2005 from http://www.who.int/whr/2001/en/.

World Health Organization (2004). *World health report 2004: Changing history.* Geneva: World Health Organization.

Wyden, R. (2000). Steps to improve the quality of life for people who are dying. *Psychology, Public Policy, and Law, 6*, 575–581.

Wynaden, D., Chapman, R., McGowan, S., Holmes, C., Ash, P., & Boschman, A. (2002). Through the eye of the beholder: To seclude or not to seclude. *International Journal of Mental Health Nursing, 11*, 260–268.

Yevich, S. (February 11, 2004). Prevention issues in the VA: Today and beyond. Retrieved February 6, 2005 from http://www.amsus.org/Sustainingmbrs/Feb04-A.ppt#312,1, VA National Center for Health Promotion & Disease Prevention.

Young, A. S., Klap, R., Sherbourne, C. D., & Wells, K. B. (2001). The quality of care for depressive and anxiety disorders in the United States. *Archives of General Psychiatry, 58*, 55–61.

Chapter 6

CONVERGENCE AND DIVERGENCE IN MENTAL HEALTH SYSTEMS

R. Paul Olson

INTRODUCTION

The purpose of this chapter is to compare and contrast the four mental health systems described in this book. I shall attempt to summarize some of the distinguishing characteristics of these systems, and add relevant information and comments to highlight both convergence and divergence in the challenges facing these countries and in the strategies they apply to organize, finance and deliver their mental health services.

It is not my intent to identify the best model among these four countries. A "one-size-fits-all" approach is neither desirable nor feasible: it is not desirable because there appears to be no "gold-standard" when it comes to health care systems generally (Graig, 1999, p. 8); it is not feasible because health care systems are shaped significantly by the particular contexts in which they function, that is, by geographic, demographic, historical, political, economic, and cultural factors. All of these factors make the adoption of one country's entire system by another country highly improbable.

For example, while many Americans are attracted to some of the features of the Canadian health care system, including its universal access to affordable health care, there are also many Americans who are wary of limitations they perceive in Canada's system, such as waiting lists for some health care services and the exclusion of most nonphysician, mental health specialists from reimbursement in the national health insurance system. Similar observations could be made about the limitations of the American system with nearly 46 million uninsured in 2006 in comparison to the universal access provided by the other countries.

In short, all health care systems are imperfect and suffer from limitations. As the Norwegian Minister of Health, Werner Christie once commented humorously: "Some people might even say that the whole health care system is futile, as the average death rate is still 100 percent" (as cited by Graig, 1999, p. 8).

All four of the systems presented in this volume manifest relative progress in particular areas toward the provision of high quality health care, affordable and accessible to all of their residents. Consequently, they all manifest particular strengths as well as limitations. I share with the other authors of this volume the intention to advance our understanding on how other industrialized nations organize and finance their mental health systems as a way to enhance our awareness of the range of what is possible. We are asking not only what is or has been, but what might be achievable, and what alternative approaches might help to improve mental health care for our countries. Particular policies and/or programs that seem to work well in one country might also work as elements to improve the performance of another country's health care system. An example is the application of selected management principles and strategies such as the "model line" approach to improve the efficiency, safety, and quality of service delivery (Spear, 2005).

A word about vocabulary. To avoid the hierarchical connotations and passivity associated with the label "patient," and the market-based connotations of the term "consumer," I prefer the terms "user" to designate those who utilize health care services, and the terms "provider" or "professional" to designate those who deliver the services.

This section begins with comparative rankings of health care systems for the year 1997 conducted by the World Health Organization (WHO, 2000). Unfortunately, these comparisons were not replicated and included in subsequent WHO annual reports. Though the data are not current, they provide relative comparisons of the health care systems for the same one year period. More current ratings are provided subsequently by our contributing authors of the four countries' *mental health* systems. Thereafter, I discuss the relationship between the criteria applied in this volume with the WHO evaluation criteria. The structure for the remaining sections is based on five of the six evaluation criteria used in this volume to compare the four countries selected: access and equity, quality and efficacy, cost and efficiency, financing and fairness, protection and participation. The sixth criterion of population relevance is addressed in the final chapter along with conclusions and recommendations. My greater familiarity with the American system, and its complex mixture of public and private policies and programs have led to more discussion of this system than the other three. Nevertheless, relevant information from all four countries has been noted on all evaluation criteria.

Because this has been a collaborative project, I have shared a copy of this chapter and the final chapter with the other contributing authors for their review and suggestions. Direct quotations from our contributing authors are noted by either quotation marks or in indented block format without quotation marks. I assume responsibility for the content of these final chapters.

WHO Rankings of Health Care Systems

Mental health systems are subsystems functioning within a country's general health care system; consequently, the strengths and limitations of the former are in part a function of the characteristics of the latter. The WHO applied a goal attainment approach to evaluate the health care systems of its 191 member nations for the year 1997. Health care systems were assessed in terms of their degree of attainment of three essential and universal goals: "... good health, responsiveness to the expectations of the population, and fairness of financial contribution" (WHO, 2000, p. xi).

"Goal attainment measures are *absolute measures*, which indicate how well a country has done in reaching different goals, but it says nothing about how that country compares to what might have been achieved with the resources available in the country" (WHO, 2000, p. 40). As a *relative measure* of their performance, health care systems were also evaluated relative to their resources, the latter indicated by per capita health expenditures. "It is *achievement relative to resources* that is the critical measure of a health system's performance (WHO, 2000, p. 40).

For the year 1997, Table 6.1 presents the rankings of our four selected countries on three primary criteria: (a) goal attainment, (b) performance, and (c) per capita health expenditures. The primary criterion of *goal attainment* consists of rankings on three goals: (a) health status, (b) responsiveness to the expectations of the population served, and (c) fairness of financing. These goals are summarized in a single, combined index of overall goal attainment. Two of the goals – health status and responsiveness – are evaluated on both their level of attainment and distribution within the population served. The distinction between level and distribution was drawn by WHO because:

> ... it is not always satisfactory to protect or improve the [level of] average health of the population, if at the same time inequality worsens or remains high because the gain accrues disproportionately to those already enjoying better health. The health system also has the responsibility to try to reduce inequalities by preferentially improving the health of the worse-off, wherever these inequalities are caused by conditions amenable to intervention. (WHO, 2000, p. 26)

The *raison d'etre* of a health care system is to protect, sustain, and improve the country's health. Consequently, the overall *health status* of a country is the first general indicator of goal attainment by which to evaluate its health care system. That country which ranks higher than others in both raising the average level of health in its population and with the smallest feasible differences (inequality) among its individuals and groups is judged to be a better health care system. If the system does not protect, sustain, and improve the nation's health status, it does not really matter how responsive or fairly financed the health care system is ranked. Attainment of this first global objective of good health was measured by WHO by estimates of mortality and disability, and by an index of health inequality. The latter was an index developed for the WHO (2000) report, but not repeated in subsequent annual reports (p. 26).

A good health care system is secondly, *responsive* to the population's expectations. A health care system can produce a high level of average health and even do so fairly, yet fail to fulfill the population's expectations about how it should be treated both physically and psychologically by providers of prevention, care, or nonpersonal services (WHO, 2000, p. 31). In brief, some health care systems are likely to be more responsive than other systems, and in a manner more fair to all residents of the country in which it functions. Indicators of an unresponsive system include inordinate waiting time to receive health care services, rudeness, arrogance, or prejudicial treatment from providers.

Defined by the WHO, responsiveness includes three subjective and four objective dimensions. Summarized as "respect for persons," the *three subjective dimensions* include respect for the dignity of the persons, the confidentiality of their personal health information, and their autonomy to participate in choices about their own health and treatments they receive or do not receive. Labeled collectively as "client orientation," the *four objective dimensions* of responsiveness include

> [a] prompt attention: immediate attention in emergencies and reasonable waiting times for nonemergencies; [b] amenities of adequate quality, such as cleanliness, space, and hospital food; [c] access to social support networks – family and friends – for people receiving care; [d] choice of provider, or freedom to select which individual or organization delivers one's care. (WHO, 2000, p. 32)

Respect for persons and client orientation contributed equally to the total responsiveness rankings by the WHO. Both respect for persons' dignity, autonomy, and confidentiality, and the dimensions of client orientation involve economic costs, especially the latter.

Although being responsive to a population's expectations is a universal goal of health care systems, hence an outcome criterion in the WHO comparisons of goal attainment, responsiveness can be considered also as a *process* measure with reference to the manner in which mental health services are delivered. Whereas the concept of quality refers directly to what services are provided and their effectiveness, and the concept of access refers to whom these services are provided, responsiveness addresses how these services are delivered and whether their delivery meets the population's expectations.

The level of goal attainment of health care systems was evaluated thirdly in terms of the goal of *fair financing*. "Fair financing in health systems means that the risks each household faces due to the costs of the health system are distributed according to ability to pay rather than to the risk of illness: a fairly financed system ensures financial protection for everyone" (WHO, 2000, p. 35).

Paying for health care can be unfair because either (a) it can expose families to large *unexpected* expenses, which have to be paid out-of-pocket at the point of service utilization, or (b) financing may be based on "... *regressive* payments, in which those least able to contribute pay proportionately more than the better-off" (WHO, 2000, p. 35). Since out-of-pocket payments are generally regressive (though not necessarily so), financial fairness is best served by more progressive prepayment strategies. The rankings of goal attainment of health care systems are summarized for each country in a single, global index of overall goal attainment. This index is a combination of the three previous rankings assigned the following weightings: Health status (disability-adjusted life expectancy) – 50%; responsiveness – 25%; fair financing – 25% (WHO, 2000, pp. 39, 149).

The WHO ranked health care systems not only in terms of absolute levels of goal attainment, but also in terms of their achievement relative to resources available to their health care system (measured in per capita health expenditures). *Relative performance* was assessed by WHO on a bipolar scale, one end of which corresponds to the most that could be expected of a health system, the other end corresponding to the least that could be demanded of the health system. The measure of relative performance asks the question: "Given the country's human capital and the resources devoted to its health system, how close has it come to the most that could be asked of it?" (WHO, 2000, p. 42). In this context, performance is construed as a measure of efficiency.

In addition to rankings of goal attainment and relative performance, the third primary criterion for comparing health care systems was the amount of *per capita health expenditures* expressed in international dollars. The rankings of goal attainment, system performance, and health expenditures are summarized in Table 6.1.

A narrative summary of Table 6.1 is provided below with rankings in parentheses. All categories ranked are described in this discussion as "standards."

Great Britain. Great Britain was ranked highest of the four countries on one of the nine standards: distribution of health status (ranking = 2). It shared the highest ranking on one standard: fairness of financing (8–11) with Norway. Britain was ranked equally good with the other three countries on one standard: distribution of responsiveness (3–38). It was ranked lowest on two of the standards: level of responsiveness (26–27) and per capita health expenditures (26).

Norway. Norway was ranked highest on three of the nine standards: overall goal attainment (3), performance

Table 6.1. *WHO Rankings of Goal Attainment and System Performance, 1997.*

Criterion	Britain	Norway	Canada	United States
I. Goal Attainment				
A. Health Status				
1. Level	14	15	12	24
2. Distribution	2	4	18	32
B. Responsiveness				
1. Level	26–27	7–8	7–8	1
2. Distribution	3–38	3–38	3–38	3–38
C. Fair Financing	8–11	8–11	17–19	54–55
D. Overall Goal Attainment	9	3	7	15
II. Performance				
A. On level of health	24	18	35	72
B. Overall health system performance	18	11	30	37
III. Health expenditures rankings (per capita expressed in international dollars)	26	16	10	1

Note: Sources are WHO (2000). Annex Tables 1, 7, & 8.
Copyright permission obtained from World Health Organization.

on level of health (18), and overall health system performance (11). Norway shared the highest ranking with two different countries on two of the nine standards: level of responsiveness (7–8) with Canada, and fairness of financing (8–11) with Great Britain. It was ranked as good as the other three countries on distribution of responsiveness (3–38). Norway was ranked lowest of the four countries on none of the nine standards.

Canada. Canada was ranked highest on one of the nine standards: level of health status (12). It shared the highest ranking with Norway on one standard: level of responsiveness (7–8), and it was ranked equal to the other three countries on one standard: distribution of responsiveness (3–38). Canada was ranked lowest on none of the nine standards.

United States. The United States ranked highest of the four countries on two of the nine standards: level of responsiveness (1) and health expenditures per capita (1). The U.S. ranked equal to the other three countries on one of the nine standards: distribution of responsiveness (3–38). It ranked lowest of these four countries on six of the nine dimensions: level of health status (24), distribution of health status (32), fair financing (54–55), overall goal-attainment (15), performance on level of health (72), and overall health system performance (37).

Because the per capita health expenditures in the U. S. are more than twice the expenditures of each of the other three countries, and the U.S. ranked lower on two-thirds of the criteria, its global index of overall goal attainment (15th) was ranked lowest among the four countries, and so was its overall health system performance (37th) relative to its health expenditures (WHO, 2000, pp. 400–404). The U.S. had the lowest rank of the four countries in efficiency, that is, in achieving the most that could be expected of the system, given its per capita health expenditures.

Another comparison can be made based upon the frequencies of WHO rankings assigned to the four countries (lowest, highest, equally highest rankings). Combining the number of highest and equally highest rankings (columns b+c in Table 6.2), and subtracting the number of lowest rankings (column a), yields a summative ranking of the four health care systems. These figures are presented in Table 6.2.

The summative rankings for 1997 suggest Norway ranked highest relative to the other three and the U.S. ranked lowest; Canada ranked second and Great Britain ranked third.

Comparable rankings of member countries of WHO have not been included in subsequent annual reports. The merit of comparing health care systems based on numerical measures of performance has been debated, but the procedure is a step toward evidence-based comparative evaluations (Murray and Frank, 2001; Navarro, 2001; Coyne and Hilsenrath, 2002; Navarro, 2002).

Table 6.2. *Frequencies of Ratings.*

	a lowest	*b* highest	*c* equally highest	*b+c*	*b+c −(a)*	Summative ranking
Norway	0	3	2	5	+5	≠1
Canada	0	1	1	2	≠+2	2
Great Britain	2	1	1	2	0	3
United States	6	2	1	3	−3	4

Note: Frequencies of rankings were obtained from previous Table 6.1. The highest summative rank = 1.

Current Expert Ratings of Goal Attainment

In the absence of replicated comparisons by the WHO of the current levels of goal attainment and performance of health care systems in general, and in *mental health* systems in particular, the authors of each chapter in this volume were invited to rate the level of goal attainment of their own mental health system in terms of the six evaluation criteria on a five point, bipolar scale used in Goal Attainment Scaling (GAS) developed by Kiresuk, Smith and Cardillo (1994). The five levels of goal attainment and two scoring systems are provided in Table 6.3.

By construing the evaluation criteria as goals, the authors' ratings of their mental health systems on these criteria serve as their estimates of the levels of goal attainment. For example, insofar as the goal is equitable access ("access and equity"), the ratings reflect the authors' evaluations of the performance of their mental health system on this dimension of outcome relative to what the author/rater expects.

Note that in this rating system, goal attainment is a *relative* measure rather than an absolute measure of outcome. In the WHO (2000) evaluation of mental health systems, goal attainment was construed as an assessment of the *absolute* level of outcome attained by the system on the goals of improved health, responsiveness, and fair financing. The concept of "performance" was used to assess outcome *relative* to the resources available to the system's functioning (i.e., efficiency). By contrast, the goal attainment ratings by our authors are relative measures, that is, they rated their mental health systems relative to how well they expected their systems to perform on the six evaluation criteria and overall in a global rating.

If the goals and levels of outcome had been set in advance of a mental health policy or program change, the GAS ratings would measure the degree of *change* that occurred relative to the amount of change expected or predicted (Kiresuk et al. 1994, p. 262). Technically, Goal Attainment Scaling requires both goals and the five expected levels of outcome for each goal be set prior to the intervention being evaluated. In this case, the mental health system is the intervention and the ratings by our authors were made post hoc, following completion of their analyses. Nevertheless, the scale allows our panel of contributing authors, who are expert in their own system, to make both separate and summative judgments of the outcomes of their mental health system in terms of goal attainment.

The conventional scores assigned to the five levels of expected outcome range from +2 for the "much more than expected level of outcome" to −2 for the "much less than expected level of outcome." Alternatively, a scale ranging from 1 to 5 can be used (as in this case) to avoid negative numbers (Kiresuk et al. 1994, p. 175). However, to be consistent with the more common scoring system, the authors' ratings from 1 to 5 are converted to the +2 to −2 scale, shown in parentheses in Table 6.4. The advantage of the +2 to −2 scoring is the availability of conversion tables

Table 6.3. *Goal Attainment Scale.*

Authors' Ratings	Conventional Scoring	*Level of Goal Attainment*
5	+2	Much more than the expected level of outcome
4	+1	Somewhat more than the expected level of outcome
3	0	Expected level of outcome
2	−1	Somewhat less than the expected level of outcome
1	−2	Much less than the expected level of outcome

Table 6.4. *Current Expert Ratings of Levels of Goal Attainment.*

Criterion	England	Norway	Canada	United States
Access & Equity	5 (+2)	4 (+1)	1 (–2)	2 (–1)
Quality & Efficacy	3 (0)	3 (0)	2 (–1)	4 (+1)
Cost & Efficiency	3 (0)	4 (+1)	2 (–1)	2 (–1)
Financing & Fairness	4 (+1)	5 (+2)	2 (–1)	1 (–2)
Protection & Participation	3 (0)	4 (+1)	3 (0)	2 (–1)
Population Relevance	2 (–1)	4 (+1)	2 (–1)	3 (0)
Global Rating	3 (0)	4 (+1)	2 (–1)	2 (–1)
Sum Scores	(+2)	(+7)	(–7)	(–5)
Average Scores	(0.29)	(+1)	(–1)	(–0.7)
T-Scores: All seven ratings	(54.5)	(65.8)	(34.2)	(38.7)

Note: The source of conventional scores (sums, averages, and T-scores) is Kiresuk, Smith, and Cardillo (1994), Table A.7, p. 277.

for sum scores and average scores. Moreover, with a sufficient number of scores distributed normally, there are conversion tables for standardized T-scores with a mean of 50 and standard deviation of 10 for up to eight goals (Kiresuk et al. Table A.1, pp. 274–278). These additional conversions are included by way of illustration in Table 6.4.

Authors were asked to rate levels of goal attainment separately for all six evaluation standards and to make a global rating of goal attainment of their country's mental health system. Ratings were made independently without knowing the ratings by other authors. These current expert ratings are provided in Table 6.4.

I acknowledge that it is difficult to summarize the levels of goal attainment with single numerical ratings, and especially since most of the six criteria, as well as the overall global rating, contain at least two dimensions (e.g., both access and equity, both financing and fairness), and one of the dimensions might be attained at a higher level than the other. For example, the level of access to mental health services within the population might be improved, but not equitably. Recognizing these limitations, I offer the following observations about the goal attainment scores from our contributing authors using the conventional scale of +2 to –2.

The goal attainment ratings in Table 6.4 reflect variability both within and among all four countries. Norway's *global rating* (+1) was "somewhat above the expected outcome," Britain's global rating (0) was "at the expected level," whereas the experts from the other two countries rated the overall level of goal attainment as "somewhat below the expected level of outcome": Canada (–1) and the United States (–1).

Moreover, of the seven ratings for each country (including the global ratings), the number of ratings at the expected level or above (scores 0, +1, or +2) varies considerably among the four countries: Norway (7), England (6), United States (2), Canada (1). Norway's ratings are nearly 1.5 standard deviations above the mean, Britain's rating is near the mean, whereas Canada and the United States ratings are roughly 1.5 standard deviations below the mean.

Relationship of WHO Categories and Present Criteria

In Table 6.5, hypothesized relationships are presented between our six evaluation criteria and the WHO standards, namely, the three universal objectives (good health, responsiveness, and fairness of financial contribution) and the four functions of health care systems (stewardship, financing, resource generation, service provision).

Access and Equity

Following a few introductory comments, this section begins with a definition of equitable access. Thereafter the four countries are compared in terms of (a) national policies relevant to equitable access; (b) policies addressing access by minorities (racial, ethnic, immigrant, children, and elderly); (c) policy implementation guidelines (regulations) and federal agencies to administer and regulate the system; and (d) work force planning, education, and training.

There are numerous factors that influence a population's access to its health/mental health system. In

Table 6.5. *Hypothesized Relationships of Present Criteria and WHO Categories.*

Present Criteria	WHO Categories	
	Objectives	Functions
Access & Equity	responsiveness	service provision
Quality and Efficacy	good health; responsiveness	service provision
Cost & Efficiency	fair financing	financing/stewardship
Financing & Fairness	fairness of financial contribution	financing and resource generation
Protection and Participation	responsiveness	stewardship
Population Relevance	good health	stewardship

Note: For discussion of the three objectives and four functions, see WHO (2000), pp. xi, 7–8, 23–25.

addition to financial factors such as the inability to afford insurance or to pay out-of-pocket for services, other barriers to access and utilization include health beliefs, cultural practices, social networks, and language barriers (Diamant et al. 2004). Different factors will be dominant within different systems and within a given system over time. Moreover, the interaction of these various factors presents a significant challenge to understanding and changing health care systems.

The complex array of factors influencing access to mental health services suggests that problems in access cannot be attributed solely to the functioning of the mental health system. Moreover, it is unrealistic to expect that "fixing" the system will automatically result in either universal access or improved mental health in the nation's population. Nevertheless, the structure and processes by which mental health services are organized, financed, and delivered are systemic factors that need to be addressed if national mental health policies are to be implemented to achieve equitable access for the country's population. One can at least contribute to improvement in a nation's mental health by improving the performance of the system through which mental health services are accessed and delivered. The World Health Organization (WHO, 2000) devoted an entire annual report to understanding and comparing the role of health care systems, predicated on the notion that improving the performance of health care systems is an essential means to improving a country's health.

Equitable Access Defined

By way of definition, we concur with Dr. Arnett's distinction between acceptability and accessibility. "*Acceptability* issues involve such matters as competing demands on the individual's time, a preference for self-managing one's problems, doubts that seeking assistance would help, fear of asking for help, language issues and attitudes toward illness, health care providers or the health system. *Accessibility* refers to practical issues such as cost (e.g., most psychological services provided by psychologists are not covered by the national health insurance [in Canada]), lack of transportation, lack of knowledge about where to seek help, and issues such as child-care or scheduling." Another distinction can be drawn between *availability* and accessibility of services. For example, mental health services may be available (present) within a community, but not accessible because of daytime hours of services when potential patients are working. Combing all three concepts, a good mental health delivery system would provide services that are available, accessible, and acceptable to the country's residents.

Access to a mental health system means a resident within a country can obtain the services they need in a timely manner, appropriate to their condition, and these services are both necessary and effective in improving their mental health. The Institute of Medicine's Committee on Monitoring Access to Personal Health Care Services defined *appropriate* access to health care as "... the timely use of personal health services to achieve the best possible health outcome" (Millman, 1993).

Access is not identical with utilization. Services may be accessible, yet for reasons other than their availability, people may not actually use the services. Nevertheless, utilization rates and patterns give some idea of accessibility to various groups within a population (e.g., Olfson and Pincus, 1994a, 1994b). Differences in utilization rates among various groups may be caused by unequal access.

Equitable access means that all residents have equal access to optimal mental health services appropriate to their condition irrespective of any demographic characteristic (e.g., age, sex, gender orientation, race, religion, income or assets, geographic location, or prior history of mental disorder). Stated negatively, equitable access means that no one encounters more barriers to their access to mental health services of optimal quality than any other members of the society. The concept of equity does not necessitate that everyone receives identical services, but it does require that everyone has equal opportunity to receive optimal and appropriate mental health services with a comparable probability of improving their condition (Daniels, 1982; Whitehead, 1992).

Two types of equity in health care have been identified by the World Health Organization: *Horizontal equity* is treating alike all those who face the same health need; *vertical equity* is treating preferentially those with the greatest needs. Both types need to be addressed to achieve the goal of reducing health inequalities. Moreover, an equitable system "... should assure not only that the healthy subsidize the sick, as any prepayment arrangement will do in part, but also that the burden of financing is fairly shared by having the better-off subsidize the less well-off. This generally requires spending public funds in favour of the poor" (WHO, 2000, p. 55).

Since the ultimate justification of a mental health system is the degree to which it protects, sustains, and improves the country's mental health, the definition of mental health (or mental disorders) provides criteria for evaluating equitable access as well as efficacy of outcome. In a mental health system characterized by equitable access, and informed by the DSM definition and criteria of mental disorders (American Psychiatric Association, 2000), every resident of the country would have equal protection under the mental health system from unnecessary suffering of distress, disability, loss of freedom attendant to their mental disorder, or impaired functioning resulting from their disorder. These defining criteria of a mental disorder can be applied as outcome criteria. In other words, a good mental health system prevents and decreases distress, disability, dysfunction, and loss of freedom for all of the members of its population in an equitable manner to the degree possible. A superior mental health system would be effective in preventing mental disorders and promoting mental health in addition to providing efficacious treatment in an equitable manner. The actual performance of a mental health system will depend on the mental health policies that define its purpose and programs.

National Mental Health Policies

A national mental health policy is a document written and endorsed by the government to express fundamental values in statements of purpose and guiding principles pertaining to the organization, delivery, and financing of mental health services in the country. Goals for improving the nation's mental health are articulated, along with prioritization among goals. Statements of need and reasonableness may be included to support the goals selected, the principles endorsed, and any programmatic change envisioned. Generally speaking, the plan for implementation, and details concerning program administration are developed in subsequent documents produced by agencies with oversight responsibility. National statements of policy answer the questions of what is intended and why.

All four countries included in this study have articulated either national mental health policies or legislation, though in varying number, content, and comprehensiveness. To place this evaluation in context, it is important to recognize that at the beginning of the twenty-first century, 40 percent of the 191 member countries of the World Health Organization had no explicit mental health policy and over 30 percent had no mental health program. "Over 90% of countries had no mental health policy that included children and adolescents. Moreover, health plans frequently did not cover mental and behavioral disorders at the same level as other illnesses, creating significant economic difficulties for patients and their families. And so the suffering continues, and the difficulties grow" (WHO, 2000, p. 3).

Regional comparisons have been made on the presence of mental health policies and legislation. The two regions encompassing the four countries in this study are the Americas (Canada, United States) and Europe (Great Britain and Norway). In a survey of countries in these regions, 62 percent of countries in the Americas and 63 percent in the European region reported the presence of mental health *policies*. Seventy-three percent in the Americas reported the presence of mental health *legislation* and 96 percent in the European region (WHO, 2001, Figure 4.1, p. 79).

The existence, content, and authority of national mental health policies significantly influence attainment of the goal of equitable access. Examples from the four countries of these policies are provided here. The reader is referred to the chapters on each country for more detailed discussion of the formulation, content, and implementation of their mental health policies.

Great Britain's National Policies. The landmark legislation that established the framework for a publicly financed and publicly administered health care service in Great Britain was *The National Health Service Act of 1946*. This was a significant reform of the previous national *insurance* program that provided limited coverage for services by general practitioners to only a segment of the population (largely low-income workers). The latter system was revised into a nationalized health care *service* (NHS), which was designed to provide (a) comprehensive coverage, (b) for everyone, (c) free to the patient at the point of service, and (d) financed publicly by general tax revenues (Anderson, 1989, p. 28). Thus, Great Britain (and England in particular) has adopted a formal, national policy of providing universal access to comprehensive health care services.

National *mental health* policy in Great Britain was given particular legislative authority as early as 1930 in the *Mental Illness Act*, and subsequently in the *Mental Health Acts* of 1959 and 1983. Targets for mental health services were outlined in *Health of the Nation* in 1992, and three *national service frameworks* articulated mental health policy for three age groups: (a) Mental Health for Adults of Working Age (1999); (b) Older People (1999), and (c) Children, Young People, and Maternity Services (2004).

Published in 1999, *A National Service Framework [NSF] for Mental Health for Adults of Working Age* has been the most significant single development in mental health policy in Britain. Accompanying that framework was a set of *Policy Implementation Guides* and a set of highly specific, prescribed service targets, which now constitute the core of national mental health policy. There are ten value-driven, guiding principles of this NSF for working adults, and seven general targets or goals. Additional legislation, an accompanying code of practice, and other mandatory procedures, such as the *Care Programme Approach*, collectively constitute national mental health policy. The reader is referred to chapter two in this volume for discussion of the most recent and comprehensive evaluation of the 1999 NSF for mental health of adults by the British National Director for Mental Health, Professor Louis Appleby.

Universal access to mental health services and also to social security benefits, sick and family benefits, and access to housing support for the mentally ill are all significant elements of Britain's comprehensive mental health policy. The general direction of change in adult mental health services in Britain over the past 20 years has been both to provide generic services more locally by dispersing the access points for services throughout the population, and to provide more specialized, and presumably more effective services for identified clinical subgroups. The move towards more specialized services has emerged as a consequence of advanced epidemiological and therapeutic methods as well as continuing specialization within various mental health professions.

One indicator of access to mental health services is the length of time one must wait to receive services. This is also one of the elements of the responsiveness of a mental health system. The WHO ratings on responsiveness ranked Great Britain the lowest of our four countries on the *level* of responsiveness (26–27), but equal to the other three in the *distribution* of responsiveness (3–38) (Table 6.1). Waiting lists for health care services are likely to be a significant cause of the lower responsiveness ratings for Great Britain (Blendon, 2002).

Norway's National Policies. Norway has a long tradition as a social-democratic, welfare state beginning in the 1930s under the dominant Labour Party. Basic ideas and values underlying the Norwegian social welfare system are: (a) social solidarity, (b) the collective and mutual responsibility of all citizens and residents in Norwegian society, and (c) an egalitarian view of distributive justice. In an economic context, these values are expressed in goals of (a) economic security, (b) economic growth, with measures designed to alleviate the problems of unemployment, (c) a skilled work force, with measures aimed at expanding and improving education, and thereby strengthening human capital, and (d) a fair redistribution of income. As a Norwegian economist described it, the basic guiding principle is "help toward self-help" (Amoako-Addo, 2005).

Universal and equal access to health care services was reaffirmed in Norway's *Law on Universal Social Welfare Insurance (Folketrygden)* passed in 1966 by its national parliament called the *Storting*. This was essentially a compulsory national insurance scheme, which authorized not only free health services, but numerous other benefits to the population (e.g., free education, old-age and disability pensions, unemployment payments, cash benefits in case of sickness, occupational injury benefits, etc.). Beginning in the 1980s, the state-regulated and centrally planned economy has been transformed into more of a deregulated, semi-capitalist economy. Thus, while nearly all hospitals remain owned by the central government, they are operated as *Health Enterprises* to compete for patients who are free to choose among hospitals throughout the country. By law all persons who are either residents or working as employees in Norway are insured under the National Insurance Scheme, hence all are entitled to medical benefits in case of sickness, cash benefits in case of either sickness or unemployment, as well as old-age and disability pensions.

All insured persons are granted free accommodation and treatment in hospitals, including medications. In theory, all inhabitants have access to the same services, and can choose where to be treated. There is no discrimination on the basis of income, work, insurance or place of residence – at least not in principle. These principles were articulated in the *Act on Specialist Health Care* and the *Act on Mental Health Care*. In the case of treatment given outside hospitals, the provisions of the *Act on Municipal Health Care* and the *National Insurance Act* apply.

The Norwegian Parliament authorized the *National Mental Health Programme* (NMHP) in 1998 to be implemented beginning 1999 through 2006 (later extended to 2008). The goals of the NMHP express the commitment of the central government to improve equality of access as well as quality and efficiency in the mental health system. All specialized health services, which include specialized mental health services, are financed by the central government, owned by the five Regional Health Authorities, and administered by the publicly financed Health Enterprises. These are all public entities. By law, everybody is entitled to the necessary treatment and care within the public service irrespective of their income.

In July, 1999, the Norwegian Parliament passed four new bills that addressed the country's health care system, with a particular focus on its mental health services. These were the *Specialized Health Services Act*, the *Mental Health Act, the Patient Rights Act*, and the *Health Personnel Act*. These national policies and authorized appropriations are intended to ensure equal access for all residents in Norway to essential health care services provided by all specialists, including mental health specialists, while protecting patient rights and creating a larger mental health work force across the country. The national health policy in Norway affirms explicitly universal access to high quality health care, including mental health care through its mandatory social insurance system.

Another central document expressing Norway's present health policy is the *Act on Health Enterprises* (2002). The purpose of all health enterprises (hospitals and specialist health services, including mental health) is to deliver specialized health care services of high quality and equitably to anyone in need.

The WHO (2000) rankings of member countries on the universal goals of responsiveness to the population's expectations ranked Norway (7–8) and Canada (7–8) equally for second/third position among our four countries on the *level* of responsiveness, and equal to the other three in the *distribution* of responsiveness (Table 6.1). One of the criteria of responsiveness is the timeliness with which health care services are offered.

Our Norwegian authors note that as an indicator of access, waiting lists for treatment *(queues)* are somewhat ambiguous because not all people with psychological distress who are in need of treatment and who would like to be treated are actually referred, especially if the waiting lists are very long. Consequently, this indicator overestimates the access when waiting lists are long, since referral is perceived to be in vain, and other options outside the professional services are tried. Prior to the NMHP, waiting time for mental health services had increased in Norway, especially for admissions to hospital wards, suggesting access to services had decreased.

Canada's National Policies. A publicly funded, universal health insurance system to cover hospital and diagnostic expenses was established initially in the Province of Saskatchewan in 1957, and extended to cover outpatient services provided by only physicians in Saskatchewan in 1962. Inpatient coverage was expanded to cover all Canadian provinces and territories by 1961 following the federal *Hospital Insurance Diagnostic Services Act of 1957*. Coverage was extended to physicians' outpatient services throughout Canada by 1972. One of the major objectives of Canada's national health insurance program was to ensure equitable access for all residents, and especially elderly people and people with chronic or congenital illnesses.

While there are over 30 federal laws that have relevance to health care in Canada, the *Canada Health Act* of 1984 is the single most important legislative authority for Canada's national health insurance program. According to this federal law, the health care system must provide (a) comprehensive coverage (b) for everyone, which is (c) accessible, (d) portable, and (e) publicly administered.

The objectives of this legislation included facilitating *reasonable access to medically necessary, insured* services for all residents of the country without financial or other barriers. The legislation established general standards of what is medically necessary, defined and affirmed patient rights, and delineated the parameters and performance standards of the national health insurance program known as *Medicare*. Unfortunately, because these standards are so general and the terms were ill-defined, government at all levels (federal, provincial and territorial) can limit access if it is deemed unreasonable, or deny requested services on grounds they are either not medically necessary, or simply not covered as an insured service. The use (and misuse) of the "medically necessary" criterion to ration psychotherapy and other mental health services has been challenged by several authors (Bennett, 1996; Berghold, 1995; Chodoff, 1998; Glaser, 1992; Koyanagi et al. 1997; Mohr, 1998; Olson, 1999; Olson and Beecher, 1999).

One of the complicating factors in Canada's system is that provinces and territories also set their own mental health policies. All of them have *Mental Health Acts* and with significant differences, for example, in the standards for involuntary hospital admission. As a consequence, there is inconsistency in policies, programs, and services across the country. The variability in mental health policies also influences variable utilization rates of mental health services among the provinces and territories. Nevertheless, universal and equitable access to all health services is established national policy in Canada, though Canada does not appear to have the extensive and prescriptive, policy implementation guidelines comparable to England.

The federal government sets and administers national principles and policies for health care services under the auspices of the office of the Minister of Health. With financial assistance from the federal government, provinces and territories assess their needs for mental health services and personnel, and they plan, finance, organize, and administer service delivery in their jurisdiction. Federal funding is contingent upon the Provinces meeting federal standards. Unlike Norway and Britain where the federal government has the primary responsibility for mental health services, the ten provinces and three territories are responsible for the administration and delivery of health care services across Canada. In other words, in both Great Britain and Norway, mental health services for the population are centralized in the national government; in Canada, they are more decentralized.

Two features of the Canadian Medicare program make it similar to the American Medicaid health insurance program for low income people: (a) the joint federal-provincial financing and (b) administration by provincial governments. One major difference is that Canada's Medicare is for all of its residents, hence more inclusive than either the U.S. Medicare or Medicaid programs. Consequently, Canadians view their national health insurance less as a welfare program than Medicaid is seen in the United States. There are some exceptions. In Canada, health and mental health services are administered by the federal government for selected segments of the population. These include the armed forces, national police, and the Aboriginal population.

Like England and Norway, Canada has waiting lists for some non-emergency health care services, including mental health services. The WHO (2000) rankings of member countries on responsiveness placed Canada (7–8) tied for second/third place with Norway (7–8) among our four countries on the *level* of responsiveness, but equal to the other three on the distribution of responsiveness (Table 6.1).

United States National Policies. In striking contrast to the comprehensive mental health policies of Great Britain, Norway, and Canada, the United States has no legislative or constitutional authority that guarantees equal and universal access to its health care system by all its citizens and residents. The constitutional rights to "life, liberty, and the pursuit of happiness" have not been interpreted to mean that Americans have a fundamental right of access to health care services, even though illnesses and injuries constitute potential barriers to achieving all three constitutional rights. There is no national policy or comprehensive legislation that establishes universal insurance coverage as an obligatory standard of health care in America, nor as an entitlement of its citizens. Consequently, when it comes to health care services, citizens do not have "equal protection under the law" from being uninsured, underinsured, or underserved.

What legislative authority that does exist at the federal level consists of an amalgam of separate laws for the creation, administration, and funding of particular programs for limited segments of the population. As observed by the President's New Freedom Commission on Mental Health (2003), with the exception of a few legislative proposals for universal health insurance (which never became law), policies have been limited to piecemeal approaches and disjointed reforms. "The so-called health care 'system' in America is a 'patchwork relic' that does not provide ready access to quality care." Four years earlier, the U.S. Surgeon General commented: "Even more than other areas of health and medicine, the mental health field is plagued by disparities in the availability of, and access to its services" (DHHS, 1999). Among the significant barriers to access are low income, lack of insurance, race and socioeconomic status, and social stigma.

Federal legislation authorizes the central government to provide both health insurance and health services for selected segments of the American population. National health *insurance* programs include Medicare for the elderly and disabled, Medicaid and the State Children's Health Insurance Program (SCHIP) for low income families, and the Federal Employee Benefit Program. Direct health care *services* are provided to other segments of the population through the Department of Defense for military personnel and families, through the Veterans Health Administration for military veterans, through federally funded Community Health Centers and Community Mental Health Centers for low income families, through the federal Bureau of Prisons for inmates in federal prisons, and through the Indian Health Service for the indigenous population. Thus, the United States public health care system at the federal level is a hybrid of both national health insurance programs (Canada) and national health services (Great Britain). A major difference is the United States programs cover limited segments of the population, whereas Canada and Great Britain provide coverage for their entire populations.

The two largest federal health *insurance* programs in the United States are Medicare and Medicaid, both enacted in 1965. Medicare provides coverage for about 42 million elderly and disabled, of whom about 36 million are the elderly (65+ years). Medicaid covers about 50 million individuals and families with low incomes. The U.S. Medicare and Medicaid programs are neither universal in scope nor comprehensive in coverage (benefits), and Medicaid is means-tested to determine eligibility based mainly on personal income and assets. The U.S. Medicare health insurance plan does cover most hospital costs (Part A), and about 80 percent of outpatient medical costs and 50 percent of approved (discounted) mental health fees for outpatient services provided by most licensed mental health specialists (Part B). Enrollees are entitled to "free" *hospital* services at the time of utilization (point of service) because they have made a contribution to Medicare insurance through a minimum of ten years employment, though up to as many as 45 years of working.

To extend access to mental health *specialist services* to local communities, and to provide care for the deinstitutionalized mentally ill, Community Mental Health Centers were also established across the country, as a result of the efforts of the National Institute of Mental Health (NIMH) created in 1949 and the federal *Mental Retardation Facilities and Community Mental Health Centers Construction Act* of 1963. The continued construction of Community Mental Health Centers was reaffirmed in 1978 by the President's Commission on Mental Health under President Jimmy Carter and in the consequent, but short-lived *Mental Health Systems Act* of 1980 (Grob, 2005).

The existence of both federal health services and several federally funded health insurance plans in the United States, along with a plethora of 50 different state funded plans for targeted segments of the American population suggests a *public* sector model of multiple, but restricted single-payer plans for some, but not for all. Segmented programs for some of these groups have been provided because they have not, and would not have equal access to health care services through private insurance paid either by their employers in the voluntary employer insurance sector, or by themselves out-of-pocket, or through individually purchased private insurance.

The small number of federal programs with limited coverage (benefits) and restricted eligibilities (access) reflects the American proclivity to rely upon the *private* sector for health insurance and for the delivery of health care services. In a system that relies upon private insurance as the primary method of financing, being uninsured is a major barrier on nearly every indicator of access to care (Diamont et al. 2005; Weissman and Epstein, 1993). Unfortunately, nearly 46 million Americans in 2006 were covered by neither public nor private health insurance with the result that access to the health care system is seriously restricted and highly inequitable because it is based on ability to pay rather than on medical need. If all Americans are equal, as the U.S. Declaration of Independence proclaimed, some are nevertheless more equal than others in their access to high quality and affordable health care services. George Orwell (1946) described such a system in the political realm in his book entitled, *Animal Farm*. The American pledge of allegiance "with liberty and justice for all" remains unrealized in its health care system.

This inequity in access in the American health care system is accentuated in its *mental health* delivery system. Among the federally funded health insurance programs there is a lack of standardization of benefits, eligibility requirements, deductible charges and co-payments for both outpatient and inpatient mental health services. Although a federal *Mental Health Parity Act* (MHPA) (PL104-204) was passed in 1996, it covered only a limited number of mental disorders and mandated coverage by employers only in companies with 51 or more employees. The MHPA does *not* require group health plans and their health insurance issuers to include mental health coverage in their benefits package. Only if they already provide a mental health/substance abuse benefit are they prevented from setting annual or lifetime dollar limits on mental health benefits that are lower than comparable limits for medical and surgical benefits under the plan (CMS, 2005). Moreover, the MHPA does not prohibit employers from increasing co-payments or limiting the number of mental health visits, nor from having a different cost-sharing arrangement, such as higher co-insurance payments for mental health benefits as compared to medical and surgical benefits. Consequently, true parity in benefits and premiums to cover mental disorders relative to coverage for medical conditions has not been achieved. Even the federally funded health insurance program for the elderly and disabled (Medicare) requires 50 percent co-payments by enrollees of the allowable fees for outpatient mental health services, but only 20 percent co-payments for outpatient medical services.

Evidence that parity has not been achieved in the private sector comes from a national survey of employers who provide health insurance. Barry et al. (2003) found more benefit limits and higher deductibles and co-payments for mental health services compared to medical services. One of the barriers to achieving parity is the perceived ambiguity of DSM-IV diagnostic criteria for determining benefit eligibility (Regier, 2003).

The *Health Insurance Portability and Accountability Act* of 1996 (HIPAA) was federal legislation passed to protect Americans from losing their health insurance when they change jobs or residences, but that protection is limited because so many were previously employed by a company that offered no health insurance. The President's New Freedom Commission on Mental Health (July 22, 2003, p. 1) concluded that instead of ready access to quality care, the system presents barriers that all too often add to the burden of mental illnesses for individuals, their families, and their communities.

The United States is ranked first and highest relative to the other three countries on the *level* of responsiveness of its health care system, partly because the 85 percent of Americans who are insured have more ready access to health care services (including some specialists of their choice), and most receive services in a timely manner. The U.S. (3–38) is ranked equal with the other three countries in the *distribution* of responsiveness among the population (Table 6.1). However, millions of Americans have delayed seeking health care because either they lack insurance to cover health care services, or they are underinsured with significant gaps in their coverage. Even with health insurance, both this author and his wife have waited up to eight weeks for a nonemergency, outpatient medical appointment with medical specialists.

National Policies on Minority Access

The heart and soul of a nation's compassion and justice are revealed in how it treats its minority populations. Many of these are the most vulnerable, including the poor and elderly, women and children, the unemployed, and mentally ill or chemically dependent. Particular attention to minorities is justified by numerous studies that have shown patterned disparities in the prevalence of health problems and diminished access to health care among racial/ethnic and lower income groups (e.g., Bhui et al. 2005; Carter-Pokras and Woo, 1999; House and Williams, 2000; Krieger, Chen, Waterman, Rehkopf, and Subramanian, 2005; Williams and Collins, 1995; Williams, Neighbors, and Jackson, 2003).

All four countries have national policies and/or laws that protect the rights of their minority populations. However, all of our contributing authors have commented on the inequity of access to their mental health system experienced particularly by racial-ethnic minorities, and by both indigenous and immigrant populations. With the failure of "civilized" countries to provide compensatory, community-based care to the deinstitutionalized mentally ill, (including psychosocial and vocational rehabilitation, housing and other social services), a growing number of them have become homeless or incarcerated in jails and prisons, especially in the United States (DHHS, 2004a; 2004b). It is important to broaden our sense of diversity to consider these additional groups besides the more commonly included racial and ethnic minorities.

Less often viewed as a minority is the small percentage of the population that serve in the armed forces and suffer the trauma of combat. Since the 9/11/01 terrorist attack in New York City, Americans have a greater appreciation for the distress and sacrifice experienced by public safety personnel, who have been christened as our "domestic warriors." Unfortunately, the constraints of space in this volume do not allow us to devote the attention that all of these groups deserve.

Minority Access in England. In England an issue of particular concern is how accessible mental health services are to its racial and ethnic minorities. The government's Department of Health has focused on what needs to be done at a national level to make access to services more equitable, and a number of documents exist which emphasize the importance of engagement with the local communities.

First of all, a key feature of the British NHS since its inception in 1946 was the provision of a comprehensive, federally funded delivery system for *all* residents, which includes minorities. Secondly, the 1983 *Mental Health Act* addressed minority access to the mental health system. Thirdly, England's *Human Rights Act* of 1998 incorporated the *European Convention on Human Rights* into British Law. Consequently, there are several legislative acts, which collectively protect patients' rights, for example, minimizing the risk of discrimination on the basis of race.

Since 1999, *National Service Frameworks* (NSF) have been written and approved to address the unique needs of not only the majority of working age adults, but also children, the elderly, and those with chronic conditions of all ages. These NSFs articulate in detail the overall policy framework with accompanying work streams and supporting evidence. For example, the *Children, Young People and Maternity Services NSF* (2004) established standards for a comprehensive child and adolescent mental health service irrespective of race, religion, gender, or income level. Moreover, special needs of children have been addressed in additional national policies such as the *1980 Education Act* and the *Children Act 2004*. All these national policies have been published by the Department of Health of the central government. The 2002 document, *Care Programme Approach for Older People with Serious Mental Health Problems*, illustrates the NHS concern for this minority. As a result of its publicly financed National Health Service, England has no uninsured minority.

Minority Access in Norway. Norway has traditionally endorsed the principle of equal access to health services, and that is a central aim of the government's national health policy. A major objective of the national health care system is to fund the delivery of health care services of high quality and equitably to anyone in need, independent of age, sex, area of living, income, or ethnic origin (*Act on Health Enterprises*, 2002).

Our Norwegian experts consider access to mental health services in Norway problematic for minorities such as immigrants, people with severe mental disorders (e.g., schizophrenia), and people with mental disorders who are incarcerated in jails and prison. Norway does not have an uninsured minority in its population because all of its citizens and residents qualify for the National Mental Health Programme.

The mental health needs of the rising immigrant population in Norway have received more attention. Many of them speak neither Norwegian nor English, and culturally sensitive mental health services are lacking. Non-Western immigrants occupy up to one-fifth of the acute psychiatric beds, yet mental health services are insufficient, especially outpatient services. The mental health needs of immigrants seeking asylum in Norway are not being met.

Minority Access in Canada. All Canadians are entitled to the "medically necessary, insured" coverage provided by the national health insurance program called Medicare, irrespective of their ethnic, cultural, or religious diversity. Although Canada is officially bilingual (English and French), the presence of more than 200 different ethnic backgrounds and multiple languages presents a challenge to develop sufficient numbers of culturally-competent mental health professionals (Statistics Canada, 2001).

One minority of particular concern in Canada is the indigenous people (North American Indians, Metis, and Inuit). It is not the provincial or territorial governments, but the federal government that is responsible for all health care for First Nations and Inuit people. In addition, the federal government is responsible for mental health services to inmates in all prisons, Canadian military personnel, and the Royal Canadian Mounted Police, many of whom reside throughout all of the provinces and territories. A higher rate of reported symptoms of mental disorders has been observed in lower ranking military personnel and those with repeated exposure to combat, and these groups are receiving increased attention to assess and to meet their needs.

The *Best Practices in Mental Health Reform* (1997) was a national policy document that focused on the two percent of the population with serious and persistent mental illnesses. The 2004 Senate Evaluation noted the inequity of access for this minority group. Two years earlier the Romanov Commission (2000) cited the Canadian Mental Health Association's observation that these deinstitutionalized patients had been essentially abandoned and warehoused in boarding houses in communities, but without community services for either treatment or other support. Both inadequate funding and the uneven distribution of mental health service personnel throughout Canada are barriers to achieving equitable access for this population and other minorities.

Canada does not have any uninsured minority because all citizens and residents qualify for the national health insurance system; however, outpatient mental health services provided by allied mental health professionals (nonphysicians) are not covered by Medicare except in hospitals and in a few community clinics. Thus, access to the latter is based on the ability to pay out-of-pocket or through private health insurance and constitutes a form of rationing of mental health services based on the ability to pay rather than need.

Minority Access in the United States. In a report entitled, *Healthy People 2010*, the United States Department of Health and Human Services (DHHS, 2000) affirmed objectives to improve the nation's health and longevity, including elimination of racial/ethnic health disparities. Objectives related to improving minority health were grounded in findings of significant disparities from several sources.

The Center for Disease Control and Prevention (CDC) has a department called the National Center for Health Statistics, Division of Data Services (NCHS). It records prevalence data and service utilization patterns among various groups as well as mortality rates. The Center reported that among African Americans, American Indians, Alaska Natives, Hispanics, and Asians and Pacific Islanders, suicide and homicide ranked among the top 15 causes of death in 1999. Preliminary data for 2000 indicated similar patterns (NCHS, 2003). According to the Surgeon General's report on mental health (DHHS, 1999), the prevalence of mental disorders is disproportionately higher among minorities, who are more likely to use the emergency room for mental health problems, but less likely to receive treatment for depression than whites (16% minorities compared to 24% whites). Only 26 percent of African-Americans with diagnosed generalized anxiety disorder received treatment for their disorder compared to 39 percent of whites with a similar diagnosis. In response to these and other similar findings reflecting inequity in access to both medical and mental health services, the U.S. Department of Health and Human Services launched a national program called *Closing the Health Gap* to provide information to people of color and to help them take charge of their health (DHHS, 2002).

The Indian Health Service (IHS) is the agency within the federal Department of Health and Human Services responsible for providing federal health services to the native population of about 1.5 million American Indians and Alaska Natives, who belong to more than 557 federally recognized tribes in 35 states. Created in 1958, the IHS grew out of inter-governmental relations between Indian tribal governments and the federal Bureau of Indian Affairs established in 1787 based on Article I, Section 8 of the Constitution, and subsequently on treaties, laws, Supreme Court decisions, and Executive Orders.

The IHS has a holistic mission: "... to raise the physical, mental, social, and spiritual health of American Indians and Alaska Natives to the highest level." Its stated goal is "... to assure that comprehensive, culturally acceptable personal and public health services are available and accessible to American Indian and Alaska Native people" (IHS, 2005a). The IHS has regional administrative offices throughout the country. Health services are provided through local health centers, health stations, hospitals, and behavioral residential centers operated by area tribes or by contracted agencies.

The medical and professional programs of the IHS include a behavioral health program, which combines services for mental health/social services and for alcoholism and drug abuse. The mission statement of the IHS Division of Behavioral Health includes the following goal: "To support the efforts of American Indian and Alaska Native communities toward achieving excellence in holistic behavioral health treatment, rehabilitation, and prevention services for individuals and their families" (IHS, 2005b).

The IHS budget for fiscal year 2004 was about $53 million for mental health and $138 million for alcohol and substance abuse services. Proposed increases for fiscal 2005 were $2.5 million (4.5%) for mental health and $3.4 million (2.5%) for alcohol and substance abuse (IHS, 2004c). Additional funding sources for health care for Native Americans are Medicaid and Medicare, and private insurance plans.

A minority group unique to the United States is the percentage of the population who are uninsured. Unlike the other three countries, the private and public health insurance schemes exclude 45.8 million Americans, which is 15.7 percent of the total population (U.S. Census, August 30, 2005). There is no accurate count of the underinsured, but estimates range from another 16 million to 30 million Americans have significant gaps in their coverage, especially for mental health and substance abuse care. Combined estimates of the underinsured and the uninsured approach 20 percent of the current total population of 297 million. The statistic of about 16 percent uninsured masks the much higher percentages of uninsured and low-income minorities.

Medicaid is America's public program for low-income residents. This is the nation's largest, single health insurance program for civilians. More than 51 million low income people – about 14 percent of Americans – were enrolled in Medicaid at some time during the year 2002 (Holahan and Bruen, 2003). Federal and states' Medicaid expenditures to fund the health care safety net of hospitals, community health clinics, and school health programs were more than $256 billion in 2002, about equal to what was spent that year on Medicare. Medicaid is the largest single insurer for treatment of people with mental disorders in both public and private sectors.

Based on an analysis of the 1997 and 1999 National Survey of American Families, Long, Coughlin, and King (2005) found that Medicaid beneficiaries' access and use of health care are significantly better than those obtained by the uninsured, and comparable to access and utilization levels of low-income people who have private insurance. Despite this evidence, the number of low income, uninsured Americans is likely to increase because of (a) the proposed and implemented cutbacks in Medicaid financing by states in fiscal crises (Smith et al. 2003), and (b) due to the substantial cuts in federal taxes under the current Administration, resulting in increased federal debt and rising interest payments, and reduced allocations to states for Medicaid.

Although the availability of public health insurance may be considered necessary to obtain full access to health care, it is not sufficient. Because of misinformation and perceived barriers to becoming insured among women, minorities, and individuals with mental health problems, about 20 percent of children who are potentially eligible for Medicaid are not enrolled (Davidoff, Garret, Maker, and Schirmer, 2000; Kenney and Haley, 2001; Seldin, Banthian, and Cohen, 1998; Stuber and Bradley, 2005). The U.S. Congress authorized the State Children's Health Insurance Program (SCHIP) as part of the *Balanced Budget Act* of 1997. This was designed to provide the states with flexible funding to create and expand subsidized coverage for some of the nation's eleven million uninsured children.

Expanding coverage for the uninsured will not ensure access to health and mental health care if providers do not accept all insured patients. California's Medicaid program (Medi-Cal) is an example of this problem. Medi-Cal had an enrollment of 6.3 million California residents at an estimated cost of almost $27 billion for fiscal year 2002–2003 (Street, 2002), making it the largest Medicaid program in the country.

But surveys of California physicians have found that a little more than half accept Medi-Cal patients (Bindman, Yoon, and Grumbach, 2003), and 56 percent of Medi-Cal patients reported in 1999 difficulty in finding doctors who were willing to treat them (Medi-Cal Policy Institute, 2000). The refusal of Medi-Cal patients by private practicing providers is an argument for increasing the supply of federally funded Community Health Centers to care for low income and Medicaid patients.

Established with federal funding in 1965, Community Health Centers (CHCs) provide primary health care predominantly for racial/ethnic minorities, low-income families, and uninsured or Medicaid enrolled individuals (Forrest and Whelan, 2000). A number of these centers provide mental health and substance abuse services. In 2001, 748 CHCs across the country delivered care at about 3,300 sites to over ten million of the nation's estimated 50 million underserved persons (Bureau of Primary Health Care, 2003). CHCs have been credited with improving access to primary and preventive care, and to improving the quality of care for vulnerable populations (Dievler and Giovannini, 1998; Frick and Regan, 2001; Politzer et al. 2001; Shi, Regan, Politzer, and Luo, 2001; Shi, Stevens, Wulu, Politzer, and Xu, 2004). Several of these CHCs also provide behavioral health services, and as of 2006, new centers will be required to do so. They will become increasingly important in the delivery of mental health services to minority groups in addition to providing expanded and supportive services (McAvoy, Driscoll, and Gramling, 2004).

The elderly population (65+ years) is covered by the federal Medicare insurance program, but individuals must pay for 50 percent of the allowable fees for outpatient mental health services either out-of-pocket or through supplemental (Medigap) policies they purchase in the private sector. Minimum premiums in 2005 for a basic supplemental policy offered in the private sector in the author's state (Minnesota) was $893/year for a nonsmoker living in a rural area. An urban, nonsmoker's annual premium was a minimum of $986/year for the least expensive basic supplemental plan (with least benefits). Because of the variable amounts of federal Medicare reimbursements to the states, the premiums paid by residents in other states also vary.

The minority population of severely and persistently mentally ill received federal attention as a result of the President's Commission on Mental Health in 1978, and in the consequent federal legislation in 1980 entitled the *Mental Health Systems Act* (MHSA) under President Jimmy Carter. While a few of the recommendations and authorizations have been implemented incrementally, both the Commission Report and the MHSA were limited under the 1981 *Omnibus Budget Reconciliation Act* under President Reagan (Grob, 2005). The Reagan Administration scaled back funding for the 2,000 Community Mental Health Clinics planned for construction in the 1980s. Only 750 were established and they have been struggling for their economic survival (Humphreys and Rappaport, 1993; Smith, 2005).

In 1990, the *Americans with Disabilities Act* became federal law and included protection for people with mental as well as physical disabilities from discrimination in employment, public accommodations, and in federally funded programs. Since the *Mental Retardation Facilities and Community Mental Health Centers Construction Act* of 1963, disabled mentally ill patients who were desinstitutionalized were supposed to be cared for in federally funded, community mental health centers and in local housing services. Provision of those services were seriously delayed and a significant proportion of the formerly institutionalized individuals became either homeless or incarcerated in regular jails and prisons. The latter were never intended to be institutions for the mentally ill, not even for the criminally insane.

The Federal Bureau of Prisons assumes responsibility for the health care services of inmates in federal prisons. According to Holloway (2005), "Even though rates of serious mental illness are higher in prisons, funding for mental health services has been reduced in many areas. Indeed, at the end of last year [2004], there were 182,000 inmates in the federal prison system alone, and only 400 doctoral-level psychologists providing services to them" (p. 48).

The Department of Defense finances and delivers medical services for active military and their dependents. In addition, it provides insurance (TRICARE) for military personnel to receive health care services in the civilian sector. Veterans and their families are provided health care services through the national network of Veterans Health Administration (VHA) hospitals and clinics. A particular division within the VHA addresses the condition of post traumatic stress disorder, which has increased among combat veterans.

The American Public Health Association (APHA) is a voluntary, nongovernmental organization of public health personnel, who have been advocates of access to high quality health care, and particularly for the prevention of disease and promotion of health. One of the principles of ethical practice (#6) endorsed by the APHA is the following: "Public health should advocate and work for the empowerment of disenfranchised community members, aiming to ensure that the basic resources and conditions necessary for health are accessible to all" (APHA, 2005).

All four countries included in this study face the challenge of providing culturally competent mental health services to their minority groups, especially to their immigrant and indigenous populations. Insofar as "a health care system is no better than the least well-served of its members" (Churchill, 1987), then all four countries have much work to do. Discrepancies in their attainment of equitable access have multiple causes identified by our contributing authors. Many of these causes are external to the mental health systems, but constitute the limiting or facilitating contexts in which they function: geographic, demographic, cultural-linguistic, economic, and political factors. Two *facilitating* factors that have emerged from this study are (a) the presence of implementation guidelines included within mental health policies or as supplementary documents to those policies, and (b) the presence of federal agencies charged with implementation and regulation.

National Policy Implementation Guidelines (Regulations) and Regulatory Agencies

A national policy promoting equitable access, especially for minorities, is a necessary, but not a sufficient condition for successful attainment of policy objectives. There is also a need for *policy implementation guidelines (regulations)* to clarify expectations and to specify standards, objectives, and procedures to ensure that the purpose of the policy is achieved. Implementation guidelines address programmatic elements such as what actions must be taken to achieve policy objectives, within which time frame and resources, who does it, and how.

Great Britain's Guidelines and Agencies. The existence and application of several regulatory guidelines appears to be a significant strength of the British mental health system. There are numerous examples, only a few of which are mentioned here: (a) Guidelines for the implementation of the *1983 Mental Health Act* were specified; (b) guiding principles and general standards were incorporated as *policy implementation guides* in the *National Service Framework for Mental Health for Adults of Working Age (1999)*, illustrated by the *Care Programme Approach*; (c) several other guidelines have been written and approved concerning provision of services to minority groups, women, early intervention in psychosis services, assertive outreach services, crisis resolution, home treatment services, and adult acute inpatient care, including the policy implementation guide for psychiatric intensive care units, and for medium and low secure services; (d) the document, *Organizing and Delivering Psychological Therapies* 2004, sets out expectations for what local services will provide; (e) the *Care Programme Approach for Older People with Serious Mental Health Problems* 2002 established standards of care for this minority group; and (f) several other legislative acts have provided implementation guidelines with regulatory standards: *The Chronically Sick and Disabled Act* 1970, *Better Services for the Mentally Ill* 1975, *Community Care Direct Payments Act* 1996, and the 2004 *Treated As People Act.* One of the tensions within the NHS is that these guidelines tend to be rather specific and prescriptive at the same time providers are being encouraged to become more autonomous.

Under various *policy implementation guides* and *the care programme approach* established by the National Health Service, all Trusts which commission and deliver health care must record the needs of those with formally identified mental health problems. The number of people on the *Enhanced Care Programme Approach* in a locality is taken as a proxy measure of mental health service needs.

To implement the National Service Frameworks, three primary federal agencies have been established: (a) the National Institute for Mental Health for England, (b) the National Institute for Clinical Excellence, and (c) the NHS Service Delivery and Organization Research and Development. In addition to these central agencies, mental health policies and regulations are issued by a total of five governmental agencies: Department of Health, Office of the Deputy Prime Minister, Department of Education, The Home Office, and the Department for Work and Pensions. As an example, in a document entitled, *Mental Health and Social Exclusion (2004)*, the Office of the Deputy Prime Minister articulated policies for all government departments and agencies to increase access for those with mental health needs to general community facilities such as education and housing, and to reduce stigma and overcome barriers to their employment.

Three other NHS entities are involved in policy implementation guidelines: the Commission for Health Improvement, the Social Services Inspectorate (SSI), and Local Implementation Teams. As an example, in 2004 the SSI published an important source document entitled, *Treated as People.*

Norway's Guidelines and Agencies. Since Parliament created the National Mental Health Programme in 1998, five Regional Health Enterprises were established in 2002 to develop the strategies, programs, and schedules to implement the national mental health objectives within the limits set by Parliament and the portion of the budget delegated by the Ministry of Health to the Regional Health Enterprises.

The objectives of the NMHP constitute guidelines about what needs to be implemented:

> (a) develop more user-oriented services; (b) strengthen municipal services, preventive care and early intervention; (c) reorganize mental health services for adults; (d) establish more places for round-the-clock treatment and acute admission; (e) expand *District Psychiatric Centres* and outpatient clinics; (f) develop child and youth mental health services; and (g) promote skill, development, education and research.

Together with the NMHP objectives, guiding frameworks for all Health Enterprises or Trusts (all hospitals and specialized health services) are provided by the central government through the Ministry of Health and Social Care, and by the Regional Health Authorities. Along with the major policy objectives, these frameworks form the basis for administration of the health enterprises, which are also owned and financed by the State. The guiding frameworks address accessibility, quality assessment and quality improvement, productivity and efficiency of specialist health services, patient rights, and financing mental health services. Managers and Executive Boards of Health Enterprises (including hospitals and mental health services) are responsible for implementation of national mental health policies.

Canada's Guidelines and Agencies. Canada's national health insurance program (Medicare) was established in 1972. *The Canada Health Act* 1984 articulated several mandatory implementation guidelines (standards) that the ten Provinces and three Territories must meet in order to receive full federal cash contributions. These standards affirmed (a) public administration, (b) comprehensiveness, (c) universality, (d) portability, (e) reasonable accessibility, (f) reporting to the federal Minister of Health on insured health care services and extended care services, (g) prohibition of balance billing for provider charges that exceed insurance coverage paid by provincial and territorial governments, (h) limitations on user charges to individuals at the point of service. These standards are applicable to mental health services as well as medical services.

In 1997, the combined federal/provincial/territorial governments developed strategies to implement *mental health* reforms. These were outlined in a discussion paper entitled, *Best Practices in Mental Health Reform* (Clark Institute of Psychiatry, 1997). The document advocated community-based interventions with implementation guidelines under the rubric of Assertive Community Treatment (ACT) to replace the system's reliance on long-term, inpatient care in psychiatric hospitals.

A framework for the types and range of mental health services administered by Provinces was illustrated in this volume for the Province of Manitoba. The list of services provided is comprehensive, but access to many of these services is restricted by the lack of reimbursements for the largely outpatient services, except those provided by physicians and/or by other mental health specialists (psychologists, social workers, occupational therapists) employed in hospitals. Dr. Arnett's view is that the present system of unequal participation by all mental health professionals mitigates meaningful and noncompetitive collaboration required to develop patient-centered, multidisciplinary and integrated care.

The committee of the federal Senate charged with oversight is the Standing Senate Committee on Social Affairs, Science and Technology. The federal agency responsible for health care is the Ministry of Health. Canada has no separate Ministry of Mental Health. About 20 years after the federal Canada Health Act, the Senate Evaluation concluded in 2004 that Canada lacks a national policy framework and strategic action plan to address the mental health needs of children and adolescents as well as the difficulties encountered by specific adult populations (e.g., indigenous, military, and inmates of correctional institutions).

Most publicly financed mental health services (predominantly inpatient) are organized through Provincial Ministries of Health, which delegate the responsibility for all health services in both institutional and community sectors to *Regional Health Authorities* (RHAs). Thus, a particular Province is divided into Regions. Ontario Province is an exception with its *Local Health Integration Networks* in lieu of RHAs.

United States' Guidelines and Agencies. There are a few examples of federal legislation that include policy implementation guidelines for the mental health system. The 1963 *Mental Retardation Facilities and Community Mental Health Centers Construction Act* provided policy implementation guidelines. *The Special Health Revenue Sharing Act* of 1974 reauthorized standards and implementation guidelines for the Neighborhood Health Centers Program started in 1965. *The Medicare Modernization Act* of 2003 included guidelines for those Americans who choose to enroll in Part D for medication coverage.

Policy implementation guidelines for enacted legislation in the United States are generally developed by various federal and state agencies authorized to implement and regulate the various segmented, insurance and health service programs. Several federal agencies administer and monitor publicly financed programs such as Veterans Health Administration, Centers for Medicare and Medicaid, Department of Health and Human Services, National Institute of Mental Health, the Substance Abuse and Mental Health Administration (SAMSHA), the Bureau of Prisons, and the Indian Health Service. In addition, *state* departments of health, human services, and commerce write regulations to implement legislation authorizing health insurance programs and plans operating in their states. For example, the Managed Care Systems Section of the Minnesota Department of Health monitors nonprofit health plans operating in the state to ensure conformity with the regulations governing their operations. For-profit managed care organizations are not allowed to operate in Minnesota, but they do in most other states.

The United States Department of Health and Human Services has articulated national goals for improvement of the nation's health in such reports as *Mental Health: A Report of the Surgeon General* (DHHS, 1999), *Healthy People 2000* (Keppel and Pearcy, 2000), and *Healthy People 2010* (DHHS, 2000), but these documents do not constitute either mandatory goals or enforceable policy implementation guidelines, and they paid little attention to the "how" of monitoring progress toward the goals (Kanarek and Bialek, 2003). The Institute of Medicine (IOM) report of January 14, 2004 reinforced the goal of universal access stated in *Healthy People 2010*, but added neither plans nor strategies for implementation. The IOM Committee acknowledged that piecemeal fixes were not feasible, and stated guiding principles that "health care coverage should be universal, continuous, affordable to individuals and families, and should enhance health and well-being by promoting access to high-quality care that is effective, efficient, safe, timely, patient-centered, and equitable" (IOM report, as cited by Ault, 2004).

The Centers for Medicare and Medicaid (CMS) is the federal agency responsible for the two largest, publicly funded insurance plans for Americans who are elderly and/or disabled, or qualify by virtue of their lower income. The previous title of this agency was the Health Care Financing Administration (HCFA) until it was renamed on June 14, 2001. The CMS has established numerous policy implementation guidelines, a prepayment system for inpatient care of various diagnostic groups (DRGs), a billing code system, and annually approved fees for outpatient mental health services and providers. The CMS issues other implementation guidelines related to such areas as patient protection, quality assurance requirements, and requirements for reporting fraud and abuse.

Another federal agency called the National Institute of Mental Health (NIMH) sponsors various research projects, including research on the epidemiology of mental disorders. The NIMH has guidelines for conducting federally funded research projects. The Substance Abuse and Mental Health Services Administration (SAMSHA) also conducts research and makes recommendations about improved services. SAMSHA is the primary federal agency that attends to those affected by severe mental illness or addictive disorders. Its discretionary grant program entitled, *Knowledge, Development and Application (KDA)*, focuses on making the best use of resources to serve people with serious mental illness, including children and the elderly. Another SAMHSA program is the Community Mental Health Services for Children, which addresses severe mental illness in the earliest stages (Chavez, 1997).

The Agency for Health Care Policy and Research (AHCPR) was established by the Omnibus Budget Reconciliation Act of 1989 to enhance quality and access to appropriate, cost-effective health care. Severe budget cuts to this agency were proposed in 1995 and again in 2003, but this federal agency has survived. The agency has been working to provide science-based information to help policymakers make decisions about how to allocate scarce health care resources. However, its role in developing policy and implementation guidelines has been sharply curtailed, symbolized by renaming it the Agency for Healthcare Research and Quality (AHRQ). A current statement of this federal agency's mission is "... to improve the quality, safety, efficiency and effectiveness of health care for all Americans" (Chesley and Clancy, 2005, p. xii). This agency is best known for its research on health expenditures, health insurance premiums, payment sources, the cost consequences of a variety of policy choices, the uninsured, and the development of practice guidelines with attention to their cost-effectiveness. Two major AHRQ initiatives are the Medical Expenditure Panel Survey (MEPS) and the Healthcare Cost and Utilization Project (HCUP).

Work Force Planning, Education, and Training

Access to all health services within a country depends significantly upon the resources allocated to the health care system. These include financial, capital, and human resources. Financial expenditures and capital investments to build and improve outpatient and inpatient facilities are discussed later. Human resources are noted here – primary care, specialist care, and administrative personnel.

Without sufficient numbers of qualified personnel distributed throughout the country proportional to both population densities and varying prevalence rates of mental disorders, residents will not receive the equal access intended by mental health policy. Consequently, there needs to be a national policy and implementation framework for work force planning, education, training, and placement.

Two key health professions in every *primary* health care system are physicians and nurses. A recent comparison of their potential availability in several countries was provided by *OECD Health Data 2005*. The data are summarized for our four countries in Table 6.6.

Table 6.6 indicates that Norway had the highest ratio of physicians (3.1 per 1,000 population) in 2003, but the difference among these four countries was at most one per 1,000 population compared to the lowest ratio for Canada at 2.1. Norway had the highest ratio of nurses (10.4/1,000), while the United States had the lowest (7.9/1,000). While the latter differences might appear to be inconsequential, they become more significant when extended to the entire population. For example, projecting these ratios to the year 2005, with a total population of about 297 million Americans, the ratio of 7.9/1000 nurses amounts to an estimated number of 2,346,300 nurses. If America had Norway's ratio of 10.4 nurses per 1,000 population, the estimated number of nurses would be 3,088,800.

Table 6.6. *Practicing Physicians and Nurses per 1,000 Population in 2003.*

	Canada	*Norway*	*UK*	*US*
Physicians	2.1	3.1	2.2	2.3(a)
Nurses	9.8	10.4(b)	9.7	7.9(a)
Totals	11.9	13.5	11.9	10.0

a. Data refer to one previous year
b. Data refer to two previous years
Note: Copyright permission obtained from OECD Health Data 2005.

Table 6.7. *Estimated Ratios of All Professionals Rendering Mental Health Services 2005.*

Country	Population(a)	Numbers (Ratios of All Professionals Primary Care (b) (Doctors + Nurses)	Specialty Care (All Professions)
Norway	4,577,000	61,789 (1:74)	18,293 (1:250) (c)
Canada	32,000,000	380,800 (1:84) (d)	81,600 (1:390) (e)
England	50,000,000	595,000 (1:84)	72,118 (1:693) (f)
United States	293,027,571	2,930,276 (1:100)	399,817 (1:733) (g)

Note: Primary care professionals include physicians (GPs) and nurses. Specialty care professionals include psychiatrists, psychiatric nurses, psychologists, social workers, counselors, occupational and rehabilitation counselors, etc. who share in common the requirement of being licensed/registered/certified following advanced educational and professional training.

a. Population estimates are for 2005.
b. Numbers of MDs and Nurses for 2005 are projected from the numbers per 1,000 population provided by these countries to OECD for 2003 (Table 6.6).
c. Full time equivalent ("man hours") of "qualified personnel" in Norway's mental health system include physicians, psychiatrists, psychologists, qualified nurses in psychiatric institutions in 2003. Norway's figure is from Table 3.6 in this volume.
d. Canadian data reported in this volume suggested a total of 272,000 physicians and nurses, considerably fewer than 380,800 estimated from the ratios reported to OECD.
e. Canada's mental health specialists count regulated professions (psychiatrists, psychologists, clinical social workers, occupational therapists) but not marriage and family therapists, addiction counselors or other counselors. Since it is unknown what percent of time the regulated professionals spend providing mental health services, the figure of 81,600 is likely to be a significant overestimate.
f. England's mental health specialists include psychiatrists, psychiatric nurses, psychologists, clinical social workers, speech and language therapists, and counselors.
g. The U.S. count of mental health specialists includes psychiatrists, psychiatric nurses, psychologists, clinical social workers, marriage and family therapists and professional counselors. Professional counselors (111,931) are the largest group and clinical social workers (100,000) the second largest.

More specific to the mental health systems of the four countries studied here are the ratios of mental health personnel to populations, which can be estimated from the numbers divided by total population size. Table 6.7 provides estimated numbers of all primary and specialty care professionals, total populations, and estimated ratios.

The ratios in Table 6.7 are admittedly rough estimates, but show a ranking of both primary health care and specialty mental health professions in the same order as the rankings of overall goal attainment of the health care systems in the same four countries by the WHO (2000). (Compare Tables 6.1 and 6.7 in this volume.) These similarities suggest that the number and ratios of Norway's primary and specialty services may be contributing factors to its higher level of overall goal attainment, and may account for the United States being ranked the lowest in both overall goal attainment and overall health system performance as well as the level of health of the population. There is substantial evidence that primary health care helps prevent illness and disease. Moreover, in contrast to specialist care, primary care is associated with more equitable distribution of health care in populations (Starfield, Shi, and Macinko, 2005).

England's Work Force Planning. The NHS policies addressing the work force include: (a) the 1975 *Better Services for the Mentally Ill*; (b) the 1999 *National Service Framework* addressing five principles for work force development; and (c) the 2003 *NSF Mental Health Services* on work force design and development. These policy statements guide the development of a culturally competent, evidence-based, inter-disciplinary, and collaborative work force composed of a wide range of skills.

England appears to sanction more professions for mental health services than other countries: psychiatrists, psychiatric nurses, psychologists, social workers, speech and language therapists, occupation therapists, physiotherapists, professional counselors, and various assistants or technicians. Professional counselors work mostly in primary care settings, whereas other psychologists work primarily in mental health specialist teams. All of these licensed/certified professions participate to varying degrees in the provision of mental health specialty services.

In addition, two distinctive roles authorized recently in Britain are (a) "gateway workers" and (b) "graduate primary care mental health workers." About 500 "gateway workers" are to be employed to work with general practitioners and primary care teams, to strengthen access to services, and to improve community triage for people who may need urgent contact with specialist services. Another 1,000 "graduate primary care mental health workers" are to be trained to deliver "brief therapy techniques of proven effectiveness" – a carefully constructed phrase indicating they will not be using counseling techniques, but structured, time-limited psychological interventions. The creation of new mental health roles reflects Britain's desire to transcend traditional professional boundaries to develop skilled people to address gaps in the mental health system, and particularly to enable primary health care centers to better manage common mental health problems.

As a result of national policy and funding for the education and training of mental health staff, between 1994 and 2003 there was a 51 percent increase in all mental health professions. Excluding counselors and the newly authorized roles of gateway workers and graduate primary care mental health workers, all other professional groups numbered 72,118 in 2003-2004 in England. Of these, qualified mental health nurses represented the very largest group (44,728), followed by occupational therapists (15,391), then clinical psychologists (6,757). The total number of psychiatric consultants in 2004 was 3,289. For a population of about 50 million in England alone, the ratio is one mental health professional to about 690 population.

Despite the significant commitment and financial support to develop the mental health workforce in England, Dr. Hall concluded that "the existing pool of potentially qualified mental health staff is simply inadequate to meet the demand for staff."

Norway's Work Force Planning. Work force planning, goals, actions, and outcome criteria were addressed in the National Mental Health Programme (NMHP) approved in 1998. Among the 14 national goals were: (a) to increase full-time equivalent providers by 2,300 during the ten-year period ending 2008; (b) to educate more medical doctors, psychiatrists, psychologists and other personnel with at least three years of professional (graduate level) education; (c) to increase personnel in the District Psychiatric Centres; (d) to increase by 50 percent private practicing psychiatrists and psychologists with "operative agreements" to provide mental health services covered by the national health insurance; (e) to educate and place 400 more professionals for outpatient treatment of children and adolescents; and (f) to increase the system's capacity to provide mental health treatment for children and adolescents for five percent of the population up to 18 years of age.

The NMHP (1998) included funding for the years 1999-2006, later extended to 2008, to increase the supply of qualified personnel by expanding and reforming education given both at graduate (university level) and undergraduate (university college) levels. By 2003 there was substantial growth in full-time equivalent personnel ("man-years") to 18,293. From 1995 to 2003, the full-time equivalent numbers of psychologists in specialized mental health services grew 100 percent to 2,134 (50 per 100,000). About 2,800 clinical psychologists worked in mental health services in both primary and specialized care, equivalent to about 62 clinical psychologists per 100,000 inhabitants, or about one clinical psychologist per 1,625 inhabitants. Comparable figures for psychiatrists are 713 psychiatrists, 15 per 100,000, or one per 6,400 inhabitants. Of approximately 890 clinical psychologists in private practice in 2003, 570 (64%) had contracts with publicly financed Health Enterprises and consequently, they were thus reimbursed by central government funds.

The NMHP enacted in 1998 recognized that mental health services must deal with problems which require a multidisciplinary team. "Consequently, another goal of the NMHP is to increase the number of mental health professionals other than psychologists and psychiatrists, with at least a three-year university college [undergraduate] education, and then make the staff better trained with more adequate knowledge for the new tasks and services." Medical psychiatrists will play a less dominant role in the NMHP with its shift to community-based treatment away from an institution-based system. This is a significant contrast with the medically dominated systems in Canada and the U.S., wherein hospitals and psychiatrists account for the largest percentage of expenditures for mental health services.

The *Health Personnel Act*, and the *Specialist Health Services Act*, both passed by Parliament in 1999, were additional central policies addressing work force shortages and equitable distribution of staff. By 2003 the distribution of mental health professions in adult mental health services were: Regional psychiatric nurses (21%), other regional nurses (14%), psychologists (6%), psychiatrists (4%), other physicians (3%), other therapist with a college education (9%), other health personnel (26%), other personnel (16%). Administrative personnel in all specialist health services (medical and psychiatric) increased by 3,000 (16%) from 1995 to 21,974 in 2003.

Our Norwegian experts believe that Norway has a greater problem supplying and distributing mental health personnel than in funding the mental health system. For example, the supply of psychiatrists and clinical psychologists is unevenly distributed geographically by virtue of their preferences for larger metropolitan areas. The uneven distribution is illustrated by variable densities of psychologists per 100,000 population, ranging from 13.3 in Oslo to only 3.0 in the northern region. Consequently, "even if the health enterprises are state owned, market mechanisms of supply [of providers] and demand [by users] play a part in the distribution of service settings and service providers, especially for private practitioners." Access to mental health services in Norway has been unequal also because of the variations throughout the country in the numbers of mental health professionals who have "operative agreements" (contracts) with publicly funded, state owned Health Enterprises.

Canada's Work Force Planning. Canada's national health insurance program (Medicare) developed without a national work force plan. The manner in which it developed privileged both hospital and physician services, and services for medical conditions over mental health conditions. One consequence of this development is that the small percent of Canadians with mental health symptoms who seek professional help (less than one-third) are most likely to contact a family physician, and these physicians treat the majority of these patients mostly with psychotropic medication. Unfortunately, a number of the 32,000 family physicians in Canada lack sufficient knowledge, training, and skills to screen and treat individuals with mental disorders and addictions. These deficiencies need to be addressed both in physicians' pre-degree training and consultation during subsequent practice. This is especially critical in Canada because only physicians are reimbursed by Medicare for outpatient health and mental health services, hence they are much more accessible than allied mental health professionals whose outpatient services are rationed by individuals' ability to pay either by private insurance (individually or employer provided) or out-of-pocket payments. About 80 percent of psychological services in Canada are *not* covered by any government program; consequently they are not equally available to Canadians at all levels of income.

Psychological consultations are also not readily available to family physicians to assist them in dealing with patients' mental health problems. This compromises the health care provided to Canadians and renders it less comprehensive than it should be and more likely, with respect to mental health issues, to be more biologically focused than is often appropriate.

Later in its development, Medicare coverage for mental health services was extended to some nonmedical, mental health professionals, but only to those working in hospitals or selected community clinics, not to private practitioners in psychology and social work providing outpatient services. "Even within hospitals, nonphysician mental health staffing is both limited and variable across jurisdictions in Canada. Thus, access to allied mental health staff in hospitals is complicated and problematic."

There are both regulated and unregulated health professionals providing mental health services in Canada. The largest single group of regulated professions providing mental health services consists of family physicians, followed by psychiatrists, psychologists, social workers, and occupational therapists (primarily in hospital settings). There is a significant number of "unregulated" personnel such as marriage and family therapists, counseling personnel, addiction counselors. The amount of mental health services provided by both regulated and unregulated professions is unknown due to the absence of a national data base. There is an estimated 4,000 psychiatrists for a full time equivalent (FTE) of 3,500 and about 5,000 psychiatric nurses.

The Canadian Senate Standing Committee on Social Affairs, Science and Technology identified human resource shortages as one of the causes for inequity in access to mental health services, especially for seriously and persistently mentally ill patients. The recently formed *Health Council of Canada* recommended in its January, 2005 report that in order to facilitate greater emphasis on health care teams and to permit more flexibility in the way team members work, legislative barriers that artificially and unnecessarily restrict the scope of practices of various health professionals should be removed.

With its aging work force, Canada will need to rely increasingly upon immigrants to fill various occupations. "Consequently facilitating the credentialing and certification processes for foreign trained professionals and skilled trades, which now can be cumbersome and problematic, will be increasingly important to Canada's economy and the well-being of its population."

As of 2004, Canada had no national data base describing Canada's human resources in mental health and administration, hence there is insufficient data to evaluate the numbers of practitioners, types of professions, or proportions of time they devote to providing direct mental health services. The absence of a national data base of personnel working in mental health areas makes it difficult to provide anything more than a very rough estimate of *administrative* personnel at all levels. One estimate of expenditures on public health administration is 6.5 percent of all public and private health expenditures for 2004. The estimated number of health service executives decreased from about 3,000 in 1994 to 2,300 in 2002.

The United States Work Force Planning. Although there is federal funding for the education and training of health care professions (especially for physicians), the United States seems to lack a coherent federal work force plan to supply the human resources required to make mental health care provided by competent practitioners accessible throughout the country. It is not for lack of national data (which is Canada's problem). A division of the U.S. Department of Health and Human Services called the Bureau of Health Professions (BHP) collects relevant data to help ensure access to quality health care professionals in all geographic areas and for all segments of society. It also monitors work force trends and protects the public through quality assurance data banks.

A division of the BHP, the National Center for Health Workforce Analysis, has developed criteria for designating geographic areas having health professional shortages in the mental health services. These policy implementation guidelines identify psychiatrists, clinical psychologists, clinical social workers, psychiatric nurses, marriage and family therapists as "core mental health professionals." Among the criteria indicating an underserved population is a core-professional to population ratio greater than or equal to 1:6000 and a psychiatrist to population ratio greater than or equal to 1:20,000 (Bureau of Health Professions, 2002).

The number of all mental health personnel reported for 2002 totaled nearly 400,000. In descending order, these numbers are 111,931 professional counselors, 100,000 clinical social workers, 88,500 psychologists, 50,000 marriage and family therapists, 40,867 psychiatrists, and 8,519 psychiatric nurses. The total number excludes vocational rehabilitation counselors, guidance counselors, pastoral counselors, and school psychologists. Counting the mental health specialties listed, the ratio to the 2002 total population of 287,941,220 was 1:719 (U. S. Census Bureau, 2005). Professional counselors, and marriage and family therapists are not all counted in other countries (notably Canada) as regulated mental health professionals. Excluding those two groups in the United States, the total number of mental health specialists was 238,069, yielding the ratio of 1:1,206 population in 2002.

In another study of the mental health work force in America, which excluded marriage and family therapists and professional counselors, Scheffler and Kirby (2003) reported that during the 1995–1999 period, the distribution of three mental health provider groups were as follows: 45 percent clinical social workers, 36 percent psychologists, and 19 percent psychiatrists. The continuing trend has been for social workers and psychologists to outnumber psychiatrists.

The National Comorbidity Survey-Replication (Wang et al. 2005b, p. 629) reported that only 41.1 percent of those with mental disorders received *any* treatment in the past 12 months. Of the treated group, the largest percentage (42%) was treated by medically trained personnel [General Practitioners (GPs) (22.8%), psychiatrists (12.3%), physicians practicing alternative medicine (6.8%)]. Psychiatric nurses were not listed.

Of these credentialed medical professionals, those with the least training in mental health treatment (GPs) treated the highest percentage (22.8%) of mental health patients. Unfortunately, on a measure of quality of care, the lowest percent of patients receiving at least minimally adequate care were patients receiving mental health care from GPs (12.7%). By contrast, the highest percent of patients receiving at least minimally adequate care was reported for patients receiving care from all mental health specialists (48.3%) (Wang et al., 2005b, p. 629, and Table 4, p. 635). The results indicate the need to add more content on the diagnosis and treatment of mental disorders to the curriculum for general practitioners along with supervised training and more collaborative consultation with mental health specialists.

Only 16 percent of treated mental health patients received their treatment from allied mental health professionals (nonpsychiatrists). Combined with 12.3 percent psychiatrists, the total percent of people with mental disorders treated by mental health specialists is 28.3 percent.

The absence of psychiatric nurses from this data implies (incorrectly) that the 8,519 personnel in this category do not provide substantial care. A congressional committee with oversight of the Department of Veterans Affairs recommended that the Veterans Health Administration establish a classification for psychiatric nurses and increase their number.

Work force planning is critical to the performance of a mental health system, partly because the quality, access, and utilization of mental health services are a function of the availability of mental health professionals. Based on analysis of claims and survey data from 1992–1999, Wei, Sambamoorthi, and Olfson (2005) found that only about 25 percent of elderly individuals receive psychotherapy for depression, and only one-third of those received therapy consistently. Availability of local providers of psychotherapy, for example, the presence of a community mental health center, was positively correlated with consistent utilization of psychotherapy. Availability of mental health services within a reasonable distance is especially important to the elderly and minority populations who are less willing to travel to specialized health care services located in regional hospitals versus accessing services provided in local hospitals (Basu, 2005). Moreover, convenient (acceptable) appointment times have been shown to reduce both failed appointments (Lasser et al. 2005) and utilization of hospital emergency services (Lowe et al. 2005), hence improving efficiency of the system.

There are differences of opinion among mental health professionals on the desired ratios of population to professionals, and whether the current and/or projected supply of mental health specialists is sufficient to meet the need. As an example, citing a 1985 estimate of 45,536 psychologists by the American Psychological Association, and a national average of 23 per 100,000, Robiner (1991) argued there was no need to continue to increase the numbers of students training to enter the profession of psychology. VandenBos, DeLeon, and Belar (1991) provided a rebuttal. Robiner and Crew (2000) and Robiner, Ax, and Stam (2002) reiterated their legitimate concerns about the work force of psychologists in health care and challenged the wisdom of basing it principally on demand. Based on the current data collected by the Bureau of Health Professions, and comparisons with the other countries in this study (Table 6.7), we believe there is a very uneven distribution and an insufficient supply of mental health professionals to meet the need for services in the United States.

The maldistribution of mental health specialists is paralleled by the geographic maldistribution of physicians in the United States, especially in rural areas. The Council on Graduate Medical Education (COGME, 1998) concluded that:

> Geographic maldistribution of health care providers and service is one of the most persistent characteristics of the American health care system. Even as an over-supply of some physician specialties is apparent in many urban health care service areas across the country, many inner city and rural communities still struggle to attract an adequate number of health professionals to provide high-quality care to local people. This is the central paradox of the American health care system: shortages amid surplus. (as cited by Rosenthal, Zaslavsky, and Newhouse, 2005, p. 1932)

Although the degree of maldistributin of physicians is partly a function of the measure of geographic access applied (Rosenthal, Zaslavsky, and Newhouse, 2005), and considerable progress has been made the past two decades, nevertheless, substantial variation in the supply of physicians across the United States remains (p. 1950).

Work force planning is an element of human resource management. It is more, however, than a technical matter of efficient placement of effective personnel. The appropriate and fair distribution of human resources throughout the population is a necessary means to achieving equality of access to the services needed. It is important to appreciate this ethical dimension of work force planning and to be clear about the ultimate goal (Burke, 1999).

Quality and Efficacy

Several factors contribute to the quality of a mental health system. Many of these factors cannot be attributed to the system per se, but to such societal factors as the level of poverty and unemployment, violence and crime, the lifestyles and the cultural values of the wider society of which the mental health system is a part. Political, economic, and environmental variables are also influential. Nevertheless, several characteristics of the mental health system itself contribute to the quality of mental health in the population. Among these are the factors identified by the WHO (2000) report on health care systems, and reflected in their definition of a system and its quality.

Definitions: System, Quality and Efficacy

The *definition of a health system is* "... all the organizations, institutions and resources that are devoted to producing health actions. A health action is defined as any effort, whether in personal health care, public health services or through intersectoral initiatives, whose primary purpose is to improve health" (WHO, 2000, p. xi). With more limited reference to mental health, this definition of a system has been adopted for the purposes of the present comparative study (discussed in chapter one).

The WHO (2000) *definition of quality* applied to a mental health care system involves both the goodness and fairness of the system's attainment of three universal goals: (a) improving the overall mental health of the population served, (b) in a system that is responsive to population expectations, and (c) financed fairly.

The Institute of Medicine (2001b) defined quality as the degree to which health services for individuals and populations increase the likelihood of desired health outcomes and are consistent with current professional knowledge (cf. Lohr, 1990). Good quality care is safe, timely, effective, and patient-centered with complementary objectives of recovery and support. Elaborating on this definition, Schuster, McGlynn, and Brook (2005) noted:

> Good quality means providing patients with appropriate services in a technically competent manner, with good communication, shared decision making, and cultural sensitivity. In practical terms, poor quality can mean *too much care* (e.g., providing unnecessary tests, medications, and procedures, with associated risks and side effects), *too little care* (e.g., not providing an indicated diagnostic test or a life-saving surgical procedure), or the *wrong care* (e.g., prescribing medicines that should not be given together, using poor surgical technique). (p. 844)

In the present study, the concept of quality addresses the question of how well the mental health system functions to protect, sustain, and improve the population's mental health status in a responsive manner. The additional criterion of fairness specified by the WHO is addressed in this study primarily in terms of the criteria of access and financing. Nevertheless, it must be acknowledged that a high quality mental health system will be one in which mental health services as a social good are distributed equitably throughout the population. Thus, a good quality mental health system would be responsive to the population's expectations to provide optimal quality services to enhance mental health *and* to do that fairly for all individuals and groups within the population. A landmark annual report by the World Health Organization was devoted to the topic of improving the performance of health care systems (WHO, 2000).

A good quality mental health system is one that provides efficacious mental health services. The concept of *efficacy* applies to mental health services actually delivered to the population. Efficacy asks the question: Did the interventions applied result in clinically significant, sustained improvement in the user's mental health? Efficacy is used here as an outcome criterion at the level of interventions. Efficacious interventions applied systematically and appropriately are essential in a mental health system of optimal quality. In general, "evidence-based" practices are preferred over trial and error procedures in order to increase the probability of improved health of the user, though truth be told, many interventions with unique individuals constitute little experiments without complete assurance of benefit and without knowing what idiosyncratic response the patient might experience or what unintended side effects could occur. This is particularly true with psychotropic medications.

Quality Indicators

There are, of course, multiple indicators of the quality of a mental health system. These can be categorized as structural, process, and outcome indicators (Donabedian, 1980).

Structural indicators are evident in both institutionalized policies and procedures as well as defined programs and subsystems with qualified personnel occupying various statuses and roles through which they perform a variety of functions. Consequently, a complete evaluation of a system's structure would assess the impact of national policies, laws, and regulations, and the organization of the roles/statuses of providers, payers, patients, families, regulators, administrators, managers, and policymakers. Structural indicators also include the financing of health care services, capital investments and facilities in which mental health services are offered.

Process indicators refer to the way in which services are organized and delivered. An example is the process by which an individual with identified mental health concerns gains access to both primary and specialty mental health services, and how long it takes. These indicators address such questions as who makes what decisions to offer which services to whom? The concepts of efficiency and productivity generally apply to the performance of the system's processes in converting inputs to outputs, or resources to services. At a clinical level, processes of care address what providers actually do in their work with clients. Do the interventions applied conform to evidence-based practices? Are they cost-effective?

The processes of health care can be evaluated in terms of their *technical quality* as either appropriate, necessary, or consistent with professional standards of competent practice. An intervention is considered *appropriate* if its expected benefits exceed its expected health risks by a wide enough margin to make the intervention or service worth doing. "A subset of appropriate care is *necessary* or crucial care. Care is considered necessary if there is a reasonable chance of a nontrivial benefit to the patient and if it would be improper [ethically unacceptable] not to provide the care" (Schuster, McGlynn, and Brook, 2005, p. 845). Practice guidelines and evidence-based practices are examples of the application of *professional standards* to delineate indicators of good quality processes of care for particular types of patients or clinical conditions.

Two examples are provided here of studies of the technical quality of processes, both of which illustrate inappropriate medication management of depression. In a multisite study of 634 patients with depression or depressive symptoms, 19 percent were treated with minor tranquilizers and no antidepressants (Wells, Katon, Rogers, and Camp, 1994). Among hospitalized elderly patients with depression, who were discharged on antidepressant medication, 33 percent were on a dose below the recommended level (Wells et al. 1994).

Process indicators of quality are not satisfactory proxy measures for outcome indicators. For example,

> The British National Health Service (NHS) has had for many years a rating system for hospitals based on how well each hospital conformed to process specifications laid down by the NHS central administration. An independent study of British hospitals [by Wright, 2003], however, found very little correlation between the NHS and patient outcomes. (Fuchs and Emanuel, 2005, p. 1404)

Despite the lack of evidence for the correlation between process and outcome, the published quality-of-care literature for the decade ending 1997 revealed there is considerably more experience with measuring processes of care than clinical outcomes (Schuster, McGlynn and Brook, 2005, p. 844).

Outcome measures can be applied at both clinical and systems levels. At a *clinical* level, outcome refers to clinically significant, sustained improvement in a client's mental health status following treatment. Indicators of change or improvement, and post-treatment levels of functioning are examples. At a *systems* level, outcome indicators refer primarily to the level of mental health and its distribution throughout the population (WHO, 2000, pp. 26–40). Levels of mental health are usually assessed from epidemiological statistics of incidence (new cases) and/or prevalence (current plus new cases) of mental illness. As noted by Mechanic (2003), prevalence statistics are ambiguous indicators of the need and/or demand for mental health services, but they constitute the more common data sets for comparisons among health care systems of different countries. About 27 member countries of the World Health Organization are participating in a standardized epidemiological survey with attention to not only prevalence, but also severity, comorbidity, age of onset, and utilization of health care and mental health care services provided by various professional groups (Kessler and Uston, 2004; WHO, 2004b).

The WHO (2000) annual report addressed outcome evaluation in terms of the degree of goal attainment by a health system of three universal objectives: (a) improving the health status of the population, (b) fair financing, and (c) responsiveness to the population's expectations about how they should be treated (WHO, 2000, pp. 23–25 and Figure 2.1). Unfortunately, this approach to outcome evaluation based on measured goal attainment has not been adopted by many member countries. Among our four countries, Great Britain and Norway are leaders in applying this approach to evaluate their mental health system. Measurable program objectives are written as elements of the policy with target dates for evaluation of goal attainment.

Quality Assurance/Quality Improvement (QA/QI) Policies

All four countries possess QA/QI policies and programs. Illustrations are provided below, including attention to the integration of mental health specialty care with primary health care services, and to ensuring the competence of mental health professionals.

Quality Assurance/Improvement in Great Britain. Great Britain has articulated *National Service Frameworks* for children, working age adults, and the elderly. All of these frameworks include standards of quality in the delivery of mental health services, and require quality monitoring and improvements. Examples include the standards for the quality of services for comprehensive child and adolescent mental health services articulated in the *NSF for Children, Young People and Maternity Services (2004)*. The *NSF for Mental Health for Adults of Working Age (1999)* expressed ten guiding principles, including the provision of high quality treatment and care which is known to be effective, acceptable, and safe. England's seven general targets included improvement in effective services for those with serious mental illness (standards 4 & 5) and reduction in the rate of suicide (standard 7), both of which should constitute priorities for most countries. These and other elements of the NSF are summarized in the document, *Journey to Recovery* (2001). The *NSF for Older People (1999)* identifies ten standards of quality mental health services for older people such as comprehensive, multidisciplinary assessment, integrated care planning, and management by competent staff in specialist services able to offer community-based support.

Complementing the NSFs are several written *Policy Implementation Guidelines*, which prescribe quality standards and quality improvement activities. Other documents published by the Department of Health, which articulate policies pertinent to QA/QI concerns, include (a) *Modernizing Mental Health Services: Safe, Sound and Supportive* (1999); (b) the *Care Programme Approach* mandating formal assessments of need for all users, a risk assessment, and an individualized care plan; (c) the *Enhanced Care Programme Approach* expressing standards for the care of those deemed to have a serious mental disorder; (d) *Safer Services*, which monitors patient safety (including suicide rates); and (e) *Organizing and Delivering Psychological Therapies (2004)*, which sets out several expectations concerning local mental health services, including offering a range of evidence-based treatments provided by professionals and agencies represented in Local Implementation Teams in each Primary Care Trust area. As of 2004, the Commission for Healthcare Audit and Inspection (CHAI) is charged with the responsibility of monitoring the performance quality of the nonfinancial elements of the NHS.

Research on the efficacy of both specific interventions and on models of service delivery is reported in the British journal, *Evidence-Based Mental Health*. The National Institute for Clinical Excellence publishes clinical practice guidelines, and the University of York publishes an *Effective Health Care Bulletin* addressing QA/QI issues.

Integrated Care. Good quality care is integrated and coordinated care. Administrative levels of the health care system are integrated within and between public and private sectors in central, regional, and local settings. Mental health services are integrated into primary health care services, and there is coordinated care between levels of intensity of services ranging from outpatient triage to inpatient and long-term care. Thus, within a good mental health system, various mental health professions and institutions would be cooperating with each other for the benefit of the patient's continuity of care.

Integrating mental health services into primary health care services and settings can provide this continuity of care, based on a more holistic approach and ease of transitions from one level of intervention to another. England has reorganized its National Health Service to emphasize primary health care, including *primary mental health care*. General practitioners (GPs) are organized as partners in Primary Care Trusts. A unique and outstanding feature of this reorganization is that "over 70 percent of GP practices have counselors attached to the practice." Two new roles have been created: (a) "gateway workers" and (b) "primary care graduate mental health workers," who will be based in primary care settings along with conventional professions such as psychiatric nurses and counselors.

In its 1997 health reform manifesto entitled, *The New NHS*, the new Labour government under Tony Blair emphasized *collaboration and cooperation* among various purchasing and service delivery organizations such as Primary Care Groups (of GPs), hospital and other specialty care Trusts, including mental health trusts (Graig, 1999, p. 171). Comprehensive, community-based care is a cardinal principle of England's national mental health policy, present since publication of *Better Services for the Mentally Ill* (1975). The *1990 NHS and Community Care Act* integrated mental health services with other social services. A publication of the Office of the Deputy Primary Minister entitled, *The Mental Health and Social Exclusion Act (2004)*, addressed the matter of integrating mentally ill patients into general community facilities.

The Department of Health's *Organizing and Delivering Psychological Therapies* (2004) articulated a comprehensive scheme to integrate mental health services ranging from community support (level 1) to tertiary specialist mental health services (level 7). Generic Community Mental Health Teams are responsible for integrating their services with primary health care services and with other specialized mental health teams. This is an expression of three movements since the 1960s: (a) deinstitutionalization, (b) community-based services, and (c) expanded range of interventions by a broader range of staff.

A major quality assessment was conducted as an element of the December 2004 evaluation of the 1999 National Service Framework for the mental health of adults. The reader is referred to discussion of results in chapter two of this volume.

Quality Assurance/Improvement in Norway. Improving the quality, as well as accessibility and productivity of mental health services is a central goal of the National

Mental Health Programme (NMHP), which has been created, funded, and administered by the central government effective 1999 through 2008. Quality improvement was reaffirmed as a central goal in the *Act on Health Enterprises* (2002).

> Since 2002, the central government through five Regional Health Authorities [RHAs] is also responsible for the provision and quality of specialist health services, including mental health/mental retardation services. The RHAs provide specialist health services through a total of 31 Health Enterprises or Trusts owned by the RHAs, or through operative agreements (contracts for services) with private service providers.

The quality of these specialist health services and hospital services is addressed through principal health policy objectives and frameworks established by the central government. Since the *Municipal Health Services Act*, effective 1984, local and country municipal boards of health are responsible for all *primary* health care, including quality assurance and quality improvement.

As an essential element in the program evaluation of the NMHP, quality assessment is conducted under the auspices of the Ministry of Health and Care Services, which has financed 15 research projects to evaluate the program. Some program evaluation projects are organized directly through the Norwegian Research Council and indirectly by financing research conducted through public universities. The Ministry of Health and Care Services has committed about US$750,000 per year for 1999 through 2008 for quality assessment and quality improvement activities.

Results from structural and process measures are reported publicly and regularly by Statistics Norway and SINTEF/Health. Patient evaluations of mental health services are conducted regularly by SINTEF/Health and published by the Directorate of Health and Social Welfare. Another research agency conducting program evaluations is the Norwegian Health Services Research Centre founded in 2004 under the Directorate for Health and Social Affairs, though it is scientifically and professionally independent. It has no role in policy formulation or implementation. The data collected by these agencies are used to improve the quality and performance of the health care services.

Efficacy of interventions is addressed in a few evidence-based guidelines that have been developed for mental health interventions, but their suitability in mental health services lacks a consensus among professionals. "Few empirical studies have dealt with actual outcomes to answer the question of whether the mental health services provided are efficacious in producing actual improvement in the mental health of those who receive the treatment. There are a few studies in selected groups." No measures of actual health outcomes are published regularly by any government agency or other independent research agency. A research group is developing quality indicators to assess mental health outcomes.

A new system of quality assurance is being implemented in the specialized mental health services with an emphasis upon measures of users' experience and satisfaction. The Ministry of Health and Care Services is the central governmental service in charge of the Norwegian health care system. It delegates national supervisory authority to the National Board of Health (NBH) to evaluate the need for health and social services, and to ensure that services are provided in accordance with adequate professional standards. At the local level, supervision is carried out by Governmental Regional Boards, which report to the NBH on matters of health and social services.

The NMHP adopted a goal-attainment strategy to evaluate the achievement of the 14 goals articulated for the program. Assessing attainment of goals is itself an outcome evaluation; however, most of the NMHP goals address structural and process variables rather than actual *outcomes* of improved mental health of the population. Perhaps some of the 15 evaluation projects will address clinical outcomes. The relative absence of outcome evaluations is not a shortcoming unique to the Norwegian system. Program evaluations based on actual treatment outcomes remains one of the major areas of development for all four of the countries included in this volume.

Integrated Care. High quality mental health care is integrated care with continuity of services and ease of transition from one level of care to the next. One of the major goals of the creation of the NMHP by Norway's Parliament was to reorganize mental health service delivery to be both community-based and integrated with primary health care services and with the education system, social services, and employment agencies. Establishment of 83 District Psychiatric Centres (DPCs) was funded to link specialized mental health services with the primary care services provided in 19 county municipalities and in many of the 434 local municipalities. One of the major functions of the DPCs is to provide consultation with the primary mental health care sector and to cooperate with the social services in the municipalities as well as psychiatric hospitals and wards. The DPCs, which will provide a full range of outpatient, inpatient, and crisis intervention, have assumed central importance within the mental health system, a position previously occupied by a smaller number of psychiatric hospitals.

In 2000, a *General Practitioner (GP) Scheme* was established by the central government to improve a better doctor-patient communication and to ensure every inhabitant has an easily accessible medical service through a regular GP. Consequently, the GP functions both as a gatekeeper to hospitals and specialist services, and also as the coordinator for comprehensive and integrated patient care.

Providers of mental health services in *primary* health care settings in Norway include (a) general practitioners, (b) psychiatric nurses, (c) general nurses, (d) school nurses, (e) school psychologists, (f) municipality psychologists, (g) social workers, and (h) offices for family advice. However, all of these professional services are not available in the smaller communities. One of the goals of Norway's national health policy expressed in the *Act on Health Enterprises* (2002) was to improve cooperation among all health and social services. Cooperation within the specialist health services was judged to be inadequate in as many as half of the institutions surveyed in 2003 by the Norwegian Board of Health.

Integration of *private and public* services is another attribute of a high quality mental health system. Private practicing psychologists and psychiatrists in Norway account for less than 20 percent of both professional groups. The majority of them have operative agreements with publicly funded Health Enterprises, hence they are reimbursed through the national health insurance system. One assignment given to the Health Enterprises is to integrate private practitioners into the public mental health system through operative agreements. The latter are like contracts to provide services consistent with quality guidelines and the terms of reimbursement. Balance billing for provider charges in excess of the approved fee is *not* allowed. In America, "accepting assignment" of Medicare's approved reimbursement rates precludes balance billing.

Norway is unique among the four countries in its vision of integrated services grounded in a holistic view of the person, which appreciates the *spiritual dimension* of life as well as the biopsychosocial dimensions. As noted by the Ministry of Health and Care Services (1998):

> A person with psychiatric disorders should not be looked upon solely as a patient, but as a human being with a body, soul and spirit. Due consideration has to be given to the human being's spiritual and cultural needs, not only to its biological and social needs. Psychiatric disorders also comprehend existential questions. The patients' needs should always be the point of departure for all treatment, and the core for all nursing. This has to be emphasized in the organization, in practice, and by the leadership in all mental health services.

Quality Assurance/Improvement in Canada. The federal government funds health research agencies such as the Canadian Institute of Health Research (CIHR) and the Social Sciences and Humanities Research Council (SSHRC) to collect data on the quality of health services. However, a report by the 1994 National Forum on Health (Health Canada, 1994) noted that Canada lacked a nationwide health information system that would maintain a standardized set of longitudinal information on health status and health system performance in order to advance a population health agenda.

The 2004 Senate Evaluation noted that the fragmentation of mental health and substance abuse services, with inadequate data collection systems, makes it ". . . virtually impossible to monitor the quality, distribution, and cost-effectiveness of mental health and addiction services other than those provided in hospitals or in primary health care settings." Quality management is impeded by the lack of a national data base of comparable data on the mental health services across Canada. There is, however, some patient satisfaction survey data available: 77 percent of those surveyed indicated they received the help they needed from the mental health system, and 82 percent said they were satisfied or very satisfied with the services.

The Canadian Council on Health Services Accreditation (CCHSA) is a national, nonprofit, nongovernmental organization (NGO) that accredits health care organizations – an expression of voluntary self-regulation. This might be parallel to the National Committee for Quality Assurance (NCQA) and the Joint Commission on Accreditation of Healthcare Organizations (JCAHO) in the United States, which function as independent, voluntary accrediting bodies of managed behavioral health organizations and hospitals.

Integrated Care. One of the indicators of good quality is the integration of the mental health system (MHS) with the primary care system (PCS). That is particularly important in Canada because 26 percent of those who consulted health professionals for symptoms of mental disorders consulted their family physicians. Unfortunately, "psychological consultations are also not readily available to family physicians to assist them in dealing with patients' mental health problems. This compromises the health care provided to Canadians and renders it less comprehensive than it should be and more likely, with respect to mental health issues, to be more biologically focused than is often appropriate.... Pharmacotherapy is the first line of treatment by physicians with regard to mental health problems."

One of the causes of the fragmentation between medical and mental health services in Canada has been its national policy. For instance, in the *Hospital Insurance and Diagnostic Services Act* (1957), inpatient psychiatric services were excluded except for some emergency hospital services. This selective financing perpetuated the mind-body split, discouraged integrated physical and mental care, and created mental health facilities separate from the "regular" health system facilities within the communities. The financing policy was a major cause for the continued development of independent psychiatric hospitals in Canada, separate from the general medical hospitals. Consequently, Canada is likely to experience considerable institutional and professional resistance to community-based outpatient mental health in primary care settings.

Integration of mental health services with primary health care services was an aim in Canada's movement away from separate psychiatric hospitals to psychiatric units within general medical hospitals within the community following the 1964 Royal Commission on Health Services. Unfortunately, resistance and inadequate resources and inefficient organization of the mental health services have resulted in high relapse rates and readmissions, homelessness, and incarceration of seriously and persistently mentally ill patients in jails.

The 2002 Romanov Commission cited the persistent fragmentation of services as a significant problem and proposed as a solution a more integrated *shared cared model*. The 2004 Senate Evaluation found that poor coordination between the mental health services and the primary care services compromises optimal quality and continuity of care, and called for increased collaboration between psychiatrists and family physicians to improve the quality of primary mental health care provided by the former and their nurses, and to improve access to psychiatric consultation as necessary. Three key principles were stated to guide this more integrative approach along with nine essential elements of support needed for an effective community-based mental health system.

> For the providers of services, the intent was (a) to increase the competence and confidence of family physicians in managing mental health problems, (b) to enhance the effectiveness of psychiatrists as consultants and supports to family physicians, and (c) to increase mutual support among psychiatrists and family physicians in managing complex mental health problems.

The *shared care model* of mental health care was seen as one important vehicle to achieve these objectives.

Some of the fragmentation within the Canadian system is due to the way it is organized. Unlike the mental health system in Norway, which has been centralized, administration of the mental health services in Canada is decentralized among its ten Provinces and three Territories (with the exception of mental health services for military, prisoners, and Aboriginals). The decentralization results in common, but also different services being provided, that is, a lack of standardization in both quality and access, somewhat similar to the multiple and diverse Medicaid programs administered by the fifty states in America.

In addition to integrating mental health services with primary health care services, there is a need to integrate mental health and addiction services, especially for dual diagnosed patients. Integration of addiction treatment services (not with mental health services) into the community and social service delivery systems began in the 1990s in Canada. The 2004 Senate Evaluation concluded the mental health and addiction services in Canada was, in fact,

> not truly a system at all; rather it is a complex array of services that are delivered through federal, provincial, territorial, and municipal jurisdictions, by private providers and self-help services initiated by individuals with mental illness and addiction themselves. Several types and levels of services are provided all of varying capacity and quality, often operating in silos, all-too-frequently disconnected from the health care system.

Thus, whereas a shared care model had been advocated by the Romanov Commission two years earlier, it appears "... a silo model of parallel, uncoordinated mental health and addiction services prevails, and mental health remains one of the least integrated aspects of health care." The fragmentation of mental health and addiction services is a barrier to the delivery of high quality services.

Dr. Arnett's conclusions concerning the quality of care are as follows:

> (a) There is no doubt that competent and high quality mental health services are available in Canada and most are satisfactory, but the fact that a majority of the 20 percent with mental disorders do *not* use the publicly funded mental health services speaks volumes about perceived dissatisfaction; (b) Canada's mental health system is not a system at all – a conglomeration of poorly coordinated services with multiple entry points,

and a serious lack of accountability and leadership; (c) the poor coordination of care compromises optimal care; (d) particular deficiencies are evident in services to children and adolescents, the elderly, and Aboriginals in rural areas [and for the seriously and persistently mentally ill]; (e) there is a significant need for more focus and funding for health promotion and disease prevention; (f) more funding for mental health services research is need; (g) there is a need for a consistent, comprehensive national MH policy across all provinces and territories; (h) a population health approach is needed to replace the narrow biological model that focuses on diagnosis and treatment in the hospital-based system dominated by physicians.

Quality Assurance/Improvement in the United States. The quality of mental health care has been an ongoing concern in the United States. In 1978, President Carter's Commission on Mental Health noted "the great gap between what we know should be done and what we do" (President's Commission on Mental Health, 1978). Largely in response to fears of compromised quality under managed care, President Clinton's Advisory Commission on Consumer Protection and Quality of the Health Care Industry published a report in 1998 on how to define, measure, and promote quality of health care. Like so many other Presidential Commission reports, it was advisory and lacked implementation guidelines. Moreover, there is ". . . no mandatory national system and few local systems for tracking the quality of care delivered to the American people. More information is available on the quality of airlines, restaurants, cars and VCRs than on the quality of health care" (Schuster, McGlynn, and Brook, 2005, p. 843; cf. p. 887).

Based on their review of published literature on quality-of-care for the decade ending 1997, Schuster et al. (2005) found a small amount of systematic knowledge available on the quality of health care delivered in the United States. Their conclusions were:

> The dominant finding of our review is that there are large gaps between the care people should receive and the care they do receive. This is true for all three types of care – preventive, acute, and chronic – whether one goes for a check-up, a sore throat, or diabetic care. It is true whether one looks at overuse or underuse. It is true in different types of health care facilities and for different types of health insurance. It is true for all age groups, from children to the elderly. And it is true whether one is looking at the whole country or a single city. (p. 846)

Overall, only about 50 percent of people actually received recommended (appropriate) health care. ". . . the majority of studies described in the tables show much room for improvement of quality" (p. 886). The authors noted that improving quality has financial implications.

> The quality of health care provided in the United States varies among hospitals, cities, and states. Whether the care is preventive, acute, or chronic, it frequently does not meet professional standards. We can do much better. The solution is not simply a matter of spending more money on health care. A large part of our quality problems is the amount of inappropriate care provided in this country. Elimination of such nonbeneficial and potentially harmful care would lead to a large savings in human and financial costs. However, there are also many examples of people who receive either too little or technically poor care; fixing these problems may increase expenditures. (Schuster et al. 2005, p. 888)

To place their conclusion in perspective, the authors granted that most people in the studies they reviewed did receive excellent care. "There is good reason to be proud of our health care system, and the evidence from international studies does not show consistent superiority elsewhere in the world. . . ." (p. 888)

The Institute of Medicine (2002b) reported there is a 15 to 20 year lag from research to practice, and even when applied, adherence to evidence-based practices is highly uneven. QA/QI strategies have been articulated by American psychiatrists (Mattson, 1992) and psychologists (Stricker and Rodriguez, 1988), but implementation of these strategies is voluntary, and a comprehensive national strategy for quality assurance in health care is lacking (U.S. GAO, 1990). Authorized by Section 1013 of the *Medicare Prescription Drug, Improvement, and Modernization Act* of 2003, the Agency of Healthcare Research and Quality (AHRQ, 2005b) launched a $15 million Effective Health Care Program to compare evidence-based medical treatments and to encourage putting them into practice.

The National Institute of Mental Health funds epidemiological research projects, including assessments of quality. The most recent example is the National Comorbidity Survey-Replication (Wang et al. 2005b), which estimated quality of care in terms of the percent of patients receiving "minimally adequate treatment."

> Minimally adequate treatment was defined based on available evidence-based guidelines as receiving either pharmacotherapy (for two or more months of an appropriate medication for the focal disorder plus more than four visits to any type of physician) or psychotherapy (eight or more visits with any health care or human service professional lasting an average of 30 or more minutes). (Wang et al. 2005b, p. 630)

One of the conclusions directly related to the quality of care was the following: "Increasing use of some modalities, most notably pharmacotherapies and physician-administered psychotherapies, has generated hope that mental disorders are being treated much more effectively than in the past" (Wang, et al. 2005b, p. 634). The conclusion favoring "physician-administered psychotherapies" does not seem to be supported by the data reported in the same study. In fact the data indicated that allied mental health professionals (non-physicians) (51.1%) had as high a percentage of patients receiving "at least minimal care" as psychiatrists (53.3%), and both groups significantly more than general physicians (12.7%). Since psychiatrists also accounted for the lowest percentage of all mental health patients treated (7.5%), nonpsychiatric mental health specialists contributed most to the combined rate of 48.3 percent of patients receiving at least minimally adequate care from all mental health specialists (Wang et al. 2005b, 630–631). Moreover, since allied mental health specialists are not licensed to prescribe psychotropic medications, but provide psychotherapy, attributing the increased effectiveness of treatment to "most notably pharmacotherapies and physician-administered psychotherapies" is both inconsistent with the data and a biased interpretation.

In the *public sector*, the federal health insurance program for the elderly and disabled (Medicare) contracts with public and private institutions to ensure quality and quality improvement in the care enrollees receive. As an example, Stratis Health is the *Quality Improvement Organization (QIO)* paid by the Medicare program to review care that enrollees receive in Minnesota (MSF, 2005, p. 82). Snyder and Anderson (2005) reported disappointing findings about the impact of QIO programs: hospitals that participate in a QIO program for Medicare patients were no more likely to show improvement on 14 of 15 quality indicators than hospitals that did not participate. The quality of QIO programs warrants further evaluation.

Federal agencies such as the National Institute of Mental Health (NIMH), the Substance Abuse and Mental Health Administration (SAMSHA) and the Agency for Healthcare Research and Quality (AHRQ) are charged with quality assurance monitoring on a national scope. Another federal agency monitoring quality for a limited segment of the population is the Veterans Health Administration (VHA). In conjunction with the Department of Defense, the National Clinical Practice Guideline Council of the VHA has been a leader in QA/QI programs and in the development of evidence-based, clinical practice guidelines (Cassidy and Nilan, 2005, June). Kizer (1999) and Greenfield and Kaplan (2004) recognized the significant improvement in the quality of health care services provided by the VHA. The Institute of Medicine (IOM, 1990) outlined a strategy for quality assurance for Medicare that awaits full application.

Continual improvement in the Indian Health Service (IHS) was authorized in 1994 through the *Indian Health Care Improvement Act Reauthorization* (PL94-437), and through regulatory updates for mental health, alcohol and substance abuse. Quality assessment is conducted through the Indian Health Performance Evaluation System (HPES). Regulations are summarized in current revisions of *Indian Health Services Manual*, with notifications provided through the *IHS Behavioral Health Newsletter* and at the Annual IHS Division of Behavioral Health Conferences (IHS, 2005).

Most federally sponsored programs have policies with respect to patient protection, in addition to policies about reimbursements paid to private practitioners (e.g., Centers for Medicare and Medicaid, TRICARE for military personnel receiving health care in the civilian sector). Departments of health, commerce, or insurance are typical *state* agencies regulating the operations of health plans in the private sector. In theory, these state agencies monitor the quality of health care services as well as financial matters; however, their regulatory powers are often limited practically, politically, and legally.

Voluntary credentialing of *private*, managed behavioral health organizations is provided by the National Committee on Quality Assurance (NCQA). The Joint Commission on Accrediting Healthcare Organizations (JCAHO) accredits private hospitals, which include psychiatric units in general hospitals and psychiatric hospitals. While there is some trend to requiring outcome data, these voluntary types of accreditation are primarily structural and process evaluations; evaluation of the actual clinical outcomes of treated patients remains secondary, if included at all.

As an example, a *process measure* was developed by the National Committee for Quality Assurance (NCQA, 1997). The NCQA is funded by employer-user fees and voluntary members of private managed care organizations, including those that specialize in managed behavioral health care (for mental health and for substance abuse disorders). Called the *Health Plan Employer Data and Information Set (HEDIS)*, this standardized survey was created to assist *employers* in selecting health plans based upon their quality ratings. Elements of the HEDIS data set have been adopted by some state departments charged with regulating the operations of managed care organizations (MCOs) in their jurisdiction, even though the HEDIS format was judged unreliable by *Consumer Reports* (1996, August). Several limitations, including the unreliability of this format led the Minnesota Health Data Institute (MHDI, 1997, October, p. 66) to reject it in favor of another survey method called Consumer Assessment of Health Plans Survey (CAHPS) (AHCPR, 1999). This instrument assesses health plan enrollees' experiences with access, service, and providers, and overall satisfaction with their health plan. CAHPS was applied in New York State to compare enrollees in Medicaid versus commercial health plans (Roohen, Franko, Anarello, Dellehunt, and Gesten, 2003). The December, 2005 special issue of *Health Services Research* was devoted to the development and evaluation of CAHPS, and included a copy of the CAHPS Hospital Survey.

The states that regulate managed behavioral health plans do not all require the use of these "consumer satisfaction surveys." As indicators of health care quality, patient satisfaction surveys are subject to response bias, leading to overestimation of the level of satisfaction in the patient population because of the differences between responders and nonresponders (Mazor, Clauser, Field, Yood, and Gurwitz, 2002). Moreover, HEDIS does *not* provide an objective, outcome evaluation of the quality of care provided by managed care organizations in terms of *clinically significant, sustained improvement* in treated patients.

Moreover, the evaluation of health plans by state regulatory bodies have been limited to structural and process indicators. As an illustration, Olson (1999) reviewed (a) the Quality Assurance Examinations (QAEs) of selected managed care organizations conducted by the Minnesota State Department of Health (MDH), as well as (b) their quality assurance plans, (c) additional action and collaboration plans, and (d) quality work plans required of the Health Maintenance Organizations (HMOs) by the MN Department of Health, Managed Care Systems Section (MDH). Olson concluded that none of these private, nonprofit HMOs operating in Minnesota were being held accountable for mental health treatment outcomes because no objective outcome data on the efficacy of mental health treatment was provided by the HMOs to the MDH, nor was such data required by the MDH, though outcome assessment was mandated by state statute. Prior to that review reported in 1997, only one multisite, clinically focused *process* study had been conducted with Medicaid patients suffering from depression. This was a retrospective record review of (a) documentation of the severity of depression, (b) percentages of patients with documented suicide risk assessment, and (c) percentage of patients on medication with a dosage in the therapeutic range. No data were collected to address the question of whether or not the treatments provided were effective in producing clinically significant and sustained improvement of the patients' depression (Olson, 1999, pp. 22–24).

A voluntary quality improvement strategy has not been fully successful in improving the U.S. system's meeting of mental health needs, nor in improving quality of care in the *private sector*. Quality assessments of managed behavioral health organizations (MBHOs) have had only marginal impact upon employers' decisions about selecting health plans. A recent study by Gabel et al. (2003) indicated that most employers do not understand or value the quality of care provided by health plans as much as they are concerned about the cost savings. The survey indicated that a very small percentage of both small and large firms were familiar with quality measures such as HEDIS and other quality monitoring groups such as the Leapfrog Group, or voluntary accreditation of managed behavioral health organizations by the National Committee for Quality Assurance (NCQA) or URAC accreditation. These findings suggest a decline in employer's concerns about quality compared to the results based on a previous employer survey conducted in 1997 by Marquis and Long (2001).

> While price remains the dominant factor driving employers' health plans contracting decisions, there is growing interest among employers to evaluate the quality of health plans and providers. In the 1997 Robert Wood Johnson Foundation Employer Health Insurance Survey, nearly 39 percent of large firms considered health plan accreditation and 52 percent considered the board certification of physicians when making contracting decisions. (Marquis and Long, 2001, as cited by Abraham, Feldman, and Carlin, 2004, pp. 1799–1800)

If employers as the purchasers of health insurance are not concerned about the quality of health care services provided, and do not communicate the results of quality evaluations to employees, the latter are less likely to make informed decisions about their participation. Based on their survey of 1,365 employees in 16 large firms in the Minneapolis-St. Paul area in 2002, Abraham et al. (2004) reported that less than one-third of employees were aware of the consumer survey results evaluating the quality of provider groups and of quality awards given by the Buyers Health Care Action Group in which their employers participated.

Integrated Care. There are three primary reasons for integrating mental health specialty care into primary care: the high utilization by people with mental disorders of primary health care services, the need and opportunity to improve the quality of care, and to establish community-based services.

Utilization data are reported by the Division of Data Services of the National Center for Health Statistics (NCHS). In the year 2000, the number of annual office visits to physicians for mental disorders was 29,939,000, of which 10,043,000 were for depression, 4.8 million for anxiety, and 2.1 million for schizophrenic disorders. The number of psychotropic drug mentions in office practice was 113,210,000. The number of short-stay hospital discharges for mental disorders was 2.1 million (NCHS, 2002). These utilization figures constitute the *first* reason for integrating mental health care into primary care settings where so many people are seen first.

Additional data from the three major epidemiological studies done in the United States the past three decades support these findings. The latest National Comorbidity Survey Replication (NCS-R) study indicated that 22.8 percent of individuals with any 12-month DSM-IV mental disorder used general medical services (primary care sector), which was about equal to the 21.7 percent who used any mental health *specialty* services (Wang et al. 2005b, p. 632). An actual increase in utilization of about five to six percent from the early 1980s occurred mostly in the primary health care (GM) sector with general physicians. These utilization figures constitute one reason for integrating mental health care into primary care settings.

The *second* reason for integrating mental health specialty care with primary health care is to improve the quality of mental health services in the primary care sector. Commenting on the increased utilization of primary care (GM) services by people with mental disorders, Wang et al. (2005b, p. 635) reported: "... the fact that only a few patients [12.7%] in the GM sector receive minimally adequate care makes these trends concerning." By contrast, the percent of patients receiving at least minimally adequate treatment from *any* mental health specialists (48.3%) was more than three times higher than from primary health care professionals (12.7%). Moreover, the percentage in the GM sector was lower than the percentage receiving at least minimally adequate care in either (a) the non-health care, human service sector (16.9%), or (b) through participation in a self-help group (16.7%) (Wang, et al. 2005b, Table 4, p. 635). The study by Druss, Rohrbaugh, Levinson, and Rosenheck (2001) supports the view that integrated medical care for patients with serious psychiatric illness improves the quality of care.

Significant improvement has occurred in the number of American children who receive treatment for mental health problems in the primary care sector. The increases have been primarily with general practitioners and pediatricians.

> From 1985 through 1999 the percentage of children's physician visits that included a mental health diagnosis nearly tripled. Virtually all of this increase consisted of visits at which psychotropic medications were prescribed.... Much of the increase in treatment over this period occurred through more frequent diagnosis and treatment of mental illness during primary care visits. More than four times as many visits to general practitioners involved a psychiatric diagnosis in 1999 than in 1985 (3,217,000 versus 757,000). This pattern is consistent with the many efforts made during this period to increase the role of primary physicians, including pediatricians, in diagnosing and treatment of mental health problems. (Glied and Cuellar, 2003, pp. 41–42)

Unfortunately, studies have also shown that primary care providers often misdiagnose mental health problems in children, missing illnesses in some and overdiagnosing others.

> When they provide drug treatment, primary care providers often underdose and undermonitor treatment, so that the outcomes are well below those attained in clinical trials. Finally, primary care providers rarely provide psychosocial treatment as an adjunct to pharmacological treatment. The average patient visit to a general practitioner including prescription of a psychotropic drug was only twenty-three minutes long – 50 percent longer than the average visit by a patient without a mental health problem. (Glied and Cuellar, 2003, p. 42)

The Bureau of Primary Health Care (BPHC) is a subdivision of the Bureau of Health Care, which in turn, is a division of the Health Resources and Services Administration within the U.S. Department of Health and Human Services. With respect to the second reason for more integrated care, the BPHC noted that primary care settings can effectively treat many mental health problems and disorders, and that studies have demonstrated that by integrating mental health staff within a primary care setting, remission rates of depression can be produced that are comparable to those seen in efficacy studies on mental health specialty care. Quality improvement interventions with either medication management or psychotherapy have been demonstrated to improve outcomes for primary care patients with depressive disorders and subthreshold depression when compared to usual care (Wells et al. 2005).

Improvement in the quality of primary care is partly a function of how primary care services are organized. Jackson et al. (2005) analyzed the organizational characteristics of primary care services in more than 200 Veterans Hospital Administration medical centers and their community-based outpatient clinics. The characteristics associated with improved patient care were found to include: (a) physicians actively involved in quality improvement, (b) use of electronic health information systems, (c) administrative authority to establish or implement clinic policies and to address staffing needs, and (d) patients actively involved in their own care.

Unfortunately, in spite of positive mental health outcomes achieved through more integrated care of mental health specialists with primary care physicians, and in spite of the fact that the prevalence of mental disorders seen in primary care settings is often greater, many of these disorders go undiagnosed by primary health care professionals, and as a result less than 33 percent of those who need treatment receive it (Bureau of Primary Health Care, 2003).

The *third* reason for integrating mental health specialty care into primary care settings is that mental health services are more likely to become more community-based. "A lack of community mental health care has led to widespread, inappropriate use of hospital emergency departments, crisis stabilization units, and institutional and residential care, including jails, prison, and juvenile justice facilities" (Bell and Shern, 2002). One of the goals embraced by the President's New Freedom Commission on Mental Health (2003) was "a life in the community for everyone." The same Commission noted that while recovery from mental disorders was a real possibility, it is frustrated by the "fragmented, disconnected and often inadequate services."

Like the other three countries included in this study, the United States mental health system has a wide range of levels of intervention provided through various independent structures from primary medical clinics to residential treatment centers. There is a lack of integration among the various levels and institutions, and a lack of easy transition and communication among them. An example is the problem of delayed discharges from state hospitals and residential treatment centers because there are no other viable alternatives for continued care within the community (Petrila and Levin, 2004).

While there is evidence for the effectiveness of specific community-based treatment programs for children with mental health problems, community-based alternatives to inpatient mental health care have not emerged to fill in the gaps for children (Glied and Cuellar, 2003). Mental health care for children involves multiple service systems including medical centers, mental health agencies, their schools and families.

> For this reason, since 1984, the centerpiece of child mental health policy has been the development of *systems of care* [italics added] that would integrate care across these diverse settings. Federal financing for this effort began with the Child and Adolescent Service System Program (CASSP) in 1984 and continued with Comprehensive Community Mental Health Services for Children and Families ($78 million in 1999). (Glied and Cuellar, 2003, pp. 46–47)

The "system of care" (SOC) approach relies on interagency coordination and places responsibility for meeting mental health needs of children and youth at the community level rather than within a single agency.

> Under such a system, the mental health sector coordinates and delivers services in conjunction with other child-serving agencies, such as juvenile justice and child welfare. The SOC also changes the types of mental health services delivered – it substitutes community-based alternatives [e.g., partial hospitalization] for expensive inpatient care. (Foster and Xuan, 2005, p. 1960)

In the SOC approach, integration among the various agencies occurs at both the administrative and operational levels. Agency representatives participate in a cross-system service planning process and mental health personnel are stationed at other agencies such as juvenile justice. The Center for Mental Health Services (CMHS) within the U. S. Department of Health and Human Services has funded the development of SOC programs since 1994. Services are financed through block grants, Medicaid, and other sources.

Evaluations of the effects of SOC programs vary according to the method of data analysis. Using a basic model of analysis of results from a quasi-experimental, multisite evaluation, Foster and Xuan (2005) reported that children and youth in SOC sites showed (a) significantly improved functioning on the *Child and Adolescent Functional Assessment Scale* (Hodges, 1990), (b) significantly increased time between treatment episodes, but also (c) significantly longer treatment episodes, and (d) nearly twice the cost compared to communities without SOC programs. However, a second analysis of the same data using a multilevel, multiprocess model yielded different conclusions more favorable to the SOC program. Compared to control communities, SOC communities showed lower risks for children and youth both entering and exiting services at a point in time, and the cost per day of treatment episode were equivalent across SOC and non-SOC sites (Foster and Xuan, 2005, p. 1964). Under both models of analysis, individuals at the SOC site stayed in treatment longer and they were less likely to return to treatment after an episode ended. The authors concluded that children and youth in the SOC program experienced substantially greater continuity of care.

According to a review by Gleid and Cueller (2003), the results of coordinated, community-based services like the SOC are mixed. "... several large studies conducted in the 1990s suggest that coordination and the development of systems of care alone are not associated with major improvements in mental health outcomes for most children" (p. 47). Ironically, in some settings coordination of care may even lead to diffusion of responsibility and inferior results. The authors concluded that the efficacy of program elements being coordinated is more important than the coordination itself.

The integration of primary health care and mental health care was an objective of President Levant of the American Psychological Association (APA) for 2005. The APA Council of Representatives endorsed a vision of integrated care of both physical and mental illnesses based on a review of evidence that physical and mental health are inseparable. Several other professional organizations have supported the APA sponsored "Health Care for the Whole Person Collaborative" (Dingfelder, 2005). All of these groups understand that a person is not divided the way health care is provided through separate medical and mental health services. This initiative would be enhanced by an even broader vision of the person as a mind/body/spirit, which underlies Norway's National Mental Health Programme. Moreover, the integration of mental health specialties with primary health care sectors would be facilitated by the development of information technology, computerized record-keeping, and national data bases for administration of mental health services.

Competence of Mental Health Professionals

Universal access to services of questionable quality provided by incompetent or unethical providers would hardly be considered a satisfactory indicator of a good health care system. The number and distribution of qualified mental health providers was cited previously as one of the factors contributing to equity of access to the health care system. As a quality assurance procedure, all four mental health systems in this study regulate mental health professions through standardized educational and training requirements for licensure, through ethical codes of conduct, and through continuing education requirements for lifelong professional development of the knowledge, skills, and attitudes which are deemed prerequisite to providing competent and ethical services. Moreover, all four countries include a range of remedial actions available to both service users and service providers if the provisions of the regulated profession are violated. Remedial actions range from mandatory, but advisory consultations to restricted or supervised practice, loss of license to practice, or in some cases, civil court action for malpractice or negligence, or criminal prosecution for malfeasance such as sexual misconduct or other exploitative actions by providers.

The education and regulation of mental health professions is critical to ensuring ethical and efficacious services, which in turn are vital to quality improvement. In a critical review of research on methods of quality improvement, Shojania and Grimshaw (2005) suggested several reasons for inadequate quality control related to providers. Cited by Fuchs and Emmanuel (2005), these are:

> Providers may not know what experts recommend; they may know but disagree with the experts; the support systems needed to comply with the recommendations may be absent; or financial incentives may be misaligned. As has been observed in many contexts, it is difficult to get people to understand something when their income depends on their not understanding it. (p. 1402)

Provider Competence in England. In England, all health care professionals are required to be registered under either an Act of Parliament (such as the General Medical Council for medical practitioners, currently regulated by the 1983 Medical Act) or under a Royal Charter (a public process not requiring direct involvement by Parliament). All physicians, psychiatrists and psychiatric nurses are licensed to practice under one of these two processes. As of 2000, all nonmedical mental health providers, including clinical, counseling, and forensic psychologists are regulated through the registration and disciplinary procedures of the new Allied Health Professions Council. Moreover, a range of mental health professions are represented in both generic Community Mental Health Teams and in other teams specializing in crisis resolution, assertive outreach, and early intervention for psychosis.

England credentials clinical psychologists as a mental health profession distinct from professional counselors. The former work more in mental health specialty settings and teams, whereas the latter work mostly in primary care settings. Clinical psychologists must obtain a Honors degree in psychology (a four-year advanced degree beyond high school), and they must work for at least two years in a related field before proceeding to clinical training. All postgraduate, professional training has been standardized at three years, leading to a doctoral degree (D.Psy. or D.Clin.Psy.). The PhD has always been retained as a research degree in England. Training standards and credentialing for the newly created role of "gateway workers" and "primary care graduate mental health workers" await development. Both roles were created to strengthen access to mental health services within primary health care settings and to specialized services.

Provider Competence in Norway. One of the principal objectives of the National Mental Health Programme approved by Parliament in 1998 was to promote skills, development, and education of competent practitioners and to encourage research into effective (evidence-based) interventions.

Mental health services provided in *primary* care settings within *local* municipalities are regulated by the *Mental Health Act* passed in 1999. Regulation of mental health *specialist* services and other specialized medical disciplines was reauthorized under the *Specialized Health Services Act* passed by Parliament in the same year. The education and training of all "qualified personnel" is regulated by the central government. These include physicians, psychiatrists, psychologists and specialty nurses in psychiatric institutions. All qualified personnel are licensed by the Ministry of Health and Social Care to treat medically and/or mentally ill patients.

The Directorate of Health and Social Welfare credentials mental health personnel. To be credentialed as a clinical psychologist to provide individual psychotherapy requires six years of graduate level (university) education with supervised practical training. One of the goals of Norway's national health policy expressed in the *Act on Health Enterprises* (2000) was to update professional skills through lifelong learning.

Though not strictly a credentialing issue, one of the particular features in the education, training, and practice of clinical psychologists and psychiatrists in Norway has been the dominance of the psychoanalytic and psychodynamic approach the past 30 years (1970–2000) especially in outpatient psychotherapy practices. Clinical psychologists became more eclectic beginning in the 1970s, and more cognitive-behavioral in the most recent decade.

One concern expressed by our Norwegian authors is the increase in self-identified "psychotherapists" without formal approval or certification.

> Especially in the large cities psychologists without a clinical specialty and people with a three-year education from a university college [undergraduate program], for instance a nurse or social worker, can open a private practice not approved or without being included in the public mental health system. The patients pay the total cost themselves to these "unregulated" private practicing psychotherapists.

Provider Competence in Canada. In Canada there are both regulated and unregulated professionals providing mental health services. Rough estimates of regulated professionals include 32,000 family physicians, 4,000 psychiatrists, 5,000 psychiatric nurses, 47,000 social workers, 16,000 psychologists, and 9,600 occupational therapists. The numbers of "unregulated" professionals are unknown, but include marriage and family therapists, counselors, addiction counselors, and others. Irrespective of their classifications, most mental health professions engage in voluntary self regulation through professional codes of ethics and practice guidelines.

In general, the *raison d'etre* for regulating the health care professions is to protect the public from harm, and to ensure a minimal level of quality of services by assessing the competence and ethics of applicants for certification or licensure. Consequently, the presence of unregulated professionals is a cause for concern in Canada just as the presence of unregulated "psychotherapists" is a concern in Norway. Unlike Great Britain, Canada's "counselors" are not regulated.

While there are many specialty certifying bodies with a national scope in Canada, the regulation of health care practitioners is constitutionally guaranteed as a provincial responsibility similar to regulation by the states in America. This is a decentralized system of regulation, which results in considerable variability in regulatory standards.

Professional self-regulation is an important element in maintaining the quality of services. For example, the Canadian Psychological Association has its own ethics committee and the Association promotes evidence-based practices. Agencies providing mental health services can pursue national accreditation voluntarily with the Canadian Council on Health Services Accreditation (CCHSA), an independent, non-profit, non-governmental organization.

With family physicians providing 25 percent or more of outpatient mental health care in Canada, it would seem appropriate to review the educational requirements for licensure and include mental health and substance abuse (MH/SA) modules and supervised field work (practica), as well as the percentage of post-licensure, continuing education credits devoted to MH/SA issues.

Provider Competence in the United States. Most graduate education programs for doctoral level clinical psychologists are four or five-year programs, including part-time field training and a one year, full-time, supervised internship. Health care professionals are licensed by each state, though there are national qualifying exams for some mental health professionals to ensure that individuals who are licensed meet at least minimal standards of knowledge, skills, and attitudes deemed requisite to competent practice (e.g., the national boards for psychologists called the Examination for Professional Practice in Psychology). Most states require one year of postdoctoral supervised employment for a psychologist to be licensed for independent, clinical practice. State licensure boards have a mandate to protect the public from incompetent and unethical conduct on the part of licensees. Various levels of sanctions are available to the state licensing boards from educational conferences to termination of licensure. Most states have continuing education requirements for mental health specialists to maintain their license. Sexual exploitation of clients by their therapist has been criminalized in a number of states.

Cost and Efficiency

Definitions

Costs. Construed solely in economic terms, cost is the monetary expenditure required to pay for a volume of services at a particular price. The formula is: [Cost = price/unit X number of units purchased]. There are both direct and indirect costs of both mental disorders and in administering and delivering mental health services.

Direct costs include the economic costs incurred to supply the elements necessary for the system to perform its functions and to achieve its goals. These would include costs for both goods (e.g., psychotropic medications) and services such as outpatient psychotherapy. Salaries, wages, and fees paid to health care providers and capital investments in facilities are presumed necessary, hence included as direct costs. Administrative costs are sometimes considered indirect costs (overhead), but belong properly to the category of direct costs because any health care system must be administered or managed to be efficient. The ratio of providers/administrators is one indicator of efficiency. Direct costs are generally measured by financial expenditures of the health care system.

Indirect costs of mental disorders are more difficult to estimate, but include loss in productivity; the use of other social service resources for housing, disability pension, vocational rehabilitation; the burden of care for family members with mental disorders; and the unnecessary pain and suffering endured because of inequitable access to affordable mental health services of optimal quality.

Efficiency. One way of construing the concept of *efficiency* is in terms of benefit/cost ratios: what volume of which type and level of service is provided at what cost? In an information processing model with the elements of Input-Processing-Output (IPO), the ratio of outputs to inputs of the system, or how well the processes convert inputs (financial, human, capital resources) into outputs (units of service) are indicators of efficiency. For example, are the mental health services purchased strategically to maximize the services offered? If so, are services offered to those with the more serious mental disorders or to a larger number irrespective of the severity of their mental disorder?

Another way of assessing efficiency is in terms of the ratio of mental health providers and administrators to the population. For example, how many mental health specialists are required to provide the mental health services needed for a population of 6,000, in which 28 percent (1,680) is the prevalence of mental disorders? Is the ratio of 1:6,000 population set by the United States Bureau of Health Professions (2002) satisfactory? And what is the number of administrators employed to manage the system relative to both the population size and to the number of direct service providers?

Efficiency can be construed in terms of *productivity*, that is, the number of units of service per provider or clients per provider. It is sometimes assessed in terms of the cost/unit of service or per capita costs of users of the service. An efficient system would avoid duplication and yield an optimal level of productivity. Group therapy, for example, has been justified over individual therapy because it increases the ratio of users to provider.

Efficiency is influenced by several system and nonsystem factors. *System factors* include: (a) the presence and implementation of national health policy addressing the cost-effectiveness of the health care system; (b) the structural organization of institutions and agencies through which the program is administered and regulated, and services are delivered; (c) work force planning, education, and training; (d) the mechanism employed to collect revenues, to pool revenues and other resources, and to purchase services; (e) the commitment and action of service personnel to provide high quality services most efficiently; (f) the cost-consciousness of service users; and (g) the effectiveness of mechanisms to limit waste, fraud, and abuse.

A primary factor in determining efficiency is the commitment of practitioners to provide cost-effective care. In a situation of competing and limited resources, it is insufficient for providers to consider the benefits of their interventions relative to only risks; providers must also consider the effectiveness relative to the costs. Cost-effective care has not been implemented on a wide scale anymore than empirically-based practices because providers have not been fully committed to either one.

Efficiency Measures and Rankings

In order to capture influences on the efficiency of performance of a health care system from nonhealth system factors, the WHO (2000) derived two measures of efficiency: (a) the performance on level of health, and (b) overall performance. The index of performance on the *level of health* (WHO, 2000, Annex Table 10, pp. 200–203) is taken as an estimate of ". . . how efficiently health systems translate expenditures into health as measured by disability-adjusted life expectancy (DALE). "DALE is estimated from three kinds of information: The fraction of the population surviving to each age, calculated from birth and death rates; the prevalence of each type of disability at each age; and the weight assigned to each type of disability, which may or may not vary with age" (WHO, 2000, Box 2.1, p. 28).

Performance on the level of health is defined as the ratio between achieved levels of health and the levels of health that could be achieved by the most efficient health system. "More specifically, the numerator of the ratio is the difference between observed DALE in a country and the DALE that would be observed in the absence of a functioning modern health system, given the other nonhealth system determinants that influence health, which are represented by education. . . ." (WHO, 2000, p. 150).

The adjustment of rankings in terms of overall educational levels of the population has been challenged (Deber, 2003), but it seems as good a proxy indicator as any other nonhealth system determinants that influence health. Moreover, including these determinants is an important step to recognizing the socioeconomic context in which health systems function.

As a more global estimate of efficiency, the rankings of *overall performance* of health systems were measured using a similar process relating overall health system achievement to health system expenditures (WHO, 2000, p. 150). The rankings of efficiency for the year 1997 are provided in Table 6.8, along with overall goal attainment rankings.

A comparison of performance on health level (column 1) with overall performance (column 2) reveals a change in these ratings of efficiency of all four countries relative to the total 191 countries ranked, but the rank order among the four remains the same on both measures. Moreover, the overall performance rankings (column 2) are higher for all four countries than rankings on performance on health levels (column 1), with the lowest ranked country (United States) much closer to the other three in overall performance.

On the rankings of overall goal attainment (column 3), all four countries are higher than most of the total group of all 191 countries that were ranked. Among the four countries, the order of rankings of Norway (highest) and the United States (lowest) are consistent with the rank orders on overall performance. Only the ranking of the United Kingdom (9) and Canada (7) on overall goal attainment have reversed from their rankings in overall performance (United Kingdom – 18, Canada – 30).

The efficiency of a health care system will be influenced by several factors, including its *method for purchasing* health care services, that is, its method for ". . . determining which investments are made and which interventions are bought, and for whom" (WHO, 2000, p. 113). The performance of the system

Table 6.8. *Rankings of Efficiency (Performance) and Goal Attainment.*

Country	Performance on health level (DALE)	Overall Performance	Overall Goal Attainment
Norway	18	11	3
United Kingdom	24	18	9
Canada	35	30	7
United States	72	37	15

Note: Sources of these data are WHO (2000). Annex Tables 9 & 10, pp. 196–203.

will depend upon the intelligent use of pooled revenues to purchase the best attainable mixture of actions to improve health and satisfy people's expectations. Thus, efficiency is a criterion of the performance of a health care system relative to the resources made available to the system.

Health Expenditures 2003

Economic estimates of both costs and efficiency require knowledge of health expenditures, including the percent of Gross Domestic Product spent on health, total health expenditures per capita, and average growth rate in total health expenditures. The source of health expenditure data cited in the previous chapters of this volume was primarily the Annex Tables of the *World Health Report 2005*, which reported figures up to 2002 (WHO, 2005b). Comparative data for 2002 are provided in Table 1.2 of this book. At the time of writing this final chapter, more recent data for 2003 became available from *OECD Health Data 2005 June 5*, which is summarized in Table 6.9.

Table 6.9 indicates that the United States has the most expensive and least efficient health care system as indicated by both (a) total health expenditures as a percent of GDP and (b) total health expenditure per capita in US$ adjusted for purchasing power parity. However, in the average growth rate in total health expenditures 1998–2003, the U.S. (4.6%) is about equal to Canada (4.2%), both of which have controlled the rate of increasing costs about one percent better than Norway (5.3%) and Great Britain (5.7%).

The percentage of the Gross Domestic Product (GDP) spent on health care depends upon the overall performance of the economy indicated by the GDP. Consequently, a country with a relatively poorer performing economy (lower GDP) can have a higher ratio of expenditures on health care. Conversely, as an economy does better overall (higher GDP), the ratio of health care expenditures to total GDP may drop (Deber, 2003). Since population size will influence the number in the work force, hence GDP, another indicator applied is the per capita health expenditures.

Great Britain's Costs and Efficiency

Costs. The OECD data for 2003 (Table 6.9) indicate that Great Britain's Gross Domestic Product (GDP) was US$1,797.9 billion. Total expenditures on health accounted for 7.7 percent of the GDP, an estimated US$138 billion, of which 83.4 percent was public expenditures (an estimated US$115 billion). Total health expenditure per capita in US$ adjusted for parity in purchasing power was $2,231. The average growth rate in total health expenditures from 1998 to 2003 was 5.7 percent.

Efficiency. On the WHO (2000) efficiency ratings of overall system performance, Great Britain (18th) ranked second among our four countries (Table 6.8). The NHS appears to have relatively *high administrative costs*. A head count of the total number of managers employed in the NHS in England yielded 130,000 (Government Statistical Service, 2004). With a population of about 50 million in England, the ratio of managers per capita in the NHS is 1:385 population. Including the entire population of the UK of about 60 million, the ratio is 1:461.

Table 6.9. *Health Expenditures 2003.*

	Canada	**Norway**	**UK**	**US**
Total Gross Domestic Product (a)	856.6	220.6	1,797.9	10,951.3
Total expenditures on health as % of GDP	9.9(b)	10.3(b)	7.7	15.0(b)
Public expenditure on health as % of total expenditure on health	69.9(b)	83.7(b)	83.4(c)	44.4
Total health expenditure per capita in US$ PPP(e)	3003(b)	3807(b)	2231(c)	5635
Average growth rate in total health expenditures, 1998–2003	4.2	5.3	5.7(d)	4.6

a. GDP is expressed in billions of US$ at current and constant prices based on exchange rates for the year 2003.
b. Estimated data.
c. Data refers to one previous year.
d. Average growth rate for 1998–2002, instead of 1998–2003.
e. PPP stands for purchasing power parity which takes into account the cost of living in each country.
Note: Copyright permission from OECD Health Data 2005.

None of the other three countries approaches such a generous ratio. The NHS is the major employer within the entire health care system in Britain. It appears to take proportionate many more managers and other personnel to administer the NHS than the health care systems in the other three countries.

There appear to be about 400 NHS entities, each with their Local Authority joint partners, providing NHS mental health services. Each has a Finance Director at the Board level, with supporting staff, and a range of support functions, such as human resources and information technology. Figures for the number of administrative positions associated only with mental health services were not reported.

Cost Containment Strategies. The costs, efficiency, and financing for adult mental health services in Britain were reported in December 2004 as elements of the comprehensive evaluation of the 1999 National Service Framework for mental health for adults. The reader is referred to chapter two of this volume for detailed discussion.

England applies largely supply-side strategies for controlling costs. Through centralized planning and ownership of health services, the expenditures for operational costs, administrative services, and capital investments are controlled administratively. Both the volume and prices of health services and goods are subject to public control rather than being left to the market place.

Norway's Costs and Efficiency

Costs. The OECD data for 2003 (Table 6.9) reported a total GDP for Norway of US$220.6 billion. Total expenditures on health accounted for 10.3 percent of GDP (an estimated US$22.7 billion), of which 83.7 percent was public expenditure (an estimated US$19 billion). Total health expenditure per capita in US$ adjusted for parity in purchasing power was $3,807. Average growth rate in total health expenditures 1998–2003 was 5.3 percent.

Estimated in terms of actual expenditures, an increasing amount of public resources are spent on the health sector in Norway. In 2003, Norway spent NOK 61 billion on specialized health services (US$ 8.6 billion at the 2003 exchange rate of 7.080), making it one of the European countries – and *the* Nordic country – with the highest level of public per capita spending on health services.

An increasing share of the total health costs has been spent on *mental health* services. For the first time in several years, the growth in costs of mental health services from 2002 to 2003 was larger than the growth in costs of general hospitals and institutions. NOK 11.1 billion was spent on the specialist mental health services in Norway (US$ 1.6 billion at the 2003 exchange rate of 7.080).

Public expenditure on health as a percent of *total* expenditure on health was equivalent for Norway (83.7%) and Great Britain (83.4%) for 2003 (Table 6.9). However, the estimated percent of total *public* expenditures spent on only mental health services in Norway is 18.2 percent, about two percent more than in Great Britain (16%). As both systems are largely financed publicly, the percentages could be taken as rough estimates of the percentages of the *total* health expenditures on mental health services in each country.

Efficiency. On the WHO (2000) efficiency ratings of overall system performance, Norway (11th) ranked highest among our four countries (Table 6.8). As a strategy to improve efficiency, Norway opted for centralization of its mental health services. Prior to the 1961 *Act of Mental Health Care*, mental health and other specialized services and hospitals had been owned and run for decades by the central government. These services were transferred to the county councils in 19 regions in 1961, but about 40 years later (2000), services were returned to central government ownership and administration. Ownership and full responsibility for these services, which are called Health Enterprises or Trusts, was assumed by the State through the Ministry of Health and Care Services (MHCS) of the central government. The public mental health system is administered through appointed managers and executive boards of the five Regional Health Authorities and 31 Health Enterprises.

The centralization of specialized services was designed to reduce variability in both access and quality of mental health specialty services in the counties and 434 municipalities, to ensure equity of access, and to improve efficiency of operational functions such as purchasing of services and supplies. Through the MHCS, the central government has a greater opportunity now to intervene in the health care system than when specialized services were owned and run by numerous counties. Nevertheless, policy prohibits the MHCS from daily micromanaging the appointed managers and executive boards of the Regional Health Authorities and Health Enterprises providing mental health and other specialty services. All local Health Enterprises are expected to operate in a cost-effective manner.

The *Act on Health Enterprises* (2002) affirmed several goals, which included coordinating procurement within and between regions; improving utilization of buildings, facilities, and equipment; increasing productivity of mental health services; and increasing both competition and cooperation regionally and locally.

One estimate of efficiency is the percentage of all qualified providers in the specialist health service involved in providing direct service. In Norway that figure is 75 percent of all full-time equivalent personnel. Full-time equivalents in administration and support services account for 25 percent.

One way to improve efficiency is to improve *productivity*. Most productivity indicators are based solely on the number of patients treated per year or "man-year," not on the outcome or result of the treatment. One of the 14 major goals of the National Mental Health Program (NMHP) approved by Parliament in 1998 was to increase by 50 percent productivity of outpatient clinics for adults (goal #9) and also for children and adolescents (goal #13).

From 1998 to 2002, the number of outpatient consultations with adults increased by 29 percent as a result of the addition of 43 percent more full-time equivalent personnel. The productivity, measured by number of consultations per full-time personnel ("man-years"), did not increase. It was stable the first three years (1999–2001), and decreased in 2001 from 1.67 to 1.54. Instead of an assumed and planned 50 percent increase, productivity in outpatient adult services decreased by 10 percent from 1998 to 2002. By contrast, there was a substantial increase in productivity in the outpatient clinics for children and adolescents in the period 1996 to 2001, and it continued in the first five years of 2000. The average level of productivity in 2001 was more than 25 percent higher than it was in 1996 due first and foremost to shorter durations of stay. This implies an average annual growth in productivity of 4.5 percent in the outpatient clinics for children and adolescents.

The public regulation of mental health services for Children and Adolescents (C&A) started with the *Mental Health Act* in 1961. Reorganization of these services occurred as a result of a new Act in 1999. A goal of the NMHP was to increase mental health services for C&A from two percent in 1998 to five percent by 2006. In 2003, 17 percent of the costs of the mental health services went to children and adolescents, an increase from 10 percent in 1990 and 13 percent in 2001.

Our Norwegian experts state that for all ages within the population, there are substantial variations in mental health services in capacity and productivity among different health regions and clinics.

> In most of the outpatient clinics there are waiting lists, and the clinics have to choose between different types of patients. Patients are often treated on a first come-first served basis, and waiting lists are regarded as a result of scarce resources. In these outpatient settings, patients with minor mental disorders requiring short-term treatment seem to be given priority as a way to increase productivity.

Days in psychiatric hospitals are also decreasing with less severe mental disorders. Presently, 20 percent of the population is considered as actual or potential patients, and very few of them are hospitalized. Community-based, outpatient services are expected to dominate the delivery system, even if 80 percent of the resources are still spent in the institutions. By contrast, Canada continues with a predominantly hospital-based mental health system, hence it is also more expensive.

Cost Containment Strategies. To contain costs, Norway does not use prior or concurrent authorizations by third parties, nor case management procedures. Nor is there any financial incentive for patients to contain costs such as requiring deductibles or co-insurance, though co-payments at the point of service may be charged by private practitioners, depending upon their contracts with Health Enterprises. These and other private sector, market-based strategies are applied in the United States. Instead, the Norwegian public mental health system employs (a) centralized planning and ownership of Health Enterprises; (b) block grants to Regional Health Authorities based on numbers of patients and service activities; (c) increased productivity of mental health services to reduce the cost per patient, and in this way increase the capacity (volume) with the same amount of expenditure; (d) free choice of hospitals and specialist services (market demand) to encourage Health Enterprises to compete on quality and efficacy as well as efficiency and productivity, but not to influence financing or cost.

It is generally less expensive to treat mental health patients with outpatient and intensive outpatient therapy than inpatient treatment. Norway's recognition of this cost savings is reflected in the 30 percent reduction in beds in mental health institutions from 1990 to 2003 (32% reduction for adults, but a 27% increase for C&As). Outpatient consultations increased 148 percent during the same period.

Despite the significant progress achieved since the central government initiated the NMHP in 1998, our

Norwegian experts noted that 80 percent of the funding for specialized mental health services for adults is still spent on inpatient treatment rather than community-based services. To meet this challenge, the government is reconsidering the distribution of resources among hospitals, District Psychiatric Centres (DPCs), and services provided by the local councils, and it will propose further expansion of the community-based services, including supported housing. During 2005 and 2006, ambulatory service teams will be organized at all DPCs.

The inadequate cooperation among mental health service units in Norway, which was cited previously under the criterion of integrated services, is also relevant to the criterion of efficiency. To become more efficient, the mental health services need to improve their cooperation and coordination.

Canada's Costs and Efficiency

Costs. The OECD data for 2003 (Table 6.9) reported a total GDP of US$856.6 billion. Total expenditure on health accounted for 9.9 percent of GDP (an estimated US$84.8 billion), of which 69.9 percent was public expenditures (an estimated US$59 billion). Total health expenditure per capita was $3,003 in US$ adjusted for purchasing power parity. The average growth rate in total health expenditures 1998–2003 was 4.2 percent in Canada.

Based on data from the Canadian Institute for Health Information (CIHI), total costs for all health care in Canada was reported in Chapter Three of this volume for 2004 at $130 billion CDN, about $4,200 per capita CDN. At the 2004 exchange rate of 1.3017, the figures are respectively US$100 billion and US$3,230 per capita. This was reported as a 5.9 percent increase in spending over 2003, and represented about 10% of Canada's GDP. However, compared to the OECD data for Canada in 2003, the increase in total health expenditures for 2004 was US$15.2 billion (from US$84.8 billion to US$100 billion) equal to an 18 percent increase. Whether the increase is 5.9 percent or 18 percent, it appears the federal and provincial governments made significant investment in their health system in 2004.

Canada does not have a national data base to track all health care expenditures, and it needs to develop one to track all mental health expenditures in particular. Five reasons these data are not available were discussed in Chapter Three of this volume. The Canadian Mental Health Association estimated that in the Province of Ontario 8.8 percent of its total health care budget on mental health services in 1998–1999. "Relative to prevalence estimates of 20 percent of the population experiencing mental disorders, the 8.8 percent of total health care budget in Ontario appears to be disproportionately low." Based on the total GDP of US$856.6 billion for 2003, 8.8 percent amounts to US $75.4 billion.

Dr. Arnett stated that the figure of 8.8 percent underestimates total mental health costs in the private sector. Counting both *direct* costs of mental health services in 1998 at $6.3 billion CDN and estimated *indirect* costs at $8.1 CDN, mental disorders constituted the third most costly health conditions in Canada, totaling 14.4 billion CDN (US$9.7 billion at the 1998 exchange rate of 1.484), and these costs continue to increase. Cost of addiction to alcohol and drugs, and costs in disability and loss of life are additional. Dr. Arnett suggested that the costs and ". . . expenditures clearly demonstrate the need for cost-effective mental health services in Canada."

Dr. Arnett identified five causes for the rising health care costs in Canada: First, the continued predominance of hospital-based mental health services, and secondly, rising costs of prescription drugs are major causes, as one might expect in this physician-dominated system characterized by a biomedical approach. Thirdly, these rising costs in turn cause the federal and provincial governments to resist diversifying services by insuring more and other mental health specialists, which only exacerbates the inefficiency by limiting outpatient services. Fourthly, integrated, collaborative relationships between family physicians and psychiatrists were recommended by the Romanov Commission (2002) and the Senate Evaluation (2004) to facilitate more efficient use of resources. In practice this model of "shared care" has been disappointing five years after it was affirmed in principle by the professional organizations of Canadian Psychiatry and Family Medicine. Fifthly, Canada has taken a lead in identifying work-life conflicts of four types as significant causes of mental health costs. These types of work-life conflicts include role overload, work to family interference, family to work interference, and caregiver strain, and create additional economic costs in lost productivity and disability payments by employers.

The most costly services (inpatient psychiatric services) continue to dominate mental health spending in Canada. In Ontario in 1998–1999, for every dollar spent on community-based mental health services, 3.5 dollars were spent on hospital-based mental health services. Funds were spent increasingly on psychiatric units in general medical hospitals and decreasingly in the independent psychiatric hospitals.

"Administrative costs are about 6.5 percent to seven percent of total health care expenditures, however, this figure underestimates administration expenses as the increasing emphasis on accountability requires line staff to spend increasing amounts of time completing forms and responding to requests for information. This time is not always captured in its entirety in estimates of administration time and costs."

Efficiency. On the WHO (2000) efficiency ratings of overall system performance, Canada (30th) ranked third among our four countries (Table 6.8). It is generally considered to be more efficient (cost-effective) to *prevent* mental illness and substance abuse than to treat these disorders. That observation was noted in 1974 by Marc LaLonde, as the federal government's Minister of Health and Welfare in a paper entitled, *A New Perspective of the Health of Canadians.* His comments have been largely ignored, and ". . . the efforts by government at all levels in Canada have been nothing short of anemic in terms of health promotion and illness prevention strategies."

Dr. Arnett concluded:

> With annual per capita expenditures on [all] health care of nearly $4,100 CDN (US$3,150 at the 2004 exchange rate of 1.3017), Canada is one of the top six spenders on health care among OECD countries. However, the country lacks and very much needs a financial data base for mental health care that would permit an accurate tracking of mental health expenditures across jurisdictions in Canada. The absence of such information makes it difficult to assess the efficiency of the mental health system.

Dr. Arnett reported the widely-held perception that mental health services are underfunded. He also noted that there is an inefficient time lag of information transfer of published research on effective clinical services and systems, and less effective treatments remain in place for an inordinate time.

Cost Containment Strategies. Canada has employed both supply-side and demand-side cost containment strategies. One of the *supply side strategies* has been to limit the *volume* of all mental health care services by restricting Medicare payments to "medically necessary, insured" conditions. The volume of inpatient services has been limited also by closing mental health hospitals and "replacing" them with fewer total psychiatric beds in general medical hospitals. Moreover, the supply of services has been restricted by insufficient funding of community-based services, resulting in high recidivism rates in general-medical hospitals. Finally, funding for graduate level work in mental health fields other than psychiatry is less than for medical education generally and for psychiatric training in particular.

There have been persistent demands over the years by the Provinces for more money from the federal government to pay for rising health care costs, and with some merit to their demands. Health care expenditures account for about 40 percent of provincial government expenditures versus about 16 percent by the federal government.

Two additional *supply side strategies* have been to limit mental health services by restricting Medicare reimbursements to physicians and by limiting budget allocations to hospitals. Initially, costs were contained by provincial governments negotiating physician fees and placing hospitals on global budgets to manage as they saw fit. More recently, provincial health ministries have expanded their roles from setting policy and priorities to mandating specific programs to be instituted by hospitals, and recommending, if not requiring specific personnel be hired. Is this increased control and micromanagement efficient? Why has it been necessary? Dr. Arnett raises the concern that government leaders may be confounding political pressures with long term health priorities.

Another major *supply-side* strategy for containing costs in Canada, supported by the dominant medical profession, has been to exclude from Medicare coverage the outpatient mental health services provided by all mental health specialists who are not physicians, including both regulated professions such as psychologists, social workers, occupational therapists, and unregulated professions such as marriage and family therapists, counselors, addiction counselors.

As one might predict, pharmacotherapy is the predominant intervention in mental health care in the Canadian system, which privileges family physicians first, psychiatrists second, and marginalizes allied mental health specialists. Our Canadian expert has argued that the primary problem underlying the Canadian mental health system is the dominance of the biomedical model and national insurance coverage of only *medically* necessary conditions treated exclusively by physicians. Dr. Arnett calls for a population-based, public health approach grounded in a broader biopsychosocial model to conceptualize mental health conditions and to justify the necessity of interventions of broader scope authorized by a wider range of mental health professions.

The major *demand-side* strategy to contain costs has been based on the population's ability to pay for private mental health services provided by nonphysician mental health specialists. About 80 percent of the costs for outpatient mental health services by psychologists, social workers and counselors must be paid out-of-pocket or by private individual or employment-based supplemental insurance. The same strategy could be viewed as a supply-side cost containment. Dr. Arnett concluded:

> Overall, given the high cost associated with mental health problems and the frequently long waiting times for services leads to one inescapable conclusion: Including (a) patient transfers from the mental hospitals to the general hospitals, (b) the near exclusive focus on the biomedical model of illness, (c) the retention of the basic illness philosophy that was embodied in the mental hospitals, and (d) minimal effort at illness prevention and health promotion, the manner in which mental health problems have been dealt with to date is both inefficient and unsustainable in the long term.

United States' Costs and Efficiency

Costs. The OECD data for 2003 (Table 6.9) reported a total GDP of US$10,951.3 billion. Total expenditure on health accounted for 15.0 percent of GDP (an estimated $1,642.7 billion), of which 44.4 percent was public expenditures (an estimated $729 billion). Total health expenditures per capita were $5,635. The average growth rate in total health expenditures from 1998–2003 was 4.6 percent.

The United States General Accountability Office (GAO, 2000) estimated that in 1997 $73 billion was spent on *mental health* services. Another $78.6 billion was attributed to indirect costs such as lost productivity. By the year 2001, spending for mental health and substance abuse (MHSA) treatment in the United States totaled $104 billion, representing 7.6 percent of all health care spending of $1.4 trillion in 2001 (Mark, Coffey, Vandivort-Warren et al. 2005, W5-133). Of the total MHSA spending, $85 billion (82%) was for mental health and $18 billion (18%) was for substance abuse in 2001. The increase in spending for mental health services alone from 1997 ($73 billion) to 2001 ($85 billion) was $12 billion. The average annual growth rate for the decade (1991–2001) was 5.7 percent for mental health and 4.8 percent for substance abuse care, compared to a rate of 6.5 percent for all health care spending. The share of total health care spending in 2001 was 7.6 percent for MHSA combined, 6.2 percent for mental health alone, and 1.3 percent for substance abuse alone (SAMSHA, 2004, as cited by Mark et al. 2005, pp. W5-135-136).

Numerous explanations have been offered for the continued, rising high costs of health care and mental health care in America. Anderson et al. (2005) noted that:

> Observers and analysts are divided about whether prices, technology, aging, waste, inefficiency, the legal system, new disease patterns, corporate consolidation, or profligate providers and consumers are chiefly to blame for the rate of climb. Nor is there much sign of consensus about how to slow the trend. The system has turned decisively toward increased cost sharing, but without any assurance that this strategy will abate growth or merely relocate the burden. (p. 903)

Efficiency. On the WHO (2000) efficiency ratings of overall system performance, the United States (37th) ranked the lowest among our four countries (Table 6.8). The authors of our chapter on the United States system wrote:

> To reduce their costs for mental health patients, most states closed their state mental health/mental retardation institutions beginning in the 1950s. It took about a decade, however, before Medicaid (1965) paid for alternative residential care facilities and small group homes to support deinstitutionalized mentally ill or retarded. Moreover, the transition to community mental health care was not only inefficient; it was a failure.

According to OECD Health Data 2005, June 05, the availability of acute inpatient beds in all hospitals in the United states in 2003 was 2.8/1,000 population, lower than Norway (3.1), Canada (3.2), and the United Kingdom (3.7). *The Mental Health Atlas – 2005* (WHO, 2005a) listed the number of psychiatric beds per 10,000 population as follows: Canada (19.3), Norway (12), United States (7.7), and Great Britain (5.8). Canada has proportionately more psychiatric beds than the United States in both mental and general hospitals, and in other settings. Nevertheless, as Mechanic (1999) noted, inefficient allocations to state mental hospitals in the United States persist. Wang et al. (2005b, p. 634) noted another cause of inefficiency, namely the overutilization of outpatient mental services by individuals with no mental disorder. They suggested that many services are being consumed unnecessarily by people without apparent mental disorders (accounting for nearly one-third of all visits).

Estimates of *administrative costs* of the U.S. health care system range widely from $159 billion to $209 billion per year. Estimates of all hospital administrative costs run at about 25 percent. The number of administrative personnel in the mental health system is unknown, but data for the health care labor force as a whole from the Bureau of Labor Statistics suggest a disproportionate increase has occurred in health administrative personnel relative to physicians and nurses. During the expansion of managed care organizations between 1970 and 1998, the number of health administrators increased more than 24 fold, while the number of physicians and other clinical personnel increased about 2.5 fold. For the same time period, total health care employment in the United States grew 149 percent, while the number of managers in health care grew 2,348 percent. If the United States reduced its health administration work force to Canada's levels (on a per capita basis), it would employ about 1.4 million fewer managers and clerical staff (cited by PNHP, 2002).

Of the two major federal health insurance programs for civilians, Medicare and Medicaid, the latter covers about 30 percent of the American population. Because Medicaid is means-tested, significant administrative costs are incurred to determine if individuals' income and assets make them eligible. Moreover, means-testing is inefficient because it encourages evasion of reported income, and it generates discontinuity of coverage as recipients move into and out of eligibility (Fuchs and Emmanuel, 2005). These findings are particularly germane to the mental health system in light of Dr. Hall's report that receiving means-tested benefits in Britain was associated with a greatly increased likelihood of having a mental illness, most likely due to lower household income of those receiving such benefits (ONS, 2003).

Typical estimates of administrative costs quoted by *private* health plans in the U.S. range from 10 to 15 percent. It is somewhat difficult to determine the accuracy of such estimates because these data are considered by many private health plans to be privileged, commercial information, and most of the health plans want to present a favorable image to regulators and the public as very efficient organizations. Moreover, the amounts that regulated health plans report to governmental agencies will vary according to the reporting formula. As an example, health maintenance organizations (HMOs) registered with the Minnesota state department of health reported average administrative costs in 1996 of only about eight percent. By contrast, an independent audit sponsored by the Minnesota Physician-Patient Alliance on 1996 financial data of the three largest HMOs operating in the state yielded an estimate closer to 31 percent, and less than 4 percent of HMO expenditures were for mental health services (MPPA, 1998). The striking difference was an anomaly in the reporting requirements, which allowed these nonprofit HMOs to count administrative personnel and support services as if they were direct health care services providers.

One of the most efficient health plans operating in the United States is not in the private sector, but in the public sector. Administrative costs of the Medicare program have been reported by the U. S. General Accounting Office (1994) to be consistently under three percent. It seems that when it comes to health care insurance, the government is a more efficient vendor, largely because it does not spend the billions of dollars on marketing, risk assessments, duplicated billing departments, nor on campaign financing and lobbying elected officials as private health corporations spend.

At the federal level in the public sector, the *Health Insurance Portability and Accountability Act* of 1996 (HIPAA) included a section on Administrative Simplification (Title 11, Subtitle F). The aim of this policy was to improve efficiency in health care delivery through standardized electronic data exchange while simultaneously protecting the confidentiality and security of health information through enforceable standards. Whether the intended efficiencies will be achieved awaits full evaluation (Turner and Foong, 2003).

A second example of improved efficiency of operations in a federal government program is the Veterans Health Administration, which reduced costs for mental health services by 21 percent from 1995–2001, largely by emphasizing outpatient mental health services.

Cost Containment Strategies. In its predominantly private sector of health care, the United States seems to have opted for *demand-side* controls of cost. This strategy of shifting costs to the users of services is rationalized by an economic *theory of moral hazard*, to wit, that possession of health insurance itself can have the paradoxical effect of producing risky and wasteful behavior. The notion seems to be that to offset this tendency toward wasteful overutilization due to third party insurance, consumers need to be given incentives to use the health-care system more efficiently by making them more responsible for a share of the costs. The theory of moral hazard is the primary justification for the Bush Administration's proposal of Health Savings Accounts. The implication is that Americans have too much health insurance; hence, broadening insurance coverage for the nearly 46 million uninsured would be aggravating the problem of wasteful overutilization. To the reader this might seem like just another example of political smoke and mirrors, if not blatant hypocrisy. Unfortunately, it has been taken seriously by some economists and politicians alike.

> Nyman, an economist at the University of Minnesota, says that the fear of moral hazard seems to lie behind the thicket of co-payments and deductibles and utilization reviews which characterizes the American health-insurance system.... The moral-hazard argument makes sense, however, only if we consume health care in the same way that we consume other consumer goods, and to economists like Nyman this assumption is plainly absurd. (Gladwell, 2005, p. 46)

Because cost is a function of both price and volume, some health policy experts argue that the major cause of rising health care costs is the price (Gilmer and Kronick, 2005, W5-143), while other health economists (McGuire and Serra, 2005) argue that it is the increasing volume due to high utilization by an aging population of expensive medical technologies and prescription medications. By and large, *managed care strategies* have controlled costs by limiting (rationing) the volume of services (e.g., number of inpatient days, number of outpatient visits) through prior, concurrent, or even retrospective utilization reviews leading to provider profiling, and more recently, through case management strategies focusing on the smaller number of high service users, especially the seriously and persistently mentally ill. A second cost-containing strategy has been to control the prices (fees) by establishing discounted fees and capitation arrangements, thereby shifting financial risk from the health plan to the provider and creating an incentive for undertreatment. According to Maxwell and Temin (2002), most American employers who pay for health insurance have not adopted managed competition as the primary method of cost-containment.

In the private sector, employers pay the greatest share of the costs of health insurance. About 55 percent of Americans receive their health insurance through their place of employment (Fuchs and Emanuel, 2005). In a survey sponsored by the United States Chamber of Commerce, about 11 percent of every payroll dollar of U. S. businesses was spent on health care benefits in 2002 (U. S. Chamber of Commerce, 2003).

Following the principle that the easiest way to contain costs is to shift them to someone else, American employers have been shifting costs for health insurance increasingly to employees. A recent example of cost-shifting by employers is the announcement by General Motors (GM) that the company would pay less for health care for unionized workers and retirees (Star Tribune, 10/18/05, p. D3). Presently, GM pays for health care for about 750,000 American wage earners, retirees, and their dependents. It is one of the major private payers for health insurance in the country, with an expenditure of $5.6 billion in 2005. With a 25 percent reduction in health care liabilities for GM's retirees, the company expects to save $15 billion over a seven-year period. Cash savings to the company are estimated at about $1 billion per year. According to the company, hourly wage earners unionized as the United Auto Workers now pay only seven percent of their health care costs, whereas salaried employees pay 27 percent. Union members will have to absorb increased costs, and retirees will have to pay for supplemental health insurance. If they cannot afford the increase, these hourly wage earners will need to rely upon their spouse's health insurance, or become uninsured and increase the demand upon public sector insurance and services. What is good for General Motors is not necessarily good for the country, even if "the business of America is business."

Although premiums leveled off during the latter half of the 1990s, double-digit inflation has returned. Based on a national, employer health benefits survey, Gabel et al. (2003) reported that the cost of health insurance to employees rose 13.9 percent from 2002 to 2003, the highest rate of increase since 1990. "Employers indicate little confidence in any future strategies for controlling health care costs" (p. 117).

In the face of rising premiums for private health insurance plans, America's voluntary, employment-based health insurance system in the private sector is unsustainable for both employers and employees alike. Although the 1990s was a decade of relative prosperity, the percentage of Americans without health insurance coverage rose over 17 percent, due largely to the decline in coverage offered by employers (Farber and Levy, 2000; Lewin Group, 1998). Based on national samples in 1989–1991 and 1998–2000, Chernew, Cutler, and Keenan (2005) determined that "more than half of the decline in coverage rates experienced over the 1990s is attributable to the increase in health insurance premiums.... Changes in economic and demographic factors had little net effect" (p. 1021).

Strategies for Rationing of Limited Resources

Every health care system must deal with both the needs and demands for health care services and simultaneously with the limited resources available to finance these services. With aging populations and high costs of both medical technology and prescription drugs, along with increased prevalence of chronic diseases including AIDS, cancer, and coronary disease (and serious mental disorders), some strategy is required for the allocation of the country's limited resources. Consequently, discussion of this topic needs to be framed not by the question of whether or not a health care system rations services, but *how* it rations its limited resources to pay for those services, and *who* makes the rationing decisions for whom? Obviously, any form of rationing within the overall health care system is likely to limit access to the mental health services as well as medical services.

At best, rationing of resources is a public policy strategy for achieving socially defined priorities and for distributing a public good fairly (WHO, 2000, pp. 58–60). It has been construed typically in a more narrow sense as solely an economic strategy for containing costs. The basic economic formula is:

Cost = (price/unit) × (number of units purchased)

The two key variables for controlling costs are therefore price and volume. Most countries attempt to ration health care services by controlling both, but there are differences in emphasis. Three basic questions to ask about rationing strategies are (a) whether they encourage achievement of national health policies and priorities, (b) whether rationing decisions are made democratically with participation by users of health care services, and (c) whether the strategies used for rationing are fair to the population served.

Three procedures for controlling the *price* of services are setting limits on charges and fees for services (price controls), capitation arrangements for larger group practices, and placing hospitals and/or large group practices on budgets. The latter two payment methods also control *volume*, which is essentially a constraint on the supply of services. "Supply constraints include limiting the number of hospital beds that could be built; controls on the diffusion of medical technology; limits on the number of physicians; limits on what specialties physicians could enter; and drug formularies" (Anderson, Hussey, Frogner, and Waters, 2005, p. 906).

"Four different ways of rationing health interventions have been identified based on both the cost of an intervention and the number of interventions rationed: (a) rationing by not subsidizing or investing in high-cost interventions; (b) rationing by not subsidizing low-cost interventions; (c) rationing *all* interventions in the same population; and (d) rationing with no regular relation to either cost or frequency, so that rationing is more severe for *some* services than for others" (WHO, 2000, p. 60). While there may be no one best way, the fourth approach is guided more by explicit priority-setting based on identified health care needs of a population, and determined less by cost or utilization rates. If the priorities are chosen by elected representatives of the stakeholders and implemented according to some appropriate and consensual criteria, rationing is a strategy that can contribute to better performance of the mental health system. Examples of explicit rationing based on criteria determined consensually are found in Norway and the state of Oregon in the United States.

Rationing in England. England rations health care largely with *supply side controls.* The central government determines the amount of money that will be allocated to the National Health Service, initially through negotiations between the Chancellor of the Exchequer, who has responsibility for overall financial affairs and approval of all public expenditure, and the Secretary of State for Health, who heads the Department of Health. Allocations are disbursed through 28 Strategic Health Authorities to various "Trusts," which commission (purchase) services from various provider groups and hospitals. The central government controls the revenue allocations for the NHS operations as well as the amount of public funding for capital investments like hospitals and medical technology (e.g., operating rooms, MRIs, CAT scans).

Limiting financial, human, and capital resources creates problems in timely access to certain services in England. Emergency and other medically necessary interventions receive top priority, hence require less waiting time. However, residents might have to wait three to four months for elective surgeries such as hip replacements, cataract removal, hernia repair, and even kidney dialysis treatment (Graig, 1999, p. 159).

> In a recent survey about access to care, about a third of the population sampled in Australia, Canada, and the United Kingdom believed waiting times to be one of their two biggest health care problems. In these countries, the average wait for nonemergency surgery was more than one month, with between a quarter and a third of respondents reporting waiting more than four months. (Blendon, 2002)

According to King and Massialas (2005), one of the major motivations for people in Great Britain to purchase private medical insurance is to guarantee faster access to inpatient care by medical specialists. The fact that nearly 12 percent of the population possessed private insurance by the end of the year 2000 (Laing and Buisson, 2001) suggests that delayed treatment in the National Health Service is a significant source of dissatisfaction for nearly seven million residents. It seems likely that the waiting time for elective treatments is a major factor that accounts for the lowest ranking of Great Britain in the level of responsiveness of its health care system: Great Britain (26–27), Norway (7–8), Canada (7–8), and the United States (1). [See Table 6.1 this chapter and WHO (2000), Annex Table 1, pp. 152–155.] Limited choice of providers is likely to be another contributing factor to dissatisfaction.

This *rationing by queue* (waiting lists) has been necessary in England due to insufficient funding of the National Health Service, but this strategy has been favored also as a more equitable way of allocating limited resources than the U.S. system of rationing based upon the ability to pay either out-of-pocket or with private health insurance (Graig, 1999, pp. 159–160). From a British perspective, *delayed* access does not equate with the *denial* of access, which so many uninsured Americans seem to experience.

The current government has recognized this problem of delayed services, and it has increased funding of the National Health Service by seven percent in each year from 2002 to 2007 to reduce waiting times through extra funding of direct health services, increasing the supply of surgical suites and physicians, improving waiting list management, and by shifting some services to the private sector (Hurst and Siciliani, 2003, as cited by Anderson, Hussey, Frogner, and Waters, 2005, pp. 908 & 913; King and Mossialos, 2005).

British policy concerning mental health services includes consideration for the timeliness as well as the quality of services. The author of our British chapter reported no data on waiting times for individuals seeking *mental health* services, but he acknowledged that reducing the delays in both outpatient and inpatient services have become prominent political targets. The fact that several policy statements guiding the NHS address the standard of timeliness suggests delays in mental health services have been a significant problem. One example is the 2004 document, *Organizing and Delivering Psychological Therapies*. This policy holds local mental health service agencies and professionals accountable to making appropriate services "accessible in a reasonable time."

Rationing in Norway. Limiting capital investments, placing hospitals and other services on budgets, and limiting funding and positions for the education and training of mental health specialists are examples of *supply-side* strategies employed by the Norwegian central government. These strategies can be employed more effectively in Norway because the mental health system has been centralized under the Ministry of Health and Social Care.

Like England, Norway engages in *de facto* rationing by prioritizing the medical necessity/urgency of various conditions and placing lower priority conditions on waiting lists for treatment. A current estimate of waiting times for mental health services is about two months. Our Norwegian experts state:

> The waiting lists in the mental health services have increased in recent years, especially for admissions to hospital wards, which suggests that accessibility to the services has decreased, even if more patients than ever before are treated. The demand for treatment has increased to a still larger extent than the offer [supply]. There is a particular shortage of acute beds in mental health services, which in turn seems to be due to insufficient capacity of intermediate and long-term facilities, which delays the discharge of patients from acute psychiatric units. The District Psychiatric Centres should help solve this problem, but they are not yet fully operational.

Since timeliness is one of the important elements of the measure of responsiveness to a population's expectations, the WHO (2000) rankings are germane to the question of waiting times. Among our four countries, Norway (7–8) was tied with Canada (7–8) for second and third place relative to the United States (1) and Great Britain (26–27) (Table 6.1). One of the goals of the *Act on Health Enterprises* (2002) was to reduce waiting times for all health services.

The *demand-side* strategy of rationing by ability to pay is not a Norwegian strategy of cost-containment in the public national health insurance system as it is in the more dominant private sector systems in the United States and Canada. However, the fact that nearly 100 percent of costs for services provided in the small private sector must be paid out-of-pocket certainly discourages demand for those services. In Norway, health care services are viewed as a public good, not as a private commodity to be purchased in the marketplace by those who can afford it.

Rationing in Canada. Canada employs both supply-side and demand-side strategies to contain costs (*Economist*, May 23, 1998). Canada has limited the overall *supply* of inpatient beds available by closing larger mental hospitals and not providing sufficient capital investments for acute psychiatric beds in general medical hospitals. Secondly, it has limited reimbursement from the national insurance scheme for outpatient mental health services largely to physicians. Thirdly, underfunding of the mental health system was identified by the 2004 Senate Evaluation as a major cause for inequitable access to mental health services, especially for seriously and persistently mentally ill patients. Underfunding was implicated as a major cause for the deficiencies in services for adults, children, and adolescents as well. With about 40 percent of provincial budgets and 16 percent of federal expenditures devoted to all health care in Canada, there is resistance by provincial governments to increase funding for health care from their revenues.

The limited funding for mental health services appears to be part of a larger pattern of nearly a decade of cost-cutting under the present federal government. A national opinion poll released in November, 2005 by Ipsos Public Affairs Research indicated that Canadians consider their government-funded health care system their number one concern. The funding cuts have resulted in too few doctors and hospital beds, both of which account for a "wait-time crisis," illustrated by reports of six to seven hours waiting to see an emergency room physician (Webster, 2005).

Maintaining long waiting lists is a way to limit demand. One of the commonalities found among Great Britain, Canada, and Norway is that they all have varying degrees of *rationing by queues* (*Economist*, May 23, 1998). According to Dr. Arnett, "about half of the adult population who need [mental health] services must wait for eight weeks or more."

These waiting lists constitute a *de facto* rationing policy expressed through limited budgetary allocations for operations, restricted capital investments in health care facilities, and in controlled funding for the education and training of mental health professionals. The long waiting times to receive health care services is a major cause of dissatisfaction among Canadians, even though the majority of residents prefer their system to any other.

On the *demand* side, Canada employs rationing based on individuals' ability to pay in the private sector, since outpatient mental health services provided by nonphysician mental health professionals are not reimbursed by the national health insurance scheme, hence individuals and/or employers must purchase supplemental private health insurance or pay out-of-pocket.

Rationing in the United States. For many Americans, rationing has a very negative connotation of arbitrary denials of health care with an associated loss of freedom to choose which interventions to receive or not to receive, who will provide it, when, where and how. Particularly in American policy debates, caricaturing proposals for publicly-financed health reforms as tantamount to rationing is standard rhetoric by the private and corporate vested interests in the status quo. What many Americans fail to realize is that the voluntary insurance system in the private sector is rationing by ability to pay rather than rationing according to medical necessity and/or prioritizing by the severity of medical conditions.

It is simply an illusion to believe the American health care system is free of rationing; it must ration health care because of the limited resources invested in the health care system, even though the U.S. per capita health expenditures are the highest in the world. In the year 2002, for example, U. S. citizens spent $5,267 per capita for all health care, which was 53 percent more than any other country (Anderson, Hussey, Frogner, and Waters, 2005, p. 904). Comparable per capita expenditures in US$ adjusted for purchasing power parity were Norway ($3,083), Canada ($2,931), and Great Britain ($2,160). Presently, the $260+ billion military actions in Afganistan and Iraq, several billion dollars for recovery from the 2005 disasters from hurricanes Katrina and Rita, the substantial tax cuts that increase both the federal debt and interest payments on the debt, and the enormous trade deficits all constitute major financial barriers to investments in the health care system. However, the federal government (taxpayers) will be required to fund Medicare at a higher level by virtue of an aging population in America expected to double to about 77 million by 2011. Reductions in Medicare benefits and cost-shifting to beneficiaries will most likely occur. That seems to be the American way.

Rationing by controls placed on the *demand* for health care services has been the dominant strategy employed in the United States. Private insurance companies are allowed to develop variable benefit packages and to set premium prices to compete with other health plans to sell their products to employers, other groups and individuals. Most individuals in both private and public health plans pay a share of the premiums, incur annual deductibles, and make limited co-payments at the point of service. The notion has been that "consumer" demand will be limited by shifting the burden of costs increasingly to consumers, hence motivating them to be more selective in their utilization of health care services.

In the United States, health expenditures in the *private sector* exceed expenditures in the public sector by a ratio of about 55 percent to 45 percent, and the major strategy for allocating health care dollars in the private sector is rationing by *ability to pay*. Access to the system is significantly influenced by one's possession of health insurance, which is paid either by individuals or by their employers. Premiums for individuals are substantially higher and their premiums are generally paid with after-tax dollars, but nearly everyone who is able is paying.

Rationing by ability to pay is itself a regressive obstacle to equitable access because people with lower incomes pay a higher proportion of their income for health care and some cannot pay at all. A recent and shocking statistic is that "... the average cost of family coverage now exceeds the average yearly income of minimum-wage Americans" (Gabel et al., 2005, p. 1237). The price of private health insurance is a major factor in explaining the rising number of uninsured Americans, which is projected to increase by about 10 million to 56 million uninsured by 2013 (Gilmer and Kronick, 2005, W5-143). Polsky, Stein, Nicholson, and Bundorf (2005) provided evidence that the higher premiums passed on to employees increases the odds that they will decline the health insurance offered by their employer and that these employees will remain uninsured. In 2001, an estimated 1.9 to 2.2 million Americans (filers plus dependents) filed for bankruptcy because of the costs of their health care, though 75.7 percent of them had insurance at the start of illness (Himmelstein, Warren, Thorne, and Woolhandler, 2005).

Rationing health care by prices means that who gets what health care services depends not only on how much those services are valued by people, but on who has the means to buy them in the marketplace. In this *market-driven rationing*, "priorities are not set by anyone, but emerge from the play of the market. As indicated, this is almost the worst possible way to determine who gets which health services. Every health system therefore confronts the question of what other means to use, when resources are inadequate to needs or wants" (WHO, 2000, p. 58).

Related to the equity of access is the question of *who decides* what should be covered, and how much users should pay. The private sector in the United States is primarily a voluntary, employment-based health insurance system. In this sector, it is the owners and executives of businesses who negotiate with health plan managers to determine benefit packages for employees, usually with limited options, if health insurance is a benefit at all. Consequently, except in some settings where employee unions provide group health insurance, rationing decisions in the private sector are made primarily by a small number of unelected corporate managers with common interests in reducing costs to increase profits in a competitive marketplace, for which managers receive substantial salaries and bonuses. A recent survey of these managers indicated they were significantly less concerned about the quality of health care services provided to their employees than the employers' cost to purchase health plans (Gabel et al. 2003).

In the *public sector*, national policy decisions are made by elected congressmen and federal government administrations, both of which are subjected to massive lobbying by very powerful and wealthy, special interest groups. In America, money is the mother's milk of politics. Campaign financing by self-serving constituents leads to inordinate access and influence upon the federal government, but results in unequal access for the population to both the health and mental health systems (Center for Public Integrity, 1995a, 1995b; Common Cause, 1992).

The major strategies for cost containment used by federal and state programs are supply-side mechanisms. Benefits and funding are limited, eligibility requirements restrict coverage to a limited segment of the population, and increasingly, federal and state programs are carving out mental health care to be managed by private health plans, including those that specialize in such care, which are called Managed Behavioral Health Organizations (MBHOs). Operating mostly as for-profit corporations, MBHOs have used strategies such as prior and concurrent utilization review to reduce the volume of mental health services, particularly inpatient mental health care, and to reduce the number of outpatient visits to their panel of preferred providers, who also must accept the health plan's discounted fee schedule, allegedly compensated with a steady volume of referrals. Miller (1966a, 1966b) commented on the "invisible rationing" procedures employed by MBHOs, namely a substantial reduction in the number of outpatient sessions resulting in "therapy ultra-lite." An extreme example is the "case rate" formula of about $325 paid to "preferred providers" by an HMO in Minnesota as the capitation rate for up to twenty sessions of outpatient psychotherapy without balance billing.

Although the United States has no formal system of patient waiting lists, its predominant method of rationing by ability to pay, coupled with high priced health care produce *de facto* delays in receiving treatment.

Delayed treatment has been documented even among low income families receiving public health services on a sliding fee scale. In a survey of a large sample of users of primary health care in the public health system in Los Angeles, 33 percent reported delaying needed medical care during the preceding 12 months, 25 percent reported an unmet need for care because of competing expenses for food, shelter, or clothing, and 46 percent had either delayed or gone without care (Diamont et al. 2004). Other studies have reported the following:

> Uninsured adults are more likely to delay seeking care than those who are insured . . ., less likely to receive preventive and screening services . . ., less likely to be referred by primary care physicians for other health services. . . . Delayed or nonreceipt of medical care may result in more serious illness for the patient, increased complications, a worse prognosis, and longer hospital stays. . . . (Diamont et al. 2004, p. 783)

In both the public and private sectors, a limited supply and uneven distribution of health care providers reduce demand because people must travel a longer distance to receive services. Fortney, Steffick, Burgess, Maciejewski, and Peterson (2005) found that reducing the distance to primary care facilities was a significant and substantial predictor of an increase in primary care visits by American Veterans 1995–1999. The distance problem was exacerbated for rural residents between 1990 and 2000, because 24.7 percent of nonmetropolitan counties lost primary care physicians, compared with seven percent of metropolitan counties (Ricketts, 2005).

An example from this author's experience indicates that this form of limited and uneven supply occurs in the United States as in other countries. The author grew up in a small town in central Minnesota, where two doctors served about 1,700 town people and more from surrounding rural areas. There was a community hospital with visiting medical specialists. When both physicians retired, the community could not find replacements, and the hospital was converted into a nursing home. The closest general medical clinic and hospital is about seven miles away in a neighboring town. The closest specialty hospitals are about 50 miles away in Minneapolis-St. Paul.

This problem of uneven distribution of health care professionals is also evident in mental health specialties. In 1997 about 20 percent of nonmetropolitan areas in the United States had no mental health professional, and of those areas designated as a "health professional shortage area," 76 percent were rural counties (Hartley, Bird, and Dempry, 1999, as cited by Ricketts, 2005).

Financing and Fairness

Financing a health care system involves three major functions: revenue collections, pooling of resources, and purchasing of services. All three functions have variable impacts upon expenditures and provider behavior. For example, the tax rate for a national health insurance program will influence total revenues available. Moreover, different mechanisms of purchasing services (paying providers) will result in different provider behaviors. An example is how a fee-for-service system will encourage delivery of high quality services responsive to legitimate population expectations, but it does less to encourage providers to contain costs or to focus on the prevention of health problems (WHO, 2000, 106).

Financing a health care system can be done publicly, privately, or by a combination of both sources. *Public* financing is generally through some tax revenues levied by the government as a part of a national health insurance scheme (Canada) or to fund a national health service (Britain and Norway). The taxes may be specified as contributions to the national health insurance plan, or the health care system may be funded from general tax revenues. *Private* financing is largely through premiums paid by employers, employees, or individuals to private insurance companies or health plans to cover most of the costs incurred for health services. Usually there are also out-of-pocket expenses such as deductibles, co-insurance, and/or co-payments at the point of service.

Fair Financing Defined

Fair financing is one of the three universal goals by which the WHO compared health care systems in its annual report on improving health care systems. "Fair financing in health systems means that the risks each household faces due to the costs of the health system are distributed according to ability to pay rather than to the risk of illness: a fairly financed system ensures financial protection for everyone" (WHO, 2000, p. 35).

A system of fair financing accomplishes two goals: First, it protects families from exposure to large *unexpected* expenses, which have to be paid out-of-pocket at the point of service utilization. Second, out-of-pocket payments will be *progressive*, in which those most able to contribute, pay proportionately more than those least able to pay. Fair financing arrangements would ensure that all citizens are not denied access to quality care because they cannot afford it.

The purpose of health financing is to make funding available, as well as to set the right financial incentives for providers, to ensure that all individuals have access to effective public health and personal health care. This means reducing or eliminating the possibility that an individual will be unable to pay for such care, or will be impoverished as a result of trying to do so. (WHO, 2000, p. 95)

The system for financing is critical because it affects both the equity and efficiency of the health care system. The most important determinant of how fairly a health system is financed is the proportion of total spending through prepayment as opposed to out-of-pocket payments. Moreover,

how these revenues are collected therefore has a great impact on the equity of the system . . . it also matters greatly how the revenues are combined so as to share risks: how many pools there are, how large they are, whether inclusion is voluntary or mandatory, whether exclusion is allowed, what degree and kind of competition exists among pools, and whether, in the case of competing pools, there are mechanisms to compensate for differences in risk and in capacity to pay. All these features affect the fairness of the system, but they also help determine how efficiently it operates. (WHO, 2000, p. 113)

Three financing functions defined. As noted previously, financing a health care system involves performance of three functions: Revenue collection, pooling of resources, and purchasing. The WHO (2000) descriptions of these functions are as follows: *Revenue collection* is "the process by which the health system receives money from households and organizations or companies, as well as from donors" (p. 95). Revenues can be collected through (a) general taxation, (b) mandated social health insurance contributions (usually based on salary rather than health risk), (c) out-of-pocket payments and (d) donations (usually to poorer countries, but also from charitable organizations to individuals). *Pooling of resources* is "the accumulation and management of revenues in such a way as to ensure that the risk of having to pay for health care is borne by all members of the pool and not by each contributor individually" (p. 96). The purpose of this insurance function is to share the financial risk associated with health interventions for which the need is uncertain. *Purchasing* is "the process by which pooled funds are paid to providers in order to deliver a specified or unspecified set of health interventions" (p. 97).

The performance of all three functions will influence the equity and efficiency of the health care system, both its absolute levels of goal attainment and its performance relative to financing afforded the system for operations and capital investment. Moreover, to protect people financially the fairest way possible, and to ensure they have access to health care services, all three interrelated functions of health system financing need to be considered: revenue collection, pooling of resources, and purchasing of interventions. While there does not appear to be a consensus on an optimal level of health care expenditure (McGuire and Serra, 2005), the fairness of financing needs to be discussed in the context of comparative health expenditure data and the proportion of public vs. private financing.

Financing the British System

On the goal of fairness of financial contribution to the health care system for the year 1997, the WHO (2000) ranked Britain (8–11) and Norway (8–11) equally, moderately higher than Canada (17–19), and substantially higher than the United States (54–55) (Table 6.1).

In Great Britain, *revenue collection* is predominantly through general taxation, though in recent years more reliance has been placed on income from national insurance contributions, and patient charges for certain categories of services (such as prescription drugs). The revenues are *pooled* centrally by the Department of Health. The funds are allocated through 28 Strategic Health Authorities to about 200 Primary Care Trusts, which *purchase* services that are *provided* through the National Health Service by individual provider Trusts (including mental health provider groups) and Local Implementation Teams.

As indicated in Table 1.2, the total expenditures on all health care by Great Britain for 2002 as a percent of GDP were 7.7 percent. As a percent of the total health care expenditures, the government spent 83.4 percent on health, which ranks Great Britain equal to Norway at 83.5 percent. The percent of the total of all *government* expenditures spent on health was 15.8 percent the same year.

The 83.5 percent of total health expenditures in Great Britain spent by the general government indicates that the National Health Service (NHS) is funded overwhelmingly by the government-collected revenues. Minor funding of health care services is provided by health insurance schemes (12%) or personal spending (Laing and Buissan, 2001). Health care in Britain is construed primarily as a social good, not as a private or commercial commodity to be bought and sold in the marketplace.

Allocations of government funding to individual Primary Care Trusts are made to cover operational costs on a "weighted capitation" basis with the goal of producing a targeted fair share for each part of the country. Since 2003–2004, the capitation formula takes into account both indicators of social deprivation and unmet need. According to the Healthcare Financial Management Association (HFMA) (2004),

> the allocation of funds considers the following components, which account for variable percentages of the total allocations (given in parentheses): hospital and community health services (82.8%); prescription drugs (14.1%); cash-limited, general medical services for GPs' practice staff, premises, and computer costs (2.5%); HIV/Aids treatment (0.7%). A fifth component term "non-cash limited general medical services" pays for health care providers who work as independent contractors, and are not directly employed by the NHS.

The process by which a Primary Care Trust (PCT) will purchase services for its listed patients is called *commissioning*. This is really a process of negotiating agreements to pay service providers to meet the health needs of a segment of the population for which the PCT is responsible. The reader is referred to Chapter Two for detailed discussion of this process and the levels of commissioning.

In general, the flow of financing for the health care system in Britain begins with the central government's collection and pooling of national insurance taxes and general tax revenues. The revenues are distributed by the central government under the auspices of the Department of Health to 28 Strategic Health Authorities (SHAs). Each of the SHAs allocates funding to the six to ten Primary Care Trusts (PCTs) for which they are responsible. The PCTs provide primary care services and purchase services from other individual provider trusts including specialist (e.g., mental health) and hospital services for the list of patients under the PCT's care. There are some initiatives and specialized services funded directly by the central government.

Capital expenditures on equipment and facilities (other than routine maintenance) are financed directly through the central government, and since 1992, secondarily through private funding. A persistent problem of underfunding of the NHS has placed budgetary limits on both capital expenditures for medical technology and operational expenditures for certain forms of treatment (Graig, 1999, p. 172). One consequence is rationing by *queues*, that is, waiting lists – a topic addressed earlier in this chapter.

The National Health Service was designed to be fairly financed by general tax revenues, and to provide health care services free to patients at the point of service. The judgment of our expert from Great Britain is that "public funding is a fair and efficient way to provide a comprehensive, high quality service, based on need, and not on the ability to pay."

Financing the Norwegian System

Partly because the tax base for revenues is the entire working population, pooled by the central government, and disbursed through publicly run institutions and services, Norway has been ranked high among the four countries on the goal of fairness of financial contribution to the health system for the year 1997. Norway (8–11) was ranked equally high with Great Britain (8–11), higher than Canada (17–19) and much higher than the United States (54–55) (Table 6.1).

In Norway, *revenue collections* for the health care system come primarily from general public revenues, and secondarily from mandated social insurance taxes. There is very little private insurance or out-of-pocket expense. The public revenues are *pooled centrally* through the Ministry of Health and Social Care, and distributed through regional authorities, which *purchase* health services from the majority of providers who are salaried employees of the government-owned Health Enterprises, or from a smaller group of private practitioners with "operative agreements" with the Health Enterprises.

As indicated in Table 1.2, total expenditures on health as a percent of GDP was 9.6 percent for Norway in 2002. *Governmental* expenditures accounted for 83.5 percent of all *total* health expenditures, which ranks Norway with Britain (83.4%) as the highest among the four countries in governmental expenditures. The Norwegian government's expenditure on health as a percent of total *government* expenditures was 18.1 percent for the same year.

The National Insurance Scheme is financed by contributions from everyone who earns an income. Employees earning NOK 23,000 (US$ 3,412 at 2005 exchange rate of 6.740) or more in gross annual wages pay about 7.8 percent of their gross wages to the National Insurance Scheme. Workers earning less than NOK 23,000 (US$ 3,412) pay no health insurance tax. The percent paid by employers ranges from zero percent to 14.1 percent of paid wages depending upon the level of economic development of the geographic region in which they operate. Norway has a progressive income tax up to 49 percent of income at higher levels, but regressive sales taxes of 23 percent (Dregni, 2005, p. 19).

A portion of these tax revenues collected and pooled by the central government is allocated to finance the mental health services. For example, for the year 2002, 31 percent of gross revenues for psychiatric institutions came from reimbursement from the National Insurance Administration, 32 percent from earmarked grants from the central government, and 23 percent reimbursement of paid sick leave, for a total of 85 percent. Norway has a publicly financed health care system.

Both the financing and delivery systems in Norway are predominantly public systems. As noted by our Norwegian authors:

> The financing system in Norway is not an insurance-based system. Only a small amount of the expense is covered by the National Insurance Scheme or by private/voluntary insurances. The public health services are financed in the same way as other State activities, by revenues for instance from the oil production, taxation on income, and VAT [value added tax]. Most providers serve as paid employees of the government-financed system [like Great Britain]. User fees, or out-of-the pocket money, play a marginal role. Private/voluntary insurance also plays a very limited role for mental health care. All mental health services are therefore in principle public services financed primarily by the government and the municipalities.

Our Norwegian authors also noted:

> There is no private sector in the mental health services in Norway. A private practitioner is part of, and incorporated into the public system, often through an operative agreement as a contracted provider, and reimbursed by the publicly financed system. Consequently, it would not be really accurate to present a public and a private sector of mental health services in Norway as if they were separate.... The financing and functioning of mental health services in Norway are therefore simple to understand and analyze: there is only one "sector" – the public one – financed by taxes and contributions from employees, self-employed persons, employers' contributions, and by contributions from the State/Government.

Moreover, expenditures are mainly channeled through publicly run institutions and services, which account for 90 percent of the total costs. About 95 percent of all funding originates from the central government in the form of grants and reimbursements for outpatient services.

The central government administers the specialist health services with the help of a New Public Management, inspired by competition in a more deregulated and competitive market. The municipalities are responsible for providing *primary* health care and social services, including primary mental health care services. These services are financed through local taxes (income tax), federal government block grants, special government reimbursement grants and fees.

To enable the NMHP to achieve its goals, the central government authorized a grant of NOK 6.3 billion (US$834 million at an exchange rate of 7.552 for the year 1998). Moreover, national subsidies earmarked for mental health operations will be increased by NOK 4.6 billion (1998 US$609 million) through 2008 compared to 1998 levels, and will not require any financing by county or local municipalities.

The Norwegian mental health system protects all of its citizens from unexpected costs due to mental disorders as well as medical conditions. The financing principle seems to be the following: Everyone contributes so that everyone can receive comprehensive health care services. Outpatient health and mental health services provided by private practitioners are not, however, free at the point of service in Norway. Co-payments for visiting a specialist (psychiatrist or psychologist) depend on the specialist's contract with the Health Enterprise. If the private practitioner has an operative agreement with the municipality or the health enterprises, the patient pays only part of the total cost for the visit. The specialist is reimbursed by the National Insurance Scheme, which covers the main part of the expenses. There are certain exemptions from cost-sharing, for example, children under the age of 18 make no co-payments for mental health services.

Our Norwegian experts believe the present problem for Norway is not first and foremost a lack of funding, but to persuade service providers to function according to the NMHP objectives and policies. Mental health specialists are not accustomed to providing services in a new kind of community and cooperative delivery system outside the institutions. There is a general lack of "ideology" or theory for this kind of community mental health approach. More money or higher funding is not likely to solve this problem. It may take a new generation of providers whose education is more community-oriented, and who are trained in listening to the patients' voice.

Financing the Canadian System

On the goal of fairness of financial contribution to the health care system for the year 1997, the WHO ranked Canada (17–19) third among the four countries included in this study, lower than Great Britain (8–11) and Norway (8–11), but much higher than the United States (54–55) (Table 6.1).

Canada's *revenue collection* for its national health insurance financing is through mandated social insurance payments deducted as payroll taxes. Private insurance and out-of-pocket payments are very small *sources* of revenues for hospital and medical services, though they account for more than 80 percent of payments for outpatient mental health services provided by nonphysicians. The public revenues are *pooled centrally* by the Ministry of Health and dispersed through the Provinces, which also collect revenues from their residents. The Provinces *purchase* or reimburse the services provided by physicians.

As indicated in Table 1.2, total health expenditures as a percent of GDP for Canada was 9.6 percent in 2002. The percentage of total health expenditures by the *government* was quite high in 2002 – 69.9 percent, ranking as the third highest of the four countries after Norway at 83.5 percent and Great Britain at 83.4 percent. The government's expenditure on health as a percent of total *government* expenditures was 15.9 percent. Canada's national health insurance system is publicly financed.

Public tax revenues collected by Provinces and Territories help to fund the health care system, in addition to federal government transfers of money and tax points to the Provinces. About 70 percent of all health care expenditures in Canada are paid by federal/provincial governments. The joint financing by the federal and provincial/territorial governments makes Canada's Medicare program more like the Medicaid program in the United States.

Under Canada's Medicare program (established nationwide in 1972), the existing fee-for-service billing arrangement for physicians was maintained, but the government became the single payer of both hospitals and physicians' charges rather than individual citizens' out-of-pocket payments or third-party reimbursements by private insurance companies. Physician fees are negotiated, and if necessary resolved through binding arbitration, hence provincial governments cannot dictate fee schedules or pay physicians whatever the government chooses to pay.

Private insurance companies have been prohibited from offering duplicate coverage provided through the national insurance plan until the Supreme Court decision in early June, 2005 (*Chaoulli* v. *Quebec Attorney General*). Dr. Arnett reported the following in a personal communication:

The Supreme Court essentially ruled that Quebec could not prohibit the purchase of private insurance for an insured service if that service was not provided by the Quebec health insurance plan in a timely manner. At this point the ruling applies only to Quebec, but one can see its applicability across Canada. Also, the Supreme Court granted Quebec's request to delay implementation of the law for a period of one year.

There are three strategies via block grants by which the federal government allocates funding to the provinces and territories for health care services: (a) transfers of cash through the Canada Health Transfer (CHT) program, (b) tax transfers to the provinces by which the federal government agrees to reduce its taxation by the exact amount it allows the provinces and territories to raise their taxes (tax points), and (c) equalization funding to redistribute wealth from financially better off provinces to provinces that are less economically advantaged. The purpose of equalization is to ensure that the provinces and territories have the financial means to provide a reasonably comparable level of services, while maintaining similar taxation levels. The federal funding is contingent upon the provinces and territories adhering to federal health policy outlined in the *Canada Health Act.*

The costs for health care were initially borne about equally by federal and provincial-territorial governments, but there has been a shift away from a 50/50 arrangement (which was never intended). In 2001, about 44 percent of provincial government spending across Canada was consumed by health care costs, in contrast to only 16 percent of all federal government expenditures on health (WHO, 2004, Annex Table 5, p. 136). In 1996, the single federal block grants called the Canadian Health and Social Transfer (CHST) gave provinces more flexibility to set their own health expenditure priorities in relation to their educational and social services. In April 2004, this CHST was separated into two new funds: The Canada Health Trust (for health care) and the Social Transfer (for education and social services). The uneven federal vs. provincial funding was adjusted in 2004 with a US$33 billion federal transfer to Provinces via the Canada Health Trust program.

Although public financing predominates in Canada's national health insurance program at about 70 percent of total health expenditures, that leaves nearly a third of health care that is financed privately. The sources of *private* funding are out-of-pocket payments, premiums paid by individuals, employees and employers to private insurance companies, and in some cases, deductible amounts or user fees paid to nonphysician mental health practitioners in the private sector. Even though balanced billing and hospital user fees have been disallowed, users must pay for selected services and supplies because some of these are not deemed "medically necessary" or are not insured by the national insurance plan.

A lack of fairness is evident in Canada's system due to the favoring of services for medical-physical conditions versus mental health conditions. The mental health system has been viewed as the "orphan" of the Canadian health care system. Underfunding and insufficient numbers of qualified personnel result in waiting lists with delays up to two months for mental health services in the public sector. Delays are reduced in the private sector for those who can afford supplemental private insurance or pay out-of-pocket for outpatient psychotherapy by nonphysician mental health specialists.

The vast discrepancy between public reimbursements to physicians (98.3%) versus nonphysician professionals (9.3%) reflects unfair financing with respect to both mental health professionals and service users, whose access to outpatient mental health services becomes based on their ability to pay rather than their need for services. "This situation creates a significant disparity in the average Canadian's access to the broad range of health care services by nonphysicians."

Financing the American System

On the goal of fairness of financial contribution to the health care system for the year 1997, the WHO ranked the United States (54–55) significantly lower than the other three countries: Great Britain (8–11), Norway (8–11), and Canada (17–19) (Table 6.1). It is noteworthy that the WHO ranked 53 countries more fair in financing their health care system than the United States. It is even more informative to know these other countries included most of the developed nations of Western Europe (e.g., France, Germany, Switzerland, England, Ireland, Belgium, Austria, Spain, Greece, Italy, Turkey), all six Scandinavian countries (Iceland, Finland, Netherlands, Norway, Denmark, and Sweden), countries from North and South America, Australia, and New Zealand, as well as some Arab countries (United Arab Emirates, Saudi Arabia, Kuwait), and even less industrialized countries of India and Bangledesh.

As indicated in Table 1.2, total health expenditures by the United States as a percent of GDP was 14.6 percent in 2002, ranking higher than Canada (9.6%) and Norway (9.6%), and nearly double Great Britain (7.7%). *Government* spending on health as a percent of *total* expenditures on health was 44.9 percent, significantly lower than Norway (83.5%), Great Britain (83.4%) and Canada (69.9%). The government's expenditure on health as a percent of total *government* expenditures was 23.1 percent in the same year, which was slightly more than Norway (18.1%), Canada (15.9%), and Great Britain (15.8%). The United States has a mixed system of financing its health care system, but predominantly private sector (55.1%) versus public sector (44.9%) financing. The percent of private expenditures on health paid out-of-pocket was 25.4 percent (lowest of the four countries), while private prepaid plans accounted for 65.7 percent (highest for all four countries).

Private Sector Financing. In contrast to the other three countries, the United States is distinguished by the predominance of private sector financing (55% versus 45% public financing). Although, there are both publicly and privately financed and delivered health care services, the major source of *revenue collection* to finance this mixed health care system is premiums paid to private insurance companies and health plans by corporate employers, employees, or by other groups and individuals in the private sector. Additional out-of pocket revenues come from deductibles, co-insurance, and co-payments at the time of service utilization, all of which are demand-side cost controls, rationalized by the economic theory of moral hazard previously discussed. Private insurance companies seek contracts with large corporations to *pool resources and risks*. Because the private sector is organized predominantly as a voluntary, employer-based system, *purchasing* of health insurance and health plan contracts is done primarily by employers, and not by employees. The private insurance companies and health plans purchase mental health services or reimburse private practitioners, who provide mental health services in solo practice, or increasingly in larger group practices and multispecialty clinics. The payment mechanisms employed include capitation arrangements, diagnostic-related payments, and fee-for-service with discounted fees. In the private sector, financing and providing health care services is a commercial arrangement with prices determined by competitive bidding – at least in theory.

In a market-based economy wherein goods and services are bought and sold, health care itself becomes a commodity of exchange, and like every other private good to be purchased, health care in America must be purchased in order to become a personal possession. The predominant mode of purchasing health care services is by owning insurance or by working for an employer who owns a policy covering employees. Thus, in the private commercial sector, health care is a commodity that becomes private property when one has the ability to pay for it. Consequently, if one's employer does not provide health insurance, or provides a policy with limited coverage with cost sharing by employees, or if one's income is too low to make private insurance premiums affordable, then one cannot expect to access the health care system except perhaps in hospitals with a mandate to provide uncompensated care when their emergency beds are not filled. Other public sector safety nets include Community Health Clinics and Community Mental Health Centers, which offer services on a sliding fee scale.

The price of health insurance, like the price of all goods and services, is presumed to be regulated and contained by the immutable law of supply and demand in a competitive system of free enterprise. However, increasing consolidations among private health plans have reduced competition among them (Robinson, 2003; see reply by Hyman and Kovacic, 2003). Moreover, competition is based primarily on price, not on the quality of services rendered.

The predominance of the private sector in the U.S. health care system is symbolized by the labels used to describe the roles people play in the system: consumers, providers, and payers. In Norway where the health care system is publicly financed, the term "consumer" is seldom applied. Because the health services are owned, financed, and run by the State, Norwegians do not see themselves in economic terms as consumers in a health care market place. Health care is not viewed as a commodity, but more as a common good belonging to the community.

The federal agency that tracks health expenditures for mental health (MH) and substance abuse (SA) care is the Substance Abuse and Mental Health Services Administration (SAMSHA). The most recent data for the decade 1991–2001 were reported by SAMSHA in 2004 (cited by Mark et al. 2005, W59-133-142). The total personal health care expenditure in 2001 was $1.4 trillion. Of this total, spending for mental health (MH) and substance abuse (SA) combined was $104 billion (7.6%); for MH alone it was $85 billion (6.1% of the total health care expenditures); and for SA alone it was $18 billion (1.5% of the total health care expenditures). Of the $104 billion spent on MHSA combined, 82 percent was spent on MH and 18 percent on SA. Public payers covered 65 percent of the total MHSA spending and private payers covered 35 percent.

The percentages and sources of MHSA expenditures financed by private and public sectors are presented in Table 6.10.

Of the 35 percent spent by private payers on mental health and substance abuse combined (MHSA), only 20 percent was paid by private insurance. About 12 percent was out-of-pocket payments made by service users, and another three percent from other private sources such as philanthropy. The percentage spent on MHSA by private insurance (20%) is lower than the most recent estimated prevalence of mental disorders at about 26 percent of the total population (Kessler, Chiu, Demler, and Walters, 2005b, p. 617), and less than half of the 55 percent of total health care spending in the private sector.

Table 6.10. *Percentages Spent on MH and SA Care and all Health Care by Payer, Calendar Year 2001.*

Payer	MHSA	MH	SA	All Health
Total Private	35	37	24	55
Out-of-pocket	12	13	8	15
Private Insurance	20	22	13	36
Other Private Payers	3	3	3	4
Total Public	65	63	76	45
Medicare	7	7	5	18
Medicaid	26	27	19	16
Other Federal	6	5	14	4
Other state & local	26	23	38	7

Note: Data source is the Substance Abuse and Mental Health Services Administration (SAMSHA) (2004), as cited by Mark et al. 2005, W5-137.

For the decade 1991–2001, the average annual growth rate in expenditures for MHSA combined in the private sector was 5.6 percent overall, 4.7 percent for private insurance, 3.7 percent for out-of-pocket, and a decline of 1.5 percent for other private sources (Mark et al. 2005, p. W5–139).

Public Sector Financing. Of the $104 billion total expenditures for MHSA combined in 2001, public payers covered 65 percent. This is about 20 percent higher than the 45 percent of all health care expenditures paid by the government. Whereas the percent of all expenditures for MHSA paid by private sources decreased by seven percent from 42 percent in 1991 to 35 percent in 2001, the percent paid by public sources increased by seven percent from 58 percent in 1991 to 65 percent in 2001. Public financing grew to become the major source of spending on MHSA services during the decade ending 2001.

Table 6.10 indicates that among publicly funded programs, Medicaid has become the largest public payer (26%) of all MHSA services, and larger than all private insurance combined (20%). For MHSA services, Medicaid expenditures (26%) for low-income families was more than three times the Medicare expenditures (7%) for elderly and disabled Americans. The combined federal and state expenditures by Medicaid increased by eight percent from 18 percent of the total MHSA spending in 1991 to 26 percent in 2001. The increase in Medicaid expenditures was about $16 billion from $10.8 billion in 1991 to $26.7 billion in 2001.

Allocating the share of Medicaid paid by the states, the percent of total MHSA spending by states was 37 percent and federal spending accounted for 28 percent. The states carry the greatest financial burden for MHSA care. Consequently, the inequity in access to state administered MHSA services may be attributed significantly to the variability among states' levels of financing.

For the year 2002, the general *government* expenditures on health were 44.9 percent of the country's *total* health expenditures. The major source of *revenue collection* to finance the *public* sector program for about 42 million elderly and disabled is the Medicare tax deducted from individual income (salaries and wages). For a married couple filing jointly and a surviving spouse, the "progressive" income tax on gross adjusted incomes projected for 2005 ranged from 10 percent tax on income up to $14,600, to a high of 35 percent on taxable incomes over $326,450 (CCH, 2005, p. 28). More specifically, a married couple with taxable income between $14,600 and $59,400 would pay $1,460.00 plus 15 percent on the amount over $14,600 up to $59,400. The 2005 Medicare tax was 1.45 percent of gross income, paid by the employee and matched with an additional 1.45 percent by the employer for a total of 2.9 percent of all wages (no limit). The amount is a tax deductible expense to the employer, but not to employees. Self-employed individuals pay the full 2.9 percent mandatory Medicare tax (CCH, 2005).

The sources of revenues for about 50 million, low-income Americans receiving Medicaid are general tax revenues collected by both the federal and state governments, derived mostly from personal income taxes paid by working adults. In the Administration's proposed 2006 federal budget of $2,178 billion, revenues from personal income taxes account for $967 billion, more than four times the revenue from taxes on corporation income ($200 billion). The remaining sources of revenue (in billions of dollars) were Social Security insurance and retirement taxes ($819), custom duties ($28), estate and gift taxes ($26), and other receipts ($42).

Pooling of risk and resources occurs both at the federal and state levels, and so does *purchasing.* Mental health services are provided through public community mental health centers, some community health centers, and public hospitals, but also by private practitioners, general or psychiatric hospitals and managed behavioral health organizations. Provider payment mechanisms include fee-for-service, diagnostic-related payments, capitation, and line item budgeting for such federal health care programs as Medicare, Medicaid, SCHIP, Federal (and state) Employee Benefits Program, Department of Defense medical services, Veterans Health Administration, and Indian Health Services.

Publicly financed health care in America does not mean the users of these services pay nothing. An example from the publicly financed Medicare program is instructive. The Kaiser Family Foundation reported that in the year 2003, Medicare beneficiaries paid an average of $3,455 in health care costs, largely in premiums, deductibles, or co-payments at the point of service (as cited by Kiplinger, 2005, p. 96). If Medicare recipients enroll in the new Part D to cover medication costs (effective January 2006), they will pay out-of-pocket an additional, annual minimum of $1,232 for coverage up to $2,250 expenses, plus 100 percent of costs for the next $2,850 spent on prescriptions. Only when an individual's total medication expenditures reach $5,100 does this plan cover 95 percent of the costs (Ibid, p. 96).

In contrast to the other three countries in this study, the United States has a predominantly private sector health care system and it is the most market-maximized. Also in contrast, the United States is the only country with nearly 16 percent of its population (45.8 million) who are uninsured. For the past decade, nearly one million per year have been added to the roles of uninsured, yet despite the persistent deterioration in the system of coverage, the public discourse is characterized by appeasing platitudes rather than real reforms to bring about distributive justice in health care access for all Americans. The apparent lack of compassion for the uninsured, underinsured, and underserved in the American health care system is appalling. It makes a mockery of the constitutional rights to "life, liberty, and the pursuit of happiness," and it makes the American pledge of allegiance to "one nation, indivisible, under God, with liberty and justice for all" seem disingenuous at best. While the other three countries have imperfect systems, unlike the United States they seem to have resolved a fundamental moral and legal issue, to wit, that health care is a human right, a right of citizenship, something to which everyone who is able is obliged to contribute, and a public good to which everyone is entitled based upon who they are and what they need, not upon what they can afford to pay.

The inability to afford health insurance is problematic for millions of Americans, but especially for those with both low income and mental disorders. Both the 1994 National Comorbidity Survey and the 2005 National Comorbidity Survey-Replication found that among people with mental disorders who received treatment, having insurance was associated with utilization of health care services, both primary health care services and mental health specialty services (Wang et al. 2005b, pp. 637–638). Having insurance was not correlated with receiving *any* type of treatment (whether in the health care or human service systems, or self-help or support groups); nor was it related to the adequacy of the treatment among the people with mental disorders who received treatment. In fact, of the people with mental disorders who received treatment, the percent receiving at least minimally adequate care was higher (21.6%) in nonhealth sectors than in general medical (primary health care) sectors (12.7%), though lower than in mental health specialty care (45.4%) (Wang et al. 2005b, Table 6, p. 637). Among people who received *any* treatment for their mental disorders, having insurance was associated with using *health care sectors* (both primary and specialty services). Nevertheless, the authors concluded that "the effects of low income most likely reflect the formidable influences of financial barriers; because insurance was controlled, these results imply that simply having insurance may not be sufficient to overcome these effects" (Wang et al. 2005b, pp. 637–638). The same NCS-R epidemiological study found low income levels to be a predictor of both the prevalence rates of mental disorders and co-morbidity of depression with another disorder (Kessler et al. 2005b, pp. 622–623).

None of the four countries reviewed in this study represents a system financed completely by private funding such as private health insurance, or out-of-pocket deductibles or co-payments. Nevertheless, the private sectors play a much larger role in the health care systems of both the United States (55.1%) and Canada (30.1%) than in either Great Britain (16.6%) or Norway (16.5%).

Protection and Participation

The mental health systems of all four countries in this study have developed policies and incorporate procedures to ensure both the participation and protection of citizens, and especially those who suffer with mental disorders. There are, however, varying degrees to which both of these standards are met. Before discussing them, we offer a few comments to indicate what we mean by these terms.

Definitions

Protection. What do citizens need to be protected from? From (a) geographic and financial barriers to access to the mental health system; (b) discriminatory policies and practices evident in a lack of parity in the benefits or costs of mental health services versus medical services; (c) financial hardship from unexpected health events or from regressive forms of financing; (d) marginal or poor quality of services; (e) incompetent and unethical practitioners; (f) denials of informed consent to treatment; (g) refusals of access to one's own health record; (h) unauthorized disclosures of confidential health care information; (i) denials of due process, especially in criminal cases and involuntary commitment; (j) social stigma and discrimination in jobs and housing; (k) social conditions that foster mental disorders and distress such as poverty, unemployment, crime, violence, abuse and neglect.

Three types of approaches can be distinguished in national legislation protecting patients' rights: (a) some countries have enacted a single comprehensive law (Norway in 1999); (b) other countries have integrated patients' rights into legislation regulating the health care system or into several health laws (Canada in 1992, USA in 1999); and (c) charters on the rights of patients are sometimes embodied in the regulations of health care establishments and have varying status as national policy (United Kingdom 1991–1995) (WHO, 2000, Box 6.7, p.132).

There is a global consensus about the rights of people with mental disorders and their right to appropriate mental health care of optimal quality at affordable cost. The *Preamble to the Constitution of the United Nations* affirmed health care as a fundamental human right, and the World Health Organization defined health as "a state of complete physical, mental and social well-being and not merely the absence of disease or infirmity" (WHO, 1946). The *European Convention on Human Rights* is another expression of this consensus (Council of Europe, 1950, 1966). Protection of human rights for mental patients in particular was affirmed in the *Declaration of Caracas* adopted on November 14, 1990 by participants in the Regional Conference on Restructuring of Psychiatric Care in Latin America (summary in WHO, 2001, p. 52).

The United Nations General Assembly Resolution 46/119 was passed in 1991 to curb the political abuses of psychiatry found in several regions of the world (Maingay, et al. 2002). While this has not been as serious a problem in our four countries, mentally ill patients have not been protected consistently and equally. A relatively high rate of involuntary psychiatric hospitalizations has been noted in Norway. Excessive seclusion and restraints in a Georgia state mental hospital in the United States was judged to be the cause of 142 deaths among its inpatients (Liberman, 1999). Continuous monitoring is required to ensure patient safety. A report by researchers with the Institute of Medicine estimated that between 44,000 and 98,000 deaths occur annually in the United States as a result of medical errors, which cost from $17 billion to $29 billion per year (Kohn, Corrigan, and Donaldson, 2000).

Participation. Individuals receiving mental health services are empowered and motivated by their genuine participation in setting treatment goals and strategies. Moreover, the perspectives of users are vital if a mental health system is to be responsive to the population's expectations, including respect for users' autonomy and other elements specified by WHO (2000, p. 32). But genuine participation means much more than answering surveys to assess "consumer satisfaction" with services received. It means ultimately that the citizens of a country participate meaningfully and fairly in the formulation and change of health care policy at local, state, provincial, and national levels. In short, we mean to commend as a criterion for evaluating a mental health system consideration of the degree to which it can be considered democratic – "of the people, by the people, and for the people."

Protection and Participation in Great Britain

Protection. Under the *Human Rights Act 1998*, which came into force in 2000, the *European Convention on Human Rights* was incorporated into British law. There are several other legislative acts which collectively protect patients' rights, for example, minimizing the risk of discrimination on the basis of race, protecting from disclosure of information given during health care consultations, and providing for compensation in case of professional negligence or malpractice. At the most basic level, the British system protects its citizens from unexpected financial burdens associated with ill health, and from regressive taxes resulting in unfair contributions to funding its health care system.

Children and adolescents are protected under *The Children, Young People and Maternity Services National Service Framework [NSF] 2004*, and complementary acts such as the *1980 Education Act* and *Children Act 2004*. These national policies set standards for comprehensive services and requirements on local health, education, and social care agencies to provide services to meet their needs. The *NSF for Mental Health for Adults of Working Age* (1999) and the *NSF for Older People* (1999) address similar protections for these age groups, along with several policy implementation guidelines (e.g., *Care Programme Approach*, the *Policy Implementation Guide for Psychiatric Intensive Care Units [PICUs] and Low Secure Environments*, and *Commissioning Arrangements for Medium Secure Services*), and other publications such as *Modernizing Mental Health Services: Safe, Sound and Supportive* (1998) and the *Journey to Recovery (2001)*. Special safeguards for High and Medium Security Psychiatric Services are provided in National Service Frameworks and Policy Implementation Guidelines, though not for low secure psychiatric services provided by the National Health Service.

Participation. The British form of democracy is a constitutional monarchy with parliamentary governance. The federal parliament consists of a nationally elected House of Commons with representatives from England,

Northern Ireland, Scotland and Wales. The House of Lords, whose members are appointed for life, serve primarily in the roles of formulating policy, advising, and recommending reforms. The political powers of the Royal Crown are highly circumscribed.

Participation by British citizens in their government is ensured by Parliamentary elections of the 645 representatives to the House of Commons. These elections must occur at least every five years. The political party with the largest percentage of popular vote becomes the ruling party in Parliament, from which the Prime Minister is selected. The administrative branch of government is headed by the Prime Minister and Cabinet of Ministers, which include the Secretary of State for Health. The latter heads the Department of Health.

At the level of policy formulation, participation of the population is through public debate of policy proposals among elected representatives in Great Britain's House of Commons. Public consultation is also required prior to any legislative changes in national health policy, though not in other acts of parliament. There are few lay people or service users on the Boards of National Health Service Trusts which commission (purchase) services, but *Acute Care Forums* ensure user participation in effective purchasing, and representatives are elected to lower level organizations of the NHS such as *Local Implementation Teams*, and *Local Authorities* and *Councils*, which contribute to social services for the population, including the mentally ill.

At the individual and clinical level, the users of mental health services generally participate in problem identification and development of treatment plans, if not intervention strategies. Most clinicians express their respect for their clients by treating them collaboratively, and by honoring informed consent and confidentiality as obligations of their professional codes of ethics.

Protection and Participation in Norway

Protection. What has been said about Great Britain's financial protection of its population seems equally true of Norway. The entire population in Norway is effectively protected from unexpected costs for mental health services and from regressive out-of-pocket payments in this publicly financed and publicly administered mental health system. That is, they are protected from making unfair financial contributions to fund the system. But like Great Britain's population, Norwegians have not been protected from an unresponsive system with long waiting lists for mental health services.

The *Act of Patients' Rights* was passed by Parliament 1999 and became effective in 2001. It was designed to give patients better quality health services and to ensure patients' trust and confidence in these services. These are the goals and reasons for granting (a) essential health assistance from the specialist health service, (b) the right to a medical examination within 30 days, (c) the right to a second examination and (d) the right to choose the hospital they will use. The *Act of Patients' Rights* is meant to protect the patient by giving information about the treatment planned, including possible risks and side effects. Patients' have the right of access to their medical records. Regional Health Authorities and Health Enterprises have the responsibility to inform mental health service providers about new laws and regulations they don't seem to know.

The Patient Ombudsman was established to meet patients' needs and to protect their interests and legal rights with respect to the health services. Any person may contact the Patient Ombudsman and request that a case be taken up for consideration. Patients are generally protected in an acceptable manner when admitted to the services, and they are seldom injured.

Among the health care services to which all Norwegian residents are entitled are (a) hospital and emergency care, (b) outpatient mental health services within 30 working days of a referral, (c) the right to choose the specialist service setting (hospital or district psychiatric centre, or treatment unit in such an institution in which the treatment is provided), though not to choose the level of treatment provided. Patients requiring long-term, coordinated health services are entitled to have an individual plan drawn up in accordance with the provisions of the *Municipal Health Service Act*, the *Specialist Health Service Act*, and the *Act on the Provision and Implementation of Mental Health Care*.

The rates of compulsory admissions for mental health treatment have been historically, relatively higher in Norway than in other countries. In 2002, approximately 40 percent of inpatients were involuntary admissions to psychiatric wards and hospitals. One of the goals of the *Act on Health Enterprises* (2002) was to reduce compulsory admissions and the use of forced treatment. According to the *Act of Patients' Rights*, health care may be provided only with the patient's informed consent, unless they are judged to be incompetent to give consent.

Participation. A fundamental element of the National Mental Health Program (NMHP) approved by

Parliament in 1998 was the emphasis placed upon the user's perspective as essential to improving services. "Participation is also vital for empowerment and for the ability to master one's own life. This is a central value and fundamental to the vision of the NMHP." According to Yaw Amoako-Addo, associate professor of economics at Buskerud University College in Kongsberg, Norway: "In the Norwegian democratic system, no drastic policy changes are introduced without a public commission and a broad consensus of the population" (Amoako-Addo, 2005, p. 20).

The participation of service users and their families occurs both on a system level and individual level. At the *systems* level, representatives from five major organizations of users of mental health services participate as a consulting group to the Ministry of Health and Social Care to ensure users' perspectives and concerns are addressed. Moreover, State funds have been earmarked to strengthen users' organizations. Also at the systems level, elected representatives serve on Regional Health Authorities (RHAs) that allocate funding and Health Enterprises that provide mental health services. The *Act on Health Enterprises* (2002) was passed to ensure the involvement of patients and the public. All Health Enterprises (hospitals and specialized services such as mental health) have a users' council. These include civic representatives, patients, and representatives from patient organizations – anyone who is not working in the health services.

The Norwegian health care system is democratic like Britain's system, but there appears to be a difference in the degree of public involvement structured into decision-making processes leading to the formulation and implementation of policy. In contrast to Britain's centrally administered NHS, primary health and welfare services are administered by locally elected bodies in the 434 local municipalities in Norway. There appears to be greater participation by the Norwegian population through elected representatives than evident in the largely appointed personnel in the British National Health Service, and much greater than in the United States system. However, mental health services are administered by the central government in Norway through Regional Health Authorities and Health Enterprises owned by the central government.

At the *individual and clinical level,* people participate in their health care decisions. Developing an individualized treatment and care plan that coordinates necessary services has become both a mandatory task for the services and a legal right for the patients. While nearly all hospitals are owned by the central government, they are to be operated as health enterprises to compete for patients who are free to choose among hospitals throughout the country. However, the geographic barriers and distance to hospitals tend to encourage utilization of the hospital nearest one's local community. The closest hospital will have a definite competitive advantage over other hospitals located at a greater distance.

A *patient list system* was designed to provide all citizens with a personal and regular general practitioner (GP). In 2000, everyone in the country was invited to choose a regular GP. Those who did not choose themselves were assigned to a GP. The purpose of this *General Practitioner Scheme* is to encourage better doctor/patient communication and to ensure easy access for every resident to medical services through a regular GP.

Protection and Participation in Canada

Protection. Like Great Britain and Norway, Canada provides financial protection to its population from unexpected costs for health care services and from regressive out-of-pocket payments in its publicly financed and administered mental health system. The Canadian national health insurance system (Medicare) has "spared many Canadians from financial ruin related to the costs of illness." Nevertheless, coverage by Medicare is generally limited to "medically necessary, insured" conditions. Moreover, Canada's government-sponsored health insurance program protects all of its residents from financial exposure to potentially crippling costs associated with illness, so long as services are rendered by the preferred providers within the system (viz., hospitals and physicians).

There is no national parity legislation that would require comparable expenditures for mental health services relative to medical services. That lack of parity is reflected in the much smaller public funding of the mental health system. The population is not protected by Medicare from the costs of outpatient mental health services provided by mental health specialists who are not physicians.

Canada has several national policies to protect the privacy rights of individuals. A *Charter of Rights and Freedoms* was included as an element of Canada's Constitution Act of 1982 to define and guarantee the personal rights and fundamental freedoms of all Canadians. Other examples include the 1983 *Privacy Act*, the 2001 *Personal Information Protection and Electronic Documents Act.* There are policies pertaining to the conditions under which disclosures can be made without consent. A 2003 review of privacy legislation for family physicians by the College of Family Physicians of Canada (CFPC) identified ten principles, all of which are based on the two foundational values of consent and confidentiality.

In addition to federal legislation, most provinces and territories have their own *Mental Health Acts*. There are considerable variations in the protection of individual rights among Provinces with different legislative and regulatory provisions.

In Canada, criminal law is the sole responsibility of the federal government. Consequently, assessment of one's mental competence to stand trial for a criminal act is under federal jurisdiction rather than provincial or territorial law. Attempted suicide was decriminalized in 1972 by the Minister of Justice, Otto Long; however, counseling or assisting suicide remains a criminal act of Section 241 of the Criminal Code of Canada with up to 14 years imprisonment. Protections of individuals' rights in civil commitment proceedings for involuntary hospitalization have legislative authority in the Provinces, but the criteria and due process procedures vary among the thirteen jurisdictions.

There has been insufficient protection of the most vulnerable people in need of mental health services in Canada. The seriously and persistently mentally ill were deinstitutionalized from psychiatric hospitals, but the number of hospital beds made available in community hospitals for psychiatric care never matched the increased need. The result has been high rates of recidivism in psychiatric units in general-medical hospitals − a "revolving door" of patients who are discharged prematurely to make room for others, and discharged without the needed follow-up support services within their community (e.g., outpatient therapy, case management, housing, vocational rehabilitation services, social security benefits).

External protections against incompetent and unethical practitioners are present for the regulated mental health professions, but not for the unregulated professions such as marriage and family therapists, counselors, and addiction counselors. Self-regulation by all the mental health professions is considered an important safeguard.

Participation. Similar to Great Britain, Canada is a constitutional monarchy with parliamentary rule. At the federal level, laws and policies must be approved by three constituencies: (a) members of the Senate, who are recommended by the Prime Minister and appointed by the Governor General, (b) the elected members of the House of Commons, and (c) by the Queen's representative called the Governor General. With few exceptions all three must approve federal legislation to become law. Unlike Great Britain, Canada is organized politically as a federation with ten Provincial and three Territorial governments, each with a Lieutenant Governor representing the royal crown. All levels of government are involved in health care services. Dr. Arnett concluded that while overall there is a satisfactory level of both participation and protection, there is also a need for federal legislation to guarantee protection of personal health information.

At an individual and *clinical* level, most mental health professionals work collaboratively to encourage participation by clients in goal setting and treatment planning. At the *system* level, participation in policy formulation and implementation is encouraged, but it does not seem to be required and monitored as comprehensively as in the Norwegian system.

Protection and Participation in United States

Protection. Unlike the other three countries, it cannot be said that the United States system protects its population from unexpected costs of health care services, nor from regressive out-of-pocket payments in its predominantly private sector system. Protection from financial distress seems better in the other three countries than for people in the United States because in the latter country, access to the health care system is contingent upon possession of health insurance which must be provided either by an employer, by some other group, or purchased by the individual. In short, access and utilization are contingent upon the ability to pay, and influenced by both levels of income and possession of insurance, as shown in the most recent epidemiological study conducted in the United States (Wang et al. 2005b). Among low income families, public coverage provides significantly greater protection from the financial burden of health care than private insurance coverage (Galbraith, Wong, Kim, and Newacheck, 2005).

The Institute of Medicine (2002a) highlighted the difficulty that the uninsured have in accessing care, and their resulting poorer health outcomes. Stuber and Bradley (2005) reported similar findings: "Without health insurance, many children lack needed access to services, which results in lower rates of immunizations, higher emergency room use, increased incidence of preventable diseases, and more common speech, hearing, and behavioral problems" (p. 525). Hargraves and Hadley (2003) reported on two cross-sectional surveys of households conducted during 1996–1997 and 1998–1999, which indicated that the lack of health insurance was the single most important factor in racial/ethnic disparities. Income differences were the second most important factor. Their results suggest that the positive effects of insurance coverage in reducing racial/ethnic disparities outweigh the benefits of alternative strategies, such as increasing physician charity care or access to emergency rooms.

At the federal level, the *Americans with Disability Act* was passed in 1990 to protect both mentally and physically disabled from discrimination in employment and housing. The 1996 *Mental Health Parity Act* was a federal initiative that requires employers with more than 50 employees, and who provide medical insurance, must also provide mental health coverage. The restricted limits on parity in the private sector contrasts with full parity in the public sector for federal employees. By Executive Order from President Clinton on June 7, 1999, the U. S. Office of Personnel Management was directed to provide parity for mental health and substance abuse coverage in the Federal Employees Health Benefits Program. That was achieved by 2001 (OPM, 1999).

The 1996 *Health Insurance Portability and Accountability Act* (HIPAA) was passed to ensure continued health insurance coverage for employees in transition between jobs, and to ensure privacy of protected health information. An example of a comprehensive consumer protection policy is the "Patient's Bill of Rights" applicable to the Federal Employees Health Benefits Plan (OPM, 1999, Nov. 3). Patient protection acts and mental health bills of rights passed by states, and state mandated reporting of neglect and abuse are further protections. Protections of patients' civil rights are provided by regulations with respect to the proceedings leading to involuntary commitments for psychiatric treatment, as well as the right to receive and/or refuse treatment, and standards under which an insanity defense can be pleaded in criminal cases.

To protect the rights of elderly, disabled, and low-income enrollees in the federal and state sponsored programs of Medicare and Medicaid, there are both federal and state government agencies (e.g., Centers for Medicare and Medicaid, state Boards of Aging, state departments of commerce and health, consumer assistance, Ombudsman offices, and legal aide services). There are also numerous voluntary, national and state advocacy groups such as the National Association of Mentally Ill, the National Mental Health Association, Elder Care Rights Alliance, and the American Association of Retired Persons, plus several other groups with a particular focus at the state and local levels. In the authors' home state, examples are the Minnesota Association for Children's Mental Health, the Mental Health Consumer-Survivor Network, and SAVE: Suicide Awareness Voice of Education.

Federal laws require hospitals to provide all Medicare patients at the patient's admission with a pamphlet entitled, *An Important Message from Medicare*. This pamphlet describes rights and responsibilities and where to go if patients have questions. Hospitalized patients have the right to be advised of their planned discharge date. If the patient thinks she/he is being discharged from a hospital too soon, she/he has the right to appeal to a local Quality Improvement Organization (QIO) authorized and funded by Medicare. A QIO may review complaints regarding quality of care issues in several Medicare certified settings including psychiatric and rehabilitation specialty hospitals and community mental health facilities (MSF, 2005).

There are various federal and state laws stipulating appeals procedures within and subsequently outside health plans, which have delayed or denied health care services. Efforts to hold Health Maintenance Organizations (HMOs) accountable for negligence or malpractice have included numerous state laws allowing individuals to file suit for damages against HMOs in state courts. The U.S. Supreme Court struck down those laws. Individuals cannot be compensated for damages, only for the treatment costs incurred. The legal moats around the citadels of the health care industry are deep and wide.

Protection from incompetent and unethical practices is provided by all of these countries through standardized educational and training requirements to obtain a license to deliver mental health services. State licensing boards have the authority to sanction their licensees, up to and including removal from national health insurance reimbursement and termination of their license to practice in the state or province.

The absence of a national, comprehensive quality assessment system in the United States is a serious deficiency because the safety of health care users is not fully protected. For example, an estimated three to four million ambulatory care visits are made each year in the United States as a result of adverse drug effects, harm, or injury resulting from the use of medications (Zhan et al. 2005).

Participation. The United States is a democratic country founded on a set of documents known as the *Declaration of Independence* (1776), *Articles of Confederation* ratified in 1781, the *Constitution and Bill of Rights* ratified in 1788, with a total of twenty-five amendments passed subsequently.

The first three articles of the Constitution define the powers, restraints, and duties of the Legislative, Executive, and Judicial branches of the federal government. The remaining articles address the relationship of the states to each other and to the federal government (Article IV), the method of amending the Constitution (V), the preempting authority of the federal Constitution and law over states (VI) and the method for ratifying the Constitution (VII). These Articles and 25 Amendments constitute the framework for the American federal system and express some of the fundamental values upon which the country was founded.

The Declaration of Independence was signed by representatives of the original colonies gathered in the first General Congress July 4, 1776. The Declaration was much more than merely a list of grievances against the tyranny of Great Britain's King over the original colonies in America. The document affirmed fundamental human rights and entitlements: "We hold these truths to be self-evident, that all men are created equal; that they are endowed by their Creator with certain inalienable rights, that among these are life, liberty, and the pursuit of happiness. To secure these rights, governments are instituted among men, deriving their just powers from the consent of the governed. . . . (*The Constitution of the United States.* 1966, p. 22). It took several decades before women and minorities would participate in the exercise of these rights, including the right to vote. Americans with mental disorders have yet to be fully included with equal treatment. In the American health care system, a *Declaration of Interdependence* is needed to ensure that the healthy and wealthy help the sick and poor.

The following discussion addresses participation at the clinical level of intervention and evaluation of mental health services, at a systems level in individual choice of insurance plans and providers, and at the level of public policy formulation.

At the *clinical level*, most therapists relate with clients respectfully by engaging them in collaborative goal-setting and treatment planning. At the *systems level*, most federal and state employees, and employees of large companies have a menu of health plan options with varying benefits and levels of premiums, deductibles, and co-payments. Employees' insistence upon choice of both plans and providers has led to the growth in popularity of preferred provider organizations (PPOs) and point of service plans (POS) over the earlier staff models of Health Maintenance Organizations ((HMOs) with a more restricted panel of health care personnel. However, in the private sector, the decision to offer any health insurance plan remains with employers who pay the bulk of the health insurance bill. The majority of employees are in companies with less than 50 workers, and if any insurance is provided, at most there is one health plan option. Increasingly, large corporations are opting for a self-insuring strategy because under a federal law, known as the Employee Retirement Income Security Act of 1974 (ERISA), they become exempt from mandated coverage under various state laws and rules, such as state parity laws requiring coverage of mental health and substance abuse treatment.

At the level of *policy formulation*, by and large the American public leaves it to their elected legislators and governmental agencies to assess the need and reasonableness of proposals to reform the health care system. While there have been examples of such legislation at both federal and state levels, the influence upon legislators by powerful interest groups who spend millions to finance politicians' campaigns and to lobby their candidates once elected, makes major reform in the public interest very difficult. One example of that at the federal level is the defeat in 1993 of President Clinton's *Health Security Act* by business interests and by the health care industry. More recently, the *Medicare Prescription Drug, Improvement and Modernization Act (MMA)* of 2003 prohibited the federal government from negotiating prices of prescription drugs under Medicare Part D. Along with health insurance and health plan corporations, private pharmaceutical companies have inordinate power. The so-called "modernization" of Medicare was basically designed to provide financial incentives to expand participation of private health plans, most of which are for-profit corporations (Gold, 2005, p. 302).

By way of summary, this review indicates our four countries vary in their performance on the five evaluation criteria: access and equity, quality and efficacy, cost and efficiency, fairness and financing, participation and protection. Their performance in addressing unmet needs for mental health services is addressed in the final chapter under the criterion of population relevance.

REFERENCES

Abraham, J., Feldman, R., Carlin, C. (2004). Understanding employee awareness of health care quality information: How can employers benefit? *Health Services Research, 39*(6), 1799–1815.

Agency for Health Care Policy and Research (AHCPR) (1999). *CAHPS 2.0 Survey and Reporting Kit.* Rockville, Maryland: U. S. Department of Health and Human Services.

Agency for Healthcare Research and Quality (AHRQ) (2005). AHRQ launches new effective health care program to compare medical treatments and help put proven treatments into practice. *Research Activities*, No. 302, Oct., p. 20. Available at www.effectivehealthcare.ahrq.gov

American Psychiatric Association (2000). *Diagnostic and statistical manual of mental disorders.* (4th ed. Text revision). (DSM-IV-TR). Washington DC: Author.

American Public Health Association (2005). *Public health code of ethics.* Retrieved September 21, 2005 from http://www.apha.org/codeofethics/ethics.htm

Amoako-Addo (2005). An expert opinion. *Viking. Magazine for the members of Sons of Norway, 102*(8), p. 20. Interview with Dr. Yaw Amoako-Addo from Norway.

Anderson, G. F., Hussey, P. S., Frogner, B. K., & Waters, H. R. (2005). Health spending in the United States and the rest of the industrialized world. *Health Affairs, 24*(4) July August, 903–914.

Anderson, Odin W. (1989). *The health services continuum in democratic states: An inquiry into soluble problems.* Ann Arbor, Mich.: Health Administration Press.

Ault, A. (2004). IOM calls for universal health coverage by 2010. *The Lancet, 363,* January 24, p. 300.

Barofsky, I. (2003). Patients' rights, quality of life, and health care system performance. *Quality of Life Research, 12,* 473–484.

Barry, C., Gable, J., Frank, R., Hawkins, S., Whitmore, H., & Pickreign, J. (2003). Design of mental health benefits: Still unequal after all these years. *Health Affairs, 22*(5), 127–137.

Basu, J. (2005). Severity of illness, race, and choice of local versus distance hospitals among the elderly. *Journal of Health Care for the Poor and Underserved, 16,* 391–405. Reprint available as AHRQ Publication No. 05-R054.

Bell, N. N., & Shern, D. L. (2002). *State mental health commissions: Recommendations for change and future directions.* [Report]. Alexandria, VA: National Technical Assistance Center for State Mental Health Planning. National Association of State Mental Health Program Directors.

Bennett, M. (1996). Is psychotherapy ever medically necessary? *Psychiatric Services, 47,* 966–971.

Berghold, L. (1995). Medical necessity: Do we need it? *Health Affairs, 14*(4), 181–219.

Bhui, K., Stansfeld, S., McKenzie, K., Karlson, S., Nazroo, J., & Welch, S. (2005). Racial/ethnic discrimination and common mental disorders among workers: Findings from the EMPIRIC study of ethnic minority groups in the United Kingdom. *American Journal of Public Health, 95*(3), 496–501.

Bindman, A., Yoon, J., & Grumback, K. (2003). Trends in physician participation in Medicaid: the California experience. *Journal of Ambulatory Care Management, 26*(4), 334–343.

Blendon, R. J. (2002). Inequities in health care: A five-country survey. *Health Affairs, 21*(3), 182–192.

Bruce, S., & Paxton, R. (2002). Ethical principles for evaluating mental health services: A critical examination. *Journal of Mental Health, 11*(3), 267–279.

Brundtland, Gro H. (2001, Oct.). Message from the Director-General. *The World Health Report 2001. Mental Health: New Understanding, New Hope.* Geneva: World Health Organization, (ix–x).

Bureau of Health Professions (2002). *Health Professional Shortage Area: Mental Health Designation Criteria.* Retrieved December 14, 2002 from http://bhpr.hrsa.gov/shortage/hpsacritmental.htm

Bureau of Primary Health Care (2003). *Mental Health Primary Care.* Retrieved January 22, 2003 from http://bphc.hrsa.gov/bphc/mental/

Burke, F. (1999). Ethical decision-making: Global concerns, frameworks, and approaches. *Public Personnel Management, 28*(4), 529–540.

Callaway, M. E., & Hall, J. (2000). Distributive justice in Medicaid capitation: The evidence from Colorado. *The Journal of Behavioral Health Services & Research, 27*(1), February, 87–97.

Campbell, A. (1995). *Health as liberation: Medicine, theology, and the quest for justice.* Cleveland, Ohio: The Pilgrim Press.

Carter-Pokras, O., & Woo, V. (1999). Health profile of racial and ethnic minorities in the United States. *Ethnicity Health, 4,* 117–120.

Cassidy, C., & Nilan, L. (2005, June). The VA/DoD Evidence-Based Practice Work Group. *Forum.* Washington DC: VA Office of Research and Development.

CCH Editorial Staff (2005). *2005 U. S. Master Tax Guide.* Chicago: CCH Incorporated. A Wolters Kluwer Co.

Center for Public Integrity (1995a). Well-healed: Inside lobbying for health care reform, Part I. *International Journal of Health Services, 25*(3), 411–453.

Center for Public Integrity (1995b). Well-healed: Inside lobbying for health care reform, Part II. *International Journal of Health Services, 25*(4), 593–631.

Chavez, N. (1997). Serving the underserved – our societal responsibility. *Professional Psychology: Research and Practice, 28*(3), 203–204. (Interview with SAMHSA Administrator, Nelba Chavez, edited by Patrick DeLeon).

Chernew, M., Cutler, D. M., & Keenan, P. S. (2005). Increasing health insurance costs and the decline in insurance coverage. *Health Services Research, 40*(4), 1021–1039.

Chesley, F. D., & Clancy, C. M. (2005). AHRQ Update: Research funding opportunities: Fiscal Year 2006. *Health Research Services, 40*(5), xi–xiv.

Chodoff, P. (1998). Medical necessity and psychotherapy. *Psychiatric Services, 49*(11), 1481–1483.

Churchill, L. R. (1987). *Rationing health care in America. Perceptions and principles of justice.* Notre Dame, IN: University of Notre Dame Press.

Churchill, L. R. (1995). *Self-interest and universal health care.* Boston: Harvard University Press. (Cited in Pediatrics, June 96, Part 1 of 2, 97(6), p. 895.)

Clark Institute of Psychiatry (1997) *Best practices in mental health reform.* Health Systems Research Unit. Author.

Common Cause (1992). Why the United States does not have a national health program: The medical-industrial complex and its PAC contributions to congressional candidates January 1, 1981 through June 30, 1991. *International Journal of Health Services, 22*(4), 619–644.

Consumer Reports (August, 1996). *How good is your health plan?* Author, pp. 28–41.

Council on Graduate Medical Education (1998). *Physician distribution and health care challenges in rural and inner-city areas,* pp. 1–74. Washington, D. C.: U.S. DHHS, Health Resources and Services Administration.

Council of Europe (1950, 1066). The European Convention on Human Rights, and its Five protocols. Strasbourg: Author. Retrieved September 27, 2005 from http://www.hri.org/docs/ECHR50.html

Coyne, J. S., & Hilsenrath, P. (2002). The World Health Report 2000: Can health care systems be compared using a single measure of performance? *American Journal of Public Health, 92,* 30 & 32–33.

Dalgard, O. S., Kringlen, E., Dahl, A. (2002). Psykiatrisk epidemiologi. (Psychiatric epidemiology). *Norsk Epidemiologi, 12*(3), 161–162.

Daniels, N. (1982). Equity of access to health care: Some conceptual and ethical issues. *Milbank Memorial Fund Quarterly, 60*(1), 51–81.

Davidoff, A., Garret, B., Maku, D., & Schirmer, M. (2000). Medicaid-eligible children who don't enroll: Health status, access to care, and implications for Medicaid enrollment. *Inquiry, 37,* 203–218.

Deber, R. B. (2003). Healthcare reform: Lessons from Canada. *American Journal of Public Health, 93*(1), 200–24.

Declaration of Caracas (1990). Adopted by the WHO Regional Conference on Restructuring Psychiatric care in Latin America. Cited in WHO (2001). *The world health report 2001. Mental health: New understanding, new hope,* pp. 52 & 84. Geneva: World Health Organization.

DHHS (1999). Department of Health and Human Services. *Mental Health: A report of the Surgeon General – executive summary.* Rockville, Md.: U.S. Department of Health and Human Services, Substance Abuse and Mental Health Services Administration, Center for Mental Health Services, National Institutes of Health, National Institute of Mental Health.

DHHS (2000). Office of Disease Prevention and Health Promotion. *Healthy People 2010.* (2nd ed.). Washington, DC: Government Printing Office.

DHHS (2002). Department of Health and Human Services. *Closing the Health Gap.* Retrieved October 2, 2002 from http://www.healthgap.omhre.gov/mental_health.htm

DHHS (2003). New Freedom Commission on Mental Health. *Achieving the promise: Transforming mental health care in America. Final report.* Rockville, Md.: Department of Health and Human Services. Publication SMA-03-3832.

DHHS (2004a). New Freedom Commission on Mental Health, *Subcommittee on Housing and Homelessness: Background Paper.* DHHS Pub. No. SMA-04-3884. Rockville, MD.

DHHS (2004b). New Freedom Commission on Mental Health, *Subcommittee on Criminal Justice: Background Paper.* DHHS Pub. No. SMA-04-3880. Rockville, MD.

Diamant, A. L., Hays, R. D., Morales, L. S., Ford, W., Calmes, D., Asch, S. et al. (2004). Delays and unmet need for health care among adult primary care patients in a restructured urban public health system. *American Journal of Public Health, 94*(5), 783–789.

Dievler, A., & Giovannini, T. (1998). Community health centers: Promise and performance. *Medical Care Research and Review, 55*(4), 405–431.

Dingfelder, S. I. (2005). A four-point plan. *Monitor on Psychology, 36*(10), 62–63.

Donabedian, A. (1980). *Explorations in Quality Assessment and Monitoring, Volume 1: The Definition of Quality and Approaches to its Assessment.* Ann Arbor, Mich.: Health Administration Press.

Dregni, E. (2005). A helping hand. *Viking,* August, 2005, 102(6), 18–19, 21.

Druss, B. G., Rohrbaugh, R. M., Levinson, C. M., & Rosenheck, R. A. (2001). Integrated medical care for patients with serious psychiatric illness: A randomized trial. *Archives of General Psychiatry, 58,* 861–868.

Economist (1998). "Waiting for Dobbo," May 23, cited by Graig (1999).

Eisenberg, L. (1999). Where is the voice of the faculty? Talk given before the American Association of University Professors, May 22, 1999. Cited in *Pediatrics,* Nov. 99, Part 1 of 2, 104(5), p. 1094.

Farber, H. S., & Levy, H. (2000). Recent trends in employer-sponsored health insurance coverage: Are bad jobs getting worse? *Journal of Health Economics, 19*(1), 93–119.

Feldman, M. A. (1998). Health care policy evaluation: A conceptual model using medical ethics. *Journal of Health and Human Service Administration, 21,* 181–198.

Forrest, C. B., & Whelan, E. M. (2000). Primary care safety-net delivery sites in the United States: A comparison of community health centers, hospital outpatient departments, and physicians' offices. *Journal of the American Medical Association, 284*(16), 2077–2083.

Fortney, J. C., Steffick, D. E., Burgess, J. F., Maciejewski, M., & Peterson, L. (2005). Are primary care services a substitute or complement for specialty and inpatient services? *Health Services Research, 40*(5), Part I, 1422–1442.

Foster, E. M., & Xuan, F. (2005). An episode-based framework for analyzing health care expenditures: An application of reward renewal models. *Health Services Research, 40*(6), Part I., 1953–1971.

Frankena, Wm. (1973). *Ethics* (2nd ed.). Upper Saddle River, New Jersey: Prentice-Hall.

Frick, K. D., & Regan, J. (2001). Whether and where community health center users obtain screening services. *Journal of Health Care for the Poor and Underserved, 12*(4), 429–445.

Fuchs, V. R., & Emanual, E. J. (2005). Health care reform: Why? What? When? *Health Affairs, 24*(6), 1399–1414.

Gabel, J., Claxton, G., Gil, I., Pickreign, J., Whitmore, H., Finder, B., Hawkins, S., & Rowland, D. (2005). Health benefits in 2005: Premium increases slow down, coverage continues to erode. *Health Affairs, 24*(5), 1273–1280.

Gabel, J., Claxton, G., Holve, E., Pickreign, J., Whitmore, H., Dhont, K., Hawkins, S., and Rowland, D. (2003). Health benefits in 2003: Premiums reach thirteen-year high as employers adopt new forms of cost sharing. *Health Affairs, 22*(5), 117–126.

Galbraith, A. A., Wong, S. T., Kim, S. E., & Newacheck, P. W. (2005). Out-of-pocket financial burden for low-income families with children: Socioeconomic disparities and effects of insurance. *Health Services Research, 40*(6), 1722–1736.

General Accountability Office (GAO) (December, 2000). *Community-based care increases for people with serious mental illness.* Washington, CD: Author. (GA)-01/224).

Gilmer, T., & Kronick, R. (2001). Calm before the storm: Expected increase in the number of uninsured Americans. *Health Affairs, 20*(6), 207–210.

Gilmer, T., & Kronick, R. (2005). It's the premiums, stupid: Projections of the uninsured through 2013. *Web Exclusives: A Supplement to Health Affairs,* vol. 24, supplement 1, January-June, W5-143- W5-151.

Gladwell, M. (2005). The moral-hazard myth: The bad idea behind our failed health-care system. *The New Yorker.* New York, pp. 44–49. Available at www.newyorker.com

Glaser, W. (1992). Psychiatry and medical necessity. *Psychiatric Annals, 22,* 362–366.

Graig, L. A. (1999). *Health of Nations: An international perspective on U.S. Health Care Reform.* (3rd ed.). Washington, D.C.: Congressional Quarterly, Inc.

Greenfield, S., & Kaplan, S. H. (2004). Creating a culture of quality. The remarkable transformation of the Department of Veterans Affairs Health Care System. *Annals of Internal Medicine, 141*(4), 316–318.

Grob, G. N. (2005). Public policy and mental illnesses: Jimmy Carter's Presidential Commission on Mental Health. *The Milbank Quarterly, 83*(3), 425–456.

Gruskin, S. (2004). What are health and human rights? *Lancet, 363,* January 24, p. 329.

Gulbinat, W., Manderscheid, R., Baingana, F., et al. (2004). The international consortium on mental health policy and services: objectives, design, and project implementation. *International Review of Psychiatry, 16*(1-2), 5–17.

Hargraves, J. L., & Hadley, J. (2003). The contribution of insurance coverage and community resources to reducing racial/ethnic disparities in access to care. *Health Services Research, 38*(3), 809–829.

Hart, S. N. (1982). The history of children's psychological rights. *Viewpoints in Teaching and Learning, 58,* 1–15.

Hartley, D., Bird, D. C., & Dempsey (1999). Rural mental health and substance abuse. In T. C. Ricketts (Ed.). *Rural health in the United States.* 159–178. New York, New York: Oxford University Press, Inc.

Health Canada (1994). *Update of the Report on the Task Force on Suicide in Canada.* Mental Health Division. Author.

Henderson, S., & Whiteford, H. (2003). Social capital and mental health. *Lancet, 362,* August 16, pp. 505–506.

Healthcare Financial Management Association [HFMA] (2004). *Introductory guide to NHS finance in the U.K.* Bristol: Author.

Himmelstein, D., Warren, E., Thorne, D., & Woolhandler, S. (2005). Illness and injury as contributors to bankruptcy. *Web Exclusives: A supplement to Health Affairs,* vol. 24, supplement 1, January-June, 2005, W5-63-73.

Hodges, K. (1990). *Child and Adolescent Functional Assessment Scale (CAFAS).* Ypsilanti, MI: Department of Psychology, Eastern Michigan University.

Holahan, J., & Bruen, B. (2003). *Medicaid spending: What factors contributed to the growth between 2000 and 2002?* Washington, DC: Kaiser Commission on Medicaid and the Uninsured.

Holloway, J. D. (2005). Striking a balance between correction and care. *Monitor on Psychology, 36*(10), 48–49.

House, J. S., & Williams, D. R. (2000). Understanding and reducing socioeconomic and racial/ethnic disparities in mental health. In B. Smedley, & S. Syme (Eds). *Promoting Health: Intervention strategies from social and behavioral research.* Washington, DC: National Academy Press, 81–124.

Humphreys, K., & Rappaport, J. (1993). From the community mental health movement to the war on drugs: A study of the definition of social problems. *American Psychologist, 48,* 892–901.

Hurst, J., & Siciliani, I. (2003, July 7). *Tackling excessive waiting times for elective surgery: A comparison of policies in twelve OECD countries.* OECD Health Working Paper. (Paris: Organization for Economic Cooperation and Development. Cited by Anderson, Hussey, Frogner, and Waters (2005, p. 908 & 913).

Hyman, D. A., & Kovacic, Wm. (2003). Monopoly, monopsony, and market definition: An antitrust perspective on market concentration among health insurers. *Health Affairs, 23*(6), 25–28.

Indian Health Service (IHS) (2004a). *Introduction.* Retrieved November 7, 2005 from http://www.ihs.gov/PublicInfo/PublicAffairs/Welcome_Info/IHSintro.asp

Indian Health Service (IHS) (2004b). *Behavioral Health Announcements: What's New. Vision and Mission.* Retrieved November 7, 2005 from http://www.ihs.gov/MedicalPrograms/Behavioral/

Indian Health Service (IHS) (2004c). IHS budget for fiscal year '05. *Behavioral Health Newsletter,* Jan., 2004, p. 4.

Indian Health Service (IHS) (2005). *Behavioral Health Initiatives and Programs.* Retrieved November 7, 2005 from http://www.ihs.gov/MedicalPrograms/Behavioral/index.cfm?module=BH&option="Activit

Insel, T. R., & Fenton, W. S. (2005). Psychiatric Epidemiology: It's not just about counting anymore. *Archives of General Psychiatry, 62,* June, 590–592.

Institute of Medicine (IOM) (1990). *Medicare: A strategy for quality assurance.* Washington, D.C.: National Academy Press.

Institute of Medicine (IOM) (2001a). *Neurological, psychiatric and developmental disorders: Meeting the challenge in the developing world.* Washington, DC: National Academy Press.

Institute of Medicine (IOM) (2001b). *Envisioning the national health care quality report.* Washington, D.C.: National Academies Press.

Institute of Medicine (2002a). *Care without coverage: Too little, too late.* Washington, DC: The National Academies Press.

Institute of Medicine Committee on Assuring the Health of the Public in the 21st Century (IOM) (2002b). Washington, DC: The National Academies Press.

Jackson, G. L., Yano, E. M., Edelman, D. et al (2005). Veterans affairs primary care organizational characteristics associated with better diabetes control. *American Journal of Managed Care, 11*(4), 225–237.

Jenkins, R., Gulbinat, W., Manderscheid, R., et al. (2004). The mental health country profile: background, design and use of a systematic method of appraisal. *International Review of Psychiatry, 16*(1–2), 31–47.

Joint Commission on Accreditation of Healthcare Organizations (JCAHO) (1992). *Accreditation manual for hospitals.* Chicago: Author.

Kanarek, N., & Bialek, R. (2003). Community readiness to meet Healthy People 2010 targets. *Journal of Public Health Management Practice, 9*(3), 249–254.

Kangas, E. E. (1997). Self-interest and the common good: The impact of norms, selfishness and context in social policy opinions. *Journal of Socio-Economics, 26*(5), 475–495.

Kenney, G., & Haley, J. (2001). *Why aren't more uninsured children enrolled in Medicaid and SCHIP?* Washington, DC: The Urban Institute. Series B, No. B-35.

Keppel, K., & Pearcy, J. (2000). Healthy People 2000: An assessment based on the health indicators for the United States and each state. *Healthy People 2000 Statistical Notes 19,* 1–31.

Kessler, R. C., Berglund, P., Demler, O., Jin, R., & Walters, E. (2005a). Lifetime prevalence and age-of-onset distributions of DSM-IV disorders in the national comorbidity survey replication. *Archives of General Psychiatry, 62,* 593–602.

Kessler, R. C., Chiu W.T., Demler, O., & Walters, E. (2005b). Prevalence, severity, and comorbidity of 12-month DSM-IV disorders in the national comorbidity survey replication. *Archives of General Psychiatry, 62,* 617–627.

Kessler, R. C., McGonagle, K. A., Zhao, S., Nelson, C. B., Hughes, M., Eshleman, S., Wittchen, H. U., & Kendler, K. S. (1994). Lifetime and 12-month prevalence of DSM-III-R psychiatric disorders in the United States: Results from the National Comorbidity Survey. *Archives of General Psychiatry, 51,* 8–19.

Kessler, R. C., & Ustun, T. B. (2004). The world mental health (WMH) survey initiative version of the World Health Organization (WHO) composite international diagnostic interview (CIDI). *International Journal of Methods in Psychiatric Research, 13,* 93–121.

King, D., & Mossialos, E. (2005). The determinants of private medical insurance prevalence in England 1997–2000. *Health Services Research, 40*(1), 195–212.

Kiplinger, K. A. (2005, Fall). *Kiplinger's retirement planning.* Washington DC: The Kiplinger Washington Editors Inc.

Kiresuk, T., Smith, A., & Cardillo, J. (1994). *Goal attainment scaling: Application, theory, and measurement.* Hillsdale, NJ: Lawrence Erlbaum.

Kizer, K. W. (1999). The 'New VA': A national laboratory for health care quality improvement. *American Journal of Medical Quality, 14*(1), 3–20.

Klein, R. (2003). Lessons for (and from) America. *American Journal of Public Health, 93*(1), 61–63.

Kohn, L. T., Corrigan, J. M., & Donaldson, M. S. (Eds) (2000). *To err is human: Building a safer health system.* Institute of Medicine.

Koyanagi, C., Burmin, I., Bevilgcqua, J. et al. (1997, March). *Defining medically necessary services to protect plan members.* Washington, DC: Bazelon Center for Mental Health Law.

Krieger, N., Chen, J., Waterman, P., Rehkopf, D., Subramanian, S. (2005). Painting a truer picture of U. S. socioeconomic and racial/ethnic health inequalities: The public health disparities geocoding project. *American Journal of Public Health, 95*(2), 312–323.

Kronick, R., & Gilmer, T. (1999). Explaining the decline in health insurance coverage, 1979–1995. *Health Affairs, 18*(2), 30–47.

Labacqz, K. (1987). *Six theories of justice: Perspectives from philosophical and theological ethics.* Minneapolis: Augsburg Fortress Press.

Laing, W., & Buisson, M. (2001). *Private medical insurance – UK market sector report 2001.* London: Laing and Buisson Publications, Ltd.

Lalonde, M. (1974). *A new perspective on the health care of Canadians: A working document.* Ottawa: Government of Canada.

Lasser, K. E., Mintzer, I. L., Lambert, A., et al. (2005, August). Missed appointment rates in primary care: The importance of site of care. *Journal of Health Care for the Poor and Underserved, 16,* 475–486.

Lewin Group, Inc. (1998). *Paying more and losing ground: How employer cost-shifting is eroding health coverage of working families.* Washington, DC: AFL-CIO.

Liberman, J. (1999). *Testimony of Senator Joseph Lieberman on Deaths and Injuries to Mental Health Patients.* Senate Appropriations Committee on Labor, Health and Human Services, and Education.

Library of Congress (2005). Thomas: Legislative information on the internet/search bills and resolutions. Retrieved September 28, 2005 from http://thomas.loc.gov/

Lohr, K. N. (Ed.) (1990). *Medicare: A strategy for quality assurance.* Washington, D.C.: National Academy Press.

Long, S. K., Coughlin, T., & King, J. (2005). How well does Medicaid work in improving access to care? *Health Services Research, 40*(1), 39–58.

Lowe, R. A., Localio, A. R., Schwarz, D. F., et al. (2005). Association between primary care practice characteristics and emergency department use in a Medicaid managed care organization. *Medical Care, 43*(8), 792–800.

Malm, U., Jacobsson, L., & Larsson, N. O. (2003). Values, system, and evidence for a reform in progress. *International Journal of Mental Health, 31*(4), 50–65.

Mark, T. L., Coffey, R. M., Vandivort-Warren, R., Harwood, H. J., King, E. C., & the MHSA Spending Estimates Team (2005). U.S. spending for mental health and substance abuse treatment, 1991–2001. *Web Exclusives: A supplement to Health Affairs,* Vol. 24, Supplement 1, January-June, W5-133–W5-142.

Marquis, M. S., & Long, S. (2001). Prevalence of selected employer health insurance purchasing strategies in 1997. *Health Affairs, 20*(4), 220–230.

Mattson, M. (Ed.). (1992). *Manual of psychiatric quality assurance: Report of the APA Committee on Quality Assurance.* Washington, D.C.: American Psychiatric Association.

Maxwell, J., & Temin, P. (2002). Managed competition versus industrial purchasing of health care among the Fortune 500. *Journal of Health Politics, Policy, and Law, 27*(1), 5–30.

Mazor, K. M., Clauser, B. E., Field, T., Yood, R. A., & Gurwitz, J. H. (2002). A demonstration of the impact of response bias on the results of patient satisfaction surveys. *Health Sciences Research, 37*(5), 1403–1417.

McAvoy, P. V., Driscoll, M. B., & Gramling, B. J. (2004). Integrating the environment, the economy, and community health: A community health center's initiative to link health benefits to smart growth. *American Journal of Public Health, 94*(4), 525–527.

McGuire, A., & Serra, V. (2005). The cost of care: Is there an optimal level of expenditure? *Harvard International Review,* Spring, pp. 70–73.

Mechanic, D. (2003). Is the prevalence of mental disorders a good measure of the need for services? *Health Affairs, 22*(5), 8–20.

Medi-Cal Policy Institute (2000). *Speaking out: What beneficiaries say about the Medi-Cal program.* Oakland, CA: Medi-Cal Policy Institute.

Miller, I. (1966a). Time-limited brief therapy has gone too far: The result is invisible rationing. *Professional Psychology: Research and Practice, 27*(6), 567–576.

Miller, I (1966b). Ethical and liability issues concerning invisible rationing. *Professional Psychology: Research and Practice, 27*(6), 583–587.

Millman, M. (Ed.). (1993). Committee on Monitoring Access to Personal Health Care Services. *Access to Health Care in America.* Washington, DC: National Academy Press.

Minnesota Health Data Institute (MHDI) (1997, Oct.). *1997 Medicaid and Minnesota care managed care member satisfaction survey. Summary report of aggregate and plan-specific comparisons.* Minneapolis, MN: Author.

Minnesota Physician-Patient Alliance (MPPA) (1998). *Managed care costs: Where do Minnesota HMOs spend our money?* Minneapolis: Author.

Minnesota Senior Federation (MSF), (2005). *Health Care Choices.* St. Paul: Author.

Mohr, P. (1998). Medical necessity: A moving target. *Psychiatric Services, 49*(11), 1391.

Murphy, M., DeBernardo, C., & Shoemaker, W. (1998). Impact of managed care on independent practice and professional ethics: A survey of independent practitioners. *Professional Psychology: Research and Practice, 29*(1), 43–51.

Murray, C., & Frank, J. (2001). World health report 2000: A step toward evidence-based health policy. *Lancet, 357,* 1698–1700.

National Alliance for the Mentally Ill (NAMI) (2005). *About NAMI.* Retrieved September 28, 2005 from http://www.nami.org/

National Committee for Quality Assurance (NCQR) (Ed.). (1997). *HEDIS 3.0: Narrative: What's in it and why it matters.* Washington, CD: Author.

Navarro, V. (2001). World health report 2000: A response to Murray and Frank. *Lancet, 357,* 1701–1702.

Navarro, V. (2002). The World health report 2000: Can health care systems be compared using a single measure of performance? *American Journal of Public Health, 92,* 31 & 33–34.

National Center for Health Statistics, Division of Data Services (NCHS) (2002). *Facts and Stats: Mental Health.* Retrieved October 25, 2002 from http://www.cdc.gov/nchs/fastats/mental.htm

National Center for Health Statistics, Division of Data Services (NCHS) (2003). *Health, United States, 2002.* Retrieved June 12, 2003 from http://www.cdc.gov/nchs/

OECD Factbook 2005. National Accounts of OECD Countries, Vol. 1, p. 265). Retrieved July 19, 2005 from http://www.oecd.org

OECD Health Data 2005. Retrieved July 19, 2005 from http://www.oecd.org

Office of Personnel Management (OPM) (1999, Nov. 3). *Patient's Bill of Rights and the Federal Employees Health Benefits Program.* Retrieved July 7, 2005 from http://www.opm.gov/insure/html/billrights.html

Office of Personnel Management (OPM) (1999, June 7). *White House Directs OPM to Achieve Mental Health and Substance Abuse Health Coverage Parity.* Retrieved July 7, 2005 from http://www.opm.gov/pressrel/1999/health.htm

Olfson, M., & Pincus, H. (1994a). Outpatient psychotherapy in the United States I: Volume, costs, and user characteristics. *American Journal of Psychiatry, 151,* 1281–1288.

Olfson, M., & Pincus, H. (1994b). Outpatient psychotherapy in the United States II: Patterns of utilization. *American Journal of Psychiatry, 151,* 1289–1294.

Olson, R. P. (1997). *Manual for setting, scaling, and rating assessment and therapy practicum goals.* Minneapolis: Author.

Olson, R. P. (1999). *A critique of Minnesota's managed mental health care with special reference to medical necessity determinations for outpatient psychotherapy: A resource document.* Minneapolis: Author.

Olson, R. P., & Beecher, L. (1999, Sept.). Medical necessity: Rationing psychiatric services. *Minnesota Physician, 13*(6), 20–26.

Office of National Statistics (ONS) (2003). *Census 2001: General report for England and Wales.* London: Author.

Orwell, G. (1946). *Animal Farm.* New York: Harcourt, Brace, and Co.

Petrila, J., & Levin, B. L. (2004). Mental disability law, policy, and service delivery. In B. L. Levin, J. Petrila, & K. D. Hennessy. *Mental Health Services: A Public Health Perspective* (2nd ed., pp. 42-71). New York: Oxford University.

Phillips, K. (2002). *Wealth and democracy: A political history of the American rich.* New York: Broadway Books.

Physicians for a National Health Program (PNHP) (2002). Power point presentation. Retrieved October 31, 2005 from http://www.PNHP.org

Politzer, R. M., Yoon, J., Shi, L., Hughes, R. G., Regan, J., & Gaston, M. H. (2001). Inequality in America: The contribution of health centers in reducing and eliminating disparities in access to care. *Medical Care Research and Review, 58*(2), 234–248.

Polsky, D., Stein, R., Nicholson, S., & Bundorf, M. (2005). Employer health insurance offerings and employee enrollment decisions. *Health Services Research, 40*(5), Part I., 1259–1278.

President's Commission on the Health Needs of the Nation (1953). Washington, DC: U.S. Government Printing Office.

President's Commission on Mental Health (1978). *Report to the President from the President's Commission on Mental Health.* 4 vols. Washington, DC: U. S. Government Printing Office.

President's New Freedom Commission on Mental Health (2003). *Achieving the Promise: Transforming Mental Health Care in America.* Available at http://www.mentalhealthcommission.gov/finalreport/fullreport.htm

Regier, D. A. (2003). Mental disorder, diagnostic theory, and practical reality. *Health Affairs, 22*(5), 21–27.

Ribines, L. N., & Regier, D. A. (Eds.). (1991). *Psychiatric disorders in America: The epidemiologic catchment area study.* New York, NY: The Free Press.

Ricketts, T. C. (2005). Workforce issues in rural areas: A focus on policy equity. *American Journal of Public Health, 95*(1), 42–47.

Roberts, M. C., Alexander, K., & Davis, N. J. (1991). Children's rights to physical and mental health care: A case for advocacy. *Journal of Clinical Child Psychology, 20*(1), 18–27.

Robiner, W. (1991). How many psychologists are needed? A call for a national psychology human resource agenda. *Professional Psychology: Research and Practice, 22*(6), 427–440.

Robiner, W., Ax, R., & Stam, B. (2002). Addressing the supply of psychologists in the workforce: Is focusing principally on demand sound economics? *Journal of Clinical Psychology in Medical Settings, 9*(4), 273–285.

Robiner, W., & Crew, D. (2000). Rightsizing the workforce of psychologists in health care: Trends from licensing boards, training programs, and managed care. *Professional Psychology: Research and Practice, 31*(3), 245–263.

Robinson, J. (2003). Consolidation and the transformation of competition in health insurance. *Health Affairs, 23*(6), 11–24.

Rodriguez-Garcia, R., & Akhter, M. N. (2000). Human rights: The foundation of public health practice. *American Journal of Public Health, 90*(5), 693–695.

Roemer, R. (1988). The right to health care - gains and gaps. *American Journal of Public Health, 78*(3), 241–247.

Roohan, P. J., Franko, S. J., Anarello, J. P., Dellehunt, L. K., & Gesten, F. C. (2003). Do commercial managed care members rate their health plans differently than Medicaid managed care members? *Health Services Research, 38*(4), 1121–1134.

Rosenthal, M. B., Zaslavsky, A., & Newhouse, J. P. (2005). The geographic distribution of physicians revisited. *Health Services Research, 40*(6), Part I, 1931–1952.

Rowland, D., Garfield, R., & Ellias, R. (2003). Accomplishments and challenges in Medicaid mental health. *Health Affairs, 22*(5), 73–83.

Scheffler, R. M., & Kirby, P. B. (2003). The occupational transformation of the mental health system. *Health Affairs, 22*(5), 177–188.

Schilder, K., Tomov, T., Mladenova, M. et al. (2004). The appropriateness and use of focus groups methodology across international mental health communities. *International Review of Psychiatry, 16*(1–2), 24–30.

Schoen, C., Doty, M., Collins, S., & Holmgren, A. (2005). Insured but not protected: How many adults are underinsured? *Web Exclusives: A supplement to Health Affairs*, vol. 24, Supplement 1, January-June, W5-289–W5-302.

Schuster, M. A., McGlynn, E. A., & Brook, R. H. (2005). How good is the quality of health care in the United States? *The Milbank Quarterly, 83*(4), 843–895. Reprinted from *The Milbank Quarterly*, 1990, 76(4), 517–563.

Securing Access to Health Care. A report on the ethical implications of differences in the availability of health services. Volume One: Report, President's Commission for the Study of Ethical Problems in Medicine and Biomedical and Behavioral Research. Alexander M. Capron, Executive Director, Washington, DC.

Seldon, T., Banthian, J., & Cohen, J. (1998). Medicaid's problem children: Eligible but not enrolled. *Health Affairs, 17*(3), 192–200.

Shi, L., Regan, J., Politzer, R. M., & Luo, J. (2001). Community health centers and racial/ethnic disparities in healthy life. *International Journal of Health Services, 31*(3), 567–582.

Shi, L., Stevens, G. D., Wulu, J. T., jr., Politzer, R. M., & Xu, J. (2004). America's health centers: Reducing racial and ethnic disparities in perinatal care and birth outcomes. *Health Services Research, 39*(6), 1881–1901.

Shojania, D. G., & Grimshaw, J. M. (2005). Evidence-based quality improvement: The state of the science. *Health Affairs, 24*(1), 138–150.

Smith, L. (2005). Psychotherapy, classism, and the poor: Conspicuous by their absence. *American Psychologist, 60*(7), 687–696.

Smith, V. R., Ramesh, R., Gifford, K., et al. (2003). *States respond to fiscal pressure: State Medicaid spending growth and cost containment in fiscal years 2003 and 2004. Results from a 50-state survey.* Washington, DC: Kaiser Commission on Medicaid and the Uninsured.

Sommers, B. D. (2005). From Medicaid to uninsured: Dropout among children in public assistance programs. *Health Services Research, 40*(1), 59–78.

Snyder, C., & Anderson, G. (2005, June). Do quality improvement organizations improve the quality of hospital care for Medicare beneficiaries? *Journal of the American Medical Association, 293*, 2900–2907.

Spear, S. J. (2005). Fixing health care from the inside, today. *Harvard Business Review, 83*(9), 78–91.

Starfield, B., Shi, L., & Macinko, J. (2005). Contributions of primary care to health systems and health. *The Milbank Quarterly, 83*(3), 457–502.

Star Tribune (2005, Oct. 18). *$1.6 billion loss for GM, but it gets health care deal.* Minneapolis: Author, p. D3.

Statistics Canada (2001). *Language Composition of Canada, Census 2001.* Retrieved December 22, 2004 from http://www12.statcan.ca/english/census01/products/highlight/languagecomposition/principal.cfm. Cited by J. Arnett, chapter four this volume.

Statistics Canada (2003). *The Canadian Community Health Survey: Mental Health and Well-Being.* Cited by J. Arnett, chapter four this volume.

Street, L. (2002). *The Medi-Cal budget: Cost drivers and policy considerations.* Oakland, CA: Medi-Cal Policy Institute.

Stricker, G., & Rodriguez, A. (Eds.) (1988). *Handbook of quality assurance in mental health.* New York: Plenum Press.

Stuber, J., & Bradley, E. (2005). Barriers to Medicaid enrollment: Who is at risk? *American Journal of Public Health, 95*(2), 525–527.

The Constitution of the United States (1966). Introduction by E. C. Smith. New York: Barnes & Noble.

The World Bank Group (June 5, 2003). Social capital for development. Cited by Henderson, S., & Whiteford, H. (2003). Social capital and mental health. *Lancet, 362*, August 16, p. 506.

Thornicroft, G., & Tansella, M. (1999). Translating ethical principles into outcome measures for mental health service research. *Psychological Medicine, 29*, 761–767.

Townsend, C., Whiteford, H., Baingana, F., et al. (2004). The mental health policy template: Domains and elements for mental health policy formulation. *International Review of Psychiatry, 16*(1–2), 18–23.

Turner, S., & Foong, S. (2003). Navigating the road to implementation of the Health Insurance Portability and Accountability Act. *American Journal of Public Health, 93*(11), 1806–1808.

United Nations General Assembly (1948). *Universal Declaration of Human Rights.* Retrieved September 21, 2005 from http://www.unhchr.ch/udhr/lang/eng.htm

United Nations General Assembly (1989, October 16). *Convention on the rights of the child.* New York: Author (UNGA document A/REW/44/25)

United Nations General Assembly (1991). *The protection of persons with mental illness and the improvement of mental health care.* UN General Assembly resolution A/REW/46.119. Available at http://www.un.org/ga/documents/gadocs.htm

United Nations General Assembly (2000). *United Nations Millennium Declaration. Resolution 55/2.* Fifty-fifth session. Agenda item 60(b) adopted the original Resolution 217 A (III). New York: Author. Retrieved September 21, 2005 from http://www.un.org/english/engtxt.shtml

United States Census Bureau (2005). *Annual population estimates.* Retrieved October 4, 2005 from http://www.census.gov/popest/states/tables/NST-EST 2004-01.pdf

United States Chamber of Commerce (2003). *The employee benefits survey.* Washington, DC: AIG Companies. Available at http://www.uschamber.com/resources/research/benefits.htm

United States General Accountability Office (U. S. GAO) (1990, Feb.). *Quality assurance: A comprehensive national strategy for health care is needed.* Briefing Report to the Chairman, United States bipartisan Commission on Comprehensive Health Care. GAO/PEMD-90-14BR, 1–32.

U. S. News and World Report, March 9, 1998, p. 48.

VandenBos, G., DeLeon, P., & Belar, C. (1991). How many psychological practitioners are needed? It's too early to know! *Professional Psychology: Research and Practice, 22*(6), 441–448.

Wang, P.S., Berglund, P., Olfson, M., Pincus, H., Wells, K., & Kessler, R. (2005a). Failure and delay in initial treatment contact after first onset of mental disorders in the national co-morbidity survey replication. *Archives of General Psychiatry, 62*, 603–613.

Wang, P.S., Lane, M., Olfson, M., Pincus, H., Wells, K., & Kessler, R. (2005b). Twelve-month use of mental health services in the United States. *Archives of General Psychiatry, 62*, 629–640.

Webster, P. (2005). Canada struggles with health care: Prime minister faces no-confidence vote. *USA Today*, Nov. 25, p. 9A.

Wei, W., Sambamoorthi, U., & Olfson, M. (2005). Use of psychotherapy for depression in older adults. *American Journal of Psychiatry, 162*(4), 711–717.

Weissman, J. S., & Epstein, A. M. (1993). The insurance gap: Does it make a difference? *Annual Review of public Health, 14*, 243–270.

Wells, K., Katon, W., Rogers, B., & Camp, P. (1994). Use of minor tranquilizers and antidepressant medications by depressed outpatients: Results from the medical outcomes study. *American Journal of Psychiatry, 151*, 694–700.

Wells, K. B., Norquist, B., Benjamin, B., Rogers, W., Kahn, K., & Brook, R. (1994). Quality of antidepressant medications prescribed at discharge to depressed elderly patients in general medical hospitals before and after a prospective payment system. *General Hospital Psychiatry, 16,* 4–15.

Wells, K., Sherbourne, C., Duan, N., et al. (2005, June). Quality improvement for depression in primary care. *American Journal of Psychiatry, 162,* 1149–1157.

White House Domestic Policy Council (1993). *The President's health security plan: The Clinton blueprint.* New York: Random House.

Whitehead, M. (1992). The concepts and principles of equity and health. *International Journal of Health Services, 22*(3), 429–445.

Williams, D. R., & Collins, C. A. (1995). U.S. socioeconomic and racial differences in health. *Annual Review of Sociology, 21,* 349–386.

Williams, D. R., Neighbors, H. W., & Jackson, J. S. (2003). Racial/ethnic discrimination and health: Findings from community studies. *American Journal of Public Health, 93,* 200–208.

World Book Encyclopedia (1980). Chicago: World Book-Childcraft International, Inc.

World Health Organization (WHO) (1946). *Preamble to the Constitution of the World Health Organization as adopted by the International Conference, New York, 19–22 June, 1946; signed on 22 July, 1946.* Retrieved September 21, 2005 from http://www.who.int/about/definition/en/

World Health Organization (WHO) (1948). *Constitution of the World Health Organization.* Retrieved September 21, 2005 from http://policy.who.int/cgi-bin/om_isapidll?

World Health Organization (WHO) (1997). *An overview of a strategy to improve the mental health of underserved populations: Nations for mental health.* Geneva, Switzerland: Author (unpublished document WHO/MSA/NAM/ 97.3).

World Health Organization (WHO) (2000). *World health report 2000. Health systems: Improving performance.* Geneva, Switzerland: Author.

World Health Organization (WHO) (2001). *The world health report 2001. Mental health: New understanding, new hope.* Geneva, Switzerland: Author.

World Health Organization (WHO) (2004a). *The World Health Report 2004: Changing history.* Geneva, Switzerland: Author.

World Health Organization (WHO) (2004b). The World Mental Health Survey Consortium. Prevalence, severity, and unmet need for treatment of mental disorders in the World Health Organization World Mental Health Survey. *Journal of the American Medical Association, 291,* 2581–2590.

World Health Organization (WHO) (2005a). *Mental Health Atlas – 2005.* Geneva, Switzerland: Author. Retrieved October 17, 2005 from http://www.who.int/mental_health/evidence/atlas/main/htm

World Health Organization (WHO) (2005b). *The world health report 2005: Make every mother and child count.* Geneva, Switzerland: Author.

Wright, O. (2003). Best hospitals have worst death rates. *Times (London),* 12 May 2003.

Wu, Z., & Schimmele, C. M. (2005). Racial/ethnic variation in functional and self-reported health. *American Journal of Public Health, 95*(4), 710–716.

Zhas, C., Arispe, I., Kelley, E., et al. (2005). Ambulatory care visits for treating adverse drug effects in the United States, 1995–2001. *Journal of Quality and Patient Safety, 31*(7), 372–378.

Chapter 7

MEETING THE NEEDS, CONCLUSIONS, AND RECOMMENDATIONS

R. Paul Olson

The sixth and final criterion our contributing authors were asked to apply was population relevance. This criterion addresses the general question about the degree to which a country's mental health system is meeting the needs of those who suffer mental disorders. This chapter begins with a definition of unmet need, followed by global estimates and the authors' views of unmet need in their respective countries. (Direct quotes from our chapter authors are indicated by either quotation marks or in block indented format without page references.) Comparisons among the four countries on the six evaluation criteria are summarized, along with additional lessons we've learned from each country's system. Thereafter, the present author draws some conclusions and provides methodological recommendations concerning comparative studies and for improving mental health delivery systems. The chapter ends with discussion of some of the current strategies for health care reform in the United States.

ADDRESSING UNMET NEEDS

Defining Unmet Need

Mechanic (2003) noted that epidemiological studies of prevalence are ambiguous and unsatisfactory measures of need, partly because indicators of the degree of disability, distress, duration, and recurrence are often masked or excluded in statistical tabulations. Some of these limitations have been addressed in the newly revised methodologies of epidemiological studies, which include estimates of severity (disability) and comorbidity (Insel and Fenton, 2005), and these additional indicators are being incorporated into current epidemiological studies in 27 countries participating in the WHO World Mental Health Survey initiative (Kessler and Ustun, 2004). Despite limitations, these studies provide us with some window into potential need, which may or may not translate into actual demand for services. "Quantifying the prevalence of mental disorders, the disabilities associated with them, and the adequacy of service provision forms the foundation for national and international mental health policy" (Insel and Fenton, 2005, p. 591). The basic indicator of unmet need is the percentage of the population with mental disorders who do not receive mental health services.

Global Estimates of Mental Health Needs

The WHO Director-General stated the following in 2001: "Initial estimates suggest that about 450 million people alive today suffer from mental or neurological disorder or from psychosocial problems such as those related to alcohol and drug abuse" (Brundtland, 2001). International studies suggest that nearly 50 percent of a population acquires a mental disorder through their lifetime, and 20 percent to 30 percent have had a mental disorder within the last 12 months (Dalgard, Kringlen, and Dahl, 2002). Moreover, it has been estimated by the WHO (2000, pp. 23-26) that in 2000, about 12 percent of the total burden of all disease was accounted for by mental and neurological disorders, projected to increase to 15 percent by the year 2020. In all age groups, for both sexes, unipolar depression was ranked as the fourth leading cause of disability (12% of all causes of disability). Six neuropsychiatric conditions ranked among the top 20 causes of the number of years lost due to disability in the world: unipolar depressive disorders, alcohol use disorders, schizophrenia, bipolar affective disorder, Alzheimer's and other dementias, and migraine. An estimated 24 percent of the patients in primary health care settings manifest mental or behavioral disorders. The Institute of Medicine (2001) reported that about 85 percent of people with mental disorders in developing countries and 46 percent in developed countries were untreated in 1990. The most recent national epidemiological study of the U.S. population (Wang et al. 2005b) reported 60 percent of people with mental disorders were untreated.

Current Versus Future Needs. The need for mental health treatment is likely to increase in the future with changing demographics, which may not be reflected in current prevalence data. As an example, comparative data compiled by the WHO (2004a, pp. 112–119) are available on the changes in percentages of populations age 60+ years from 1992 to 2002. The data are summarized for the four countries included in this study in Table 7.1.

The statistics reported suggest relatively stable percentages of elderly (60+ years) for the decade ending 2002. The most noticeable changes are the 1.0 percent decline in Norway in contrast to the 1.3 percent increase in Canada. The averages of all four countries suggest that about 18 percent of the populations are elderly, and that over the decade there was no significant change in that proportion.

What the statistics do not show is the very rapid growth in the proportion of elderly that will occur within the forthcoming decade. For example, estimates of the "graying of America" project a significant rise in the percentage of elderly as "baby boomers" (born soon after the end of World War II) begin retiring. One estimate is that the 36 million Americans who are 65 years and older and receiving Medicare in 2005 will more than double within six years to 77 million in 2011. "With the baby-boomers streaming down the pipeline in unprecedented numbers, the need and the cost of care will only go up" (Kiplinger, 2005, p. 102). Any estimate of potential and future unmet need must take into account the very significant change in demographics that is likely to occur. The need for geriatric mental health services will increase markedly in the next decade. A failure in appropriate work force planning will only exacerbate the unmet needs for mental health services among the elderly.

Unmet Need in Great Britain

The overwhelming majority of mental health services in England are provided through the National Health Service, which collects regular statistics on prevalence data of DSM and ICD-10 categories of mental disorders, service utilization data, and data from systematic surveys using measures such as the *Cardinal Needs Measure* (Marshall et al. 1995) and the *Camberwell Assessment of Need* (CAN) measure (Slade, Loftus, Phelan, Thornicroft, and Wykes, 1999), including an adaptation to assess the need for the elderly (CANE).

Point prevalence estimates of the need for services are that 10 percent of children and 16 percent of adults suffer from a mental disorder at any one time. Among those receiving disability benefits, 866,000 adults report their primary condition is a mental disorder. Hazardous drinking is present among 26 percent of adults and illicit drug use among 11 percent. There are more than 4,700 suicides in England and Wales each year, though the overall rate of suicide is falling. One in ten older people aged 60–74 years living in private households in the UK will have a common mental disorder such as anxiety, depression, or phobia. Up to 670,000 have some form of dementia, five percent of people over 65, and 10 to 20 percent of people over 80. Elderly with lifelong mental disorders, combined with physical disability can become extremely isolated and neglected. The 11 percent non-Caucasian, minority population in the UK (about 6.5 million) are unevenly distributed geographically, and that presents a challenge to the equitable provision of culturally competent mental health services. A significant (but unknown) portion of the increasing population of refugees and asylum seekers in Britain have traumatic histories, but understanding their needs is complicated by the fact that their English language skills may be poor, and some may be illiterate in their own language.

Table 7.1. *Changes in Percentages of Populations Age 60+ Years, 1992 to 2002.*

Country	1992	2002	% Change
Great Britain	21.1	20.8	–0.3
Norway	20.6	19.6	–1.0
Canada	15.8	17.1	+1.3
United States	16.4	16.2	–0.2
Mean, 4 countries	18.5	18.4	–0.1

Note: Source is WHO (2004a). Annex Table 1, pp. 112–119.

Based on a conservative point prevalence rate of 26 percent of adults and children with mental disorders, of the total population of about 50 million in England, 13 million are estimated to be in need of mental health services. The percent of people with mental disorders *not* receiving full and appropriate mental health services varies by treatment setting. For primary care settings the range of unmet need is from 50 percent for severe disorders to 80 percent for moderate mental disorders. For mental health specialist care settings, the comparable range is from 30 percent to 60 percent (Hall, J., personal communication December 24, 2005). The unmet need for mental health services is greatest in the primary care settings for both severe and moderate mental disorders. The average unmet need for mental health care is 65 percent in primary care and 45 percent in specialist care settings. About 25 percent of consultations with family physicians (GPs) concern mental health issues.

Improving access to mental health services among minorities and other subgroups has been a target of national policy since 2003, especially with reference to those at high risk for suicide and in need of acute inpatient treatment. Dr. Hall observed:

> Improvements in psychiatric epidemiology have led to increased recognition of subgroups in the population with high levels of need that may not have been previously recognized (eating disorders being the obvious example). These subgroups may either be distributed relatively similarly across the country, or they may be very sensitive to variations in local demography, such as ethnic origin and levels of social deprivation.

Recognition of the unmet need led to detailed guidelines from the Department of Health (DoH), articulated in a 2004 document entitled, *Organizing and Delivering Psychological Therapies*. The DoH expects local services to meet several standards, such as providing evidence-based treatments accessible within a reasonable time to meet the psychotherapeutic needs of the range of groups and settings in the service area. Key functions and interventions to be offered by qualified staff were identified for seven levels of care: support by the wider community (level 1); voluntary, self-help and independent sector provisions (level 2); primary mental health care (levels 3 & 4); generic and specialized community mental health teams (level 5); local specialist inpatient and residential services (level 6); and tertiary specialist mental health services (level 7). ". . . particular policy attention has been paid to the provision of psychological therapies in the NHS because this area of intervention has shown the greatest gap between demand and provision since the mid-1990s."

To meet the needs of serious and complex mental disorders that are either very small in volume, or present high levels of clinical risk, the NHS developed guidelines for high and medium secure services. "The category of low-secure tertiary services is not specifically covered in the National Service Frameworks or in any of the Policy Implementation Guidelines, and the lack of low-secure inpatient services, and the associated community support and advice, may constitute a significant gap in provision."

There is a continuous needs assessment that has become a part of the decision-making process for the allocation of NHS funds. The process by which the NHS determines its purchasing of health care services is called "commissioning."

> Commissioning consists of a conventional cycle of (a) assessment of the needs of a given population, (b) comparing that assessment with current levels of provision to identify gaps, and (c) prioritizing desired services in the light of government priorities. Thus, effective commissioning depends on an accurate understanding both of local demography and epidemiology, and of high-need subgroups within the population.

In 2005, national guidance was provided for the 300 mental health commissioners who participate in the commissioning decisions of Primary Care Trusts. The detailed guidelines appeared in *The Commissioning Friend for Mental Health Services* (National Primary and Care Trust Development Programme, 2005).

Another indicator of unmet need in Britain has been its persistent waiting lists for certain health care services. The reader will recall that waiting time for health care services is one element in the WHO indicator of the performance of a health care system termed "responsiveness." Among the four countries, Britain was ranked lowest in responsiveness in 1997 (see Table 6.1, this volume). Since 2004, reducing waiting times for both outpatient and inpatient mental health appointments has become a specific target of the Commission for Healthcare Audit and Inspection (CHAI). England is increasing capital investments in treatment facilities and equipment to reduce the waiting time for health care services.

One of the more significant needs identified by Dr. Hall is the shortage of qualified mental health staff: "the existing pool of qualified staff is simply inadequate to meet the demand for staff." The shortage of qualified mental health specialists is also a problem in Norway, and more of a problem than financing.

Unmet Need in Norway

Based on epidemiological studies in Norway, *point prevalence* is estimated at 15–20 percent of the population have some sort of psychological distress, and that the majority of these are in need of treatment. About 15 percent of the population represents most of the psychiatric morbidity. Our Norwegian experts estimated the following:

> Based on a total population of 4,577,000 in January 1, 2004, and a conservative estimate of 15% of the population with psychological distress, an estimated 687,000 inhabitants have a reduced mental health. An increasing share is asking for treatment and care. Approximately 180,000 were actually in contact with the specialized mental health services in 2003, which is 4% of the total population, and about 25% of those with some sort of psychological distress or disorders. This figure suggests that more than 10% of the total population in Norway, or about 500,000 people with disorders or distress, do not receive treatment in the specialized mental health services.

As interpreted by this editor, among the 15 percent of the population in Norway with some sort of psychological distress or disorder, about 75 percent did *not* receive treatment from the specialized mental health services. The percentage with psychological distress or disorders who received some treatment in the primary health care sector is unknown.

In 1998, only about two percent of the population below 18 years of age was offered mental health services. The NMHP goal was to increase that to five percent by 2006. The rate increased to 2.9 percent in 2002. "There is a great 'gap' between the number of patients in need of treatment estimated from epidemiological studies, and the number actually treated in Norway. Though more people than ever before actually are treated, the 'gap' has widened in recent years due to increased acceptance and demand."

Unmet need is most evident among the elderly, immigrants, and people with severe mental disorders. There continues to be "severe shortcomings" in the provision of living arrangements, supportive care, and treatment possibilities provided in local communities, especially for chronically ill patients. The continued shortage of beds in acute psychiatric units or wards in both general medical and psychiatric facilities results in long waits. Insufficient numbers and types of alternatives in intermediate and long-term facilities are some causes of the back-up in acute units. The length of waiting lists for acute psychiatric units for children and adolescents as well as adults varies with the health region and county. An unintended result is *de facto* inequity in access to acute inpatient mental health services.

There was a growing awareness in Norway of unmet needs for mental health services in the 1990s. A 1996/1997 government document, *White Paper on Mental Health Issues*, provided a clear picture of multiple deficiencies. The legislative response by Parliament in 1998 was to create and fund the National Mental Health Programme (NMHP) effective in 1999 to 2006, later extended to 2008.

By 2003, 71 of 83 District Psychiatric Centres (about 85%) had been established. The remaining 12 will be developed in the coming years. These centres have full responsibility to provide inpatient, outpatient, crisis intervention for their geographic catchment area. "Unfortunately, other institutions have been closed down at a much faster rate than planned, reducing the total number of beds available." Institutional beds for acute psychiatric care are especially deficient in number and distribution throughout the country.

Of the 14 objectives of the NMHP, seven (50%) were attained at or above the targeted level by 2002. Progress toward the targeted levels of improvement seems considerable on 12 of the 14 goals (86%). Nevertheless, unmet need is evident in the relatively slower progress on the goal of increasing institutional beds (a) for children and adolescents, (b) for people who are sentenced to treatment, and (c) on the goal of increasing by 50 percent the productivity of adult outpatient mental health services.

A conclusion by our Norwegian authors:

> Despite noteworthy progress since the NMHP was initiated in 1999, services are lacking in several respects. Community-based services, provided by the municipalities, are not sufficiently developed to meet requirements. Cooperation between services and coordination of services on the individual level are also lacking in several respects. As a result, the pressure on specialized services, especially acute services, becomes unnecessarily high, leading to unnecessary waiting and to misplacement of patients in institutions. Despite the development of community-based services and a policy of deinstitutionalization, 80 percent of the resources in specialized services for adults are still spent on inpatient treatment, in many cases providing services to patients primarily in need of community-based services.... Cooperation with users and relatives on an equal basis has still to be considerably improved....

Epidemiological estimates of the need for mental health services do not equate with actual demand for those services. Prevalence rates of 15–20 percent of the population with mental disorders or distress in Norway are higher than peoples' own judgment of their need for treatment. Studies in Norway based on self-rated mental health indicate that about 10 percent of the population have worries, are depressed or anxious. The actual demand for mental health services is therefore less than 20 percent. Moreover, the demand increases partly as a function of the increased supply of services, as the population becomes more aware of how to deal with problems of mood disorders, anxiety, and deviant behavior.

It is important to remember that Norway has essentially a publicly financed and publicly administered mental health system. Even centrally organized, mental health systems in wealthy countries face the persistent challenge of unmet needs of the population. This raises the question of whether public financing and administration is either a necessary or sufficient condition for optimal performance of a mental health system in meeting its population needs for mental health services. It also raises a deeper philosophical question: Is there some limitation within human nature itself that limits the perfection of the systems humans create?

Unmet Need in Canada

As estimates of the need for mental health services, Canada has a prevalence range of about 10 percent (12-month) to 20 percent (lifetime) of the population. The lower estimate comes from the 2002 *Canadian Community Health Survey: Mental Health and Well-Being* (Statistics Canada, 2003), which found an annual rate *(period prevalence)* of 10.6 percent of mental disorders and substance abuse among the 37,000 Canadians ages 15+ years, who were surveyed with the World Mental Health-Composite International Diagnostic Interview (WMH-CIIDI) (WHO, 1990). The interview yields diagnostic evaluations consistent with definitions of mental disorders used in DSM-IV (American Psychiatric Association, 1994).

A larger figure for *lifetime* prevalence comes from a *Report on Mental Illnesses in Canada* (Health Canada, 2002):

> Approximately 20 percent of Canadians will experience a mental health disorder in their lifetime. The costs for mental illnesses doubled from $7 billion Canadian Dollars (CDN) in 1993 to $14 billion CDN in 1998, just five years later. Thus, the need for cost-effective comprehensive, patient-focused, accessible, and high quality mental health services is compelling and pressing.

As an approximate estimate of need, Dr. Arnett cited the prevalence rate of mental disorders in the population of about 20 percent. At the current population of about 32 million, the estimated number of people with mental disorders is about 6.4 million in need of mental health services. In the *Canadian Community Health Survey: Mental Health and Well-Being* (Statistics Canada, 2003), less than one-third of Canadians reporting symptoms suggestive of a mental disorder or substance abuse problem reported contacting any health professional about their issues. The estimated unmet need for mental health services is about 70 percent or 4.5 million, comparable to the estimate for Norway (75%), but higher than England with average estimates of 65 percent unmet need in primary mental health care and 45 percent in specialty care for people with both moderate and severe mental disorders. Only about one-fourth to one-third of Canada's population with mental disorders or psychological distress received mental health specialist services.

Dr. Arnett identified the following subjective and objective barriers to equitable access to mental health services in Canada:

> (a) inadequate funding for mental health services; (b) a shortage of qualified mental health professionals; (c) the uneven distribution of mental health professionals across the country, and especially in more rural and remote areas; (d) greater attention given to short-term acute psychiatric care than care for the seriously and persistently mentally ill; (e) access limited by individuals' ability to pay in the private sector; (f) a virtual monopoly over government reimbursement by the medical establishment to the exclusion of other mental health professions for outpatient mental health services; (g) the continued dominance of a medical model of mental disorders, and biological interventions (psychopharmacology) restricts access to a wider range of psychosocial interventions; and (h) social stigma (i.e., being afraid to ask for professional help or fearful of what others might think if one did so).

That the ability to pay for mental health services delivered privately would function as a financial barrier to receiving mental health care in Canada is somewhat surprising because the system is largely (70%) publicly financed (Table 1.3), and user fees and balanced billing were disallowed by the 1984 *Canada Health Act*. So why are there any private payments at all in this national health insurance system? One significant answer is found in its national policy, which excludes allied mental health professionals in the private sector from reimbursement by Medicare for outpatient services.

Dr. Arnett writes:

> Presently, the mental health system in Canada does not comprehensively meet the mental health service needs of Canadians. There is good evidence that the system is under-resourced in urban areas and even less accessible in the more remote and northern areas of Canada, particularly for Canada's Aboriginal populations. The mental health system is largely institutionally-based and there are inadequate community services. These limitations have not changed much over the years in spite of provincial government promises. Mental health services are poorly coordinated and there is little linkage between primary care, mental health services, housing, income support, etc. In general there is a significant absence of strong leadership. The underlying philosophy that guides the development of clinical services, particularly in health care institutions, is typically based on a biomedical and illness model of mental health problems for which pharmacotherapy is the mainstay of treatment. Although there does not appear to be a major public revolt aimed against the current mental health system in Canada, the system is used by only about one-third of those experiencing mental health problems.... Overall, and in spite of years of reform, the fundamental components of the institutionally-based mental health system appear to be similar to the way they were prior to reform, except smaller. The fundamental biomedical model has remained intact and may in fact have strengthened.

Among Dr. Arnett's recommendations are the following: (a) address the unmet needs of minorities, children and adolescents, elderly, Aboriginal, rural and remote residents, and the severely and persistently mentally ill; (b) develop a suicide prevention program; (c) encourage psychologically-based services; (d) make a conceptual shift from biologically-based, medically necessary treatments to a broader biopsychosocial model of mental disorders and interventions.

To these recommendations we add that to implement the above changes (especially c & d) nonphysician, mental health professionals will have to organize politically with citizens to influence policymakers through legislation or litigation to change the discriminatory policy expressed in the exclusion of their outpatient mental health services from reimbursement by the publicly funded, national health insurance plan. Politics involves the exercise of power. There is presently in Canada a serious imbalance of power in the mental health system that privileges hospitals and physicians, with the result that the country's ability to meet it's population needs for mental health services is compromised. There needs to be protections against discrimination for all mental health professionals as well as protections of the population. Indeed, establishing greater equality of opportunity among all mental health professions is very likely to lead to improved equity of access for the Canadian population. It would seem they deserve no less, if the public good is to supersede private physician interests.

To place this discussion in a comparative context, and to anticipate discussion of the United States, we close this section with a quotation from David Mechanic: "Comparisons with health insurance in Canada suggest that mental health care there is distributed in closer correspondence to need than in the United States. This misallocation requires corrections through fairer insurance coverage and appropriate administration of a parity benefit" (Mechanic, 2003, p. 18).

Unmet Need in the United States

Based on both the percentages and large numbers of people with untreated mental disorders, there is very significant unmet need for mental health services in the United States. Three national epidemiological studies support this conclusion: (a) the Epidemiological Catchment Area (ECA) study of the 1980s funded by the National Institute of Mental Health (Robins and Regier, 1991), (b) the National Comorbidity Survey (NCS) a decade later (Kessler et al. 1994), and most recently, (c) the National Comorbidity Survey Replication (NCS-R) (Kessler et al. 2005a, 2005b; Wang et al. 2005a, 2005b). These studies indicate that mental disorders are highly prevalent in the general population. The average *period prevalence* of the three studies is 28 percent for 12-month mental disorders, while the most recent study revealed a *lifetime prevalence* of 46.4 percent. With a current total population of about 297 million Americans in 2005, the projected numbers are 83 million for 12-month mental disorders and 136 million for lifetime prevalence. The prevalence of mental disorders in the United States appears to be significantly higher than in the other three countries included in this study, all of which have significantly lower per capita expenditures on health than the United States (Table 1.3).

Moreover, in the most recent NCS-R study, nearly 60 percent of those diagnosed with a disorder in the previous 12 months were rated as "serious" (22.3%) or "moderate" (37.3%) rather than "mild." The estimated 60 percent of people with mental disorders having moderate or serious levels of impairment amounts to about 17 percent of the current total population. Thus, even if mildly impaired people with mental disorders are eliminated in estimating the need for treatment, with a total current population of about 297 million in 2005, the number of Americans with 12-month mental disorders with moderate and serious impairment is projected at about 50 million (Kessler et al. 2005b, pp. 619–620), a number equal to the entire population of the second largest country (England) included in this study.

The most recent NCS-R survey supports the views expressed by the Surgeon General's report (DHHS, 1999) and the President's New Freedom Commission on Mental Health (DHHS, 2003) that mental health care in America is ailing.

> Over a 12-month period, 60% of those with a disorder (of which 60% were rated serious or moderate) receive no treatment. For those with impulse control and substance abuse disorders, nearly half of all lifetime cases have never been treated. Among those with any of the disorders who do report obtaining care, only 32.7% report service that meets criteria of minimally adequate care. Moreover, the unmet need for treatment continues to be greatest in traditionally underserved groups, including elderly persons, racial-ethnic minorities, those with low incomes, those with no insurance, and residents of rural areas. (Wang et al. 2005b, p. 629)

Compared with the other three countries, the estimated unmet need expressed in percentages is somewhat lower in the United States (60%), but the total number in America is much larger due to the greater total population. The majority of people with mental disorders in all four developed countries do not receive mental health services.

There is some encouragement in the increasing percent of Americans with mental disorders who receive some form of treatment: from 19 percent (ECA) to 25 percent (NCS) to 41 percent (NCS-R) (Wang et al. 2005b, p. 629). These estimates, however, suggest that the majority of Americans with mental disorders remain untreated (ECA – 81%, NCS – 75%, NCS-R – 59%). Finally, the delay in initial treatment contact of a minimum of six years up to 23 years, with a median of nearly a decade, results in an unnecessary burden of untreated mental disorders (Wang, et al. 2005a, p. 603). David Mechanic (2003) reached the following conclusion:

> U. S. psychiatry over the past fifty years has been a deviant instance of the important medical principle that first priority should be given to people with the most severe illnesses and greatest needs. Studies have repeatedly found that psychiatric care, particularly at the outpatient level, is disproportionately used by people who are better insured and better educated. (p. 18)

One of the serious consequences of unmet needs for mental health services is an increased use of illicit drugs for self-medication (Harris and Edlund, 2005), which contributes to the high prevalence rates (45%) of co-morbidity among people with mental disorders (Kessler et al. 2005b, p. 617). Thus, timely screening and treatment of mental health problems may prevent the development of substance use disorders among those with mental disorders. Prevention of substance use disorders is itself important, partly because the unmet need for treatment of substance abuse in the United States is no better. The Office of National Drug Control Policy estimated that in 1996, only about two million of the 4.4 to 5.3 million Americans (less than half) in need of treatment for substance abuse received such treatment, even though the cost-effectiveness of outpatient programs had been established (Mojtabai and Zivin, 2003).

Access to mental health treatment for American children improved from five percent in 1987 to 7.7 percent in 1998; however, the proportion receiving treatment remains less than the estimated 11 percent of children with mental health impairment (Glied and Cuellar, 2003).

> The delivery and financing of child mental health services have greatly improved the past decade: The out-of-pocket burden of financing mental health care has fallen; more children have health insurance that covers mental health services; the evidence base for service provision has expanded; and more children are receiving effective therapies today than ever before. Despite these successes, problems remain. Most children still do not have access to effective therapies, and for many children with very serious problems, mental health service systems still have no solutions available. (p. 48)

The largely ineffective, and costly inpatient care for severely ill children in the 1980s has diminished, "... but the evidence-based community alternatives to these services do not yet exist in most places, and the limited availability of specialty services leaves some children with few options" (Glied and Cuellar, 2003, p. 48).

Reasons for the unmet need in the United States mental health system are legion: (a) the lack of parity in the provision of mental health services under both public and private insurance plans; (b) benefit limitations in health insurance and behavioral carve-outs; (c) inefficient management of mental health benefits; (d) budget cuts in publicly funded programs at both federal and state levels; (e) the continued presence of stigma and discrimination; (f) lack of information about services available and about patient rights; (g) the failure of users of mental health services and their families to engage in effective advocacy and lobbying; (h) the selfish interests of providers who want to create higher demand, yet not treat the underserved; (i) the rising costs to employers for health insurance, which they are passing on to employees; (j) the profiteering by health plans, insurance companies, pharmaceutical companies and extravagant compensation paid to their executives; (k) the political and economic power of these companies to finance campaigns and lobby their elected representatives for favorable legislation; (l) the lifestyle behaviors of tobacco, alcohol, and other drug abuse; (m) increasing co-morbidity of substance abuse and mental disorders without appropriate treatment strategies to address both issues simultaneously. In addition, numerous historical-cultural and political-structural explanations have been provided by Vladeck (2003).

Ironically, the impaired mental health of people can be a cause for their unmet need. Gaskin and Mitchell (2005) found that about 11 to 14 percent of children with special health care needs have unmet care needs during a given year. Germane to the present study is the finding that the mental health problems of both the children and their caregivers are barriers to obtaining care. More specifically, *caregivers* with symptoms of depression were 26.3 percent more likely to report an unmet need for their children, 67.6 percent more likely to report an unmet hospital or physician need, and 66.1 percent more likely to report an unmet mental health care need. Moreover, caregivers of *children* who manifested poor adjustment were 26.3 percent more likely to report their child had an unmet need and 92.3 percent more likely to report an unmet mental health care need. Most of the children in this study were African-Americans living in urban areas.

One of the major causes of unmet need is the failure of the American system to provide insurance for its entire population. An increasing number of Americans are uninsured, numbering 45.8 million (15.8%) (U.S.Census, 2005, August 30). The number of uninsured Americans is larger than the total population of Canada (32 million), and nearly equal to the total population of England (50 million). Kronick and Gilmer (1999), and Gilmer and Kronick (2001, 2005) have established that the rising cost of health insurance accounts for the continued rise in the number of uninsured Americans: "It's the premiums stupid. . . ." Applying their empirically supported model to predict national health spending, the authors project that ". . . the number of nonelderly uninsured Americans will grow from forty-five million in 2003 to fifty-six million in 2013" (Gilmer and Kronick, 2005, p. 1 W-143). The projected increase is about eleven million more uninsured, roughly one million per year over the decade ending 2013. By August 2005, the U.S. Census Bureau reported the number had increased to 45.8 million, which is lower than projected; however, as a conservative estimate, another 16 million Americans ages 19 to 64 were *underinsured* in 2003 (Schoen et al. 2005, p. W5-289). Kennedy (2003) reported that the U.S. Census Bureau estimated in December, 2003 that in the course of a year, 30 million more Americans will be underinsured, including gaps in their coverage for mental health services. The rising number of uninsured Americans is a serious problem because the uninsured receive less care, suffer more, and are substantially more likely to die than those who are insured (IOM, 2002).

Many of the uninsured have become marginalized and suffer unnecessarily both from their untreated diseases, including mental disorders, and from an inordinate share of the burden for financing the health care system. As a proportion of their income, those with less pay more.

> Half of the uninsured owe money to hospitals, and a third are being pursued by collection agencies. . . . The death rate in any given year for someone without health insurance is twenty-five per cent higher than for someone with insurance. Because the uninsured are sicker than the rest of us, they can't get better jobs, and because they can't get better jobs they can't afford health insurance, and because they can't afford health insurance they get even sicker. (Gladwell, 2005, p. 44)

Limits placed on government insurance programs may be one of the significant factors in the rising number of uninsured Americans. For example, welfare reform in 1996 replaced the long-term Aid To Families with Dependent Children with the Temporary Assistance to Needy Families (TANF) program, which emphasizes leaving welfare for paid employment. However, 50 percent of former TANF recipients and 15 to 30 percent of their children become uninsured after the expiration of the transitional Medicaid coverage they received for one year after leaving TANF (Hartley, Seccombe, and Hoffman, 2005).

The very high number of uninsured Americans is partly a consequence of the dominant *actuarial model* of health insurance underlying "risk adjustment" practices. How much you pay in premiums is in large part a function of your individual condition and medical history, or the history of the group to which you belong and through which you receive insurance.

Hence, premiums vary to compensate for the fact that some people are at greater risk than others for illnesses, injuries, or death, and consequently they have to pay more.

Another view of insurance is found in countries like Canada, Germany, and Japan, and other industrialized countries with universal health care. They view health insurance as *social insurance*, whose function is to help equalize financial risk between the healthy and the sick (Gladwell, 2005, pp. 48–49). In other words, health insurance is not private property to be possessed solely by an individual, nor by subgroups within the population, the cost of which varies with their personal or group medical history; rather, health insurance is a social good and a means to protect all members of a society equally against the financial shock of serious illness anyone could experience at any time, though perhaps with varying probability. The underlying principle is that the healthy have an obligation to help the sick, just as the wealthy have an obligation to help the poor. In this model, social health insurance is a way to achieve greater equality through fairer financing of universal coverage for the country's entire population.

The employment-based health insurance system in the United States has functioned as a quasi-social insurance program. As Fuchs and Emanuel (2005) observed: "Ever since World War II, the cornerstone of U. S. health care finance has been employer-based insurance. Today such insurance still covers approximately 55 percent of the population, but with declining coverage and loss of community rating [of insurance risk] its role as quasi-social insurance has greatly eroded in recent decades" (p. 1400).

The link between financial (insurance) protection and universal access has been established empirically. What has been written about ensuring universal access to maternal, newborn, and child health care applies equally to mental health care:

> For services to be taken up, financial barriers to access have to be reduced or eliminated and users given predictable financial protection against the costs of seeking care: universal access has to go with financial protection. Only then can health services be made universally available on the basis of need rather than on the basis of people's ability to pay, and households and individuals protected from financial hardship or impoverishment. (WHO, 2005d, p. 137)

Another financial cause for unmet health and mental health needs in America seems to be rooted in the dominant economic theories used to rationalize federal policy. One of these is the economic *theory of moral hazard*, to wit, that having insurance leads to the insured taking undue risks. From this perspective, the cost of health care is high because Americans are overinsured, and consequently, consume medically unnecessary care. As an example, about one-third of Americans who utilize mental health services have no diagnosed mental disorder (Wang et al. 2005b, p. 634). To reduce excessive consumption of health care services, overinsured Americans need to bear more risk via deductibles, co-payments, and sharing more of the premiums. The same theory functions as a barrier to reducing the number of uninsured Americans (Gladwell, 2005), and these tools of cost sharing mitigate achievement of greater efficiency and equity in the health care system (Galvin, 2005, p. W5-1; Lindroth, LoSasso, and Luried, 2005).

Another reason for the unmet need and persistent inequality is the economic interpretations of liberty and equality that dominate the American value system. The meaning of liberty (freedom) has been interpreted at various times in the country's history to mean freedom from political tyranny, from poverty, and from discrimination in voting, housing, education, and employment, but not freedom from unnecessary suffering due to untreated mental disorders or medical illness because one is uninsured. More fundamentally, even the term "equality" has been interpreted consistent with a capitalist ethos of free enterprise to mean "equality of opportunity," *not* the egalitarian meaning of distributive justice. The all too easy (and unspoken) inference is that those who are not successful in this society have themselves to blame – they simply have not taken advantage of the opportunity. Although some exceptions have been made to correct conditions of the "disadvantaged," it is a short step to blaming the victims for the conditions they experience, including poverty. Despite political rhetoric to the contrary, America has become a nation with an ever-widening gap between rich and poor, and more unequal in material wealth than any other industrialized nation. Moreover, the inordinate influence of wealthy individuals and corporations upon government has transformed American democracy into a plutocracy (Phillips, 2002).

By way of summary, the global estimates by the WHO (2001, 2005d) of significant unmet need for mental health services are supported by our study of the four developed countries of Great Britain, Norway, Canada, and the United States. Especially pressing needs are evident in all four countries among their minority populations, including those with severe and persistent mental disorders. National policies and programs must address the needs of these groups and particularly the rising numbers of elderly people with mental disorders.

Concluding Observations

This section begins with discussion of some of the limitations and challenges of this comparative study, followed by observations about contextual factors affecting the performance of mental health systems, characteristics of the mental health systems, summary comparisons on the six evaluation criteria, and highlights of lessons learned from the four countries included in this study. The chapter ends with methodological recommendations, and recommendations for improving the performance of mental health systems generally, and strategies for reforming the American system in particular.

Limitations and Challenges

This book is the result of more than a year's work by contributing authors. It has been a very significant challenge for all of us to acquire the information necessary both to describe our country's mental health system and to address the evaluation criteria adopted for comparative study. Preparation for each one of the chapters has required selection by the authors from the enormous amount of information about their complex systems. The limited space for each country has made selections necessary, and many relevant details have been omitted.

A second limitation is that data have not been reported in equal proportions from all four countries on all of the evaluation criteria, nor in all of our comparisons. That has made comparisons seem at times like "apples versus oranges." The data that have been reported are also subject to various interpretations. None of our authors claims to be representative of a consensus or "official" view of their mental health systems. Readers are invited to draw their own conclusions, which may or may not agree with any of us involved in this review.

A third limitation is a function of our selected sample for comparative case study. All four countries are wealthy, urbanized, industrialized economies and political democracies. Generalizations about their mental health systems are not likely to be directly applicable to developing countries as the World Health Organization has observed (WHO, 2000).

Fourthly, our study is less comprehensive than the framework applied for both the development and evaluation of mental health policy presented by Townsend et al. (2004). Neither were our authors asked to create a "mental health country profile" according to the design and evaluation specifications developed by the International Consortium on Mental Health Policy and Services (Gulbinat et al. 2004; Jenkins, et al. 2004; Schilder et al. 2004). The latter more comprehensive approach warrants application to developed countries as well as the developing countries where it has been applied, including about a dozen countries from six WHO regions. It is our hope that some of the extensive information presented in this volume might be used to assist the completion of that type of comprehensive and standardized evaluation for comparisons of the levels of goal attainment and performance of mental health systems in our developed countries relative to their unique contexts, resources, provision, and outcomes.

Given the aforementioned limitations (and others our readers will help us appreciate), some general observations can be made, first about the context in which these mental health systems operate, and second, about the systems themselves. Contextual factors include the geographic and demographic characteristics of these countries, their political, economic, and general health care systems.

Contextual Factors

Geography and Demographics. All four of these countries face *geographic challenges* as they attempt to provide equitable access to mental health services throughout their countries. Combined with variable population densities, and the limited supply and uneven distribution of mental health specialists, none of these four developed countries can be said to have met their country's need for mental health services.

Comparative statistics on populations, geographic area, and population densities are provided in Table 7.2.

A comparison among the four countries reveals very significant differences in the geographic areas occupied by these four countries. Moreover, there are equally vast differences in population sizes, which result in a very wide range in population densities. The marked differences in population sizes suggest substantial variation in the total numbers of people who will need mental health services in each of these countries. The considerably larger range in population density from 1,000/sq.mi. in England to 8/sq.mi. in Canada suggests that access to mental health services is likely to vary considerably as a function of the degree to which the population is concentrated or

Table 7.2. *Population Estimates, Geographic Area, and Population Density.*

Indicator	England	Norway	Canada	United States
Current Population	50,000,000	4,577,000	32,000,000	297,273,627
Area (sq. miles)	50,364	125,182	3,852,000	3,615,122
Population density per square mile	1,000	36	8	81

Note: Population density equals the estimated population divided by the total area of each country in square miles, the latter retrieved from the *World Book Encyclopedia (1980)*. U.S. population is based on U.S. Census Bureau's estimate for 2005.

dispersed. Even though populations in all four countries are more urban than rural, and all of them have a relatively efficient public transportation infrastructure, it would seem that Canada and Norway especially, and secondarily the United States would face greater challenges in distributing and delivering mental health services to their populations than England with its very high density population, and high concentration in a few major metropolitan areas. Thus, while these countries share a common challenge to distribute services equitably, the geographic challenge varies considerably among them. Any comparative evaluation should take account of these differences.

Although the total populations in all four countries are relatively stable, the demographics in all of these countries are changing. Their populations are becoming increasingly heterogeneous with a growing percentage of elderly. All four countries face the challenge of providing equitable access to culturally competent mental health services for their racial-ethnic, indigenous, and immigrant minorities, and increasingly for the elderly. Children and adolescents, and the seriously and persistently mentally ill, the poor, and in the United States, the uninsured and underinsured are additional minorities whose mental health needs are not being met. The mental health needs of both military personnel and their families as well as prison populations warrant more attention in all four countries.

Political Systems. Political systems have significant influence over the formulation and implementation of national mental health policy, and upon the shape and performance of their mental health systems. Public participation in mental health policy formulation and implementation can be considered a defining characteristic of a good quality mental health system. A truly democratic mental health system is preferred to a system fragmented by self-serving stakeholders with inordinate power over the system. The society's cultural values and polity are significant factors in the development of a good mental health policy.

Parliamentary systems of government are characteristic of Great Britain, Norway, and Canada, all of which have been ranked as countries with health care systems that perform better than the United States with its bicameral legislative branch, separated from executive and judicial branches of government. There is a systemic inefficiency in the United States polity with two separate, elected houses in Congress, each generating hundreds of bills per year, each bill being addressed by several overlapping committees. Moreover, a very small number of legislators control which bills will be heard both by their committee and by the larger elected body of representatives or senators. The final form of federal legislation is often decided in House-Senate conference committees by a smaller group of powerful legislators from both houses. The cumbersome political process is itself a barrier to the development of a coherent, comprehensive, national mental health system.

The political systems of Great Britain, Norway, and Canada are democratically constituted to enable the legislative and executive branches to enact the policies and programs that the population has elected representatives to implement. In contrast, the American political system offers generous opportunities to powerful special interests to obstruct, delay, or sabotage legislation even if it has the support of the majority of the population (Klein, 2003). That observation need not result in a kind of cynical fatalism, but it challenges notions of naive optimism about accomplishing health care reform within the American political system. Advocates of health care reform need to appreciate both the political constraints as well as the possibilities for change even as they embrace a bolder vision of a national health insurance program (Oberlander, 2005; cf. the Jan., 2003 issue of *The American Journal of Public Health*).

By contrast, in the other countries included in this study, the "Senate" or "House of Lords" functions primarily to study social, economic, and political problems, and to make informed recommendations to the single "House" of elected representatives. The result seems to this author to be superior mental health policy formulation and more efficient implementation. Not being elected, the "Senates" in parliamentary systems are less beholden to lobbying by special interests, and less dependent upon their campaign contributions, which are made contingent on a responsive U.S. Senator who needs their money to be reelected. The influence of special interests upon elected federal officials in America helps to explain why proposals for national, universal health insurance have been rejected repeatedly. Its all about politics... but also about economics.

Economic Systems. As advanced industrialized nations, all four countries have strong economies, though their Gross Domestic Products vary considerably. Expressed in billions of US$ at current prices and exchange rates for the year 2003, the GDPs are: United States – $10,951.3, UK – $1,797.9, Canada – $856.6, and Norway – $220.6 (OECD, 2005). The GDP per capita figures for 2003 expressed at current prices in US dollars are provided in Table 7.3.

As a measure of the country's wealth, GDP per capita for 2003 ranges from $27,100 in Canada to $48,300 in Norway. For the same year, current purchasing power ranges from $29,900 in the United Kingdom to $37,600 in the United States. Per capita purchasing power in Norway is about $500 less than in the United States due largely to the high prices of goods and services in Norway. Canada ranks third and Great Britain is a close fourth in current purchasing power.

Table 7.3. *GDP Per Capita, 2003 at Current Prices in US Dollars.*

Country	Based on current exchange rate	Based on current purchasing power
Canada	27,100	30,500
United States	37,600	37,600
Norway	48,300	37,100
United Kingdom	30,200	29,900

Note: Source is OECD (2005). *OECD Factbook 2005. National accounts of OECD Countries, vol. 1. Gross domestic product per capita for OECD countries.* Retrieved 7/19/05 from http://www.oecd.org/dataoecd/48/5/34244925.xls. Copyright permission obtained from OECD.

While all four countries have organized and productive economies, the ways in which they organize their means of production and distribute goods and services among their populations vary considerably. The four countries can be viewed on a continuum from the most market-minimized economy (Great Britain) to the most market-maximized economy (United States), with Norway closest to Great Britain and Canada closest to the United States (Anderson, 1989, as cited by Graig, 1999). Is it mere historical coincidence that among these four countries, the one that has been ranked lowest in goal attainment and performance of its health care system is also the country with a predominantly capitalist economy? The free enterprise system of the predominantly private sector economy in America has the least amount of regulation and greatest reliance upon market forces of supply and demand to determine both the price and volume of goods and services, including mental health services. The three other countries studied in this volume have a much more comprehensive welfare system with a greater role of central or even decentralized government in financing, if not owning mental health services (England and Norway), in administering the mental health system (England, Norway, and Canada), and in assuming responsibility for the delivery of mental health services (England and Norway).

In this respect, Norway's experience is instructive. Over several decades, the responsibility for mental health services in Norway changed from the central to county government, back to the central government. Norway learned that centralizing mental health services is more efficient and effective in reducing regional variability in access, quality, and cost. Canada and the United States suffer significant deficiencies in the equal distribution of access to optimal mental health services due partly to their decentralized approaches. Canada's Medicare for its entire population of 32 million is administered and partly financed by its ten Provinces and three Territories in a manner similar to the Medicaid program in the United States, which is administered by the 50 states for about 50 million low income people. Both programs suffer significant inconsistencies and widely ranging inequalities in access to mental health services. In the United States, the significant duplication characteristic of 50 different state administrations of variable Medicaid programs results in further inconsistencies and inefficiencies, not to mention the duplication compounded by the legion of private insurance policies and health plans operating within states and nationally. Moreover, because Medicaid is means-tested, significant administrative costs are incurred to determine initial and continued eligibility of beneficiaries.

By contrast, the efficiency of the federally financed and centrally administered Medicare program for about 42 million elderly and disabled Americans has been documented by the United States General Accounting Office (1994, p. 25) to have administrative costs less than three percent. Although implemented through various private fiscal intermediaries and carriers to cover inpatient and outpatient services respectively, there is more consistency in the coverage under this federal program than under Medicaid, which is administered by the states. It would seem that one rational and efficient solution is to transfer Medicaid to the centralized financing and administration at the federal level with a formula for equitable allocation of federal funds to the states based on demographics, epidemiological data on mental disorders, and utilization rates. One strategy is to allocate funding to the states as Norway provides to its Regional Health Authorities. The current bill introduced in the U.S. House of Representatives for national health insurance (House file 676) would fold Medicaid into "Medicare for All," and administer the former under the current and/or expanded Medicare administration.

We have been discussing the economic context in which mental health systems function. This context needs to be considered for another major reason. A country with a growing population falling into *poverty* is a country that will face an increasing prevalence of mental disorders. There is consistent evidence that the poor are among those at greater risk for developing mental disorders, and they are less likely to receive mental health services (e.g., Krieger, Chen, Waterman, Rehkopf, and Submramian, 2005; Wang et al. 2005a, 2005b). Moreover, there is evidence that access to regular health care services is a function of the level of poverty as well as the degree of urbanization in the county in which one resides (Litaker, Kovoukian, and Love, 2005; Litaker and Love, 2005).

In the United States, the poor represent a disproportionate number of the uninsured, though most of the uninsured are employed in low income jobs. A poignant portrayal of the plight of the poor was the disproportionate number of poor African Americans who could not escape the ravages of Hurricane Katrina August 2005 because they could not afford to own automobiles, public transportation infrastructures and vehicles were significantly damaged, and government provisions for their rescue were inadequate.

Another significant element of the economic context in which mental health systems function is *international globalization*. International agencies such as the World Bank, the International Monetary Fund, and the World Trade Organization have been instrumental in promoting free trade in global, deregulated markets. Along with that, they have promoted managed competition, user fees in the delivery of health care services, privatization, and reductions in public health services (Light, 2000; Ruger, 2005). Some international free trade agreements would limit government agencies from regulating public health services in their own country, and foster participation of multinational corporations in administering programs and institutions, such as public hospitals and community health centers, currently managed in the country's public sector (Shaffer, Waitzkin, Brenner, and Jasso-Aquilar, 2005). The impact of "free trade" agreements upon mental health systems has not been fully evaluated, though the exodus of nurses from less developed countries has been cited as one negative impact.

The General Health Care System. Another important context of mental health systems is the country's overall health care system. The four countries in this study vary from those which have a more centralized, publicly financed and publicly administered health care system (Great Britain and Norway) to mixed public-private systems in which the public sector is dominant (Canada) or in which the private sector dominates in a market-maximized system (United States). Reforms and improvements of the mental health system in each of these countries may well necessitate broader reforms in the overall health care system. For example, a medically dominated health care system like Canada's must be changed if nonmedical health care professionals are to be able to provide mental health services and to be reimbursed by the national health insurance system. Canada might benefit from "any willing provider" legislation adopted by some American states (Ohsfeldt, Morrisey, Nelson, and Johnson, 1998), and comparable inclusive policies from the other countries to expand their services by eliminating the privileged position of psychiatrists and also general practitioners, who have even less mental health training than allied mental health professionals.

Health care systems are what many people love to hate. At one level, legitimate complaints about access, quality, and cost are expressed by people in all countries, though in varying proportions. At another level, people encounter their health care system usually when they are in pain, ill, or injured, and consequently also anxious. Finally, encounters with potentially life-threatening conditions confront us all with our mortality, which many would just as soon deny. These psychological factors, however, must not detract from genuine concerns about the overall goal attainment and performance of health care systems. None of the four mental health systems has met their population's need for mental health services, though distinctions have been drawn in the level of goal attainment on such criteria as the population's health status, the responsiveness of the system to the population's expectations, and fairness of financing. On these absolute measures of goal attainment, and on performance relative to financial resources available to the system, the WHO (2000) has ranked Norway the highest and the United States the lowest among the four countries included in this study.

By way of summary, an evaluation of a mental health system needs to take into account the unique and variable characteristics of each country, which influence the shape and performance of its mental health system. These contextual factors are geographic, demographic, political and economic, and especially the way the health care system in general is financed, organized, and delivered. In addition, there are aspects of the mental health system per se which also warrant evaluation.

Mental Health Systems

Discussion of the mental health systems of our four countries begins with some observations about their developmental stages. Thereafter I discuss the roles of national mental health policies and guidelines, and offer summary observations about the six evaluation criteria.

Common Developmental Stages. We find common trends in the historical development of mental health systems in all four countries: (a) At the beginning of the twentieth century, there was an initial isolation, if not neglect of people with mental disorders in understaffed and overcrowded asylums, which were characterized by custodial care or "treatments" lacking substantial evidence for their efficacy or safety (e.g., hydrotherapy, insulin coma, lobotomies); (b) a period of deinstitutionalization followed in the mid-twentieth century with an emphasis upon active treatment within the individual's community in psychiatric units located in general-medical hospitals; (c) rising costs of mental health care led to strategies to contain costs, notably by reducing the number of inpatients and inpatient days, with increased use of neuroleptic medications and/or outpatient psychotherapy and psychosocial rehabilitation; (d) the number of outpatient mental health visits per user has generally declined; (e) a movement away from "schools" of psychotherapy to more eclectic and multidisciplinary team approaches has occurred. In addition, there has been (f) standardization of graduate level training for mental health specialties; (g) evolution of ethical codes of practice and treatment guidelines for cost-effective practices; (h) an increased specialization within mental health professions; (i) increased professionalism with certification/licensure at either the federal or state levels; (j) a more recent emphasis upon the integration of specialty mental health services within primary health care settings; (k) increased research on evidence-based practices; and (l) yet a relative lag in information transfer from research to practice.

Some of these trends in the development of mental health systems may be partly a function of the evolution of health care systems in general. The World Health Organization identified three generations of health system reform that have occurred during the twentieth century.

> The first generation saw the founding of national health care systems, and the extension to middle income nations of social insurance systems, mostly in the 1940s and 1950s in richer countries and somewhat later in poorer countries. . . . A second generation of reforms. . . saw the promotion of primary health care as a route to achieving affordable universal coverage. . . . In general, both the first-generation and second-generation reforms have been quite supply-oriented. Concern with demand is more characteristic of changes in the third generation currently underway in many countries, which include such reforms as trying to 'make' money follow the patient' and shifting away from simply giving providers budgets, which in turn are often determined by supposed needs. (WHO, 2000, pp. 13–17)

In describing these developmental stages of health care systems, the WHO also discerned a pattern: "This development can be sketched as a gradual convergence towards what WHO calls the 'new universalism' – high quality delivery of essential care, defined mostly by the criterion of cost-effectiveness, for everyone, rather than all possible care for the whole population or only the simplest and most basic care for the poor. . . ." (WHO, 2000, p. 15)

The implicit criteria of a good health care system are (a) universality, (b) cost-effectiveness, (c) high quality, and (d) the provision of essential health care services. These criteria are relevant to the evaluation of mental health systems, so long as "essential" services are not defined narrowly as "medically necessary."

Our readers are invited to consider the stage of health system reform their own country has attained. Simply asking the question in light of this developmental framework leads to insights about both what is desirable and what might be possible to achieve in the mental health sector.

National Mental Health Policies and Programs. According to the *Mental Health Atlas – 2005* (WHO, 2005a), Great Britain, Norway, and Canada have formulated a national, comprehensive mental health *policy*. By definition, a *mental health policy* is "... a specifically written document by the Government or Ministry of Health containing the goals for improving the mental health situation of the country, the priorities among those goals, and the main directions for attaining them" (WHO, 2005b, p. 2). The policies in all three countries address all essential areas of advocacy, promotion, prevention, treatment and rehabilitation. The United States lacks such a comprehensive mental health policy at the national level, though it has a substance abuse policy like the other three countries. All four countries have laws governing protection of the civil rights of people with mental disorders.

Despite the absence of a national mental health policy, the United States has funded public mental health *programs*, but these have been less comprehensive and less inclusive than Great Britain and Norway. Canada has yet to implement its national mental health policy in a comprehensive, national mental health program. By definition, a national *mental health program* "... indicates what has to be done to achieve policy objectives, who has to do it, during what time frame and with what resources" (WHO, 2005b, p. 5).

All four countries have mental health programs for selected minority groups and for the elderly. Three countries (Norway, Canada, United States) have mental health programs for refugees, for people affected by disasters, and for children. Two countries (Canada and United States) have mental health programs for their indigenous populations. Based on these system elements of mental health programs, Great Britain was rated as lacking mental health programs for the largest number of subgroups in its population: refugees, disaster affected people, indigenous groups, and children.

All four countries have articulated national policies for all age groups and for most minority groups, though some are more comprehensive and have a broader consensus than others; however, the procedures through which these policies have been developed vary considerably. Moreover, the countries vary in the degree to which they have comprehensive guidelines for implementing policies.

A national policy promoting equitable access, especially for minorities, is a necessary, but not a sufficient condition for successful implementation of policy objectives. There is also a need for *policy implementation guidelines (regulations)* to clarify expectations and to specify standards, measurable objectives, and procedural strategies and time frames to ensure that the purpose and objectives of the policy are achieved. Great Britain and Norway seem to this author to be more advanced than the other two countries in national guidelines for policy implementation.

What follows are summary comparisons among the four countries on the six evaluation criteria selected for this study.

Summary Comparisons on Evaluation Criteria

Access and Equity. Three of the four countries have national policies which establish universal access to health care. The absence of either legislative or constitutional authority in the United States ensuring universal access is one of the factors that accounts for the growing number and significant percentage of Americans who were uninsured in 2005 (45.8 million, 15.8% of the total population). All four countries struggle with the challenge of providing equal access to culturally competent mental health services for their minority populations. Access to community-based services by the severely mentally ill is a common and persistent problem in all four countries.

Quality and Efficacy. The WHO (2000) compared the health care systems of its member countries on three universal criteria (goals): Health status of the population (level and distribution), responsiveness to the population's expectations (level and distribution), and fair financing. These criteria were incorporated into a global ranking of the systems' goal attainment. Among our four countries, the WHO (2000) evaluation of health care systems for the year 1997 ranked Norway highest (3) on overall goal attainment, followed by Canada (7), Great Britain (9), and the United States (15) (Table 6.1).

Our contributing authors were asked to rate the overall levels of goal attainment of their mental health system relative to their own expectations and knowledge of both the prevalence of mental disorders and the delivery of mental health services in their country. The order of these ratings were: Norway (1) at somewhat more than the expected level of outcome, Britain (0) at the expected level, with Canada (–1) and the United States (–1) both somewhat less than the expected level of outcome.

All four countries provide mental health facilities in the primary health care sector as well as community mental health services. Unlike the other three countries, the United States provides neither mental health treatment in primary care for severe mental disorders, nor adequate training facilities for primary care personnel in mental health (WHO, 2005a). One potential model for primary mental health care of the seriously mentally ill is the Chronic Care Model to improve the quality of care for conditions such as depression (Bonomic, Wagner, Glasgow, and VonKorff, 2002; ICIC, 2003; Pearson et al. 2005). All four countries are making significant efforts to integrate mental health specialty services into primary health care settings. Great Britain is a leader with 70 percent of general practitioners reporting affiliations with counselors.

All four countries credential mental health specialists, such as psychiatrists, psychiatric nurses, psychologists, and clinical social workers, but marriage and family therapists, counselors, and addiction counselors are unregulated in Canada and so is the title of "psychotherapist" in Norway.

Cost and Efficiency. As an estimate of the efficiency of health care systems, the WHO (2000) assessed performance relative to health expenditures. On overall performance, Norway (11) was ranked highest, followed by Great Britain (18), Canada (30), and the United States (37) (Table 6.1). By a large margin, the United States is the most expensive health care system in the world, and the least efficient among our four countries. Duplication of administrative services and personnel among multiple private and public health insurance schemes in the United States, plus its decentralized administration of Medicaid contribute significantly to systemic inefficiencies. During the era of managed care (from 1970 to 1998), administrative personnel in the American health care system increased about 15 times greater than the increase of physicians and nurses (PNHP, 2000). The bureaucracy in the private sector has become a major drain on health care dollars. Comparing the two most publicly financed programs, the proportion of administrative positions in Britain's National Health Service seems to be much higher than in the Norwegian system.

Financing and Fairness. On the criterion of fairness of financial contribution to the health care system, Britain (8–11) and Norway (8–11) perform better than Canada (17–19) and all three significantly better than the United States (54–55) (Table 6.1). According to the WHO (2005a), the primary (though not exclusive) method of financing mental health care is either tax-based (Great Britain and Canada) or social insurance (Norway); however, our Norwegian experts have noted that financing from the national health insurance scheme is much less than from other general taxes and revenues. The United States is unique in relying primarily upon private health insurance. Thus, with the exception of the U. S. system, the primary source of funding mental health services is public rather than private (see Table 1.3).

All four countries allocate public funds to a mental health budget, though the amounts vary as a proportion of total health expenditures ranging from about six percent in the United States to about 18 percent in Norway. The amount spent on mental health in all four countries is less than expected based upon (a) their reported prevalence rates of mental disorders within their populations, and upon (b) their estimates of significant, unmet mental health needs. To place these observations in perspective, the WHO (2000) reported that about 20 percent of member countries surveyed spent less than one percent of their total health budget on mental health. Global resources for people suffering both mental and neurological disorders are grossly insufficient, and have not improved since the 2001 survey by the WHO (2005c).

Reforms in the method of financing mental health services may be necessary to improve the system's performance. As Fuchs and Emanuel (2005) observed:

> The experience of the past 40 years shows that without major changes in finance, past efforts to improve organization and delivery have not had widespread success.... Tangible incentives will be required to get physicians and hospitals to change their practice patterns. Although finance reform is certainly not a sufficient condition for major improvement in organization and delivery, it is probably a necessary one. (pp. 1409–1410)

Protection and Participation. Among the four countries, Great Britain and Norway seem to provide greatest protection from financial hardships associated with all forms of illness, including mental disorders. The United States seems to provide financial protection least well for significant segments of its population, notably the uninsured, underinsured, and other minorities.

All four countries have national policies, legislation and/or regulations which are intended to protect people with mental disorders from discriminatory treatment or other violations of their civil rights pertaining to involuntary civil commitments and criminal cases invoking an insanity defense. Informed consent, confidentiality of records, and access to one's health record are protected within all four countries. Licensure boards regulate most of the mental health professions with a mandate to protect the public. These boards have the power to sanction mental health professionals, up to and including termination of their license to practice.

Although all four countries have a democratic polity, the level of public participation in policy formulation seems greater in Norway, followed in decreasing order by Great Britain, Canada, and the United States. At the clinical level, there seems to be a common commitment among mental health practitioners in all four countries to empower their clients by involving them in treatment planning with informed consent and respect for confidentiality.

Population Relevance. This criterion was included to provide our authors with the opportunity to make a more global assessment of how well their mental health system is meeting the needs of their population with mental disorders. The authors from all four countries have concluded that their own mental health system is not meeting their country's need for mental health services. Table 7.4 below gives some comparative data reported for these countries in our four chapters. The estimates have been reviewed by our contributing authors, and in some cases, modified from our initial approximations.

The above data seem to support the conclusion based on other standardized, international epidemiological studies. Compared with other countries that participated in the WHO-WMH Survey Initiative, the NCS-R prevalence estimates for the United States are consistently higher than in these other countries (Kessler et al. 2005b, 624). That fact suggests the other countries are performing better in protecting, sustaining, and improving the mental health status of their population.

One explanation for its poorer performance is that mental health expenditures as a percentage of total

Table 7.4. *Comparative Statistics.*

Indicator	Great Britain	Norway	Canada	United States
Per capita total health expenditures(a)	2,301	4,033	2,222	5,274
Mental health expenditures as a % of total health expenditures(b)	16%	18.2%	8.8%	6.1%
12-month prevalence(c)	16%	15%	10.6%	26.2%
Life-time prevalence	10–20%	20–25%	20%	46.4%
% people with mental disorders or psychological distress treated in primary health care(d)	25%	na	26–50%	22.8%
% people with mental disorders or psychological distress treated in mental health specialist services(e)	33%	25%	8%	28.3%
Estimated ratio of mental health specialists to population(f)	1:693	1:250	1:390	1:733
% people with mental disorders or with psychological distress not receiving *any* treatment (g)	67+%	na	70%	59%

a. For 2002, at average exchange rate in US$. From WHO (2005), Annex Table 6, pp. 200–203.
b. Estimated by our chapter authors, excluding substance abuse. The U. S. estimate is for the year 2001 (Mark et al. 2005, p. W5-133). Including substance abuse, the U. S. estimate is 7.6%.
c. Data are from the most recent epidemiological studies from each country. Figures for Great Britain and Norway are point prevalence estimates ("at any one time"). Canada's 12-month prevalence is for ages 15+ years.
d. Primary health care refers to general medical settings serviced by general (family) physicians and nurses.
e. Mental health specialists counted by all four countries include psychiatrists, psychiatric nurses, psychologists, and clinical social workers. U.S. estimates have ranged from 6% (DHHS, 1999) to the higher 28.3% reported in the most recent NCS-R epidemiological study (Kessler et al. 2005a, 2005b). The Norwegian estimate refers to about 26% of the 15% of the population with mental disorders or psychological distress treated in mental health specialist services.
f. Excluding marriage and family therapists, and professional counselors, the U.S. estimate would be closer to 1:1,200.
g. Estimated by our chapter authors based on national epidemiological studies.

health expenditures is lowest in the United States (6.1%). Moreover, the percentage of people with mental disorders or psychological distress treated in specialized mental health services in the United States (28.3%) is only slightly higher than Norway (25%) and lower than Great Britain (33%), despite the much higher per capita total health expenditures in the United States. Nevertheless, the percent of people with mental disorders or psychological distress treated in the United States (28.3%) is significantly higher than Canada (8%), where nonphysician mental health professionals are excluded from participating in the national health insurance system.

Meeting a population's need for mental health services requires a sufficient supply of mental health specialists distributed across the country proportional to demographics and regional prevalence rates. The estimated ratios of mental health specialists to the populations presented in Table 7.4 were derived from figures reported (and reviewed) by our chapter authors. Another estimate of work force ratios for four mental health specialties was reported recently in the *Mental Health Atlas – 2005* (WHO, 2005a). The results are summarized in Table 7.5.

These data suggest considerable variations in the ratios of selected mental health professions among these four countries. Among the four listed mental health specialties, the predominant specialties in each of the four countries are: Great Britain – psychiatric nurses (104); Norway – psychologists (68); Canada – psychiatric nurses (44); and United States – social workers (35.3). Counting only the medical specialties of psychiatrists and psychiatric nurses, the combined numbers per 100,000 are Great Britain (115), Norway (62), Canada (56), and the United States (20.2). Excluding social workers, for whom data was not reported for Norway and Canada, and adding the three remaining mental health specialties, the numbers in descending order are Norway (130), Great Britain (124), Canada (91), and the United States (51.3). All four countries face continued challenges in supplying sufficient numbers of qualified mental health specialists distributed evenly throughout their population.

Assessing the meaning and implications of so much information about these four mental health systems has been a formidable challenge, yet essential to understanding how they function, what seems to be working well and what doesn't in various systems. Mental health policy cannot be totally data-driven, but it should be evidence-based to help identify the need and demand for mental health services in a population, those interventions that are cost-effective, and the systems that do well in attaining the three universal goals of all mental health systems: (a) improved mental health for the entire population, (b) responsiveness to the population's expectations, and (c) fair financing. These four countries have been found to vary in their overall goal attainment (see Table 6.1) in part because they vary in how well the mental health systems perform the four functions necessary to attaining the three universal system goals. The four functions are: (a) stewardship (oversight), (b) financing (collecting, pooling and purchasing), (c) creating resources (investment and training), and (d) delivering services (provision of mental health services) (WHO, 2000, p. 25). Overall, it appears to this author that Great Britain, Norway, and Canada are better mental health systems than the United States on most evaluation criteria.

Some Additional Lessons

Aside from the comparative evaluations summarized above, it seems fruitful to ask what we might learn from each of these four mental health systems. Each country manifests particular strengths that will be highlighted here. From **Great Britain** we can learn how to integrate mental health professionals into primary health care settings. Recall that 70 percent of general practitioners reported they worked closely with counselors. The other three countries do not seem to have achieved that level of integration in primary health care settings either with counselors or other mental health specialists.

Great Britain has developed a multimeasure approach to assessing the need for mental health services.

Table 7.5. *Mental Health Specialists Per 100,000 Population.*

Mental Health Specialty	Great Britain	Norway	Canada	United States
Psychiatrists	11	20	12	13.7
Psychiatric Nurses	104	42	44	6.5
Psychologists working in mental health	9	68	35	31.1
Social workers working in mental health	58	na	na	35.3

Source: WHO (2005a). *Mental Health Atlas – 2005.* Geneva: Author.

To complement objective measures of prevalence and utilization rates, subjective measures of need from surveys of potential service users have been used to provide valid self-reports of their perceived need or desire for mental health services.

Researchers in Great Britain have also investigated the influence of employment conditions on mental health. In their analysis of British civil servants aged 35–55 years in 1985–1988, Ferrie et al. (2005) reported strong associations between self-reported job insecurity and both poor, self-rated health and minor psychiatric problems.

In the late 1980s and early 1990s, the Conservative Thatcher government instituted market-based reforms based on managed competition, but by 1996 these reforms were rejected as costly and inefficient, undermining the public health, and requiring more government regulation and monitoring to check the inequalities in access to what became a two-tier system of health care. These results from Britain's experiment with privatization and managed competition supported the conclusions of British researchers, who found little evidence for the alleged benefits of managed competition (Light, 1995, 1997; Robinson and Steiner, 1998; cf. *Journal Health Politics, Policy, and Law*, 2000, vol. 25, no. 5 on competition in health care markets).

Additional lessons from Britain about financing a health care system are (a) health care should be free at the point of service because co-payments create inequities and raise barriers to access; (b) an insurance-based health care system costs more to operate and is more inequitable than a public system financed by mandatory and progressive taxes on income; (c) primary care providers need to be provided incentives to treat patients requiring long term care (such as the seriously and persistently mentally ill) and others in underserved areas; (d) the cost of prescribed drugs can be controlled by limiting both profits and the proportion of revenues companies can spend on marketing (Light, 2003).

Among the lessons to be drawn from **Norway** are the changes that country made in the organization of its mental health system. Prior to the early 1960s, mental health services were essentially owned and operated by the central government. A transfer was made to county municipalities by the *Hospital Act* in 1970, but was reversed in 2002 with implementation of the *National Mental Health Programme* approved by Parliament in 1998. The change from (A) centralized to (B) decentralized back to (A) centralized administration of the mental health system is analogous to the three phases of a quasi-experimental design (an A-B-A reversal design), though admittedly lacking repeated and standardized measurements. The reasons for the reversal should be taken seriously in any proposals for reforming a mental health system.

Among the complaints that led to the return to central administration were the inconsistency and variability in access and quality of mental health services administered by nearly 20 county municipalities. The Norwegians adopted centralized financing and administration of mental health specialty services to produce a more standardized and equitable system for delivering high quality care. Presently the American system is much less standardized and much more inequitable, especially in the federal/state financed program for those of low income (Medicaid), which is administered differently by the 50 states. When one takes into account hundreds, if not thousands of private health insurance policies and health plans, the variability is enormous. The same rationale that has led to the establishment of "best practices" in clinical interventions is applicable to standardizing health insurance for everyone to ensure equitable access to high quality, affordable care.

Another lesson from Norway pertains to the vital role of work force planning. Even when mental health services are state-owned and most mental health professionals are educated, trained, and salaried through public financing, practitioners need to be motivated by incentives to accept positions throughout the country if access is to become more evenly distributed. Without redistribution of personnel according to population density and prevalence rates, it is unlikely that a national policy authorizing universal access will be fully implemented or that the needs for mental health services will be met equitably, and especially in rural areas. In a democratic society, one can expect providers to exercise their freedom to choose where they want to live and work based on several factors besides the concerns of policymakers about the population's equity of access. One cannot presume that social interest will necessarily overcome personal preferences.

From **Canada** we can learn about the challenges of delivering health care services to a widely dispersed population, and how a national reform in health care can begin not at the federal level, but at the province/state level. Canada's social insurance program began in one Province (Saskatchewan). From there it was extended to the nation. A comparable beginning in the United States would be to establish a social insurance program within one or more of the

50 states. Though defeated in Oregon, similar proposals have emerged recently in state legislative bodies in California, Minnesota, and New Mexico.

A second lesson from Canada related to reforming a system is to change one major component at a time. There will be too much resistance to overcome if people attempt to change both how mental health services are delivered and the mode of payment to providers at the same time that changes are made in the method of financing the system (Vladeck, 2003). Canada instituted its national health insurance program without changing the mode of payment to physicians, which was, and largely remains a fee-for-service system.

We must also learn from the Canadian system about the serious risks of nationalizing a health care system that has historically privileged inpatient medical care. The exclusion from reimbursement by Canada's Medicare of outpatient mental health services provided by both regulated mental health professionals (e.g., psychologists, clinical social workers) and unregulated professions (e.g., marriage and family therapy, addiction counselors) is a seriously flawed, inefficient, and discriminatory system rationalized by Canada's national health policy. That such a small minority of health care professionals (psychiatrists) relative to the larger supply of other mental health specialists can continue to dominate the system is itself a major cause for unequal access, rising costs, and marked inefficiency of the Canadian system. As always, it is the patients who suffer from unmet needs.

There is both irony and hypocrisy evident in the discriminatory policy of excluding nonmedical mental health professionals from Medicare reimbursement in Canada. The medical profession initially opposed establishment of the publicly financed health insurance system in Saskatchewan on grounds that it would give the government monopolistic power and control. A work strike by physicians lasting three weeks was unsuccessful in defeating the proposal of the publicly financed, single-payer system and its extension to the entire country. However, the same medical professionals, including family physicians and psychiatrists, seem to have no compunction about maintaining their monopoly power over the provision of mental health services. The politics within mental health services is a central issue, that is, who has the power and who uses it to influence decisions about which services will be insured and provided by whom to whom, when, where, and how.

Canada is a leader in identifying work-life conflicts as significant causes of distress and mental health costs. These types of work-life conflicts include (a) role overload, (b) work to family interference, (c) family to work interference, and (d) caregiver strain. Collectively these work-life conflicts create additional economic costs in lost productivity and disability payments by employers and tax payers who finance a public health insurance system. Organizations could benefit from psychological consultation about policies and programs that promote mental health in the workplace.

Another twofold lesson about financing can be learned from Canada. First, in a national health insurance system, health care allocations can be cut for several years in order to balance the federal budget. Secondly, with effective advocacy of elected representatives, a parliamentary government can authorize increased expenditures. In 2004, the Canadian federal government approved a plan to pump an additional $35 billion over the next decade into the public health system, which costs about $22 billion annually (Webster, 2005).

We can learn from Canada that when sufficiently funded, a federally financed system administered at the provincial (state) level, which reimburses private practitioners via fee-for-services, can function efficiently, effectively, and fairly to provide universal access to a consensually defined set of health care services, while simultaneously ensuring quality and containing costs (Deber, 2003). Government involvement in health care planning, financing, and administration of health care services based on need provides an efficient alternative to unchecked competition and market forces of supply and demand that result in so many uninsured residents in the United States being left out and left behind. According to an early comparison by the United States General Accounting Office (1991), if the United States had reduced its administrative costs for its health care system to the Canadian level (at that time less than 2%), the United States could afford to cover its entire uninsured population. A publicly financed, single-payer system is more efficiently administered than a plurality of private insurance plans with so much wasted duplication of common functions. Moreover, in a publicly financed system, expenditures on risk assessment, marketing, and lobbying become "medically unnecessary."

Fair financing can be achieved (as in Canada) through a universal health insurance tax, which maximizes the pooling of risk throughout the population so no one becomes uninsurable. A universal health insurance tax can also avoid the gaps in coverage found in America's voluntary, employment-based financing.

One more lesson from Canada. A national health insurance program can be guided by a small number of principles. Canada has just five fundamental principles: Public administration, comprehensive benefits, universal coverage, portability, and reasonable accessibility.

From the **United States** we can learn that *responsiveness* to a population's expectations is influenced significantly by the experienced freedom of individuals to choose their health plans and providers, as evident in the growing popularity of Preferred Provider Organizations (PPOs) over Health Maintenance Organizations (HMOs) (Gabel et al. 2005, p. 1278). Moreover, the timeliness with which they receive the good quality services they want or need to restore and improve their health is another significant factor contributing to satisfaction or dissatisfaction. Among the 191 member nations of the World Health Organization, the United States was ranked number one in its *level* of responsiveness to population expectations, in contrast to Norway (7–8), Canada (7–8), and Great Britain (26–27); however, all four of them ranked equally in the *distribution (fairness)* of responsiveness within their populations (WHO, 2000, p. 184; cf. Table 6.1 this volume).

One of the persistent challenges for the other three countries has been reducing the waiting times for health care services. *De facto* rationing by long waiting lists is no more acceptable than rationing by ability to pay. The outcome is the same – a delay in services. Like justice, services delayed are services denied if people are discouraged from seeking treatment. Although there is evidence of delays in treatment in the United States, especially for indigent patients (e.g., Friedman, Lemon, Stein, and D'Aunno, 2003), waiting times in America are less of a problem than in the other three countries that ration by queues.

Reducing waiting lists for mental health services of questionable or inconsistent quality would not be considered progress. The United States is a leader in the development of empirically-based treatment guidelines to improve the quality of mental health services. With the Department of Defense, the National Clinical Practice Guideline Council of the Veterans Health Administration has developed more than 27 clinical practice guidelines, and others have been developed by both the American Psychiatric Association (2003, 2004), the American Psychological Association (1981, 1986, 1987, 1995, 1998, 2003; cf. Bass et al. 1996), by the Committee on Ethical Guidelines for Forensic Psychologists (CFP, 1991), and several more by the federal Agency of Healthcare Research and Quality (AHRQ).

A negative lesson can be learned from the United States Medicaid program, which is the largest single insurer of mental health services in the country in both the public and private sectors. Medicaid is financed by both the federal and state levels of government, and administered by the states. In federated systems like the United States (and also Canada), there is continual debate about how much of the public health care bill should be paid by the federal government versus provincial/state governments. A plurality of payers (the federal government and several provinces or states) within the public sector seems to foster cost shifting. "The first law of cost containment states that the easiest way to control costs is to shift them to someone else" (Deber, 2003, p. 22). The result is unaccountability and a chronic and fruitless blame game. Like most games people play, someone usually gets hurt.

All four countries are challenged by rising costs. As indicated by per capita health expenditures, the United States has had greatest difficulty in achieving cost containment, despite its experiment with managed competition (Enthoven, 1993), perhaps because of it. Voluntary risk pooling among multiple, private for-profit health plans and insurance companies is unlikely to yield universal coverage because these private corporations need only avoid a small number of high users of health care services to reduce costs and increase their profits, leaving high-risk individuals uninsurable and shifting the costs of their care to the public sector (i.e., to taxpayers).

In lieu of price controls, the major cost-containment strategy adopted in the American health care system and mental health system has been control of the *volume* of services. Drastic reductions in inpatient psychiatric hospitalizations and inpatient days have occurred along with severe limits on the number of outpatient mental health visits under the control of managed behavioral health organizations (MBHOs). In disregard of the evidence for a dosage effect in psychotherapy, with optimal improvement for the largest percentage of patients at about 25 sessions (Howard, Kopta, Krause, and Orlinsky, 1986; Kopta, Howard, Lowry, and Beutler, 1992, 1994), the number of sessions in the preferred modality called "brief therapy" seems to have been reduced to a model of very abbreviated, crisis intervention (Miller, 1966a). This trend is significant because MBHOs were estimated to enroll about 164 million Americans in 2002, an increase from 70 million in 1993. Depending on various definitions of managed care, estimates of covered workers in firms carving out mental health benefits to specialized MBHOs range from 36 percent in HMOs, PPOs, and POS plans, to 66 percent when stand-alone utilization review and case management services are included (Barry et al. 2003, pp. 132–133).

Employer mandated health insurance coverage was a controversial element in the 1993 reform proposed by the Clinton Administration, which was defeated without so much as a House or Senate floor vote. The United States continues with a largely voluntary, employment-based health insurance system in the private sector. Job-based health insurance was estimated to cover about 175 million Americans, including 160 million active workers and their dependents, three million early retirees, and twelve million Medicare eligible retirees. But this voluntary system has gaping holes. An estimated 59 percent of the nation's firms have three to nine workers, and of these small firms, just over half offer health insurance coverage (Gabel et al. 2003, pp. 117, 123). This is one explanation for the finding that among the uninsured in America (about 46 million in 2005), approximately 80 percent are from families whose head of household is employed.

We cannot countenance the shocking inequality in access of uninsured Americans to their health care and mental health systems. A country that leaves nearly 46 million (about 16%) of its citizens and residents uninsured cannot be commended as the best system in the world – it hardly qualifies as a civilized society. Presently, there seems to be no unified, influential constituency in the United States to bring about social justice in the health care system, though there are a number of citizen advocacy groups that have been formed (e.g., CMHR, 2005; Healthcare-NOW, 2005; UHCAN, 2005a). The United States seems to lack a consensus of values that would serve as the moral foundation for universal health care: community, equity, and respect for human dignity (Brown, 2003).

Methodological Recommendations

This study of four mental health systems leads to some methodological recommendations about the measures of need, evaluation criteria, evaluation strategies, information technology and transfer, and future studies.

Objective and Subjective Indicators of Need

Any judgments about access and unmet need involve prior estimates of the need for mental health services, and these estimates are dependent upon the procedures and measures applied. These measures can be objective or subjective.

A basic methodological question that has arisen in this study is this: "What is the most valid indicator of the "need" for mental health services? Objective measures such as prevalence and utilization rates have been the primary measure applied by most countries. David Mechanic's (2000) critique is a legitimate one: many epidemiological studies have been tabulations of the numbers of mental disorders without appreciation for the severity of the disorders. An attempt has been made to address that shortcoming in the most recent methodology employed in the National Co-morbidity Study Replication (NCS-R) (Insel and Fenton, 2005; Kessler, et al. 2005a, 2005b). Including estimates of mild, moderate, and serious mental disorders based on reported levels of impairment, age of onset, co-morbidity, the burden of disease, and adequacy of treatment (or unmet need) are improvements over earlier studies of prevalence, and this NCS-R methodology has been adopted in epidemiological studies in 27 other countries under the aegis of the World Health Organization in its World Mental Health Survey Initiative (Insel and Fenton, 2005, p. 591).

Another type of "objective" indicator of the need for mental health services, closer to actual demand, is utilization rates. Nevertheless, measured by insurance claims data or patient registries, utilization data can tell us only about the number, types, and durations of mental health services, not about those who need the services, but have not used them. There have been estimates that only about 40 percent of Americans with mental disorders actually receive help from *any* health care professional, and about half of that percentage receives any help from mental health specialists.

Whether the studies record prevalence or utilization data, such "objective" studies seem to equate prevalence or utilization with need, and need with demand. I concur with Mechanic (2000) that subjective, randomized surveys of populations with self-identified mental health "needs," and queries about their desire/demand for mental health services seem as important as any of the "objective" measures.

One of the strengths of the British system is that multiple methods are employed to estimate need, including epidemiological and service utilization measures, systematic surveys by trained interviewers, and specific measures to obtain data from groups of users or potential users of mental health services. Great Britain uses surveys of potential users of mental health services within its population as a subjective indicator of need for mental health services. We can learn from that country's experience about population survey methods and consider adoption of the validated measures of need applied in those surveys. The latter are illustrated by the *Cardinal Needs Measure* and the *Camberwell Assessment of Need* measure, which have proven useful for examining the needs of low volume – high risk users, low volume and high cost service users, and for sampling with high volume user groups.

Aside from measures used to estimate need, in general "measurement provides the foundation on which health decisions are made. Poor measurement quality can affect both the quality of health care decisions and decisions about health care policy" (Morgan, Teal, Reddy, Ford, and Ashton, 2005, p. 1573). Stated positively, measuring performance and outcomes is essential for continuous quality improvement (Meehan, 2005, p. 1571). Health service researchers will find helpful measurement resources from the National Library of Medicine's National Information Center on Health Services Research and Health Care Technology (NICHSR, 2005; Witener, Van Horne, and Gauthier, 2005).

Evaluation Criteria

There are many more methodological questions to be addressed, not the least of which is how to assess the interaction effects of so many complex variables such as access, cost, and quality, as they influence one another and the performance of mental health systems generally. Future research on mental health systems should apply some of the criteria for evaluating health care systems outlined by the WHO about five years ago to facilitate comparative evaluations (WHO, 2000). We have mentioned the three universal goals of (a) protecting, preserving, and promoting the country's health status, (b) responsiveness to the population's expectations, and (c) fair financing, and the four functions, performance of which is prerequisite to attaining the goals of health care systems generally (stewardship, investment in resources, financing, and service provision). Attainment of these goals and performance of these functions seem to us to be necessary evaluation criteria, but perhaps not sufficient for a comprehensive evaluation.

The criteria selected for comparing the countries in this volume emerged from the editor's review of some of the relevant literature. There is a need to reach wider agreement as to whether these and/or other criteria should be applied in future studies, and how they can be measured validly and reliably. In this regard, the *mental health policy template* (Townsend et al. 2004) and the *mental health country profile* (Jenkins et al. 2004) developed by the International Consortium on Mental Health Policy and Services are instructive. Both procedures have been applied to several developing countries. They warrant application to developed countries as well. The *Mental Health Atlas – 2005* produced by WHO (2005a) is an illustration of mental health profiles.

Evaluation Strategies: Goal-Attainment Outcome Evaluations

Many of the evaluation strategies applied in the past have focused on the structural and process variables within health care systems to the exclusion of actual outcomes. The most fundamental question to ask about a mental health system is the degree to which it protects, sustains, and improves the mental health of its entire population and whether it does so fairly. This is a question of both the level and distribution of actual mental health outcomes.

One of the generally accepted outcome criteria is patients' improved quality of life (QOL) following treatment. The recent review by Wyrich et al. (2005) indicates the need to develop a consensus about methodology for determining *clinically significant improvement* in patients' QOL.

Measuring improved quality of life of treated clients is one approach to evaluating the effectiveness of interventions provided within a mental health system. This approach needs to be complemented by application of another criterion, namely the comparative cost-effectiveness of various interventions. Stated another way, evidence-based practices are not the same as value-based practices. The former address clinical criteria of quality, whereas the latter address economic criteria. In order for a mental health system to function efficiently, the interventions applied must be cost-effective (Newman, 2005).

To permit both accurate interpretation and replication, cost-effective analyses need to include clear descriptions of (a) the intervention, (b) the alternative compared, (c) the target population, and (d) the study's perspective. Rosen et al. (2005) found all four data elements were present in only 20 percent of abstracts in published journal articles on cost-effectiveness from 1998 through 2001. And in an analysis of over 500 cost-utility studies conducted in the United States, Neumann et al. (2005) found that among the *Healthy People 2010* priorities, depression, bipolar disorder, and substance abuse disorders were underrepresented.

At a clinical level, good quality treatment is characterized by clear and individualized treatment goals and appropriate, cost-effective interventions to attain these goals. Similarly, good quality mental health systems require clear goals and measurable objectives set collaboratively with goal-attainment evaluated regularly and reliably, and with results fed back into the system to foster continuous quality improvement. At this level, program evaluation based on actual treatment outcomes remains one of the major areas of development for all four of the countries included in this volume.

In a "consumer-driven" mental health system, a typical indicator of outcome is patient (i.e., customer) satisfaction. The use of patient satisfaction surveys to evaluate either outcomes or quality of mental health services is questionable. Although patient satisfaction is associated with the technical quality of care for common mental disorders, the strength of association is only moderate, hence insufficient to take satisfaction measures as a proxy indicator of technical quality (Edlund, Yound, Kung, Sherbourne, and Wells, 2003). Moreover, the differences between responders and nonresponders result in inflated estimates of satisfaction (Mazor, Clauser, Field, Yood, and Gurwitz, 2002).

One useful strategy is to evaluate outcomes in terms of the level of attainment of measurable goals. This goal-oriented outcome evaluation is a comprehensive and systematic approach that awaits application to mental health systems in particular. Two of the four countries in this study (England and Norway) seem to be more advanced than others, both in building a consensus to support well-defined, measurable goals articulated in national health policies, and in conducting systematic and systemic program evaluation based on goal attainment. We are impressed particularly with the process used to develop and evaluate Norway's National Mental Health Programme (NMHP). The need for reform was identified in the *White Paper 1996–1997*. That led to articulation of fourteen goals of the NMHP. These were not platitudes or mere rhetoric, but goals with expected outcomes specified in measurable terms with target dates, several of which included quantitative indicators (e.g., "increase by 50 percent productivity of outpatient clinics for adults"). Federal funds were allocated for about 15 research projects to evaluate the system's goal attainment and other impacts from its inception in 1998 through 2008.

A goal-attainment outcome evaluation is a strategy advocated and illustrated by the WHO in its annual report in 2000 on the performance of health care systems. Unfortunately, that evaluation strategy has not been replicated systematically to allow continuous, comparative evaluations among the 191 member countries to enhance mutual learning about what works well, what doesn't seem to work, and why or why not. It may be that the data set required for such evaluation is overwhelming, or that countries, which contribute financially to the WHO, don't like to be compared, especially if results challenge their illusions about being among the best health care systems in the world. Comparisons can be made, however, from standardized evaluations of individual countries provided recently by WHO (2005a).

A goal-attainment strategy was developed by Kiresuk, Smith, and Cardillo (1994) to evaluate outcomes in the mental health field. It was applied initially at the individual case level to evaluate outcomes of psychotherapy provided to a variety of clients by a heterogeneous group of providers in a community mental health center, who could not agree on universally acceptable outcome criteria consistent with their diverse psychotherapeutic approaches. Although developed initially to evaluate the outcomes of mental health treatments, goal-attainment scaling (GAS) has been applied to evaluate outcomes in several other fields, including education, medical residency training, rehabilitation, and program administration (Kiresuk et al. 1994, p. xv, 61–104). Olson (1997) applied GAS to evaluate practica training outcomes for doctoral candidates in clinical psychology. Spano, Kiresuk, and Lund (1977; as cited by Kiresuk et al. 1994, p. 95) reported on a comprehensive and computerized, goal-oriented evaluation system including goal-attainment scaling to assess outcomes in a department of social services at the University of Minnesota Medical School. Thus, GAS has been applied at the individual client level, program and departmental level, and it could be applied at the systems level.

A unique feature of this outcome evaluation strategy is that goals are set collaboratively at the beginning with five expected levels of outcome on a bipolar scale from "much more than the expected outcome" to "much less than the expected outcome." Goal attainment is scored after the intervention is applied for formative and/or summative evaluations of the change that occurred relative to the predicted or expected level of change. By including levels of expected outcome set in advance, the procedure incorporates relevant and realistic evaluation criteria and the expectations of stakeholders in the goal-setting process.

A goal-attainment procedure has been applied to evaluate the National Health Service in Britain and the National Mental Health Programme in Norway, but without setting multiple levels of expected outcome, though quantitative targets have been included. Insofar as population expectations are included, the additional step of setting five levels of expected outcome in advance could ensure that the responsiveness of the new program will be assessed. Basically, one follows the steps of problem identification, goal-setting (with five levels of expected outcome), implementation of the solution (health care program) followed by evaluation by relevant stakeholders (goal-attainment scoring).

Information Technology and Transfer

Prerequisite to providing the information needed to make policy decisions is the development of an information technology system to monitor the volume and types of mental health services, the quality, costs, responsiveness and goal attainment of the mental health system. According to the *Mental Health Atlas – 2005* (WHO, 2005a), all four of our countries conduct epidemiological studies to assess the prevalence of mental disorders, and all four have information technologies to provide annual reports on mental health services, though Canada and the United States seem to have made less progress in monitoring the quality of health care.

There is a priority need for an information technology system to support the development of a national policy and program to monitor and report the safety of patients as well as improving the quality of health care in the United States. A report by researchers with the Institute of Medicine estimated that between 44,000 and 98,000 deaths occur annually in the United States as a result of medical errors, with estimated costs ranging from $17 billion to $29 billion per year (Kohn, Corrigan, and Donaldson, 2000). The absence of a national system to provide a comprehensive assessment of quality of health care for the nation is a major reason for the small amount of systematic knowledge in this area. "Even though health care is a huge industry that affects the lives of most Americans, we have only snapshots of information about particular conditions, types of surgery, and locations of care" (Schuster, McGlynn, and Brook, 2005, p. 846).

One of the reasons for the lack of implementation of information technology in clinical practices is the manner in which health care is organized and delivered. For example, in America, more than half of all physicians are in practices too small to afford electronic medical record systems, which have been shown to reduce both medical errors and costly variations in the way health care is provided (Regenstreif, 2005).

In the two-year period, 2004 and 2005, the federal Agency for Healthcare Research and Quality awarded a total of about $165 million in grants for demonstration projects to implement health information technology systems. Several of these grants have been awarded to small and rural committees and for targeted populations such as ethnic minorities, immigrants, and patients with chronic diseases to improve coordinated and safer patient transitions between health care settings, timeliness of follow-up services, and to reduce medical errors and unnecessary, duplicated testing (AHRQ, 2005).

Equally important is to speed up the transfer of knowledge from academic centers of research to both clinicians and policymakers. There is a lack of transfer of methodologies of outcome assessment (Crombie, 2003; Ogles, B., Lambert, M., and Masters, K. 1996; Wiger and Solberg, 2001) to regulatory agencies charged with the responsibility of monitoring the quality of health plans. All four countries need to move to results-oriented outcome appraisals, rather than continuing to focus exclusively upon structural or process evaluations.

One further consideration. The United States health care system spends much more money on medical technology for patient care (e.g., drugs, MRIs, and other devices) than it spends to achieve equity in the delivery of existing services. An analysis of mortality rates from 1991 to 2000 led Woolf, Johnson, Fryer, Rust, and Satcher (2004) to conclude that achieving equity may do more to improve the health of the American population than perfecting medical technology.

Future Studies

We think we have asked some of the right questions in this comparative study. The evaluative criteria are certainly relevant to compare performances by mental health systems. We haven't been able to provide definitive answers or precise data from all four countries in identical formats pertinent to all of the evaluation criteria: access and equity, quality and efficacy, cost and efficiency, financing and fairness, protection and participation, and population relevance. Nevertheless, we have obtained sufficient information from our panel of experts to make informed judgments, and for us and our readers to draw some meaningful comparisons.

Future studies might address the interaction of the multiple factors and criteria pertinent to deciding which clinical and system-wide interventions to finance and provide (WHO, 2000, p. 55). Are some criteria more important than others in deciding how a mental health system is organized, financed, and delivered? Should mental health services be delivered publicly, privately, or by both sectors simultaneously? What can be done to improve the population's access to affordable mental health care of optimal quality? What are the principles, processes, and procedures that should guide decisions about rationing of scarce resources? Who decides that, how, and for whom? Is mental health a public good or a private commodity?

Additional questions to be addressed in future studies are Light's (2003) seven challenges (dilemmas) faced by all health care systems:

1. How does one reconcile the need for regional or national coordination with the ability to respond to local needs?
2. How does one reconcile urban with rural needs and the problem of maldistribution?
3. How does one devise a national health care system, and yet honor and foster the energies, creativity, and resources of the voluntary sector?
4. How does one reconcile public accountability with professional autonomy and expertise?
5. How shall primary care be integrated with specialty and hospital care?
6. How shall individualistic principles and patterns of practice be reconciled with national standards and a national system?
7. How is a system to reconcile a focus on the patient with a focus on community and population health?

Based upon his analysis of the four-volume report by the President's Commission on Mental Health established by President Jimmy Carter in 1977, and the short-lived *Mental Health Systems Act* that followed in October, 1980, Grob (2005) noted that the issues and dilemmas addressed then remain relevant today. Expressed as pertinent policy questions, they include the following:

> Should priority be given to individuals with serious and persistent mental illnesses, compared with those with less serious problems? Is it possible to minimize efforts to shift costs within a federal system composed of three levels of government [federal, state, and local]? Should legislators and policymakers concentrate on incremental changes, or should they seek a system-wide change? Can strictly health concerns be distinguished from broad environmental and social determinants? Should mental health policy remain independent of, or part of our general health policy? (pp. 449–450)

Continuity of Care. An important indicator of quality care in mental health services addressed in this study is their integration into the primary health care sector. Implicit in this criterion is another standard, namely, continuity of care. Continuity in outpatient mental health services is important because discontinuity might place clients at risk for poor clinical outcomes, and lead to inappropriate and costly utilization of hospitals and emergency rooms, and in the case of seriously mentally ill individuals, jails or prisons. Future program and system evaluations could apply some of the measures of continuity of care developed for clients in public mental health systems (Fortney et al. 2003).

Measures of Trust. Improved continuity of care is likely to help enhance a population's trust in their mental health system and providers. Even if mental health services are available and accessible, individuals' decisions both to seek treatment and to follow professional recommendations depend upon their level of trust in their health care system, in the health care professions generally, and more specifically in their individual provider (Hall, Camacho, Dugan, and Balkrishnan, 2002). A recent study by Mollborn, Stepnikova, and Cook (2005) indicated that patients' with lower levels of trust in their physician are more likely to report unmet health care needs. Consequently, an important goal of any mental health policy is to improve the population's level of trust in its mental health system and in mental health professions "... to facilitate the formation of vulnerable interpersonal relationships without extensive knowledge about [the provider's] individual personal characteristics" (Hall et al. 2002, p. 1431). Replication of the measures of trust used with primary health care providers with mental health specialists is an area for future research.

Processes of Care. The present study has compared the performance of mental health systems of four developed countries on variables such as access, quality, cost, financing, and service delivery. Future studies might make cross-national comparisons based on the actual processes of care, defined as what a mental health provider actually does when seeing a patient. The quality and efficacy of clinical practice, which are major elements of the process of care, are of particular interest for the improvement of mental health outcomes. To assess quality of care, clinical vignettes can provide accurate measures of actual clinical practice in a more valid manner than either retrospective reviews of patient records or comparisons of structural elements such as training and staffing ratios of providers. Moreover, research documenting high quality processes of care, particularly the use of efficacious clinical practices, is likely to improve the population's trust in the mental health system (Peabody, Tozija, Munoz, Nordyke, and Luck, 2004), though the ultimate criterion is actual treatment outcomes: Do treated patients experience clinically significant, sustained improvement in their mental health following treatment? Numerous outcome as well as process measures for quality improvement have been reviewed by the American Psychiatric Association (1998, 2006).

Improving the Performance of Mental Health Systems

The annual report on mental health by the World Health Organization made ten general recommendations to improve mental health care: (a) provide treatment in primary care settings, (b) make psychotropic drugs available, (c) give care in the community, (d) educate the public, (e) involve communities, families and consumers, (f) establish national policies, programs and legislation, (g) develop human resources, (h) link with other sectors (e.g., education, labor, welfare, the law and nongovernmental organizations), (i) apply mental health indicators to monitor community mental health; (j) support more research into both biological and psychosocial aspects of mental health (WHO, 2001, pp.110–112). These recommendations continue to be valid and relevant to improving the performance of mental health systems in the four developed countries included in this study.

This author endorses the ten recommendations for action made by the WHO (2001, pp. xi–xiii), especially the emphasis upon the provision of mental health services in primary health care and community-based facilities, which was articulated in the *Declaration of Caracas* written by the countries participating in the Regional Conference on the Restructuring of Psychiatric Care in Latin America (WHO, 2001, p. 52). I believe improvements in mental health services need to occur, and can occur in the following areas: (a) integrating mental health specialty care into primary health care, (b) national policy formulation on quality assessment and quality improvement, (c) prevention and promotion, (d) overcoming stigma, (e) stewardship, (f) mental health policy training, (g) value clarification, and (h) mental health and human rights.

Integrating Mental Health Specialty Care into Primary Health Care

A Health Care System Based on Primary Care. By definition, a primary health care system (PHS) provides the majority of care to the population. The PHS consists of two major domains: (a) *Structural characteristics* include health system financing, distribution of resources, physician inputs, accessibility, and longitudinality [continuity of care]; (b) *primary practice features* include first contact, coordination, comprehensive care, longitudinality, and a family and/or community orientation. Based on this multidimensional definition of a PHS, Mackinko, Starfield, and Shi (2003) proposed a scale to monitor health reform efforts intended to improve primary care. Following their review of 18 OECD countries' primary health care systems 1970–1998, the authors concluded that (1) "... a strong primary care system and practice characteristics such as geographic regulation, longitudinality, coordination, and community orientation were associated with improved population health, and (2) despite health reform efforts, few OECD countries improved essential features of their primary care systems as assessed by the scale..." (p. 831).

Although income inequality has been shown to be a more powerful influence on mortality rates than the presence or absence of primary health care providers (Shi et al. 2005), there is empirical evidence that the supply of physicians is positively associated with the overall performance of the primary health care system in a large sample of urban counties in the United States as indicated by a reduction in the number of preventable hospitalizations (Laditka, Laditka, and Probst, 2005). There is also substantial evidence that primary health care helps prevent illness and disease generally, and in contrast to specialty care, primary care is associated with more equitable distribution of health in populations (Starfield, Shi, and Macinko, 2005). Moreover, access to regular primary care improves coordination, continuity, and comprehensiveness of health care (Seid and Stevens, 2005). For these and other reasons, a strong primary health care system is vital to the overall performance of a health care system.

Unfortunately, establishing primary care in rural areas is a challenge most countries have not met. As an example, Americans living in rural areas account for about 20 percent of the total population, but less than 11 percent of the country's physicians, hence rural residents have lower access to a regular primary care provider (Ricketts, 1999). Geographic distance to a primary care clinic has been shown to be a significant barrier to access for preventive, acute, and chronic medical care (Arcury et al. 2005), and especially among minorities and the elderly (Basu, 2005).

Primary Mental Health Care. The above discussion makes the point that integrating mental health services into a primary health care sector requires that the latter is effective and functioning throughout the population. To the degree a country strives for community-based mental health care, integrated into the primary health care sector, the guiding principles articulated by the World Health Organization are relevant: (a) an early and appropriate diagnosis and effective intervention; (b) continuity of care, (c) a wide range of services, (d) partnerships with patients and families, (e) involvement of the local community, and (f) integration into primary health care (WHO, 2001, pp. 54–59). Moreover, we can concur with their call for the balanced combination of three fundamental ingredients of comprehensive mental health services: psychotherapy, pharmacotherapy, and psychosocial rehabilitation (WHO, 2001, p. 59). Providing social services, supplemental and disability income, transportation, and affordable housing or assisted living are also vital.

A common pattern across the four countries in our study is that a variable, but small percentage of people with mental health/substance abuse problems actually receive treatment from mental health *specialists*. Estimates by our chapter authors range from eight percent in Canada, 25 percent in Norway, 28 percent in the United States, to 33 percent in Great Britain (Table 7.4). By far, the majority of such individuals consult first their family physician/general practitioner, and in the United States another significant segment first consult their clergy. In England, Norway, and Canada, the family physician has been given a prominent role as a gate keeper to both inpatient and specialist services, and the role of coordinator of care. Although having primary care physicians serve as gatekeepers does yield minor cost-savings (Pati, Shea, Rabinowitz, and Carrasquillo, 2005), the major justification for primary mental health care is to improve the quality of care by making it more integrated, continuous, and community-based.

Given the significant percentage of people with mental disorders treated first by general practice physicians, which is an intentional policy in some of these countries, it would seem that resources and regulations pertaining to education, licensure, and continuing education should lead to more academic content, supervised training, and ongoing consultations to enhance the knowledge, skills, and positive attitudes of these primary health care professionals consulted most frequently by people with mental disorders and psychological distress. This seems even more critical in the United States based on the NCS-R results, which indicated that of the people with mental disorders who sought treatment, the largest group they consulted were general-medical providers (GPs) (22.8%), who also manifested the lowest percent of patients (12.8%) receiving at least minimally adequate treatment (Wang et al. 2005b, p. 629). The high prevalence of depression and well-documented deficiencies in recognition and reporting of depression by primary health care providers makes this an important area of quality assessment and quality improvement (Spettell et al. 2003).

Another significant group of providers, who tend to be slighted in the mental health primary care sector is clergy. In an analysis of the National Co-morbidity Survey conducted 1990–1992 with a sample of 8,098 Americans, Wang, Berglund, and Kessler (2003) found that 23.5 percent of Americans who sought treatment for mental disorders in 1986–1991 did so from a clergy member.

> Although there has been a decline in this proportion between the 1950s (31.3 percent) and the early 1990s (23.5 percent), the clergy continue to be contacted by higher proportions than psychiatrists (16.7 percent) or general medical doctors (16.7 percent). Nearly one-quarter of those seeking help from clergy in a given year have the most seriously impairing mental disorders. The majority of these people are seen exclusively by clergy, and not by a physician or mental health professional. (p. 647)

Wang, Gerglund, and Kessler (2003) concluded that "... while the clergy continue to be a frequent point of contact in the U. S. mental health delivery system, additional efforts may be needed to optimize their role" (pp. 667–668). Among their recommendations are additional training in mental health issues, including suicide prevention, additional training in pastoral counseling, and facilitating timely referrals.

Working more closely with better trained clergy throughout the country may be one solution to a problem in the United States, namely, that many states do not have comprehensive, primary health care programs, and an increasing number of states are experiencing budget deficits that may lead to reductions in existing programs (Wilensky, Rosenbaum, Hawkins, and Mizeur, 2005), though the Bureau of Primary Health Care projects an increase in federally funded Community Health Centers as primary care safety nets for underserved populations (Bureau of Primary Health Care, 2003, 2004; Shi, Stevens, Wulu, Politzer, and Xu, 2004). The number of clergy dispersed throughout local communities is an untapped human resource.

Mental Health Specialists Working in Primary Care Settings. More effective consultative relationships between GPs and mental health specialists is clearly warranted and recognized by all of our authors. Moreover, placement of mental health specialists within primary health care settings seems vital if these mental health systems are to attain higher levels of integrated care. In this regard, the finding that 70 percent of England's general practitioners have "counselors" associated with their practice is both exemplary and instructive. In the public sector in the United States, uniting community mental health centers with neighborhood health centers in the same location may be a way to enhance more integrated, cost-effective, primary mental health care. Potential settings for employment of mental health specialists are federally funded community health centers, personal health centers, hospital-based and free-standing medical clinics, and public/private partnership clinics (Diamant et al. 2005). Pastoral counseling centers and counseling programs in churches are additional settings.

A variety of financial arrangements could facilitate such multidisciplinary cooperation. In the private health sector, arrangements can vary from simply renting office space and sharing overhead, to salaried or contractual arrangements, partnership, or incorporation. Legislation restricting such multidisciplinary arrangements constitute legal and financial barriers to effecting more integrated care in the private sector. Adding clergy and/or pastoral counselors would be even more comprehensive, assuming a country could affirm in its mental health policy a holistic vision of the person as a multidimensional unity of mind/body/spirit, illustrated by Norway and in the United States, by the Indian Health Service.

Mental Health Specialists as Consultants. Mental health service professionals need to learn how to function as effective consultants with primary health care providers. Consulting is more than sharing expert knowledge to assist in problem-solving; it requires genuinely collaborative, mutually respectful relationships, and effective interpersonal skills. Consulting and supervision have been recognized as distinct competencies by the National Council of Schools of Professional Psychology, and these competencies are included in the curriculum of several professional psychology schools in the United States, which train clinical psychologists. Much more needs to be done in this area in all four countries.

A Biopsychosocial Model. With the advances in germ theory, genetics, microbiology and neuroscience research and technology, most health care professionals would affirm there are biological determinants of both health and mental disorders (e.g., Bortz, 2005). The error is not in affirming biological causes, but in assuming in all cases that they are the primary cause to the exclusion of other predisposing, precipitating, and reinforcing causes.

To encourage a more integrated approach, a narrow biomedical model of mental disorders and substance abuse conditions as exclusively brain-body dysfunctions needs to be broadened into a more comprehensive biopsychosocial model, and ideally to include the spiritual dimension of meaning and existential concerns. A biopsychosocial model of health was adopted by the World Health Organization in 1946 (WHO, 1946) and has not been amended, yet more than 50 years later, predominantly biologically-oriented systems prevail in mental health systems such as Canada dominated by physicians.

A broader socioeconomic model of mental disorders is particularly needed to complement both the biological and psychological models that localize etiology in the individual's brain or psyche. For example, there is considerable research that suggests inequity in the distribution of health is a function of broader social and economic inequalities (e.g., Evans, Whitehead, Diderichsen, Bhuiya, and Wirth, 2001; Hyder, 2004), hence not merely due to inequalities in access to the health care system. Braverman, Egeter, Cubbin, and Marchi (2004) proposed an approach to studying these "social disparities in health," that is, differences in health associated with different levels of social advantage or position in a socially stratified society.

Zimmerman's (2005) empirical model of utilization of children's mental health services included multiple determinants. Receiving mental health services was predicted to be a function of (a) level of symptoms, (b) socioeconomic status (SES), (c) health insurance status, (d) traumatic events, (e) the child's genetic background, and (f) demographic characteristics (e.g., gender of the child, birth order, and family structure). The SES and health insurance variables were less powerful predictors than gender, birth order, and race, and the presence of a father in the family with negative attitudes toward mental health services. These predictors are examples of social determinants of health and mental health, which argue for a broader conceptualization than the biomedical model provides (Thomas, Fine, and Ibrahim, 2004). The Communities Regeneration Initiative in England (Parry and Judge, 2005) and the Community Action Model in America (Lavery et al. 2005) are examples of approaches designed to address socioeconomic determinants of health inequalities.

National Policy on Quality Assessment and Improvement

Prerequisite to improving a country's mental health system is a national policy on quality assessment and quality improvement. "Policy to improve performance requires information on the principal factors which explain it. Knowledge of the determinants of health system *performance*, as distinct from understanding what determines health *status*, remains very limited" (WHO, 2000, p. 44).

What are the necessary and sufficient conditions to produce a mental health system that can be judged as a good system? The answer provided by WHO (2000) is the satisfactory performance of four functions common to all health care systems: (a) stewardship (oversight), (b) creating resources (capital investments and training of personnel), (c) financing (collecting, pooling, and purchasing), and (d) delivering services (WHO, 2000, Figure 2.1, p. 25). Satisfactory performance of these four fundamental functions of the health care system are presumed to be necessary to achieving the three universal goals of health care systems (a) good health for the population, (b) responsiveness to the population's expectations, and (c) fair financing. The common finding of unmet needs among all four systems reviewed in this volume suggests that all four major functions of the mental health system must be addressed for quality improvement and goal attainment: stewardship, investment, financing, and service delivery. Satisfactory performance of one function is not sufficient; improvement in all four functions is necessary. Thus, national mental health policies obligating universal access to optimal quality mental health services are necessary, but insufficient if the system does not make the equally necessary investments to develop and distribute human resources with relevant competencies.

Publicly financed systems based on progressive income taxes, health insurance taxes, or on general tax revenues seem to be necessary to pool both revenues and risk most efficiently and fairly, but that is insufficient to ensure universal access to high quality mental health care. Additional necessary elements include strategic allocation of revenues through purchasing and rationing to achieve priorities; workforce planning and funding; public education and information about both the nature of mental disorders and treatment possibilities; a network of social support for patients receiving community-based treatment; an active treatment/recovery ideology; a commitment to evidence-based practices; a shift away from an exclusive biological model to a biopsychosocial-spiritual model with appreciation for the individual's "quality of life;" a change in education of mental health professionals to emphasize primary mental health care and interdisciplinary cooperation; and effective mental health promotion and prevention programs.

A rational approach to formulating national mental health policy and evaluating the impact of policy reforms is another necessary condition. The approach taken by the International Consortium on Mental Health Policy and Services is a viable model. Typical steps in this approach include: (a) reviewing the current mental health country profile (a standardized format for recording and reporting the mental health situation of a country); (b) determining gaps in this evidence-based profile and designing ways in which to fill them; (c) outlining a new, revised country profile; (d) drafting the outline of a policy that leads from the current to the desired profile; (e) designing a strategy for policy implementation, monitoring and evaluation; (f) beginning the implementation of that strategy. This approach is not linear, but a continuous process of revising a country's mental health policy or program in light of comprehensive and standardized data collected regularly (Gulbinat et al. 2004, p. 14).

Prevention/Promotion

The mental health systems in all four countries in this volume have not maximized a basic principle of cost-containment and public health: It is less expensive to prevent mental disorders than to treat them later. Prevention of mental disorders and promotion of mental health need to be a priority funded by public and private sources to help reduce the growing demand for mental health services, and to improve efficiency by reducing costs of treatment. This public health perspective seems vital to improve the mental health status of any population. Practitioners who are trained to diagnose and treat mental disorders, and whose income depends upon the continued demand for their services, are less likely to provide leadership in prevention than patient advocacy groups and public health agencies and associations.

Overcoming Stigma

Racism, sexism, and ageism are destructive forms of prejudice and discrimination resulting in segregation and inequality, and in violation of human rights and human dignity. The segregation and neglect of the minority of the population who experience mental disorders is an expression of both prejudice and discrimination. Among the people suffering stigma and discrimination to the greatest degree are the seriously and persistently mentally ill, and chronically and severely addicted individuals, many of whom became homeless or imprisoned following the period of deinstitutionalization, which each of our four countries experienced. Based on the principle that we treat the worst first, it is this subgroup that deserves greatest attention. They are people of all ages, men, women, and children of all races and color, who suffer protracted distress and disability with a marked loss of freedom associated with their mental disorders. The World Association for Psychosocial Rehabilitation focuses on this population through its conferences and journals, the *International Journal of Psychosocial Rehabilitation*, and the English version, the *International Journal of Mental Health*.

Stewardship is Fundamental

Among the four essential functions performed by mental health systems, stewardship is the most important – more important that the other three: input production, financing, and service provision. Stewardship is preeminent because it influences the performance of all other functions, and consequently, attainment of the universal goals of improved mental health, responsiveness to a population's expectations, and fair financing.

The ultimate responsibility for the overall performance of a country's health care system, including its mental health system must always lie with the country's elected government if the health care needs of all of its citizens are to be addressed equally and democratically.

> Stewardship has recently been defined as a 'function of a government responsible for the welfare of the population, and concerned about the trust and legitimacy with which its activities are viewed by the citizenry.' It requires vision, intelligence and influence, primarily by the health ministry, which must oversee and guide the working and development of the nation's health actions on the government's behalf. (WHO, 2000, p. 119)

It appears to this author that the governments of Great Britain and Norway have advanced farther than Canada and the United States in the performance of this central function of stewardship. In both the United States and Canada, mental health programs have been the subject of countless reviews at various levels of government for decades. Nevertheless, what Dr. Arnett stated about Canada applies equally to the United States: "While there have been changes in programs and advances made, many of the recommendations have never been implemented in spite of kind words said about them by policymakers." It is discouraging to witness the continued gap between rhetoric and reality. It seems that commissioning a study and then ignoring the results is a way of creating an appearance of being responsive without being genuinely and fully responsible. Political smoke and mirrors will not bring justice to our mental health system. This is a failure of leadership, but also a failure of the citizenry to hold their leaders accountable.

It will be up to the citizens of each country to find the leaders with the vision, intelligence, and influence to bring about improvements in their mental health systems. We need leaders with wisdom as well as compassion, and a passion for social justice. Martin Luther King, Jr. expressed these traits in his recognition that "Of all forms of inequality, injustice in health care is the most shocking and inhumane." Leaders will be needed who are also skilled in fostering coalitions and partnerships in team-based approaches (Umble et al. 2005).

Mental Health Policy Training

Mental health specialists are potential leaders as well as stakeholders in the mental health system, along with its users, all payers, and citizens whose taxes finance the system. All constituents have a vested interested in influencing mental health policy, but few receive an education relevant to policy formulation and implementation, or training to become leaders in the performance of the stewardship function. Professional schools educating future mental health specialists should provide courses on mental health systems, and provide concentrations or certification programs for future practitioners to become informed and more involved in the formulation and implementation of mental health policy.

Value Clarification

Fundamentally, whether a democratic society provides universal access to high quality, affordable mental health services depends upon the values the population seeks to actualize. Cultural values are reflected in the health care policies and programs of all four countries in this study. While they share in common a respect for human rights consistent with the United Nations charter, the values of mutual responsibility, egalitarianism, and social welfare are predominant in Great Britain and Norway, less so in Canada and least present in the United States. Churchill (1995) observed:

> ... the U.S. health care system is flawed principally because we have never asked what its goals are. So long as that fundamental moral question remains unanswered, no amount of political or economic tinkering will fix the system's problems. If we carefully examine the present workings of our system, we would have to conclude that its goals are two: maintain the prerogatives of physicians and the well-being of the private insurance industry. Such goals hardly represent an exercise in moral choice, and ... are morally indefensible.

Ends and Means Are Values. The goals of a mental health system and the strategies chosen to attain the goals are not merely technical, economic, or political decisions. These are normative judgments about ends and means. For example, implicit in the goal of universal access to the mental health system is a value judgment that including everyone is good in a moral sense, and a moral obligation of society. Insofar as this end justifies the means of financing and delivering mental health services, it reflects a teleological theory of moral obligation with the implicit principle of *beneficence:* We ought to do the good. In this case, the good we ought to do is to provide mental health care for everyone. When we affirm that a mental health system is good on other grounds besides the ends or goals it achieves, we are invoking a deontological theory of moral obligation based on duty, illustrated by the principle of *justice:* Our duty is to do the good fairly. A mental health system can be justified ethically on either teleological or deontological grounds or both. Another justification is an agapist ethic grounded theologically (Frankena, 1973; UHCAN, 2005b).

To ask whether a mental health system delivers services to everyone is to affirm implicitly the ethical principle of *universalism.* To ask whether or not services are delivered equally and financed fairly is to affirm the ethical principle *justice.* Both fair financing and universal access are ethical principles by which a society selects the means to achieve the ends of protecting and enhancing the health and dignity of everyone. Thus, financing a mental health system cannot be reduced to a matter of dollars; ultimately it is about human dignity. Health economics must be grounded in social ethics and guided by humanitarian values. A similar conclusion was reached by Eisenberg (1999): health as a social good cannot be allocated effectively or equitably by the invisible hand of the market. Americans have been slow to recognize this fundamental moral insight.

Ranking Competing Values. Clarification of values is necessary when a plurality of values are endorsed, since they are likely to compete for allegiance. Clarification among the desired ends or goals of a mental health system can be accomplished by a rank ordering. Table 7.6 illustrates a rank ordering of quality above cost from (1) high quality-low cost to (4) low quality-high cost. A similar ranking could be done for the values of equity and efficacy to help clarify priorities.

Social Capital. The norms that underlie a mental health system are elements of what the World Bank defines as *social capital:* "... the norms and networks that enable collective action" (The World Bank Group, June 5, 2003). In contrast to human, financial, or material capital, social capital is a cohesive force within a society which may not be directly measurable, but is expressed in a psychological sense of community, collective efficacy, community competence, even neighborhood cohesion.

Having social capital is assumed beneficial for health policy formulation, and hypothesized as a factor contributing to mental health, though the latter is debated (Henderson and Whiteford, 2003, p. 506). Nevertheless, one explanation for persistent injustice and inequity in health care systems is a deficit in social capital and the absence of a communitarian ethic to subsume a private morality. The values of social solidarity and mutual responsibility are expressions of the

Table 7.6. *Ranking of Values: Quality above Cost.*

		Quality	
		High	Low
Cost	Low	1	3
	High	2	4

ranking of the public good over private gain, and of social interest over self-interest. These are value judgments, which are also expressed in a society's allocation of resources to its mental health system.

Health Expenditures Reflect Value Judgments. Value judgments and moral decisions are expressed in the allocations of resources. As McGuire and Serra (2005) noted recently, "growth of health care expenditure is a normative issue reflecting the value judgments expressed by a given country." This is not, however, merely a judgment about the value-added benefit of a particular intervention relative to its cost; rather, it raises much more fundamental questions about the value of human life, whether social equality is as important as personal liberty, whether the common good supersedes individual rights and privileges, whether enhancing social welfare matters more than protecting private profits, whether health insurance is a private property or functions as social insurance so the healthy help the sick and the wealthy help the poor, whether cooperation trumps competition, whether human need should triumph over corporate greed. Answers to these ethical questions influence health expenditures and the allocation of human and material resources.

Evaluation Criteria Are Values. None of the criteria by which we have compared mental health systems can be considered either value-neutral or value-free. To the contrary, a criterion like "equitable access" is a value-laden concept. Moreover, the choice of a measure of health inequity, including the units of analysis and time, have ethical implications (Asada, 2005). The first and principal recommendation on ethics in medicine reported in 1983 by President Carter's Commission on the Study of Ethical Problems in Medicine and Biomedical and Behavioral Research was that "... society has an obligation to assure equitable access to health care for all its citizens. Equitable access, the Commission said, requires that all citizens be able to secure an adequate level of care without excessive burdens" (*Securing Access to Health Care*, 1983, as cited by Roemer, 2000, p. 242). Equitable access involves the principle of justice.

The Ethical Principle of Justice. Justice in health care continues to be a major civil rights issue in the twenty-first century. It always has been a matter of human rights. The United Nations charter recognized this more than 50 years ago. Yet for millions of people with mental disorders, this right continues to be denied, even in advanced, industrialized countries like the four examined in this study.

There are several theories of justice, as there are different theories of moral obligation. The latter answer the question of what actions are right and what we ought to do. Theories of justice address questions about participation in decision-making and due process, about respect for the dignity and worth of individuals, liberty and equality, and human rights (Labacqz, 1987).

One of the theories of justice relevant to the issue of access to health care is *distributive justice*, which focuses on the question of how social resources, wealth, and power should be allocated in society. "The main premise is that distribution should be just. Resources must be distributed according to rules, and these rules must promote fairness, equity, and impartiality" (Callaway and Hall, 2000, p. 88). Insofar as mental health services are considered a social good, theories of distributive justice are relevant.

Aspects of a particular mental health system may be justified by one, or more than one theory of distributive justice. For example, using capitation financing to increase access to care may correspond to an *egalitarian* view of distributive justice, while improvements in service delivery and in the quality of outcomes may correspond to a *utilitarian* view. Results from several empirical studies of the Colorado Medicaid system were interpreted by Callaway and Hall (2000) as illustrations of these alternative theories. In contrast to both an egalitarian and utilitarian approach, the authors recommended the fair-opportunity rule as a useful principle for determining the just distribution of health care services.

Recent regional and international initiatives to reduce injustice in health care systems have been summarized by Casas-Zamora and Ibrahim (2005). A few examples are provided here, first at the *regional level*. The WHO Regional Office for Europe (EURO, 1998) made eight recommendations to reduce health inequalities, including ensuring access to, and utilization of effective health care and prevention services by socially disadvantaged and vulnerable groups. The Pan American Health Organization made serious efforts from 1996 to 2002 to reduce health inequities within and between countries in that region.

At an *international level*, a Global Health Equity Initiative was begun in 1996, which led to the Global Equity Guage Alliance to monitor health inequalities and to promote equity within and between societies. The International Society for Health Equity, founded in 2000, includes researchers and advocates of health equity. The WHO initiated a Global Health Survey in 2001 to help monitor socioeconomic inequalities in health based on the 1998 World Health Assembly resolution addressing this issue.

Value Resources. A consensus of values pertinent to protecting those who suffer with mental disorders has been expressed at international, regional, and national levels.

A review of international and regional declarations of human rights would allow individuals to assess the degree to which their mental health systems conform to these humanitarian values of civilized societies. Examples include the United Nations General Assembly documents (1948, 1989, 1991), World Health Organization documents (1948, 1997, 2000, 2000a, 2001), regional declarations such as the European Convention on Human Rights (Council of Europe, 1950, 1966) and the Declaration of Caracas (1990), and other international documents affirming the rights and protections of those with mental disorders (WHO, 2001, pp. 52–53, 82–84, 125–126.) The rights of children to health and health care were affirmed by the United Nations in the 1959 Declaration of the Rights of Children, and reaffirmed in the U.N. Convention on the Rights of the Child in 1989 (as cited by Roberts, Alexander, and Davis, 1991). Additional resolutions adopted by the U. N. General Assembly include the Declaration on the Rights of Disabled Persons, the Declaration on the Rights of Mentally Retarded Persons, the Principles for the Protection of Persons with Mental Illness and for the Improvement of Mental Health Care, the Declaration of Caracas, and the Delcaration of Madrid. A more complete listing of United Nations and WHO documents pertinent to mental health standards and legislation that respect and protect the rights of people with mental disorders was provided by Freeman, Pathare, Drew, and Funk (2005, Annex 2, pp. 155–164).

Of particular relevance is the Universal Declaration of Human Rights, adopted by the United Nations General Assembly in 1948 and reaffirmed in the United Nations Millennium Declaration in 2000 (U. N. General Assembly, 2000). It expressed an international consensus on thirty inalienable rights. Article 25 stated specifically: "Everyone has the right to a standard of living adequate for the health and wellbeing of himself and his family, including food, clothing, housing, and medical care and social services. . . ." The 1948 Constitution of the World Health Organization affirmed human rights as the foundation of health: "The enjoyment of the highest attainable standard of health is one of the fundamental rights of every human being without distinction of race, religion, political belief, economic or social condition" (WHO, 1948). Subsequent international conventions have extended those rights to include women and children, access to food, safe water, and a secure environment, and the human right to the highest attainable standard of physical and mental health.

Examples of value statements at the *national level* include the framework for evaluating Britain's National Health Service provided by Thornicroft and Tansella (1999). They articulated a set of nine ethical principles for translation into outcome measures for program evaluation purposes. The definitions were extended and operationalized by Bruce and Paxton (2002).

The White House Council on Domestic Policy (1993) articulated several values and principles that informed the *President's Health Security Plan*. These values were presented as ". . . fundamental national beliefs about community, equality, justice, and liberty. These convictions anchor health reform in shared moral traditions" (p. 11). Among the principles and values cited were universal access, comprehensive benefits, choice, equality of care, fair distribution of costs, personal responsibility, intergenerational justice, wise allocation of resources, effectiveness, quality, effective management, professional integrity and responsibility, fair procedures, and local responsibility (pp. 11–13). Though the *Health Security Plan* was defeated, the values endorsed remain a valid, ethical foundation for public health and mental health policy. They affirm the common good over self-interest as normative (Kangas, 1997).

Two additional documents from the United States Administrative branch are (a) the *President's Commission on Health Needs of the Nation* (1953), which asserted: "access to the means for the attainment and preservation of health is a basic human right" (p. 3, as cited by Roberts, Alexander, and Davis, 1991, p. 22); and (b) the report by the *White House Conference on Children* in 1970, which affirmed their right to be healthy (Hart, 1982).

Finally, citizen advocacy groups have articulated values and goals as foundations for health care reform (e.g., Healthcare-NOW, 2005; National Alliance for the Mentally Ill, 2005; UHCAN, 2005c). In response to the national citizen health care access campaign, the Congressional Universal Health Care Task Force sponsored a *Health Care Access Resolution*, which articulates fourteen principles by which to measure the impact of 50+ bills presently before Congress addressing health care reform. Grounded in moral as well as medical and economic imperatives, a *just health care system* (and by implication, a just mental health system) is envisioned as (a) affordable; (b) cost efficient; (c) comprehensive; (d) promotes prevention and early intervention; (e) ensures parity for mental health and other services; (f) eliminates disparities in access to quality health care; (g) addresses people with special health care needs and underserved populations in both rural and urban areas; (h) promotes quality and better health outcomes; (i) emphasizes the need for adequate numbers of qualified health care caregivers, practitioners, and providers to guarantee timely access to quality care; (j) promotes adequate and timely payments to guarantee access to providers; (k) includes a strong network of health care facilities, including safety net providers; (l) continuing of coverage and care; (m) allows maximum consumer choice of health care providers and practitioners; and (n) it is a system easy to use for patients, providers, and practitioners with reduced paperwork (UHCAN, 2005c).

Other resources for developing an ethical framework for national mental health policy formation and implementation include statements made by professional associations and professional codes of ethics. Several years ago, the American Medical Association articulated values expressed as principles for a health policy agenda (Balfe, Boyle, Brocki, and Lane, 1985; Boyle, 1987). More recently, the American Public Health Association articulated six principles and 24 goals to reform the American health care system (Fein, 2003). The principles are (a) universal and equitable coverage, (b) comprehensive benefits and quality health care, (c) affordable and equitable financing, (d) simplified administration and sensibly organized work, (e) accountability, and (f) a strong public health system. Feldman (1998) provided a conceptual model for evaluating health care policy based on medical ethics. Olson (2000a, 2000b) applied the ethical principles of the American Psychological Association as criteria and goals for health care reform. Barofsky (2003) called for a Declaration of Patients' Rights, with reference to their quality of life, as a social contract between clinicians and their patients. The listing of values and ethical principles in the mental health policy documents among the four developed nations reviewed in this volume constitute additional important resources, along with the list of competing values in the interface between mental health services and the wider community (Malm, Jacobson, and Larsson, 2003).

One more major, but neglected source of values to inform mental health policy is the wisdom and compassion embraced by the world's great religions. Human dignity and mutuality are common themes, as are calls for liberation from oppression and injustice (Olson, 2002). The right to life implies the right to health care to protect and sustain life. Several American denominations have expressed theologically grounded policies affirming justice in health care (UHCAN, 2005b). These sources may help to provide moral and ethical foundations for mental health policy. A primary ethical foundation is linking mental health with human rights.

Mental Health and Human Rights

Comparison of these four health care systems has raised important ethical questions. The most basic is whether health care is valued like a commodity to be bought and sold in a competitive market place, or if health care is a universal human right and a fundamental right of citizenship. Three of the countries seem to have resolved this question by affirming universal access to optimal health care as a human right of all their citizens and residents. The United States appears to remain morally ambivalent.

Nuwayhid (2004) noted that tangible progress in occupational health in developing countries can be achieved only by linking health to the broader context of social and economic justice. Abrams (2001, 2005) suggested that this link needs to be established for minorities in developed countries like the United States such as migrant farm workers. Another population that warrants attention is the disproportionate number of both legal and undocumented immigrants in the United States who are uninsured (Prentice, Pebley, and Sastry, 2005).

Rodriguez-Garcia and Akhter (2000) made a persuasive argument that human rights are the foundation of a public health care system designed to protect, sustain, and improve a population's health. A similar argument can be made as a moral obligation and foundation for a country's mental health system. Indeed, an analysis of mortality rates from 1991 to 2000 led Woolf, Johnson, Fryer, Rust, and Satcher (2004) to conclude that advancing human rights by achieving equity in the health care system may do more to improve the health of the American population than perfecting medical technology.

To affirm an obligation implies that we ought to fulfill it. A corollary of this principle is that people to whom we are obligated have a right to expect us to fulfill our duty to them. Thus, complementing a theory of moral obligation is a theory of human rights (Frankena, 1973). Gruskin (2000) noted the human rights implications of health policies and practices, and that insufficient attention has been paid to the implications of health care systems for human rights. Thus, principles guiding the financing, organization and delivery of mental health services function as moral principles of obligation defining what we should do and what people have a right to expect and claim. Roemer (2000) discussed the moral, social, legal, and constitutional grounds for the right of all Americans to health care. Roberts, Alexander, and Davis (1991) presented humanitarian, ethical, and legal arguments that children have a right to health and access to health care. The authors noted: "Despite assertions of concern for children, the United States has yet to commit itself to assuring children's physical and mental health" (p. 18).

Among all human rights, freedom is one of the most universally acclaimed. It is both legitimate and helpful to construe mental health as an element of human freedom – freedom from the distressing and disabling effects of mental disorders. An implication of this view is that the provision of mental health services is a matter of liberating people from their lack or loss of the freedom to be healthy. A corollary is that inequalities in access to the mental health system constitute a form of oppression – the denial of the freedom of weaker members of society by those who hold power within and over the system (Campbell, 1995).

By construing mental health as an element of freedom, the failure of the United States health care system to include all Americans can be considered a violation of the constitutional right to liberty. Moreover, with an estimated 18,000 Americans dying each year due to lack of insurance coverage (IOM report, as cited by Ault, 2004), Americans' constitutional right to life is being violated. Finally, the unnecessary suffering of the 60 percent of people with untreated mental disorders is a violation of their constitutional right to pursue happiness. All three rights are affirmed by the U. S. Constitution: the right to "life, liberty, and the pursuit of happiness."

In a constitutional democracy, or for that matter, a constitutional monarchy with parliamentary rule, one way to effect fundamental change is through amendments to the constitution and bill of rights. That is not the easiest path to reform, but it is a viable path, since basic human and civil rights, which are constitutionally guaranteed, provide citizens the opportunity for redress through their judicial system on constitutional and legal grounds. Unfortunately, there appears to be no government agency or even private advocacy group, such as the American Civil Liberties Union, which presses this constitutional case as grounds for social justice in the American health care system. Since the United States is a member of the United Nations, perhaps the U. N. Commission on Human Rights could apply pressure based on the U. N. Declaration of Human Rights and other documents cited previously. Yamin (2005) cited numerous international declarations, treaties, and covenants that reflect consensual norms that serve as a basis of appeal under international law for the right to health and health care, including mental health care. "The framework that international human rights offers with respect to health shifts the analysis of issues such as disparities in treatment in the United States from questions of quality of care to fundamental matters of democracy and social justice, as well as suggesting avenues for accountability" (Yamin, 2005, p. 1156).

There is a relentless logic expressed in the U. S. Constitution. It claims that the state exists for the sake of the people, and that the privilege of life under its domain is equitable and universal. Democratic values are affirmed "in the name of the people" (Roemer, 1988). That is also a vision for a democratic and just mental health system. A good and fair mental health system will finance, organize, and deliver high quality affordable health care in the name of the people – ". . . of the people, by the people, and for the people."

A value consensus will be required for Americans to affirm a national policy of universal access to affordable health care of optimal quality for both physical and mental disorders. Lacking that consensus and the vision that a comprehensive mental health policy can provide, it seems very likely that the problem of the uninsured and underinsured in America will remain and only worsen. It has been worsening for uninsured people with mental disorders, especially for the severely and persistently mentally ill who have become homeless or incarcerated in jails and prisons. And so their suffering continues. Americans have much to learn from other countries about achieving justice in health care. There is also a great deal to be learned from our fellow Americans involved in current social movements to reform our health care system.

Reforming the American System

Depending upon one's diagnosis and theory of the etiology of the systemic disorder of unmet need in the health care sector, various remedies have been proposed. Examples of recommendations relying primarily upon *private* sector reforms are (a) health savings accounts (promoted by the Bush Administration and justified by the moral hazard theory), (b) tax deductions for premiums paid by individuals comparable to deductions received by employers for health insurance costs, and (c) encouraging competition among health plans. Attempts have been made by employers and health plans to reduce their costs by reducing the demand for services through (d) cost-shifting mechanisms such as a higher share in premiums, co-insurance, co-payments, and higher deductibles for selected conditions.

With some success over a five-year period ending in the last decade, specialized managed behavioral health organizations (MBHOs) have experimented with prior and current utilization reviews, and more recently, case management strategies with high-cost users to contain the costs to the employers who purchase their management services. Unfortunately, employers' concerns about the quality of those behavioral health services have been secondary to their cost, and the return of high and rising premiums is one major reason that about 40 percent of all employers offer no health insurance plans. Since the year 2000, premiums paid by employers increased by 73 percent, at an average of 12.4 percent per year (Gabel et al., 2005, pp. 1275–1277). It appears that turning over the financing and management of the delivery of mental health services to for-profit corporations, and the conversion of not-for-profit health plans and hospitals to for-profit organizations under the mantle of managed competition is not a cost-effective strategy in America (Hall and Conover, 2003) anymore than it was in Britain's experiment with managed competition (Light, 1995, 1997). In fact, most American employers who pay for health insurance have not adopted managed competition as the primary method of cost-containment (Maxwell and Temin, 2002).

Since the Clinton proposal to provide universal access to America's health care system failed in 1993, the approach to health care reform in the *public sector* has been in incremental steps despite evidence for decades that a growing number of Americans see the need for major reforms (e.g., Blendon et al., 1990; Citizens Health Care Working Group, 2005; Coalition for a National Health Program, 2005; Healthcare-Now, 2005; MHDI, 1995, 1997; Newman, 1988; UHCAN, 2005a, 2005b, 2005c; *U.S. News and World Report*, March 9, 1998, p. 48), including many health care professionals (Benedict and Phelps, 1998; Murphy, DeBernado, and Shoemaker, 1998; PNHP, 2005; Rothbaum et al. 1998; Sleek, 1998; *Star Tribune*, December 7, 1997; Tucker and Lubin, 1994;). Moreover, "... taken as an overall strategy, there is little evidence that incremental reform has improved U. S. health care" (Fuchs and Emanuel, 2005, p. 1408).

There have been occasional efforts to effect major reform of the American health care system. A national health insurance plan to ensure universal access to affordable health care was proposed about six times in the past century – during the First World War, during the Depression, during the Truman and Johnson Administrations, in the Senate in the 1970s, and during the Clinton Administration in 1994. Each time the efforts have been defeated by powerful lobbying from groups with economic self-interest in maintaining the status quo.

> A common goal of all comprehensive reform proposals is universal coverage, providing every American with health insurance. The proposals differ in how extensive the change from the current system would be, how providers of care would be reimbursed and how money would be raised to fund the system. (Fuchs and Emanuel, 2005, p. 1404)

Comprehensive reforms have been proposed at the federal level, such as a constitutional amendment to make equal access to optimal health care a civil right. In the United States, a constitutional amendment would require confirmation by two-thirds of the states. An alternative is to pass federal legislation with national service frameworks as Britain has done to authorize universal access to its National Health Service. For several years there has been a growing movement for federal legislation to establish a national health insurance system in the United States, which would publicly finance health care services delivered in both the public and private sectors (e.g., UHCAN, 2005a). This author favors it, though with serious reservations about the control of a health care system by a Congress presently beholden to special interests.

An interim strategy might be to legislate federal standards and utilize existing and increased block grants to the states contingent upon their implementation of the standards, modeled after the U. S. Medicaid program. While that strategy might overcome the current and persistent Congressional gridlock over health care reform, it would also result in a wide range of state programs with disparities in access to appropriate mental health services. The latter problem persists in America's Medicaid program administered by the states, in Canada's program administered by the Provinces, and similar disparities among county administered programs led Norway to centralize the mental health services. Nevertheless, successful reforms at the state level to achieve universal access may become the foundation for later federal reform. The Canadian national health insurance program began in a single province.

There is a current initiative in the U.S. Congress (House File 676) to establish a national health insurance program called "Medicare for All." The Congressional Budget Office concluded in a 1991 report that ". . . a single-payer system – that is, an improved Medicare for All program – would save approximately $100 billion per year. Economists estimate that this $100 billion could provide coverage for all of the uninsured and substantially help the underinsured" (as cited by Congers, 2003).

A current barrier to covering the uninsured in America is the projected costs of covering the elderly who will qualify for the federal Medicare insurance program in the coming decades. With the new drug benefit added to Medicare in 2006, the predicted costs of this federal insurance program will consume 3.3 percent of the U. S. GDP and 7.5 percent by 2035. The major factors contributing to the escalating expenditures are (a) the rapid increase in Medicare enrollees 65+ years of age from 36 million to 77 million by 2011; (b) the open-ended entitlement that ignores the cost/benefit ratios of medical technologies; (c) reimbursement of physicians by fee-for-service, which encourages medically *un*necessary treatment (Fuchs and Emanuel, 2005). A fourth major factor is price inflation of prescription drugs. The Medicare Board of Trustees predicted recently that the Medicare Hospital Insurance Trust Fund (Medicare Part A) would be depleted by 2019. "Short of massive increases in taxes or a slowdown in spending growth, Medicare is headed for financial failure" (as cited by Fuchs and Emanuel, 2005, p. 1401).

Long-term forecasting of health care expenditures is fraught with uncertainties, as illustrated by the high-medium-low scenarios in traditional accounting projections of Medicare costs. Utilizing an alternative, stochastic time series model, which accounts for fertility and mortality rates, and per capita health spending in the United States, Lee and Miller (2002) predicted that Medicare expenditures in 2002 amounting to 2.2 percent of the GDP will rise to eight percent of GDP by 2075, due equally to both population aging and to increased spending per beneficiary. The expected shortfall in federal funding for Medicare Parts A & B over the next 75 years is about twice as large as the projected imbalance in the Social Security system, which has been the focus of the current Bush Administration. To fund the projected expenditures for Medicare alone, the mandatory payroll taxes would have to be raised by four percent beginning 2002 (Lee and Miller, 2002, p. 1384). The authors grant that "many forces will influence the future trajectory of health expenditures in the twenty-first century: new medical technologies, policies regarding access to care, the costs of services, the health status of the population, population aging, and the growth of the economy" (p. 1366).

Despite the vagaries of long-term predictions of the costs of expanding "Medicare for All," as of August 2005, 51 U. S. Representatives had become co-sponsors of this bill. Including this one, there were about 50 bills before the 2005 Congress related to health care, with several addressing issues of access, quality, cost, and patient rights. It remains to be seen whether the national steering committee for the federal bill expanding Medicare (House File 676) will mobilize sufficient grass roots support of frustrated and/or angry citizens to overcome the resistance of the health care industry. As of August, 2005, among health care professionals, the Physicians for a National Health Plan had endorsed the current federal bill.

Endorsement from providers does not equate with a political movement required to pass legislation. Based on his interview with Donald Berwick, President of the Institute for Healthcare Improvement in Boston, Galvin (2005) wrote: "A leading champion of health care quality sees the slow pace of improvement in the American health care system as evidence of a failure of provider leadership and concludes that external pressure will be necessary to move the system toward meaningful change" (p. W5–1). The wider community of citizens is potentially the most potent source of external pressure for change. Ensuring that members of the community have the opportunity for input in the development and evaluation of public health policies and programs is also one of the principles of ethical practice endorsed by the American Public Health Association (2005). A second principle is to obtain the community's consent for the implementation of public health policies and programs.

A landmark federal bill (PL 108–173) was passed by Congress in 2003. Section 1014 of that law established a Citizens' Health Care Working Group (2005) to engage in a nationwide public dialogue about improving the health care system in order to provide every American with the ability to obtain quality, affordable health care coverage. The citizens' group was charged with addressing four major questions: (a) what health care benefits and services should be provided? (b) how does the American public want health care delivered? (c) how should health care coverage be financed? (d) what trade-offs are the American public willing to make in either benefits or financing to ensure access to affordable, high-quality health care coverage and services? Following extensive community meetings to address these questions, interim recommendations will be developed and circulated to the public for comment in the Spring of 2006. A final set of recommendations will be submitted to the President, and then to Congress for hearings. The foundation for dialogue is *The Health Report to the American People*, available at http://www.citizenshealthcare.gov.

Another national mental health advocacy coalition, which has articulated principles and recommendations for mental health reform, is the Campaign for Mental Health Reform (CMHR, 2005). Composed of 16 national organizations, including the American Psychiatric Association and the American Psychological Association, the CMHR (2005a) issued a July 2005 report entitled, *Emergency Response: A Roadmap for Federal Action on America's Mental Health Crisis*. The report outlined seven action steps to fulfill the aims the President's New Freedom Commission on Mental Health (2003). The seven steps are:

1. Maximize the effectiveness of scarce resources by coordinating programs and making systems "seamless" to consumers.
2. Stop making criminals of those whose mental illness results in inappropriate behavior.
3. Make Medicaid accountable for the effectiveness of the mental health services it pays for.
4. Prevent the negative consequences of mental disorders by getting the right services to the right people at the right time.
5. Invest in children and support and value their families' role in making treatment decisions.
6. Promote independence by increasing employment, eliminating disincentives for economic self-sufficiency and ending homelessness.
7. Address the mental health needs of returning veterans and their families.

The CMHR published this call for immediate federal action partly in response to the Administration's federal budget for FY2006, which seems to ignore the findings and recommendations of the report released July 2003 by the President's New Freedom Commission on Mental Health, and due to ". . . the disregard [the budget] shows for the urgent need to address unmet mental health needs in America. . ." (CMHR, 2005b).

Citizens in several states have proposed a number of strategies to achieve affordable health care for all of their own state residents. Examples include a state initiative in Oregon to establish a publicly financed, *single payer system*. The proposal failed in a 2003 ballot, due in part to the $1.3 million spent on television ads and direct mailings by opposing insurance and hospital holding companies (HCA-O, 2005). Fund-raising has begun to place the measure on the 2008 ballot in Oregon. A similar proposal was introduced in the 84th legislative session in Minnesota in January 2005 (House File 481), and California has a bill for a single payer system (Senate File 40) as well as New Mexico (Health Security for New Mexico). *Mixed public/private expansion proposals* are illustrated by the Dirigo Health Plan passed June 2003 by the state of Maine. The New York City Health Security Act of August 17, 2005 proposed an *employer mandated* health insurance system. Some *state constitutional amendments* have been proposed to establish health care as a right for all residents (e.g., the Massachusetts Health Care Constitutional Amendment). There are proposals to study financing universal health care (New Jersey Health Access Study Commission), and other public education and task forces. A listing of state and local organizations advocating for health care justice is available from UHCAN (2005d) at http://www.uhcan.org/files/states/statelinks.html.

As a strategy to attain universal health insurance for all Americans, Bodenheimer (2003) proposed public discussion to find common ground by focusing first on the goals of a new health care system, and secondly on the gap between the goals and present reality. The goals inform principles which function as criteria by which to evaluate proposals for the means to achieving the goals. Bodenheimer (2003) proposed five principles to achieve five goals of (a) universal access (b) to high quality care, (c) provided equally, (d) at reasonable cost, (e) by friendly caregivers. Sigerist (2003) added the goals of prevention, comprehensive coverage, and salaried physicians in lieu of both fee-for-service and capitation methods of payment. These and other goals, along with the previously mentioned reform initiatives reflect the growing awareness of the continued unmet needs of Americans for health care, including mental health care. Health services research, as illustrated by the present volume, helps to identify the treatment gap, and provides some creative ways of closing it. Awakening the nation's conscience will be required to implement the changes needed.

REFERENCES

Abrams, H. K. (2001). A short history of occupational health. *Journal of Public Health Policy, 22*(1), 34–80.

Abrams, H. K. (2005). Linking health to social justice. *American Journal of Public Health, 95*(7), 1090.

Agency of Healthcare Research and Quality (AHRQ) (2005, October). AHRQ awards over $22 million in health information technology implementation grants. *Research Activities, 302,* 2–3. Silver Springs, Maryland: Author. (AHRQ Pub. No. 05-0107).

American Psychiatric Association (2003). *Evidence-based practices in mental health care.* Arlington, VA: American Psychiatric Publishing, Inc.

American Psychiatric Association (2004). *American Psychiatric Association practice guidelines for the treatment of psychiatric disorders: Compendium 2004.* Arlington, VA: American Psychiatric Publishing, Inc.

American Psychiatric Association (2006). *Improving mental healthcare: A guide to measurement-based quality.* Arlington, VA: American Psychiatric Publishing, Inc.

American Psychiatric Association (1998). *Outcomes assessment in mental health treatment: A Compendium of articles from psychiatric services.* Arlington, VA: American Psychiatric Publishing, Inc.

American Psychological Association (APA, 1986). *Guidelines for computer-based tests and interpretations.* Washington, D.C.: Author.

American Psychological Association (APA, 2003). *Guidelines for psychological practice with older adults.* Washington, D.C.: Author.

American Psychological Association, Committee on Professional Standards (APA, 1981). *Specialty guidelines for the delivery of services.* Washington, D.C.: The American Psychological Association.

American Psychological Association Committee on Professional Standards (APA, 1987). *Specialty guidelines for the delivery of services by clinical psychologists.* Washington, DC: Author.

American Psychological Association Committee on Professional Practice and Standards (APA, 1998). *Guidelines for psychological evaluations in child protection matters.* Washington, D.C.: American Psychological Association.

American Psychological Association Task Force on Psychological Intervention Guidelines (APA) (1995). *Template for developing guidelines: Interventions with mental disorders and psychological aspects of physical disorders.* Washington, DC: Author.

Arcury, T. A., Gesler, W. M., Preisser, J. S., Sherman, J., Spencer, J., & Perin, J. (2005). The effects of geography and spatial behavior on health care utilization among the residents in a rural region. *Health Services Research, 40*(1), 135–155.

Asada, Y (2005, August). A framework for measuring health inequity. *Journal of Epidemiology and Community Health, 59,* 700–705.

Ault, A. (2004). IOM calls for universal health coverage by 2010. *The Lancet, 363,* January 24, p. 300.

Balfe, B., Boyle, J., Brocki, S., & Lane, K. (1985). A health policy agenda for the American People: Phase I: The principles. *Journal of the American Medical Association, 254* (17), 2440–2448.

Barofsky, I. (2003). Patients' rights, quality of life, and health care system performance. *Quality of Life Research, 12,* 473–484.

Barry, C., Gable, J., Frank, R., Hawkins, S., Whitmore, H., & Pickreign, J. (2003). Design of mental health benefits: Still unequal after all these years. *Health Affairs, 22*(5), 127–137.

Bass, L. et al. (1996). Guidelines for the practice of psychology: An annotated bibliography. *Professional conduct and discipline in psychology.* Washington, D. C.: American Psychological Association.

Basu, J. (2005). Severity of illness, race, and choice of local versus distance hospitals among the elderly. *Journal of Health Care for the Poor and Underserved, 16,* 391–405.

Benedict, J., & Phelps, R. (1998). Introduction: Psychology's view of managed care. *Professional Psychology: Research and Practice, 29*(1), 29–30.

Bodenheimer, T. (2003). The movement for universal health insurance: Finding common ground. *American Journal of Public Health, 93*(1), 112–115.

Bonomi, A. E., Wagner, E. H., Glasgow, R. E., & VonKorff, M. (2002). Assessment of chronic illness care (ACIC): A practical tool to measure quality improvement. *Health Services Research, 37*(3), 791–820.

Bortz, W. M. (2005). Biological basis of determinants of health. *American Journal of Public Health, 95*(3), 389–392.

Boyle, J. (1987). Health policy agenda for the American people. *Journal of the American Medical Association, 257,* 1199–1210.

Braverman, P. A., Egeter, S. A., Cubbin, C., & Marchi, K. S. (2004). An approach to studying social disparities in health and health care. *American Journal of Public Health, 94*(12), 2139–2148.

Brown, L. D. (2003). Comparing health systems in four countries: Lessons for the United States. *American Journal of Public Health, 93*(1), 52–56.

Bruce, S., & Paxton, R. (2002). Ethical principles for evaluating mental health services: A critical examination. *Journal of Mental Health, 11*(3), 267–279.

Brundtland, Gro H. (2001, Oct.). Message from the Director-General. *The World Health Report 2001. Mental Health: New Understanding, New Hope.* Geneva: World Health Organization, (ix–x).

Bureau of Primary Health Care (2001). *User Manual: Uniform Data System.* Bethesda, MD: Author.

Bureau of Primary Health Care (2004). *Uniform Data Set (UDS Data).* Retrieved on October 10, 2005 from http://bphc,hrsa.gov/uds/data.htm

Callaway, M. E., & Hall, J. (2000). Distributive justice in Medicaid capitation: The evidence from Colorado. *The Journal of Behavioral Health Services & Research, 27*(1), February, 87–97.

Campaign for Mental Health Reform (CMHR, 2005a). *Emergency Response: A Roadmap for Federal Action on America's Mental Health Crisis*. Retrieved November 11, 2005 from http://www.mhreform.org/

Campaign for Mental Health Reform (CMHR, 2005b). *Budget Brings More Broken Promises*. Retrieved November 11, 2005 from http://www.mhreform.org/news/2-8-05budget.htm

Campbell, A. (1995). *Health as liberation: Medicine, theology, and the quest for justice*. Cleveland, Ohio: The Pilgrim Press.

Casas-Zamora, J. A., & Ibrahim, S. A. (2005). Confronting health inequity: The global dimension. *American Journal of Public Health, 94*(12), 2055-2058.

Churchill, L. R. (1995). *Self-interest and universal health care*. Boston: Harvard University Press. (Cited in *Pediatrics*, June 96, Part 1 of 2, 97(6), p. 895.)

Citizens Health Care Working Group (2005). *The Health Report to the American People*. Retrieved November 11, 2005 from http://www.citizenshealthcare.gov/

Coalition for a National Health Program (2005). *The United States National Health Insurance Act* (HR676). Retrieved September 28, 2005 from http://www.cnhp.us/

Committee on Ethical guidelines for Forensic Psychologists (CFP, 1991). Specialty guidelines for forensic psychologists. *Law and Human Behavior, 15*(6), 655-665.

Congers, Rep. John (2003). A fresh approach to health care in the United States: Improved and extended Medicare for all. *American Journal of Public Health, 93*(2), 193.

Consumer Reports (August, 1996). *How good is your health plan?* Author, pp. 28-41.

Council of Europe (1950, 1966). *The European Convention on Human Rights, and its Five protocols*. Strasbourg: Author. Retrieved September 27, 2005 from http://www.hri.org/docs/ECHR50.html

Crombie, I. K. (2003). *Research in health care: Design, conduct and inequity in the distribution of disease*. Indianapolis, IN: Jossey-Bass, an imprint of Wiley.

Dalgard, O.S., Kringlen, E., & Dahl, A. (2002). Psykiatrisk epidemiologi. (Psychiatric epidemiology). *Norsk Epidemiologi, 12*(3), 161-162.

Deber, R. B. (2003). Healthcare reform: Lessons from Canada. *American Journal of Public Health, 93*(1), 20-24.

DHHS (1999). Department of Health and Human Services. *Mental health: A report of the Surgeon General – Executive summary*. Rockville, Md.: U.S. Department of Health and Human Services, Substance Abuse and Mental Health Services Administration, Center for Mental Health Services, National Institutes of Health, National Institute of Mental Health.

DHHS (2003). New Freedom Commission on Mental Health. *Achieving the promise: Transforming mental health care in America. Final report*. Rockville, Md.: Department of Health and Human Services. Publication SMA-03-3832.

Diamont, A. L., Hays, R. D., Morales, L. S., Ford, W., Calmes, D., Asch, S. et al. (2004). Delays and unmet need for health care among adult primary care patients in a restructured urban public health system. *American Journal of Public Health, 94*(5), 783-789.

Edlund, M. J., Young, A. S., Kung, F. Y., Sherbourne, C. D., & Wells, K. B. (2003). Does satisfaction reflect the technical quality of mental health care? *Health Services Research, 38*(2), 631-645.

Eisenberg, L. (1999). Where is the voice of the faculty? Talk given before the American Association of University Professors, May 22, 1999. Cited in *Pediatrics*, Nov. 99, Part 1 of 2, *104*(5), p. 1094.

Enthoven, A. (1993). The history and principles of managed competition. *Health Affairs (Supplement), 12*, 24-48.

Evans, T., Whitehead, M., Diderichsen, F., Bhuiya, A., & Wirth, A. (2001). *Challenging inequities in health: From ethics to action*. New York, New York: Oxford University Press.

Feldman, M. A. (1998). Health care policy evaluation: A conceptual model using medical ethics. *Journal of Health and Human Service Administration, 21*, 181-198.

Fein, O. (2003). Rekindling reform: Principles and goals. *American Journal of Public Health, 93*(1), 115-117.

Ferrie, J. E., Shipley, M. J., Newman, K., et al. (2005, April). Self-reported job insecurity and health in the Whitehall II study: Potential explanations of the relationship. *Social Science and Medicine, 60*, 1593-1602.

Fortney, J., Sullivan, G., Williams, K., Jackson, C., Morton, S., & Koegel, P. (2003). Measuring continuity of care for clients of public mental health systems. *Health Services Research, 38*(4), 1157-1175.

Frankena, Wm. (1973). *Ethics* (2nd ed.). Upper Saddle River, New Jersey: Prentice-Hall.

Freeman, M., Pathara, S., Drew, N., & Funk, M. (2005). *WHO resource book on mental health, human rights, and legislation*. Geneva: World Health Organization.

Friedman, P. D., Lemon, S. C., Stein, M. D., & D'Aunno, T. A. (2003). Accessibility of addiction treatment: Results from a national survey of outpatient substance abuse treatment organizations. *Health Services Research, 38*(3), 887-903.

Fuchs, V. R., & Emanuel, E. J. (2005). Health care reform: Why? What? When? *Health Affairs, 24*(6), 1399-1414.

Gabel, J., Claxton, G., Gil, I., Pickreign, J., Whitmore, H., Finder, B., Hawkins, S., & Rowland, D. (2005). Health benefits in 2005: Premium increases slow down, coverage continues to erode. *Health Affairs, 24*(5), 1273-1280.

Gabel, J., Claxton, G., Holve, E., Pickreign, J., Whitmore, H., Dhont, K., Hawkins, S., & Rowland, D. (2003). Health benefits in 2003: Premiums reach thirteen-year high as employers adopt new forms of cost sharing. *Health Affairs, 22*(5), 117-126.

Galvin, R. (2005). A deficiency of will and ambition: A conversation with Donald Berwick. *Web Exclusives: A Supplement to Health Affairs, 24*, Supplement 1, January-June, W5-1 to W5-9.

Gaskin, D. J., & Mitchell, J. M. (2005). Health status and access to care for children with special health care needs. *Journal of Mental Health Policy and Economics, 8*, 29-35.

Gilmer, T., & Kronick, R. (2001). Calm before the storm: Expected increase in the number of uninsured Americans, *Health Affairs, 20*(6), 207-210.

Gilmer, T., & Kronick, R. (2005). It's the premiums, stupid: Projections of the uninsured through 2013. *Web Exclusives: A Supplement to Health Affairs, vol. 24, Supplement 1,* January–June, W5-143- W5-151.

Gladwell, M. (2005). The moral-hazard myth: The bad idea behind our failed health-care system. *The New Yorker.* New York, pp. 44–49. Available at www.newyorker.com.

Grob, G. N. (2005). Public policy and mental illness: Jimmy Carter's Presidential Commission on Mental Health. *The Milbank Quarterly, 83*(3), 425–456.

Gruskin, S. (2004). What are health and human rights? *Lancet, vol. 363,* January 24, p. 329.

Gulbinat, W., Manderscheid, R., Baingana, F., et al. (2004). The international consortium on mental health policy and services: Objectives, design, and project implementation. *International Review of Psychiatry, 16*(1–2), 5–17.

Hall, M. A., Camacho, F., Dugan, E., & Balkrishnan, R. (2002). Trust in the medical profession: Conceptual and measurement issues. *Health Services Research, 37*(5), 1419–1439.

Hall, M. A., & Conover, C. J. (2003). The impact of blue cross conversions on accessibility, affordability, and the public interest. *The Milbank Quarterly, 81*(4), 509–542.

Harris, K. M., & Edlund, M. J. (2005). Self-medication of mental health problems: New evidence from a national survey. *Health Services Research, 40*(1), 117–134.

Hart, S. N. (1982). The history of children's psychological rights. *Viewpoints in Teaching and Learning, 58,* 1–15.

Hartley, H., Seccombe, K., & Hoffman, K. (2005, August). Planning for and securing health insurance in the context of welfare reform. *Journal of Health Care for the Poor and Underserved, 16,* 536–554.

Health Canada (2002). *Report on Mental Illnesses in Canada.* Ottawa, Canada.

Health Care for All-Oregon (HCA-O) (2005). Retrieved September 28, 2005 from http://www.healthcare-now.org/

Healthcare – NOW (2005). *Health care for all people is all-American.* Retrieved September 28, 2005 from http://www.healthcare-now.org/

Henderson, S., & Whiteford, H. (2003). Social capital and mental health. *The Lancet, 362,* 505–506.

Howard, K., Kopta, S., Krause, M., & Orlinsky, D. (1986). The dose-effect relationship in psychotherapy. *American Psychologist, 41,* 159–164.

Hurst, J., & Siciliani, I. (2003, July 7). *Tackling excessive waiting times for elective surgery: A comparison of policies in twelve OECD countries.* OECD Health Working Paper. Paris: Organization for Economic Cooperation and Development.

Hyder, A. (2004). The standard of care debate: Conceptual clarifications. *American Journal of Public Health, 94*(12), 2048.

Improving Chronic Illness Care (ICID) (2003). *Model Components: Overview of the Chronic Care Model.* Retrieved October 27, 2005 from http://www.improvingchroniccare.org/change/model/components.html

Insel, T. R., & Fenton, W. S. (2005). Psychiatric Epidemiology: It's not just about counting anymore. *Archives of General Psychiatry, 62,* 590–592.

Institute of Medicine (IOM) (2001). *Neurological, psychiatric and developmental disorders: Meeting the challenge in the developing world.* Washington, DC: National Academy Press.

Institute of Medicine Committee on Assuring the Health of the Public in the 21st Century. (IOM, 2002). Washington DC: The National Academies Press.

Jenkins, R., Gulbinat, W., Manderscheid, R., et al. (2004). The mental health country profile: Background, design and use of a systematic method of appraisal. *International Review of Psychiatry, 16*(1–2), 31–47.

Kangas, E. E. (1997). Self-interest and the common good: The impact of norms, selfishness and context in social policy opinions. *Journal of Socio-Economics, 26*(5), 475–495.

Kennedy, Sen. Edward (2003). Quality, affordable health care for all Americans. *American Journal of Public Health, 93*(1), 14.

Kessler, R. C., Berglund, P., Demler, O., Jin, R., Walters, E. (2005a). Lifetime prevalence and age-of-onset distributions of DSM-IV disorders in the national comorbidity survey replication. *Archives of General Psychiatry, 62,* 593–602.

Kessler, R. C. Chiu W. T., Demler, O., Walters, E. (2005b). Prevalence, severity, and comorbidity of 12-month DSM-IV disorders in the national comorbidity survey replication. *Archives of General Psychiatry, 62,* 617–627.

Kiplinger, K. A. (2005, Fall). *Kiplinger's retirement planning.* Washington D.C.: The Kiplinger Washington Editors Inc.

Kiresuk, T., Smith, A., & Cardillo, J. (1994). *Goal attainment scaling: Application, theory, and measurement.* Hillsdale, NJ: Lawrence Erlbaum.

Klein, R. (2003). Lessons for (and from) America. *American Journal of Public Health 93*(1), 61–63.

Kohn, L. T., Corrigan, J. M., Donaldson, M. S. (Eds.) (2000). *To err is human: Building a safer health system.* Washington, D. C.: Institute of Medicine.

Kopta, S., Howard, K., Lowry, J., & Beutler, L. (1992, June). *The psychotherapy dosage model and clinical significance: Estimating how much is enough for psychological symptoms.* Paper presented at the Society for Psychotherapy. Berkeley, CA.

Kopta, S., Howard, K., Lowry, J., & Beutler, L. (1994). Patterns of symptomatic recovery in psychotherapy. *Journal of Consulting and Clinical Psychology, 62,* 1009–1016.

Koyanagi, C., Burmin, I., Bevilgcqua, J., et al. (1997, March). *Defining medically necessary services to protect plan members.* Washington, D.C.: Bazelon Center for Mental Health Law.

Krieger, N., Chen, J., Waterman, P., Rehkopf, D., & Subramanian, S. (2005). Painting a truer picture of US socioeconomic and racial/ethnic health inequalities: The public health disparities geocoding project. *American Journal of Public Health, 95*(2), 312–323.

Kronick, R., & Gilmer, T. (1999). Explaining the decline in health insurance coverage, 1979–1995. *Health Affairs, 18*(2), 30–47.

Kuder, A., & Kuntz, M. (1966). Who decides what is medically necessary? In A. Lazarus (Ed.). *Controversies in managed mental health care.* Washington, D.C.: American Psychiatric Press (pp. 159-177).

Labacqz, K. (1987). *Six theories of justice: Perspectives from philosophical and theological ethics.* Minneapolis: Augsburg Fortress Press.

Laditka, J. N., Laditka, S. B., & Probst, J. C. (2005). More may be better: Evidence of a negative relationship between physician supply and hospitalization for ambulatory care sensitive conditions. *Health Services Research, 40*(4), 1148–1166.

Lavery, S. H., Smith, M. L., Esparza, A. A., Hruslow, A., Moore, M., & Reed, D. F. (2005). The community action model: A community driven model designed to address disparities in health. *American Journal of Public Health, 95*(4), 611–616.

Lee, R., & Miller, T. (2002). An approach to forecasting health expenditures, with application to the U. S. Medicare system. *Health Services Research, 37*(5), 1365–1386.

Light, D. W. (1995). Homo Economicus: Escaping the traps of managed competition. *European Journal of Public Health, 5*, 145–154.

Light, D. W. (1997). From managed competition to managed cooperation: Theory and lessons from the British experience. *Milbank Quarterly, 75*, 297–341.

Light, D. W. (2000). The sociological character of markets in health care. In G. L. Albrecht, R. Fitzpatrick, & S. C. Scrinshaw (Eds.). *Handbook of social studies in health and medicine* (pp. 394-408) England: Sage.

Light, D. W. (2003). Universal healthcare: Lessons from the British experience. *American Journal of Public Health, 93*(1), 25–30.

Light, R. C., LoSasso, A. T., & Lurie, I. Z. (2005). The effect of expanded mental health benefits on treatment initiation and specialist utilization. *Health Services Research, 40*(4), 1092–1107.

Litaker, D., Koroukian, S. M., & Love, T. E. (2005, June). Context and healthcare access: Looking beyond the individual. *Medical Care, 43*(6), 531–540.

Litaker, D., & Love, T. E. (2005). Health care resource allocation and individuals' health care needs: Examining the degree of fit. *Health Policy, 73*, 183–193.

Maciuko, J., Starfield, B., & Shi, L. (2003). The contribution of primary care systems to health outcomes within Organization for Economic Cooperation and Development (OECD) countries, 1970–1998. *Health Services Research, 38*(3), 831–865.

Malm, U., Jacobsson, L. Larsson, N. O. (2003). Values, system, and evidence for a reform in progress. *International Journal of Mental Health, 31*(4), Winter, 2002-3, 50–65.

Mark, T. L., Coffey, R. M., Vandivort-Warren, R., Harwood, H. J., King, E. C., & the MHSA Spending Estimates Team (2005). U.S. spending for mental health and substance abuse treatment, 1991-2001. *Web Exclusives: A Supplement to Health Affairs, Vol. 24, Supplement 1,* January–June, W5-133 – W5-142.

Marshall, M., Hogg, L. L., Gath, D. H., & Lockwood, A. (1995). The cardinal needs schedule - modified version of the MRC needs for care assessment schedule. *Psychological Medicine, 25*, 605–617.

Maxwell, J., & Temin, P. (2002). Managed competition versus industrial purchasing of health care among the Fortune 500. *Journal of Health Politics, Policy, and Law, 27*(1), 5–30.

Mazor, K. M., Clauser, B. E., Field, T., Yood, R. A., & Gurwitz, J. H. (2002). A demonstration of the impact of response bias on the results of patient satisfaction surveys. *Health Services Research, 37*(5), 1403–1417.

Mechanic, D. (2003). Is the prevalence of mental disorders a good measure of the need for services? *Health Affairs, 22*(5), 8–20.

Meehan, S. (2005). Health services research: Critical measurement issues. *Health Services Research, 40*(5), Part II, 1571–1572.

Miller, I. (1966a). Time-limited brief therapy has gone too far: The result is invisible rationing. *Professional Psychology: Research and Practice, 27*(6), 567–576.

Minnesota Health Data Institute (MHDI)(1997, October). *1997 Medicaid and Minnesota Care Managed Care Member Satisfaction Survey: Summary Report of Aggregate and Plan-Specific Comparisons.* Minneapolis, MN: Author.

Minnesota Health Data Institute (MHDI) (1995, December). *Evaluation Report.* Minneapolis, MN: Author.

Mohr, P. (1998). Medical necessity: A moving target. *Psychiatric Services, 49*(11), 1391.

Mojtabai, R., & Zivin, J. G. (2003). Effectiveness and cost-effectiveness of four treatment modalities for substance disorders: A propensity score analysis. *Health Services Research, 38*(1), Part I, 233–259.

Mollborn, S., Stepanikova, I., & Cook, K. S. (2005). Delayed care and unmet needs among health care system users: When does fiduciary trust in a physician matter? *Health Services Research, 40*(6), Part I, 1898–1917.

Morgan, R. O., Teal, C. T., Reddy, S. G., Ford, M. E., & Ashton, C. M. (2005). Measurement in Veterans Affairs health services research: Veterans as a special population. *Health Services Research, 40*(5), Part II, 1573–1583.

Murphy, M., DeBernado, C., & Shoemaker, W. (1998). Impact of managed care on independent practice and professional ethics: A survey of independent practitioners. *Professional Psychology: Research and Practice, 29*(1), 43–51.

National Alliance for the Mentally Ill (NAMI) (2005). *About NAMI.* Retrieved October 3, 2005 from http://www.nami.org/template.cfm?Section=About_Nami

National Information Center on Health Services Research and Health Care Technology (NICHSR) (2005). *NICHSR mission.* Retrieved October 19, 2005 from http://www.nlm.nih.gov/nichsr/nichsr.html

National Primary and Care Trust Development Programme (2005). *The Commissioning friend for mental health services: A resource guide for health and social care commissioners.* London: National Institute for Mental Health.

Neumann, P. J., Rosen, A. B., Greenberg, D., et al. (2005). Can we better prioritize resources for cost-utility research? *Medical Decision Making, 25*, 429–436.

Newman, R. (1998, Sept./Oct.). Public opinion of managed care has switched radically in recent years. *The National Psychologist, 7*(5), 1 & 3.

Newman, P. J. (2005, July). The arrival of economic evidence in managed care formulary decisions: The unsolicited request process. *Medical Care, 43*(7S), II-27–II-32.

Nuwayhid, I. A. (2004). Occupation health research in developing countries: A partner for social justice. *American Journal of Public Health, 94*, 1916-1921.

Oberlander, J. (2005). *The Politics of Health Reform: Why Do Bad Things Happen to Good Plans?* Retrieved September 28, 2005 from http://www.healthaffairsorg/Web Exclusive/2206Oberlander.pdf

OECD Factbook 2005. National Accounts of OECD Countries, Vol. 1, p. 265). Retrieved July 19, 2005 from http://www.oecd.org/dataoecd/48/5/34244925.xls. Text citation is OECD (2005).

Ogles, B., Lambert, M., & Masters, K. (1996). *Assessing outcome in clinical practice.* Boston: Allyn and Bacon.

Ohsfeldt, R. L., Morrisey, M.A., Nelson, L., & Johnson, V. (1998). The spread of state "any willing provider" laws. *Health Services Research, 33*, 1537–1562.

Olson, R. P. (1997). *Manual for setting, scaling, and rating assessment and therapy practicum goals.* Minneapolis: Author.

Olson, R. P. (1999). *A critique of Minnesota's managed mental health care with special reference to medical necessity determinations for outpatient psychotherapy: A resource document.* Minneapolis: Author.

Olson, R. P. (2000a). Some forgotten principles in health care reform: Part I. *Minnesota Psychologist, 49*(2), March, 22–25.

Olson, R. P. (2000b). Some forgotten principles in health care: Part II. *Minnesota Psychologist, 49*(3), 17–19, 21.

Olson, R. P. (Ed.) (2002). *Religious theories of personality and psychotherapy: East meets West.* New York: Haworth Press.

Olson, R. P., & Beecher, L. (1999, Sept.). Medical necessity: Rationing psychiatric services. *Minnesota Physician, 13*(6), 20–21.

Pati, S., Shea, S., Rabinowitz, D., & Carrasquillo, O. (2005). Health expenditures for privately insured adults enrolled in managed care gate-keeping vs. indemnity plans. *American Journal of Public Health, 95*(2), 286–291.

Parry, J., & Judge, K. (2005). Tackling the wider determinants of health disparities in England: A model for evaluating the new deal for Communities Regeneration Initiative. *American Journal of Public Health, 95*(4), 626–628.

Peabody, J. W., Tozija, F., Munoz, J. A., Nordyke, R. J., & Luck, J. (2004). Using vignettes to compare the quality of clinical care variation in economically divergent countries. *Health Services Research, 39*(6), Part II, 1951–1970.

Pearson, M. J., Wu, S., Schaefer, J., Bonomi, A., Shortell, S. M., Mendel, P. J. et al. (2005). Assessing the implementation of the chronic care model in quality improvement collaboratives. *Health Services Research, 40*(4), 978–996.

Phillips, K. (2002). *Wealth and democracy: A political history of the American rich.* New York: Broadway Books.

Physicians for a National Health Program (PNHP). *About PNHP.* Retrieved September 9, 2005 from http://www.pnhp.org/about/about_pnhp.php

Prentice, J. C., Pebley, A. R., & Sastry, N. (2005). Immigration status and health insurance coverage: Who gains? Who loses? *American Journal of Public Health, 95*(1), 109–116.

President's New Freedom Commission on Mental Health (2003). *Achieving the promise: Transforming mental health care in America.* Available at http://www.mentalhealthcommission.gov/finalreport/fullreport.htm

Regenstreif, D. I. (2005). Medicare's cost crisis: Solutions are within our grasp. *Health Affairs, 24*, suppl. 2, W5-R90-R93.

Ricketts, T. C. (Ed.) (1999). *Rural Health in the United States.* New York: Oxford University Press.

Roberts, M. C., Alexander, K., & Davis, N. J. (1991). Children's rights to physical and mental health care: A case for advocacy. *Journal of Clinical Child Psychology, 20*(1), 18–27.

Robinson, R., & Steiner, A. (1998). *Managed health care.* Philadelphia, PA: Open University Press.

Rodriguez-Garcia, R., & Akhter, M. N. (2000). Human rights: The foundation of public health practice. *American Journal of Public Health, 90*(5), 693–695.

Roemer, R. (2000). The right to health care – gains and gaps. *American Journal of Public Health, 78*(3), 241–247.

Rosen, A. B., Greenberg, D., Stone, P. W., et al. (2005, July). Quality of abstracts of papers reporting original cost-effectiveness analyses. *Medical Decision Making, 25*, 424–428.

Rothbaum, P., Bernstein, D., Haller, O., Phelps, R., & Kohout, J. (1998). New Jersey psychologists' report on managed mental health care. *Professional Psychology: Research and Practice, 29*(1), 37–42.

Ruger, J. P. (2005). The changing role of the World Bank in global health. *American Journal of Public Health, 95*(1), 60–70.

Schilder, K., Tomov, T., Mladenova, M., et al. (2004). The appropriateness and use of focus groups methodology across international mental health communities. *International Review of Psychiatry, 16*(1–2), Feb./May, 24–30.

Schoen, C., Doty, M., Collins, S., & Holmgren, A. (2005). Insured but not protected: How many adults are underinsured? *Web Exclusives: A Supplement to Health Affairs, vol. 24, Supplement 1,* January-June, W5-289–W5-302.

Schuster, M. A., McGlynn, E. A., & Brook, R. H. (2005). How good is the quality of health care in the United States? *The Milbank Quarterly, 83*(4), 843–895. Reprinted from *The Milbank Quarterly, 76*(4), 517–563.

Seids, M., & Stevens, G. D. (2005). Access to care and children's primary care experiences: Results from a prospective cohort study. *Health Services Research, 40*(6), Part I, 1758–1780.

Shaffer, E. R., Waitzkin, H., Brenner, J., Jasso-Aguilar, R. (2005). Ethics in public health research. *American Journal of Public Health, 95*(1), 23–34.

Shi, L., Macinko, J., Starfield, B., Politzer, R., Wulu, J., & Xu, J. (2005). Primary care, social inequalities, and all-cause, heart disease, and cancer mortality in US counties, 1990. *American Journal of Public Health, 95*(4), 674–680.

Shi, L., Stevens, G. D., Wulu, J. T. jr., Politzer, R. M., & Xu, J. (2004). America's health centers: Reducing racial and ethnic disparities in perinatal care and birth outcomes. *Health Services Research, 39*(6), 1881–1901.

Slade, M., Loftus, L., Phelan, M., Thornicrift, G., & Wykes, T. (1999). *The Camberwell assessment of Need.* London: Gaskell.

Sleek, S. (1998, March). Despite managed care, psychologists are committed to independent practice. *Monitor,* p. 23. Washington, D.C.: American Psychological Association.

Spettell, C. M. Wall, T. C., Allison, J., Calhoun, J., Kobylinski, R., Fargason, R., & Kiefe, C. I. (2003). Identifying physician-recognized depression from administrative data: Consequences for quality measurement. *Health Services Research, 38*(4), 1081–1102.

Star Tribune (Dec. 7, 1997). *The Wellness Gap.* Star Tribune, Dec. 7, 1997. Minneapolis: Star Tribune.

Starfield, B., Shi, L., & Macinko, J. (2005). Contributions of primary care to health systems and health. *The Milbank Quarterly, 83*(3), 457–502.

Statistics Canada (2003). *The Canadian Community Health Survey 1.2. Mental Health and Well-Being.* Ottawa, Canada.

Thomas, S. B., Fine, M. J., & Ibrahim, S. A. (2004). Health disparities: The importance of culture and health communication. *American Journal of Public Health, 94*(12), 2050.

Thornicroft, G., & Tansella, M. (1999). Translating ethical principles into outcome measures for mental health service research. *Psychological Medicine, 29,* 761–767.

Townsend, C., Whiteford, H., Baingana, F. et al. (2004). The mental health policy template: Domains and elements for mental health policy formulation. *International Review of Psychiatry, 16*(1–2), 18–23.

Tucker, L., & Lubin, W. (1994). *National survey of psychologists. Report from Division 39, American Psychological Association.* Washington, D.C.: American Psychological Association.

Umble, K., Steffen, D., Porter, J., Miller, D., Hummer-McLaughlin, K., Lowman, A., & Zelt, S. (2005). The national public health leadership initiative: Evaluation of a team0-based approach to developing collaborative public health leaders. *American Journal of Public Health, 95*(4), 641–644.

United Nations General Assembly (1948). *Universal Declaration of Human Rights.* Retrieved September 21, 2005 from http://www.unhchr.ch/udhr/lang/eng.htm

United Nations General Assembly (1989, October 16). *Convention on the rights of the child.* New York: Author (UNGA document A/REW/44/25)

United Nations General Assembly (1991). *The Protection of Persons with Mental Illness and the Improvement of Mental Health Care.* UN General Assembly resolution A/REW/46.119. Available at http://www.un.org/ga/documents/gadocs.htm

United Nations General Assembly (2000). *United Nations Millennium Declaration. Resolution 55/2.* Fifty-fifth session. Agenda item 60(b) adopted the original Resolution 217 A (III). New York: Author. Retrieved September 21, 2005 from http://www.un.org/english/engtxt.shtml

U. S. News and World Report, March 9, 1998, p. 48.

United States General Accounting Office (1994). *Health care reform: Proposals have potential to reduce administrative costs. Report to the chairman, Committee on Government Operations, House of Representatives.* Washington, DC: Author (GAO/HEHS-94-158).

United States General Accounting Office (1991). *Canadian health insurance: Lessons for the United States. Report to the Chairman, Committee on Government Operations, House of Representatives.* Washington, DC: Author.

Universal Health Care Action Network (UHCAN) (2005a). *Making health care work for all campaign.* Retrieved September 28, 2005 from http://www.uhcan.org/files/national/nationalaction.html

Universal Health Care Action Network (UHCAN) (2005b). *Faith communities working for health care justice.* Retrieved September 28, 2005 from http://www.uhcan.org/faith/

Universal Health Care Action Network (UHCAN) (2005c). *Health care access campaign: Support the health care access resolution.* Retrieved September 28, 2005 from http://www.uhcan.org/HCAR/

Universal Health Care Action Network (UHCAN) (2005d). *Brief summary of current and recent state strategies to achieve affordable health care for all.* Retrieved September 28, 2005 from http://www.uhcan.org/files/states/strategiesforhe.html

Vladeck, B. (2003). Universal health insurance in the United States: Reflections on the past, the present, and the future. *American Journal of Public Health, 93*(1), 16–19.

Wang, P. S., Berglund, P. A., & Kessler, R. C. (2003). Patterns and correlates of contacting clergy for mental disorders in the United States. *Health Services Research, 38*(2), 647–673.

Wang, P.S., Berglund, P., Olfson, M., Pincus, H., Wells, K., & Kessler, R. (2005a). Failure and delay in initial treatment contact after first onset of mental disorders in the national co-morbidity survey replication. *Archives of General Psychiatry, 62,* 603–613.

Wang, P.S., Lane, M., Olfson, M., Pincus, H., Wells, K., & Kessler, R. (2005b). Twelve-month use of mental health services in the United States. *Archives of General Psychiatry, 62,* 629–640.

White House Domestic Policy Council (1993). *The President's health security plan: The Clinton blueprint.* New York: Random House.

Whitener, B. L., Van Horne, V., & Gauthier, A. (2005). Health service research tools for public health professionals. *American Journal of Public Health, 95*(2), 204–207.

Wiger, D., & Solberg, K. (2001). *Tracking mental health outcomes: A therapist's guide to measuring client progress, analyzing data, and improving your practice.* Edison, New Jersey: John Wiley.

Wilensky, S., Rosenbaum, S., Hawkins, D., & Mizeur, H. (2005). State-funded comprehensive primary medical care service programs for medically underserved populations: 1995 vs. 2000. *American Journal of Public Health, 95*(2), 254-259.

Woolf, S. H., Johnson, R. E., Fryer, G. E., Rust, G., Satcher, D. (2004). The health impact of resolving racial disparities: An analysis of US mortality data. *American Journal of Public Health, 94*(12), 2078-2081.

World Bank Group (2003, June 5). Social capital. Cited by Henderson, S., & Whiteford, H. (2003). Social capital and mental health. *Lancet, 362*, August 16, 505-506.

World Health Organization (WHO) (1946). *Preamble to the Constitution of the World Health Organization as Adopted by the International Conference, New York, 19-22 June, 1946; signed on 22 July, 1946.* Retrieved September 21, 2005 from http://www.who.int/about/definition/en/

World Health Organization (WHO) (1948). *Constitution of the World Health Organization.* Retrieved September 21, 2005 from http://policy.who.int/cgi-bin/om_isapidll?

World Health Organization (WHO) (1997). *An overview of a strategy to improve the mental health of underserved populations: Nations for mental health.* Geneva, Switzerland: Author (unpublished document WHO/MSA/NAM/97.3).

World Health Organization (WHO) (2000a). *The world health report 2000. Health systems: Improving performance.* Geneva, Switzerland: Author.

World Health Organization (WHO) (2000b). *Women's mental health: an evidence-based review.* Geneva, Switzerland: Author. (unpublished document WHO/MSD/MHP/00.1).

World Health Organization (2001). *The world health report 2001: Mental health: New understanding, new hope.* Geneva, Switzerland: Author.

World Health Organization (2004a). *The world health report 2004: Changing history.* Geneva, Switzerland: Author.

World Health Organization (2004b). The World Mental Health Survey Consortium. Prevalence, severity, and unmet need for treatment of mental disorders in the World Health Organization World Mental Health Survey. *Journal of the American Medical Association, 291*, 2581-2590.

World Health Organization (2005a). *Mental Health Atlas - 2005.* Geneva, Switzerland: Author.

World Health Organization (2005b). *Mental Health Atlas - 2005. Global and Regional Results.* Retrieved October 17, 2005 from http://www.who.int/mental_health/evidence/atlas/Global%20and%20Regional%20Results.htm

World Health Organization (2005c). *New WHO mental health atlas shows global mental health resources remain inadequate.* Retrieved October 17, 2005 from http://www.who.int/mediacentre/news/notes/2005/np21/en/print.html

World Health Organization (2005d). *The world health report 2005: Make every mother and child count.* Geneva, Switzerland: Author.

Wyrich, K. W., Bullinger, M., Aaronson, N., et al. (2005, March). Estimating clinically significant differences in quality of life outcomes. *Quality of Life Research, 14*, 285-295.

Yamin, A. E. (2005). The right to health under international law and its relevance to the United States. *American Journal of Public Health, 95*(7), 1156-1161.

Zimmerman, F. S. (2005). Social and economic determinants of disparities in professional help-seeking for child mental health problems: Evidence from a national sample. *Health Services Research, 40*(5), Part I, 1514-1533.

INDEX

Page numbers followed by letter "t" indicate tables; numbers followed by "f" indicate figures.

9/11/01 terrorist attacks, 243

A

ability to pay, 280, 281, 282, 288, 291, 295, 310
acceptability (defined), 237
access (defined), 233, 237
accessibility (defined), 237
achievement relative to resources, 232
ACT (Assertive Community Treatment), 157, 158, 249
activities
  meaningful, 47, 51, 52, 95, 205
activities of daily living, 34, 45, 85
activity therapies, 73
Act of Mental Health Care (Lov om Psykisk Helsevern) (1961) (Norway), 93
Act of Patients' Rights, 1999 (Norway). *See Patient Rights Act, 1999* (Norway)
Act on Health Enterprises, 2002 (Norway), 85–86, 240, 244, 259, 260, 268, 273, 280, 293, 294
Act on Mental Health Care (Norway), 110, 240
Act on Municipal Health Care (Norway), 110, 240
Act on Specialist Health Care (Norway), 109–10, 240
Act on the Provision and Implementation of Mental Health Care (Norway), 128, 293
actuarial model of health insurance, 313–14
acupuncturists, Canadian, 160
acute inpatient care in Canada, 158, 169, 174, 179, 280–81
acute inpatient care in Great Britain, 54, 61, 66, 248, 308
acute inpatient care in Norway
  admission, 94, 248
  beds, 51, 280, 309
  and DPCs (District Psychiatric Centers), 121
  services, pressure on, 113, 116–17
acute inpatient care in United States, 205, 216, 262, 276
ADA *(Americans with Disabilities Act)*, 206, 217–18, 247, 296
addiction counselors. *See* substance abuse: treating
addiction services. *See* substance abuse: treating
addictive substances. *See* alcohol abuse; drug abuse; substance abuse
ADHD (attention deficit hyperactivity disorder), 144, 220
administrative costs (defined), 269
administrative personnel, 17, 19, 250
administrative personnel, British, 57–58
administrative personnel, Canadian, 161
administrative personnel, Norwegian, 108
administrative personnel, U.S., 208, 277
adolescents
  mental disorders of, 16
  mental health policy on, 238
  mental health services for, 10
  mental needs of, 316
adolescents, British
  mental disorders of, 30, 31t
  mental health policy for, 39, 40, 239, 244, 257
  mental health services for, 40, 75
adolescents, Canadian
  addictive treatment for, 169
  mental disorders of, 143, 144–46, 144t, 174
  mental health needs of, 249, 311
  mental health services for, 145, 158, 170, 173, 174, 180, 181, 262, 281
  protection of, 292
  suicide rate of, 149
adolescents, Norwegian
  mental disorders of, 90
  mental health services for, 93, 95, 96, 105–6, 107, 108, 112, 113, 122, 123, 125, 126, 248, 273, 309
adolescents, U.S.
  mental disorders of, 190, 192, 193t, 205
  mental health services for, 189, 195, 201, 201t, 266–67
adults, older. *See* older people (60+ years)
adults of working age (18-59)
  mental disorders of, 16
  mental health services for, 10
adults of working age (18-59), British
  mental disorders of, 30–32, 31t, 32t, 307, 308
  mental health policy for, 39–40, 41–43, 44f, 239, 244, 257, 272
  mental health services for, 44, 66–67, 308
  protection of, 292
adults of working age (18-59), Canadian
  mental disorders of, 143, 144–48, 145t, 146t, 174
  mental health services for, 145–46, 170, 173, 174, 180, 281
  suicide rate of, 149
adults of working age (18-59), Norwegian
  mental disorders of, 88–90
  mental health services for, 94, 96, 103, 108, 112, 123, 273, 274, 309
adults of working age (18-59), U.S.
  mental disorders of, 190
  mental health services for, 189, 201, 201t
"adverse selection" risk, limiting, 206
affective disorders, 206
  See also bipolar affective disorders
African Americans
  children, 313

353

demographics of, 186
health care services for, 210–11
Hurricane Katrina impact on, 318
mental disorders of, 245
mental health services for, 211
suicide and homicide rates of, 245
after-care facilities and follow-up care, 18, 111, 112, 116, 205
Agency for Healthcare Research and Quality (AHRQ), 212, 250, 262, 263, 326, 330
age transitions, 54, 75
aging populations, 279, 307, 316
　in United States, 278, 281, 307, 343
agoraphobia, 34
AIDS, 59–60, 92, 197, 279, 285
Aid to Families with Dependent Children, 313
alcohol abuse
　deaths related to, 9
　global statistics on, 306, 307
　mental disorder classification, 7
　national breakdown of, 8, 16
alcohol abuse in Canada, 147–48, 149, 169, 274
alcohol abuse in Great Britain, 30, 32, 307
alcohol abuse in Norway, 88, 90–91, 103, 114, 129, 144
alcohol abuse in United States, 191, 206, 245, 313
Alcoholics Anonymous, 200
Alcohol Use Disorders Identification Test (AUDIT), 147
allied health care providers. *See* nonphysician health care providers
Allied Health Professions Council (England), 38, 267
Ally, Glenn, 207
Alzheimer's disease, 8, 115, 186, 193, 307
American Association of Retired Persons, 296
American Civil Liberties Union, 341
American College of Nurse Practitioners, 189
American Medical Association, 221, 340
American Medical Student Association, 221
American Nurses Association, 189
American Psychiatric Association, 213, 326, 332, 344
American Psychological Association

(APA), 189, 213, 219, 220, 255, 267, 326, 340, 344
American Public Health Association (APHA), 189, 247, 340, 343
Americans with Disabilities Act (ADA), 206, 217–18, 247, 296
Animal Farm (Orwell) (1946), 242
anorexia, 144
antidepressants, 133, 149, 212, 257
antiparkinsonian drugs, 133
antipsychotics, 133, 209, 210
antisocial personality disorder, 129, 147, 192
anxiety disorder
　in elderly, 34, 307
　prevalence in Canada, 143, 144, 146
　prevalence in Great Britain, 31
　prevalence in Norway, 87, 88, 89, 105, 131, 134, 147
　prevalence in United States, 192
　treating, 182, 212, 220, 245, 265, 310
Appleby, Louis, 64, 67, 239
Appleby Evaluation of British mental health services, 2004, 63–64, 64t, 65
appropriate access (defined), 237
appropriate intervention (defined), 257
Arab countries, health care in, 288
armed forces personnel and veterans. *See* military personnel and veterans
Aspergers syndrome, 53
Assertive Community Treatment (ACT), 157, 158, 249
Assertive Outreach teams, 49, 51
assisted living, 333
Association of Academic Health Centers, 189
asylums. *See* mental hospitals and asylums
Asylums Act of 1808 (England), 46
asylum seekers. *See* refugees and asylum seekers
attention, prompt, 233
attention deficit hyperactivity disorder (ADHD), 144, 220
AUDIT (Alcohol Use Disorders Identification Test), 147
Australia, health care in, 30, 279, 288
availability (defined), 237

B

Balanced Budget Act, 199
Bangladesh, health care in, 288
Basic Supplemental Insurance, 216
Beck Depression Inventory (BDI), 66, 89
Bedlam (Bethlem) hospital, 45
behavioral disorders
　in Canada, 144
　in Norway, 90, 90t, 93
　statistics on, 8
　term usage, 7
　in United States, 194, 195
behavioral dysfunction, 7
behavioral therapy, 105, 169
behaviorial health services, 246, 342
benefit/cost ratios, 269
benefits, comprehensive
See also type of benefit, e.g.: sick benefits
benefits, comprehensive in Great Britain, 45
benefits, comprehensive in United States, 15
Bentall, Richard, 73
Berwick, Donald, 343
Better Services for the Mentally Ill, 1975, 248
between-client group services transitions, 54
billing, health care-related, 152, 156, 248, 260
binge eating disorder in Canada, 144
biological dysfunction, 7
biomedical model of mental illness and health, 104–5, 171–72, 173, 174, 178, 179–80, 181, 261, 262, 274, 275, 276, 311, 334, 335
See also psychiatry: medical model of
biopsychosocial model of mental illness and health, 5, 20, 30, 104–5, 172, 174, 182, 260, 275, 311, 332, 334–35
bipolar affective disorders
　disability due to, 307
　national breakdown of, 8, 15
　prevalence of, 88, 111, 143, 195
　studies on, 204, 328
　treatment of, 87, 114
Blair, Tony, 258
block grant health care funding, 109, 110, 161, 287
Blue Cross standard option, 199
Blunt, Matt, 198
BMI Healthcare, 54

Bolter, John, 207
Bondevik, Kjell Magne, 111
brain-body dysfunctions, 334
brief therapy, 71, 252, 326
Britain
    demographics, 11t, 24, 316t
    overview, 24–26, 292–93
Broadmoor Hospital (England), 53
bulimea, 144
BUPA, 54
Bureau of Health Professions (BHP), 254
Bureau of Indian Affairs, 245
Bureau of Labor Statistics, 277
Bureau of Primary Health Care (BPHC), 265, 333
Bush, G.W., 188, 196, 208, 209–10, 223, 277, 342
Buyers Health Care Action Group, 264

C

CAHPS (Consumer Assessment of Health Plans Survey), 264
California, health care reform in, 222, 325, 344
California, health insurance in, 246
Camberwell Assessment of Need (CAN) measure, 37, 60, 307, 328
Camberwell Assessment of Need for the Elderly (CANE) measure, 37, 307
Cambridgeshire and Peterborough Mental Health Partnership NHS Trust, 62
CAMHS (child and adolescent mental health service). *See* adolescents: mental health services for; children: mental health services for
Campaign for Mental Health Reform (CMHR), 344
Canada
    demographics, 11t, 138–39, 141–42, 316t
    overview, 138–42, 295
Canada Health Act of 1984, 142, 150–51, 156, 161, 174, 181, 240, 248, 287, 310
Canada Health and Social Transfer (CHST), 162, 287
Canada Health Transfer (CHT), 161, 162, 287
Canada Health Trust, 287
Canada Social Transfer (CST), 162
Canadian Alliance on Mental Illness and Mental Health, 174
Canadian Assistance Plan (CAP), 162
Canadian College of Health Service Executives (CCHSE), 161
Canadian Council on Health Services Accreditation (CCHSA), 160, 260, 268
Canadian Institute for Health Information (CIHI), 143, 160, 161, 163, 274
Canadian Institute of Health Research (CIHR), 143, 180–81, 260
Canadian Mental Health Association (CMHA), 162, 169, 173, 177, 181, 244, 274
Canadian Psychological Association, 268
Canadian Register of Health Service Providers in Psychology, 160
Canadian Royal Commission on the Future of Health Care in Canada, 169, 174
Canadian Senate Standing Committee on Social Affairs, Science, and Technology, 167–68, 169, 170, 171, 173, 174, 180, 181, 249, 253
Canadian Supreme Court, 153
cancers, 9, 279
cannabis, 148
capital funding, 60
capitation payments, 211, 222, 278, 279, 282, 288, 290, 338, 344
Cardinal Needs Measure, 37, 307, 328
cardiovascular conditions, 9
caregivers
    access to, 145
    adequate number of, 340
    of children, 40, 313
    groups, 49
    program participation of, 95
    rights of, 43
    service delivery, participation in, 66, 77
    strain on, 149, 150, 169–70, 274, 325
    support for, 41, 44, 45, 75
    teaching and training of, 106
care of the sick, history of, 26
care pathways and transitions
    in Great Britain, 47, 53–54, 74, 75, 76
    in Norway, 130, 133–34
care planning and management, integrated, 44

Care Programme Approach (CPA), 41, 44, 50, 69–70, 239, 248, 258, 292
Care Trusts, 68
Carter, Jimmy, 187, 242, 247, 262, 331, 338
case management, 209
cash-limited general medical services, 59
CASSP (Child and Adolescent Service System Program), 266
CBT (cognitive behavior therapy), 169, 220, 268
CCHSA (Canadian Council on Health Services Accreditation), 160, 260, 268
CCHSE (Canadian College of Health Service Executives), 161
Center for Disease Control and Prevention (CDC), 245
Center for the Advancement of Health, 189
Centers for Medicare and Medicaid Services (CMS), 195, 197, 249–50, 263
cerebral palsy, 198
CFPC (College of Family Physicians of Canada), 153, 154, 295
CHAI (Commission for Health Care Audit and Inspection), 63, 258, 308
Chaoulli v. Quebec Attorney General (2005), 287
character analysis, 104
CHCs (Community Health Centers), 242, 246, 289, 290, 333–34
CHI (Commission for Health Improvement), 43, 63, 70, 71, 248
Child and Adolescent Service System Program (CASSP), 266
child care, 145
Child Guidance Clinic (Oslo, Norway), 96
child psychiatry, 96
children
    health care for, 339, 341
    mental disorders of, 16
    mental health needs of, 316
    mental health policy on, 238
    mental health services for, 10, 18, 334–35
    rights of, 339, 341
    sexual abuse of, 6
children, British
    education of, 40

mental disorders of, 30, 31t, 307, 308
mental health policy for, 39, 40, 239, 244, 257
mental health services for, 40, 75, 308
parents and carers, support of, 40
in poverty, 40
protection of, 42, 292
special needs of, 40
children, Canadian
mental disorders of, 144, 144t
mental health needs of, 249, 311
mental health services for, 158, 170, 173, 174, 180, 181, 262, 281, 320
in poverty, 172, 180
children, Norwegian
health care for, 85
mental disorders of, 90
mental health services for, 93, 95, 96, 105–6, 107, 108, 112, 113, 122, 123, 124, 125, 126, 248, 273, 286, 309, 320
rights of, 127
children, U.S.
emotionally disturbed, 205
health care services for, 210–11, 215, 295
health insurance for, 12–13, 197, 211–12, 246, 312 (*see also* SCHIP (State Children's Health Insurance Program))
mental disorders of, 190, 192, 193t, 220
mental health services for, 189, 199, 201, 201t, 205, 211–12, 220, 250, 265, 266–67, 312, 320, 344
minority, 313
in poverty, 194
Children Act 2004 (England), 40, 244
chiropractic care, 222
Christie, Werner, 231
Chronically Sick & Disabled Act 1970 (England), 43, 248
Chronic Care Model, 321
chronic fatigue services, 47
chronic illness, 34, 35, 279
chronic mental disorders, 132
CHST (Canada Health and Social Transfer), 162, 287

CHT (Canada Health Transfer), 161, 162, 287
CIDI (Composite International Diagnostic Interview), 88, 310
CIHI (Canadian Institute for Health Information), 143, 160, 161, 163, 274
Citizens Advice Bureau, 49
Citizens' Health Care Working Group, 342, 343
civil commitment legislation, 16
Civil Rights Act, 1964, 217
civil wars, 70
clergy, mental health issues, involvement in, 333, 334
client orientation, 233
clinical interventions, best practices in, 324
clinical interventions, evaluating, 52–53
clinical level outcomes, 257
clinical psychologists, British, 47, 56, 252
clinical psychologists, Canadian, 159
clinical psychologists, Norwegian, 107
clinical psychologists, U.S., 269
Clinton, Bill, 15, 187, 215, 223, 262, 296, 297, 327, 342
CMHA (Canadian Mental Health Association). *See* Canadian Mental Health Association (CMHA)
CMHR (Campaign for Mental Health Reform), 344
CMS (Centers for Medicare and Medicaid Services), 195, 197, 249–50, 263
Coalition for a National Health Program, 342
cocaine, 148
cognitive behavior therapy (CBT), 169, 220, 268
cognitive dysfunctions, 131
cognitive impairment in older people, 43
cognitive therapy, 105
College of Family Physicians of Canada (CFPC), 153, 154, 295
Colorado, health insurance in, 338
Commission for Health Care Audit and Inspection (CHAI), 63, 258, 308
Commission for Health Improvement

(CHI), 43, 63, 70, 71, 248
commissioning, 60–62, 285, 308
Commission on Mental Health (U.S.), 31, 187, 242, 246–47, 262, 331
Committee on Ethical Guidelines for Forensic Psychologists, 326
Committee on Monitoring Access to Personal Health Care Services, 237
common good *versus* self-interest, 339
community-based health services, Canadian, 142
Community Care Direct Payments Act, 1996, 248
community competence, 337
Community Health Centers (CHCs), 242, 246, 289, 290, 333–34
community health services in Great Britain, 59, 285
community hospitals in United States, 208
community mental health centers
in United States, 17, 201, 202–3, 204, 209, 210, 242, 289, 290, 334
community mental health clinics in United States, 247
community mental health services and support
in Canada, 157, 158, 167, 168, 169, 171, 176, 179, 180, 244, 261, 274, 275, 295, 311, 321
in Great Britain, 46, 48–49, 48f, 51, 54, 72, 73–74, 77, 258, 321
in New Zealand, 219
in Norway, 94, 99, 102, 106, 110, 111, 113, 116, 130–33, 259, 273, 286, 309, 321
primary care, integration into, 333
for severely mentally ill, 320
social support, 335
in United States, 189–90, 195, 198, 201, 202–3, 204–5, 209, 265, 266, 267, 276, 296, 321
as WHO recommendation, 332
Community Mental Health Services for Children (program), 250
community mental health teams, 48, 49, 50–51, 54, 64–65, 258, 267, 308
community nurses, 49

co-morbid conditions, 35, 43, 76, 115, 169–70, 191–92, 193, 206, 257, 261, 291, 306, 312, 327
competence to stand trial, 141, 155, 171, 295
Composite International Diagnostic Interview (CIDI), 88, 310
Comprehensive Community Mental Health Services for Children and Families, 266
conduct disorders. *See* behavioral disorders
Congressional Universal Health Care Task Force, 339–40
constitutional amendments, 341, 342, 344
Consumer Assessment of Health Plans Survey (CAHPS), 264
consumer choice, 15
Consumer Operated Services Program (COSP), 217, 221
Consumers Union, 189
continuing education requirements, 267
continuity of care, 331, 333, 340
continuous care residences, Norwegian, 85
Conyers, John, 221, 222
CORE system, 66
corporations' expenditure on health, 12
cost-containment mechanisms, 17–18, 283, 319
   in Canada, 167, 275–76
   in Great Britain, 67–68, 272
   in Norway, 273–74, 280
   in United States, 215, 277–78, 282, 326, 342
   See also health care services: rationing
cost (defined), 269, 279
cost sharing, 123–24, 276, 286
cost shifting, 278, 281, 326, 342
counseling and counselors, 252, 334
counseling and counselors, British general practitioners, affiliation with, 321, 323
   in primary care, 47, 50
   publicly funded, 39
   work settings of, 268
counseling and counselors, Canadian coverage for, 275, 276

number of, 160, 268
private, 169
unregulated status of, 295, 321
counseling and counselors, Norwegian and primary care consultation, 95
counseling and counselors, U.S., 207, 212
CPA (Care Programme Approach). *See* Care Programme Approach (CPA)
crime and criminals
   See also mentally ill: assaults by; prisoners
crime and criminals, Canadian
criminal behavior, increase in, 168, 176
   mental health status of, 141, 155, 171, 295
crime and criminals, Norwegian, mental health status of, 129
Criminal Code of Canada, 155, 158
Criminal Code Review Board (Canada), 158
crisis
   defined, 50
   houses, 51
   intervention, 49, 95, 158, 169, 259, 309, 326
   resolution, 42, 51, 248, 267
   services, 50–51, 54, 158, 168
Crisis Resolution teams, 49
critical incident stress debriefing, 158
CST (Canada Social Transfer), 162
cultural competency, 244, 307, 320
custodial care *versus* active treatment
   in Canada, 168
   in Norway, 99, 102, 104, 111
   in past practice, 319
   in United States, 204

D

DALE (disability-adjusted life expectancy), 233, 270
DALYs (disability-adjusted life years), 9
danger criteria, 98
day services for mental patients
   expenditures for, 19
   in Great Britain, 49, 51, 73
   in Norway, 11, 95, 96, 106, 110, 111, 112, 113, 122
deaths
   addiction as cause of, 9, 90–92, 91t
   AIDS-related, 92
   causes of, 330
   health care access impact on, 340
   health insurance, lack as cause of, 341
   income, low as factor in, 332
   infant, 208
   mental disorders, associated with, 9, 16, 90, 90t, 178, 181, 274
   risk of, 6
   suicide as cause of, 33, 34, 90
Declaration of Caracas (1990), 292, 332, 339
Declaration of Madrid, 339
Declaration of Patients' Rights, 340
Declaration of the Rights of Children, 339
Declaration on the Rights of Disabled Persons, 339
Declaration on the Rights of Mentally Retarded Persons, 339
deinstitutionalization of mental patients, 336
   in Canada, 162–63, 167, 168, 169, 295
   in Great Britain, 45, 46, 258
   in Norway, 94, 99, 100–101, 102–3, 113, 120, 309
   in past practice, 319
   in United States, 195, 203, 204–5, 210, 219, 247, 276
   See also mental hospitals: alternatives to
demand-side cost containment strategies, 276, 277, 280, 281, 288
dementia
   disability related to, 307
   in elderly, 16, 30, 31, 34, 35t, 54, 115, 186, 307
   prevalence of, 30, 31, 35t
   WHO statistics on, 8
dentistry in Great Britain, 44
dentistry in United States, 222
Department for Education and Skills (England), 38
Department for Work and Pensions (England), 38, 45, 248
Department of Defense health services, 189, 196, 198, 199–200,

204, 208, 213, 242, 247, 263, 290, 326
Department of Education (England), 248
Department of Health and Human Services (HHS), 6, 7, 187, 195, 200, 216, 222, 249, 265, 266
Department of Health and Social Security (England), 46
Department of Health (England), 38
   access, equitable, focus on, 244
   financing by, 60
   leadership of, 26, 29, 279, 293
   mental health services guidelines, 69–70, 73, 308
   and NHS Trusts, 28
   policies and funding, 62, 68, 284
   publications, 53, 258
   publications of, 39, 44, 47
   regulations issued by, 248
   residential placements, recommendations for, 52
   revenue distribution through, 285
   role of, 41
   service targets specified by, 42
   surveys required by, 65
   treatment outcome measuring, involvement in, 66
Department of Veterans Affairs Special Committee on Post-Traumatic Stress Disorder, 204
depression
   in adolescents, 205
   in caregivers, 313
   cost of, 149, 178
   diagnosing, 333
   in elderly, 34, 35, 115, 255, 257, 307
   general practitioner treatment of, 105
   as mental disorder, 7
   physical symptoms resulting from, 201
   prevalence (Canada), 143, 144, 149
   prevalence (Great Britain), 307
   prevalence (Norway), 88, 89, 131, 134, 146–47
   prevalence (U.S.), 195, 205, 291
   preventing, 202
   in prisoners, 129
   studies on, 328
   treating, 7, 68, 87, 182, 195, 202, 212, 255, 257, 264, 265–66, 321
   See also manic depression; unipolar depression
developing countries, mental health services in, 315
developing countries, occupational health in, 340
developmental disabilities, 198
developmental disorders, 195
deviant behavior, 7, 87, 106, 131, 310
Diagnostically Related Groups (DRGs), 197, 250
Diagnostic and Statistical Manual of Mental Disorders. See DSM-IV-TR *(Diagnostic and Statistical Manual of Mental Disorders)*
Diagnostic and Statistical Manual of the American Psychological Association (DSM-III), 190, 191
Diagnostic Interview Schedule (DIS), 190
diagnostic-related payments, 288, 290
diagnostic tests, 151
Dingell, John, 196
direct costs (defined), 269
Directorate for Health and Social Affairs (Norway), 108–9
Directorate of Health and Social Welfare (Norway), 108–9, 109n, 110, 119, 120n27, 127, 130, 259, 268
direct payments to clients, 43, 45, 51, 68, 76
direct service personnel in mental health services. *See under* mental health professionals and workers
Dirigo Health Plan, 344
disabilities associated with mental disorders
   consequences of, 34
   cost of, 19, 123, 131, 149, 177, 178, 190, 274
   dimension of, 6, 7
   managing, 188
   prevalence of, 9–10, 16, 92, 92t, 182, 306–7, 311–12
   protection from, 238
   risk of, 6, 51
   support for persons with, 77, 198, 218
disabilities in elderly, 35, 43, 186, 307
disability-adjusted life expectancy (DALE), 233, 270
disability-adjusted life years (DALYs), 9
disability benefits
   in Canada, 325
   in Great Britain, 29, 45, 307
   importance of, 333
   in Norway, 92, 92t, 103, 123, 131
   in United States, 13, 190, 194, 203
disability (defined), 217–18
disability insurance in Canada, 177
disabled persons, British, services, reimbursement for, 43
disabled persons, health insurance for, 19
disabled persons, Norwegian, services for, 101
disabled persons, U.S.
   health insurance for, 189, 197, 242, 243, 250, 318
   legal rights of, 206, 296
disaster affected people, African American, 318
disaster affected people, mental health services for, 320
discrimination, protection against
   in Great Britain, 38, 41, 42
   monitoring of, 18
distress, mental (symptom), 6, 7
distributive justice, 338
District Health Authorities (England), 77
District Psychiatric Centres (DPCs) (Norway), 95–96, 102, 104, 106, 110, 112–13, 114, 121, 126, 130, 248, 259–60, 274, 280, 309
doctor-patient communication, 260, 294
doctors
   See also family doctors; general practitioners (GPs)
doctors, British
   in administration, 58
   number of, 250t, 251t
doctors, Canadian
   compensation for, 156, 159, 164, 166–67, 275, 287, 288, 325
   number of, 141, 160, 250, 250t,

251t, 281
  status of, 311, 325
doctors, medical in mental health services, 108, 132, 173, 249, 253
  See also psychiatrists
doctors, Norwegian
  compensation for, 281
  education and training of, 268
  number of, 250, 250t, 251t
  in psychiatric institutions, 98
doctors, U.S.
  compensation for, 343
  information technology of, 330
  of minority groups, 211
  number of, 250t, 251t, 255, 277
  psychotherapy administered by, 263
  status of, 337
Douglas, Tommy, 155, 174
Down's syndrome, 198
DPCs (District Psychiatric Centres) (Norway). *See* District Psychiatric Centres (DPCs) (Norway)
Draft Mental Health Bill (2004), 39
DRGs (Diagnostically Related Groups), 197, 250
drug abuse
  deaths related to, 9
  mental disorder classification, 7
  national breakdown, 8, 16
  prevalence of, 306
drug abuse in Canada, 147, 148, 149, 169, 274
drug abuse in Great Britain, 30, 31, 35, 307
drug abuse in Norway, 88, 90, 91–92, 114, 129
drug abuse in United States, 206, 245, 313
drugs
  development of, 198
  expenditures for, 193–94, 194t, 222
  formularies, 279
  imported, 196
  safety, 196
  See also specific drug category, e.g.: psychotropic medications
drug therapy. *See* pharmacotherapy
DSM-III (Diagnostic and Statistical Manual of the American Psychological Association), 190, 191

DSM-IV-TR *(Diagnostic and Statistical Manual of Mental Disorders)*, 7, 30, 144, 192, 218, 238, 243, 265, 307, 310
dual disorders. *See* co-morbid conditions
due process, 291, 295, 338
dynamic psychotherapy, 220
dysfunctions, 7, 131, 334
dysphoria, 7, 53

E

Early Intervention in Psychosis (EIP) Teams, 51
eating disorders
  in Britain, 52, 53, 62, 308
  in Canada, 144
  in Norway, 95, 131
  in United States, 205
ECA *(Epidemiological Catchment Area)* study. *See Epidemiological Catchment Area* (ECA) study
economic justice, 340
economic self-interest, 342
economic self-sufficiency, 344
economic systems, 317–18
ECPA (Enhanced Care Programme Approach), 41, 43, 50, 248, 258
ecstacy (drug), 148
education, access to
  in Canada, 158, 169, 170
  in Great Britain, 49
  in United States, 203
Education Act, 1980 (England), 40, 244
efficacy (defined), 256
efficiency
  defined, 256, 269
  factors in, 269–70
  measures and rankings of, 270–71
egalitarian view of distributive justice, 338
Elder Care Rights Alliance, 296
elderly adults (60+ years). *See* older people (60+ years)
electroconvulsive therapy, 104, 105, 168
electronic medical records, 330
emergency medical treatment, 44
emergency social work duty teams, 51
emotional disorders, 7, 195, 205

empirically supported interventions (ESI), 213
  See also evidence-based treatments (EBT)
empirically validated treatment (EVT), 213
  See also evidence-based treatments (EBT)
Employee Retirement Income Security Act of 1997 (ERISA), 16–17, 218, 297
employer-provided health plans, 16–17
employment benefits, 203
employment in Canada
  assistance, 157, 159, 168, 169, 170, 176
  downsizing, 150
employment in Great Britain
  assistance, 29, 48, 49, 51, 52
  conditions, 324
  mental illness impact on, 71
  promoting meaningful, 42
employment in Norway
  agencies, 94, 259
  assistance, 96, 132, 134
  statistics, 84
employment in United States
  assistance, 190, 344
  following mental treatment, 212
  of mentally impaired, 218
  obstacles to, 195
end of life care, costs of, 208
end-stage renal disease (ESRD), 197
Enhanced Care Programme Approach (ECPA), 41, 43, 50, 248, 258
entitlements, 196, 199, 217, 223
epidemiological approach to need assessment, 37
Epidemiological Catchment Area (ECA) study, 190, 191, 192, 193, 311, 312
epidemiological studies, 8
epilepsy, 8, 16
Equal Employment Opportunity Commission (EEOC), 218
equality, 338
equality of care, 15
equalization funding, 161, 287
equitable access as mental health system evaluation criterion, 338
equitable access (defined), 237–38
equity, types of, 238

ERISA (Employee Retirement Income Security Act) of 1997, 16–17, 218, 297
ESRD (end-stage renal disease), 197
Established Programs Funding (EPF), 161–62
ethnic and national groups. *See* minorities, cultural and ethnic
European Community, 25, 45
European Convention on Human Rights, 38, 244, 292, 339
evaluation criteria (of mental health system)
    universal health care access, 18, 319, 337
    as values, 338
evidence-based mental health programs
    community alternatives, 312
    guidelines, 259, 263, 326
    health-promoting, 72
    policy initiatives, 75
    practices, 256, 257, 262, 268, 319, 328, 335
evidence-based treatments (EBT), 4, 77, 105, 212–13, 258, 262, 308
evidence informed practice (EIP), 213
    See also evidence-based treatments (EBT)
existential therapy, 105
extended family, 131
extended health care services, 151, 152, 248
eye care in United States, 222
eye examinations, payment for in Great Britain, 44

F

fair financing (defined), 283–84
fair-opportunity rule, 338
Families USA, 189
families with dependent children, health insurance for, 197
family advice, offices for, 260
Family Benefit (England), 45, 239
family doctors, British
    central role of, 29
    free consultations with, 44
    mental health issues, involvement in, 30, 71, 76, 308, 333
    "sick notes" from, 45
    staff and associates of, 49

family doctors, Canadian
    associations for, 153, 154
    compensation for, 156, 159
    mental health issues, involvement in, 146, 156–57, 170, 171, 253, 260–61, 269, 333
    number of, 268
    status of, 275
family doctors, mental health issues, involvement in, 6, 333
    See also doctors: psychotherapy administered by
family doctors, Norwegian, mental health issues, involvement in, 105, 333
family doctors, U.S., mental health issues, involvement in, 200, 201, 212, 220, 265, 283
family psychiatry, 93
family psychoeducation, 220
family self-help, 157
family services, offices for, 105
family therapists, 160, 206, 254, 268, 275, 295, 321
family to work interference, 149, 150, 274, 325
family violence, 202
Federal Bureau of Prisons, 247, 249
Federal Employees Health Benefits Program, 189, 196, 199, 208, 242, 290, 296
Federal/Provincial/Territorial Advisory Network on Mental Health (ANMH), 157
fee-for-service, 200, 209, 222, 283, 287, 288, 290, 325, 343, 344
financing systems, national breakdown of, 14
First Steps program, 198
follow-up and after-care, 18, 111, 112, 116, 205
Food Stamps, 196
Ford, Gerald, 202
forensic psychiatry, 129
forensic psychology and psychologists, 219, 326
forensic services, 53, 62, 158, 159
for-profit organizations, 52, 342
for-profit versus nonprofit hospitals, 209, 222
for-profit versus nonprofit mental health care providers, 205–6
freedom

liberty (value), 338, 341
    loss of, 6, 7, 238
    mental health as element of, 341
free trade agreements, 318
Freud, Sigmund, 104, 105
Frist, Bill, 196
functioning as mental health dimension, 7

G

gap between rich and poor, 314
GAS (Goal Attainment Scaling), 235–36, 235t, 329
gatekeepers, 260, 333
gateway workers, 252, 258, 268
Gaustad Asylum (Oslo, Norway), 93
gender differences
    in caregiver access, 145
    for depression, 143, 144
    for eating disorders, 144
    of inpatients, 103
    in mental disorder prevalence (general), 31, 31t, 144, 147, 147t, 192
    for personality disorders, 144
    for phobias, 144
    in suicide rates, 33, 90, 91f
gender dysphoria, 53
General Accounting Office (GAO), 194, 195
general government expenditures, 11, 11t, 12
General Medical Council (England), 38
General Motors (GM), 278
General Practitioner (GP) Scheme, 260
General Practitioner Scheme, 294
general practitioners (GPs)
    mental health issues, involvement in, 6
    See also doctors; family doctors; internists; nurse practitioners; pediatricians
general practitioners (GPs), British
    after hours services of, 51
    autonomy of, 61
    contract for, 59
    funding for, 285
    mental health issues, involvement in, 39, 57, 62, 321, 323
    organization of, 258

role of, 29
general practitioners (GPs), Canadian
    status of, 318
general practitioners (GPs), Norwegian
    access to/choosing, 87
    mental health issues, involvement in, 87, 94, 98, 104, 105, 106, 134–35, 260
    mental health specialists as, 130, 134–35
    role of, 85
    services, paying for, 123
general practitioners (GPs), U.S.
    mental health issues, involvement in, 200, 254, 265
generic community mental health teams, 50–51
generic drugs, 194
Georgia, mental health care in, 292
gestalt therapy, 105
Girl Interrupted (Kaysen), 205
Global Equity Guage Alliance, 338
Global Health Equity Initiative, 338
global network of expertise, 3
Goal Attainment Scaling (GAS), 235–36, 235t, 329
Governmental Regional Boards (Norway), 119
government health expenditures. *See* public health expenditures
gross domestic product, 11, 12, 19, 271, 317, 317t
gross domestic product, British, 26, 271, 271t, 284
gross domestic product, Canadian, 141, 164, 165t, 176, 176t, 271t, 274, 287
gross domestic product, Norwegian, 83, 96, 121, 122, 124, 271t, 272, 285
gross domestic product, U.S., 187, 214, 214t, 271t, 276, 288, 343
group and individual insurance plans, 17
group homes for mental patients, 204, 276
group therapy, 269
guidance counselors, 207

H

Hall, Emmett, 168
hallucinogens, 148
Harvard University, 190
Hastert, Dennis, 196
HCC (Health Council of Canada), 175
health, level of, 270
health, promoting, 167, 171, 172, 174, 175, 178, 180, 247, 262, 276, 332
health, socioeconomic aspects of, 172, 335, 339
health action (defined), 255–56
Health Authorities (England), 58
Health Care Access Resolution, 339–40
health care as human right, 291, 292, 339, 341
Health Care Commission (England), 68
Healthcare Cost and Utilization Project (HCUP), 250
Healthcare Financial Management Association (HFMA), 285
Health Care Financing Administration (HCFA), 195, 197, 250
health care fraud, 196
health care justice, 21
Healthcare-Now, 342
health care providers and professionals
    British, 38, 285
    Canadian, 142, 159–60, 164, 175, 245, 287, 318
    education and training of, 250
    number of, 250, 340
    U.S., 187, 207, 211, 255, 277, 283
health care reform
    in Canada, 158, 175, 176, 222, 223, 324, 343
    in Great Britain, 27, 40, 258, 324, 342
    mental health reform, prerequisite for, 318
    in Norway, 84, 86–87
    primary care reform, 332
    professional input on, 20, 21
    stages of, 319, 320
    in United States, 15, 221–23, 281, 306, 316, 327, 339, 341–44
health care services
    access and equity of, 15, 236–37, 279, 283, 284, 318, 327, 330, 332, 337, 338–39, 340 (*see also* universal health care access)
    attitudes toward, 318–19
    cost-effectiveness of, 270, 319
    cost of, 5
    delivery of, 231, 319, 330
    distribution of, 5, 15
    efficiency of, 284
    fair financing of, 232, 233, 283–84
    financing of, 250
    goal attainment, 232, 270, 284, 319
    integrated approach to, 6
    national, founding of, 319
    performance of, 232, 270–71, 284, 319, 329, 335
    psychological aspects of, 318–19
    purchasing of (*see* purchasing of health care services)
    quality of, 233, 319, 330, 340
    rankings, international, 231, 232–34
    rationing, 278–79
    regional differences in, 338
    responsiveness of, 232–33
    trends in, 319
    utilization of, 257, 279, 338
    waits and treatment delays, 233
    See also mental health services; primary health care; specialized health services
health care services, British
    access and equity of, 324
    administration of, 25–26, 27, 28–29, 30
    agencies, 76
    cost and efficiency, 271–72
    delivery of, 24, 25, 28, 29–30
    fair financing of, 284–85, 287, 288
    financing of, 25, 26, 29–30, 58–62, 77, 324
    goal attainment, 234t, 270t
    history of, 26–27
    overview of, 10
    performance of, 234t, 270t
    ranking of, 233, 234
    rationing, 279–80
    responsiveness, 239, 280, 308, 326
    waits and treatment delays, 239, 279, 280, 285, 308
    workers, 58
health care services, Canadian
    access and equity of, 142, 151, 152, 155–56, 241, 248, 326
    administration of, 167, 177, 241, 248, 275, 325
    delivery of, 241, 324

fair financing of, 284, 285, 286–88, 325
goal attainment, 234t, 270t
overview of, 10, 142–43
performance of, 234t, 270t
ranking of, 234
rationing, 280–81
responsiveness, 234, 241, 326
standards for, 150, 151–52
waits and treatment delays, 231, 279, 281
health care services, Norwegian
access and equity of, 82, 84–85, 109–10, 239–40, 244
administration and structure of, 85–87, 119
consent to, 128–29
fair financing of, 284, 285–86, 287, 288
goal attainment, 233, 234t, 270t
overview of, 10
performance of, 233–34, 234t, 270t
productivity and efficiency of, 248, 273
quality of, 248
ranking of, 233–34
rationing, 279, 280
responsiveness, 234, 240, 326
waits and treatment delays, 280
health care services, U.S.
access and equity of, 189, 190, 196, 200, 223, 241, 242, 243, 246, 282, 295–96, 339, 340, 342, 343, 344
administration of, 209, 276–77, 325
cost of, 344
crisis in, 194, 196
delivery of, 185, 187, 199, 242, 277, 344
fair financing of, 234, 284, 285, 287, 288–91, 339, 344
goal attainment, 234, 234t, 270t
performance of, 234t, 270t
policy, 194
quality of, 208, 250, 262, 296, 339, 343, 344
ranking of, 234
rationing, 280, 281–83, 326
responsiveness, 234, 243, 326
utilization of, 281
waits and treatment delays, 243, 282–83, 326

Health Centers, federally funded, 201, 202, 212
See also Community Health Centers (CHCs)
Health Council of Canada, 253
Health Council of Canada (HCC), 175
health (defined), 5, 292
Health Development Agency (England), 63
Health Districts (in Great Britain), 27
health enterprises (Norway), 86, 95, 106, 110, 117, 118, 121, 124, 130, 239–40, 248, 253, 260, 272, 273, 285, 286, 293, 294
health expenditures
achievement relative to, 270
mental health portion of total, 9
national breakdown of, 4, 11t, 12–14, 19, 271
optimal level of, 284
rising, 215, 223, 275, 276
value judgments, reflection of, 338
See also out-of-pocket health expenditures
health expenditures, British, 11t, 44, 58–62, 271, 271t, 272, 284, 285, 287, 288, 321
health expenditures, Canadian, 11t, 140, 163–67, 163t–164t, 165t–166t, 173, 176–77, 176t–177t, 181, 271, 271t, 275, 287–88, 294, 321
health expenditures, Norwegian, 11t, 121–22, 121t, 167, 271, 271t, 272, 284, 285, 287, 288, 321
health expenditures, U.S., 11t, 26, 167, 196, 200, 208–9, 213–14, 214t, 215, 216–17, 250, 262, 271, 271t, 276, 281, 282, 288, 289t, 321, 323, 343
health information system, 142, 260, 266
health insurance
access to (*see* health care services: access and equity of; universal health care access)
barriers to, 237
co-pays and deductibles, 10, 17, 19, 283
coverage, 341
premiums, 10, 17, 19

private, 283
as social good, 314
health insurance, British
co-pays, 324
private, 54, 60, 279–80
schemes, 58, 284
health insurance, Canadian
administration of, 151
coverage requirements, 151 (*see also* medical necessity standard)
national, 222, 240–41, 287, 288, 324–25, 326, 343
overview of, 10, 21, 30, 150
portability, 142, 151, 152, 156, 248, 326
private, 173, 174, 176–77, 245, 253, 276, 281, 287
psychologist participation in, 17
public, 325
supplementary, 177
See also Medicare (Canada)
health insurance, Norwegian
co-pays and deductibles, 106, 123, 273
coverage, 109–10, 239–40
versus other countries, 10, 30
private, 286
reimbursements, 106, 109
standardizing, 324
See also National Insurance Scheme (Norway)
health insurance, U.S.
co-pays and deductibles, 197, 198, 199, 208, 215, 216, 222, 243, 278, 281, 288, 290, 291, 342
cost of, 278
drug coverage, 19, 194, 215, 262, 343
employer-based, 208, 215, 263–64, 278, 282, 288, 289, 296, 297, 312, 325, 327, 342, 344
evaluation of, 264
expenditures for, 19
gaps in, 262
hospital-based, 222
lack of (*see* uninsured persons, U.S.)
limiting, 277–78
national, 240–41, 281
national (proposed), 197, 221–22, 316, 317, 318, 342
nonprofit health plans, 249
as political issue, 196

portability, 222
premiums, 208, 215, 313–14, 342
prepaid, 200
private, 185, 199, 205, 208, 209, 210, 215, 216, 218, 222, 242, 243, 245, 277, 280, 281, 282, 288–89, 289t, 290, 291, 295, 297, 312, 317, 321, 325, 326, 337
public, 240–41, 281, 312, 321
research on, 250
state-level, 249
See also uninsured; *specific type of insurance, e.g.:* Medicare (U.S.)
Health Insurance Portability and Accountability Act (HIPAA), 196–97, 217, 218–19, 243, 277
health interventions, rationing, 279
Health Maintenance Organization (HMO) Act, 1973, 218
Health Maintenance Organizations (HMOs). *See* HMOs (Health Maintenance Organizations)
Health of the Nation Outcome Scale (HoNOS), 66
Health Partners, 209
Health Personnel Act, 1999 (Norway), 24, 87, 240, 252
Health Plan Employer Data and Information Set (HEDIS), 213, 263–64
health policy
citizen impact on, 292
formulating, 337
implementing, 270
rationing impact on, 279
health policy, British, 239
health policy, Canadian, 142, 150–56, 174, 240–41, 248, 261, 325
health policy, Norwegian, 239–40, 268
health policy, U.S., 195, 196–200, 241–42, 249–50, 297, 340
Health Professions Act (Alberta), 160
Health Report to the American People (http://www.citizenshealthcare.gov), 344
health research in Canada, 143
Health Resources and Services Administration, 265
Health Savings Accounts, 277, 342
Health Security Act, 1993, 223, 297

health status
British, 233
promoting, 328, 335
U.S., 234, 343
health system (defined), 255–56
healthy life expectancy
in Canada, 10, 11t
in Great Britain, 10, 11t
in Norway, 10, 11t
in United States, 10, 11t
Healthy People 2010 (DHHS, 2000), 190, 245, 249, 328
hearing aid practitioners, Canadian, 160
help lines, 51, 158
heroin, 148
HFMA (Healthcare Financial Management Association), 285
high secure services, 42, 53, 292, 308
HIPAA *(Health Insurance Portability and Accountability Act)*, 196–97, 217, 218–19, 243, 277
Hispanics, mental health services for, 211
Hispanics, suicide and homicide rates of, 245
HIV/AIDS, 59–60, 92, 197, 279, 285
HMCs (Hospital Management Committees), 27
HMOs (health maintenance organizations), 199, 209, 215, 217, 218, 264, 277, 282, 296, 297, 326, 327
home care and help services
British, 42, 43, 51, 248
Canadian, 151, 168
Norwegian, 85, 93, 102, 120, 132
homelessness, ending, 344
homeless persons
mental health services for, 74
mentally ill as, 168, 169, 176, 195, 204, 210, 243, 247, 261, 336, 341
minorities as, 243
home nursing in Norway, 85
Home Office (England), 38, 248
homicides
mental illness, history, link to, 38
reviews following, 66
U.S. rates of, 245
HoNOS *(Health of the Nation Outcome Scale)*, 66

Hoover, Herbert, 203
Hopkins Symptom Checklist (HSCL-25), 88–89
horizontal equity, 238
Hospital Act, 1970 (Norway), 87, 93, 324
hospital and community health services, British, 59
Hospital Insurance and Diagnostic Services Act (1957) (Canada), 155, 157, 240, 261
hospitalization
alternatives to, 49, 74
partial, 199, 203
hospitalization, preventable, 332
Hospital Management Committees (HMCs), 27
hospital rating systems, 257
hospital recidivism rates. *See* readmissions, inpatient and hospital recidivism rates
hospitals, Canadian
administration of, 156
cost coverage for, 151, 164, 166
deinstitutionalization impact on, 163
mental health units in, 167, 168, 169, 180
nonmedical services in, 157, 167, 174, 180
hospitals, general, 6, 17
hospitals, Norwegian, 93, 115, 121, 122, 240
hospitals, U.S., 208, 209, 222, 263
household out-of-pocket health expenditures. *See* out-of-pocket health expenditures
housing assistance, 333
in Canada, 157, 158, 168, 169, 170, 176, 179, 295, 311
in Great Britain, 34, 45, 48, 52, 239
for minorities, 243
in Norway, 95, 113, 132, 134
in United States, 190, 194, 203
HPES (Indian Health Performance Evaluation System), 263
human life, value of, 338
human resources, 17
Human Rights Act 1998 (England), 38, 244, 292
human rights and health, 291, 292, 339, 341

human rights and mental health 99, 291, 292, 332, 338, 340–41
human services, 200, 201
Hurricane Katrina, 318
hydrotherapy, 168, 319
hypnotics and tranquilizers, 133

I

ICD-10 *(International Statistical Classification of Diseases and Related Health Problems)*, 7, 8, 30, 307
ICP (integrated care pathway), 54
immigrants
    See also refugees and asylum seekers
immigrants, mental health services for, 18, 247, 316
immigrants to Canada
    demographics, 138, 139, 141–42
    health care services for, 151–52
    as mental health professionals, 253–54
    suicide rate of, 148–49
immigrants to Great Britain, mental health needs of, 45, 65
immigrants to Norway
    demographics, 82
    mental health needs of, 114–15, 244, 309
immigrants to United States
    demographics, 186
    economic conditions of, 202
    mental health services for, 211
    uninsured, 240
income, decreasing and mental illness, 34
income, low as death risk factor, 332
independence, promoting, 41, 42, 95, 233, 344
India, health care in, 288
Indian Health Care Improvement Act, 200, 263
Indian Health Performance Evaluation System (HPES), 263
Indian Health Service (IHS), 189, 196, 198, 200, 208, 242, 245, 249, 263, 290, 334
Indian Self-Determination Act, 200
indirect costs (defined), 269
Individual Plan, 106, 126, 128
individual provider Trusts, 59
individual-society conflict, 7
infant mortality, 208

infections, 9
information technology, 75, 208, 330
inhalant drugs, 148
Inouye, Daniel K., 207
inpatient health care in Canada, 325
inpatient health care in Great Britain, 279
inpatient mental health care
    in Canada, 151, 161, 180, 249, 274, 275, 280
    expenditures for, 19, 250
    in Great Britain, 41, 44, 46, 47, 48f, 51, 54, 74, 75, 77, 258, 280, 308
    in Norway, 96, 97, 98, 101n15, 103–4, 111, 113, 114n24, 115–16, 116n, 117, 120, 122, 259, 273, 309
    in United States, 203, 205, 206, 215, 242, 266, 277, 282, 312, 326
    See also mental hospitals and asylums; psychiatric nursing homes; residential mental health care
Input-Processing-Output (IPO) information processing model, 269
insanity defense, 296
insomnia, primary, national breakdown of, 8, 16
Institute for Clinical and Health Excellence, 71
Institute for Healthcare Improvement, 343
Institute of Medicine (IOM), 185, 208, 220, 237, 249, 256, 262, 263, 292, 295, 307, 330
insulin-coma treatment, 104, 168, 319
integrated care pathway (ICP), 54
intensive case management teams, 158
interest groups. *See* special interest groups
intergenerational justice, 15, 339
intermediate care, 44
international comparative studies, 3
International Consortium on Mental Health Policy and Services, 3, 315, 328, 335
international globalization, 318
international politics, 70
International Society for Health Equity, 338–39
International Statistical Classification of Diseases and Related Health Problems (ICD-10), 7, 8, 30, 307
internists, 6
internists, U.S., 200
interpersonal relationships, 195
interventions, efficacy of, 259
    See also treatment outcomes, measuring
intravenous drugs, 148
Inuit (Canadian aboriginal people), 139, 142, 149, 244
involuntary commitments to mental institutions, 291, 322
    in Canada, 154, 168, 178, 241, 295
    in Great Britain, 34, 38, 41
    in Norway, 85, 98–99, 112, 120, 127, 129, 292, 293
    in United States, 219, 296
involuntary mental treatment
    in Canada, 154, 176, 178–79
    in Great Britain, 39
    in Norway, 98, 99, 112, 120, 129, 293
    in United States, 219
Iraq-Afghanistan conflict, 204
irrational thinking, 7

J

Jobcentre Plus Network (England), 29, 49
Johnson, Lyndon, 197, 202, 342
Johnson, Norine, 189
Joint Commission on Accreditation of Healthcare Organizations (JCAHO), 260, 263
Joseph Rowntree Foundation, 63
Journey to Recovery (Dept. of Health, 2001), 42
justice (ethical principle), 337, 338–39, 340, 341
juvenile facilities, 266

K

Kaysen, Susan. Girl Interrupted, 205
Kennedy, John, 202, 205
King, Martin Luther, Jr., 215, 336
Kucinich, Dennis, 221

L

LaLonde, Marc, 172, 188, 275
Lancashire Quality of Life Interview, 65
Lang, Otto, 155
language barriers, 237
Law on Poverty, 1845 (Norway), 93
Law on Universal Social Welfare Insurance (Folktrygden), 1966, 239
Layard, Richard, 73
L.C., Olmstead v., 1999, 206
Leapfrog Group, 213, 264
learning difficulties, counseling for, 106
learning disabled and disabilities
  See also terms beginning with mental-retardation
learning disabled in Great Britain
  hospitals for, 27
  services for, 29, 55, 56, 62
Levant, Ron, 189
Levitt, Michael, 216
liberty (value), 338, 341
Lieberman, Joseph, 205
life expectancy at birth
  in Canada, 10, 11t
  in Great Britain, 11t
  in Norway, 11t
  in United States, 10, 11t, 208
  See also DALYs (disability-adjusted life years); disability-adjusted life expectancy (DALE); healthy life expectancy
lifetime prevalence (defined), 8
Living and Treatment Centres, 102
  See also psychiatric nursing homes
Lloyd, W.S., 155
lobotomy, 104, 168, 319
Local Authorities, public health services of, 27, 28, 29, 38, 41, 45, 48, 49, 272, 293
Local Health Integration Networks (LHINs) (Canada), 157, 249
Local Implementation Teams (LITs), 38, 42, 248, 258, 284, 293
Local Practitioner Committees (LPCs), 27
loneliness, 35
long-stay accomodations
  in Canada, 151, 157
  in Great Britain, 51–52
  in Norway, 102, 103, 110, 113–14, 117, 280, 309
  See also residential mental health care

long-term health care in Great Britain, 324
long-term health care in United States, 222
long-term mental health care
  in Canada, 159
  in Great Britain, 49, 258
  in Norway, 95, 126, 135
Louisiana Academy of Medical Psychology, 207
Low-Risk Drinking Guidelines (Canada), 147
low secure services, 42, 53, 248, 292, 308
Lunacy Act of 1845 (England), 46

M

Maine, health care reform in, 344
malignant diseases, 9
managed behavioral health organizations (MBHOs), 209, 213, 215, 263, 264, 282, 290, 326–27, 342
managed care organizations (MCOs), 16, 213, 249, 264, 277
managed care plans, 17, 205, 210, 212, 215, 218, 278, 321
managed competition, 326, 342
manic depression, 34, 201
Manitoba, health services in, 175
Manitoba, mental health services in, 158–59, 249
market-driven rationing of health care, 282
marriage therapists, 160, 206, 254, 268, 275, 295, 321
Massachusetts Health Care Constitutional Amendment, 344
McDermott, Jim, 221
McLean Hospital (Belmont, Mass.), 205
MDH (Minnesota State Department of Health), 264
Mechanic, David, 311, 312, 327
Medicaid, 12, 16, 189, 194–95, 196, 197–98, 199, 204, 205, 208, 210, 211, 215, 216, 222, 223, 241, 242, 245, 246, 261, 264, 266, 276, 277, 287, 288t, 290, 296, 317, 318, 321, 324, 326, 338, 342, 344

Medi-Cal, 246
medical clinics, 6, 17
medical conditions
  cost of, 286
  severity of, 281
medical errors, 292, 330
medical ethics, 340
Medical Expenditure Panel Survey (MEPS), 211, 212, 250
medical malpractice reform, 196
medical necessity standard, 16, 150, 151, 179–80, 181, 222, 240, 241, 244, 275, 280, 288, 294, 319, 325
medical personnel, 6
medical practitioners, British, 56
medical records, access to, 127
Medical Research Council (England), 63
medical sector, general, 201
medical services, general, 59
medical technologies
  advances in, 194
  cost of, 279, 330, 343
  health, impact on, 340
  utilization of, 278
Medicare (Canada), 17, 155–56, 157, 159, 161, 164, 171, 173, 174, 175, 179, 181, 241, 245, 248, 253, 275, 287, 294, 310, 317, 325
Medicare Modernization Act (MMA), 197, 249, 297
Medicare (U.S.)
  administrative costs of, 277
  billing, restrictions on, 260
  care quality, monitoring through, 263
  consumer protection through, 218, 296
  co-payments for, 243, 290
  coverage gaps in, 198
  drug coverage through, 19, 194, 215, 262, 343
  eligibility for, 16, 327
  expanding, 221–22, 318, 343
  expenditures, 195, 246, 343
  funding and cost of, 12, 13, 208, 216–17, 281, 290
  implementation of, 205
  mental health coverage through, 189, 289t

Native Americans, funds for, 245
other insurance programs compared to, 199
payment policies of, 206
policies, decisions affecting, 196
popularity of, 223
recipients, number of, 186, 194, 307, 343
reform of, 197, 297
scope and coverage of, 216–17, 242
states, impact on, 210
medications. *See* drugs
medium secure services, 42, 53, 248, 292, 308
memory deficit disorders, 115
mental asylums. *See* mental hospitals and asylums
mental disorder (defined), 4, 6–8
mental disorders
  biological approach to (*see* biomedical model of mental illness and health)
  biopsychosocial model of (*see* biopsychosocial model of mental illness and health)
  causes of, 72, 171, 174–75
  classification of, 7, 30, 192, 307 (*see also* DSM-IV-TR *(Diagnostic and Statistical Manual of Mental Disorders)*; ICD-10 *(International Statistical Classification of Diseases and Related Health Problems)*)
  costs of, 59, 149, 150, 150t, 172, 177, 181, 190, 193–94, 194t, 195, 269, 275, 276, 286, 310
  defined, 238
  diagnosing, 5, 6, 7, 103–4, 103t, 265, 266
  employment, impact on, 71
  etiology of, 5, 7
  freedom from, 341
  gender differences in, 31, 31t, 144, 147, 147t, 192
  impact of, 8–10, 15–16
  managing, 72
  medical and surgical care associated with, 198
  versus physical disorders, 134
  preventing, 5, 6, 20, 44, 72, 238, 275 (*see also* prevention and early intervention)

  risk factors for, 30, 34, 70, 277, 291, 318
  severity of, 71, 72, 257, 269, 306, 327
  social justice for people with, 20
  socioeconomic aspects of, 334
  suicide, link to, 34
  treated *versus* untreated, 19, 87
  treating, 5, 6, 7, 182, 187, 265, 275, 291, 335
  treatment priorities, 114–15, 206
  See also neuropsychiatric disorders; *type of disorder, e.g.:* schizophrenia
mental disorders, prevalence of, 257, 266, 306–7, 321, 327, 330
  in Canada, 143–48, 144t, 145t, 146t, 147t, 174, 322t
  in Great Britain, 30–37, 31t, 32t, 33t, 35t, 307, 308, 322t
  in market economies, 190, 191t
  in Norway, 88–90, 88t, 89t, 114, 309, 310, 322t
  versus physical diseases, 190, 191t
  versus professionals to treat, 250
  in United States, 190–94, 192t, 193t, 311–12, 322t
mental health
  defined, 6, 238
  factors contributing to, 337
  improving, 256
  international aspects of, 70, 72 (*see also* immigrants; refugees and asylum seekers)
  models of (*see* biomedical model of mental illness and health; biopsychosocial model of mental illness and health)
  monitoring community, 72, 75–76, 332
  promoting, 6, 20, 41, 44, 71, 73, 188, 238, 335–36
  as public good *versus* private commodity, 331
  research, 72, 76, 180–81, 332
  social aspects of, 70
Mental Health Act, 1959 (England), 39, 239
Mental Health Act, 1961 (Norway), 87, 98, 273
Mental Health Act, 1983 (England), 34, 38, 39, 41, 69, 239, 244, 247
Mental Health Act, 1999 (Norway), 87, 96, 240, 268

Mental Health Act, 2001 (Norway), 98
Mental Health Association (MHA), 217
Mental Health Atlas – 2005 (WHO, 2005a), 328, 330
Mental Health Bill (proposed) (England), 69, 71
Mental Health Bills of Rights, 217, 218, 296
mental health care reform
  in Canada, 176, 179–82, 249, 311
  in Great Britain, 40, 46, 72–78, 258
  in Norway, 94, 324, 343
  recommendations for, 20, 21, 231, 327–32
  requirements for, 318
  in United States, 187–88, 220–23, 344
mental health charities, British, 46, 47, 54
Mental Health Consumer-Survivor Network, 296
mental health country profile, 3, 4, 315, 328, 335
mental health epidemiology. *See* mental disorders, prevalence of
mental health expenditures, 14, 321
mental health expenditures, British, 67, 67t, 322t
mental health expenditures, Canadian, 167, 173, 174, 177–78, 181, 281, 294, 322t
mental health expenditures, Norwegian, 96–97, 121, 122–23, 122t, 321, 322t
mental health expenditures, U.S., 195, 276, 289–90, 289t, 321, 322t
mental health laws and legislation
  in the Americas, 238
  British, 27
  Canadian, 150, 154–55, 160–61
  European, 238
  Norwegian, 121
  WHO recommendation, 332
  See also specific piece of legislation, e.g.: Mental Health Act, 1983 (England)
mental health nurses, British, 252
mental health parity, principle of, 340
Mental Health Parity Act, 196–97, 215, 217, 218, 242–43, 296
mental health parity legislation, 16, 209–10, 216

mental health policy
    defined, 238, 320
    ethical principles for, 340
    evaluating, 235, 315
    goals of, 331
    impact of, 238
    lack of, 9, 238
    mental disorder definition impact on, 7
    performance, impact on, 238
    planning and implementing, 3–4, 19, 250, 306, 315, 317, 323, 331, 335, 340
    template, 328
    training in, 332, 336
mental health policy, British, 39–44, 70–71, 72, 75, 239, 247–48, 258, 280, 308, 316, 320, 322
mental health policy, Canadian, 150–56, 173, 176, 180, 182, 241, 248–49, 262, 295, 310, 316, 320, 322
mental health policy, Norwegian, 92–99, 129–30, 240, 248, 316, 320, 322, 324
mental health policy, U.S., 189, 194–200, 249–50, 316, 320, 322
mental health practice guidelines, 69–70, 73, 118, 212, 213, 268, 322, 326
mental health professionals and workers
    competence of, 267, 334
    distribution of, 17
    education and training of, 267, 270, 319, 335
    human resources, developing, 332
    regulation of, 267, 321, 322
    requirements for, 17
    services of, 270
    specialist-population ratio, 269, 323, 323t
    See also under type of professional, e.g.: psychiatrists
mental health professionals and workers, British
    administrative personnel, 57–58
    competence of, 267–68
    direct service personnel, 55–57
    education and training of, 72, 268
    employment and funding for, 62, 77
    number of, 50, 251t, 308
    recruiting, 75
    types of, 56t, 251–52
mental health professionals and workers, Canadian
    administrative personnel, 161
    allied health/nonphysician, 245, 275, 276, 281, 288, 294, 310, 311, 318, 323, 325
    certification and licensing of, 268, 269
    competence of, 268–69
    cultural competency of, 244
    distribution of, 244, 310
    education and training of, 281
    nonmedical, 178
    number of, 159–60, 251t, 254, 310
    qualifications of, 180
    recruiting, 253–54
    regulation of, 160–61, 179, 253, 268, 295
    services, access to, 249
mental health professionals and workers, Norwegian
    administrative personnel, 108
    certification and licensing of, 107, 118, 119
    competence of, 268
    education and training of, 96, 98, 112, 126, 280
    number of, 107–8, 107t, 108t, 113, 251t, 308
    recruiting, 112, 125, 126, 252–53, 324
    services, access to, 240
    in transition, 132, 133
mental health professionals and workers, U.S.
    administrative personnel, 208, 277
    allied health/nonpsychiatrist, 263
    certification and licensing of, 217, 269
    competence of, 269
    education and training of, 203, 296
    number and distribution of, 206–8, 251t, 255, 283
    recruiting, 204
    regulation of, 296
mental health program (defined), 320
mental health programs, 16, 332
    See also evidence-based mental health programs
mental health resources
    allocation of, 15, 19, 59
mental health services
    access and equity, 18, 20, 21, 232, 236–37, 237t, 240, 256, 267, 269, 279, 316, 317, 320, 330, 331, 338, 341
    administration of, 240, 317
    components of, 5–6, 14
    consumer-driven, 329
    cost and efficiency, 18, 19, 20, 21, 232, 237, 237t, 269, 319, 328, 330, 331, 337, 337t
    defined, 6
    delivery of, 4, 6, 8, 17, 237, 317, 323, 331, 337, 338, 341
    economic aspects of, 3, 317–18
    evaluating, 8–9, 14–15, 16, 18–20, 21, 63–64, 64t, 65, 315, 319, 328 (*see also* evaluation criteria (of mental health system))
    fair financing of, 5, 19, 20, 21, 232, 233, 237t, 238, 256, 257, 320, 323, 328, 330, 335, 336, 337
    financing of, 4, 6, 8, 17–18, 237, 237t, 240, 323, 331, 335, 337, 341
    in geographic and demographic context, 315–16, 316t
    geriatric (*see* older people (60+ years): mental health services for)
    goal attainment, 236t, 257, 319, 320, 323, 328–30, 336
    history and evolution of, 319
    in industrial versus developing countries, 315
    need indicators and assessment, 15–16, 306–7, 327
    organization of, 237, 341
    performance of, 237t, 256, 279, 319, 328, 331, 332–41
    population relevance, 18, 19–20, 21, 232, 237t, 306, 330
    protection and participation, 18, 19, 20, 21, 232, 237t
    quality and efficacy, 18, 20, 21, 232, 237t, 240, 255, 256–57, 320–21, 329, 331, 335, 337, 337t
    ratings, 232, 235–36, 257
    recommendations (*see* mental health care reform: recommendations for)

responsiveness, 237t, 256, 257, 320, 323, 328, 330, 335, 336
specialized, 240
staffing of (see mental health professionals and workers)
utilization of, 18, 37, 257, 306, 327, 334–35
mental health services, British
   access and equity, 64–65, 64t, 73, 74, 76, 236t, 308
   adminstration and structure of, 42, 67, 76–77
   advocates for, 70, 72
   components of, 46–48, 48f
   cost and efficiency, 64t, 66–68, 236t, 272
   delivery of, 28, 29, 45–58, 66, 72, 316
   evaluating, 52–53, 63–72, 323, 336
   fair financing of, 64t, 68, 72, 236t, 321
   financing of, 42, 61–62, 71, 73, 77, 78
   flexibility and appropriateness of, 76
   gaps in, 320
   goal attainment, 236t, 257, 320, 329–30
   history and evolution of, 45 46, 70
   integration of, 258
   local, 258
   need indicators and assessment, 30–37, 41, 43, 47, 73, 76, 307–8, 323–24, 327–28
   population relevance, 64t, 70–72, 236t, 322t
   (private practice) partnerships, 54–55, 62
   protection and participation, 64t, 68–70, 236t
   quality and efficacy, 64t, 65–66, 236t, 257–58
   ratings, 235t, 236, 236t
   responsiveness, 321, 330
   specialized, 44, 47, 52–53, 54, 57, 64–65, 72, 239, 308
   utilization of, 66–67, 71, 307, 322t, 323
   waits and treatment delays, 280
mental health services, Canadian
   access and equity, 142, 154–55, 167, 169, 170, 173–75, 178, 179–80, 236t, 241, 244–45, 249, 261, 281, 310, 311, 317, 325
   administration of, 180, 261
   barriers to, 145
   cost and efficiency, 167, 176–78, 181, 236t, 260, 274–76, 310, 325
   delivery of, 156–61, 316, 325
   evaluating, 167–79, 323, 336
   fair financing of, 178, 181, 236t, 288, 321
   financing of, 159, 161–67, 168, 169, 174, 175, 241, 261, 325
   goal attainment, 236t, 320
   history and evolution of, 168
   hospital-based, 176, 274
   insurance coverage for, 311
   integration of, 169, 170, 176, 179, 180, 249, 260–62, 311
   need indicators and assessment, 143–50, 310–11
   nonmedical, 173, 174, 175, 178, 181
   performance of, 275
   population relevance, 167, 171, 179, 181–82, 236t, 322t
   protection and participation, 167, 178–79, 181, 236t
   quality and efficacy, 167, 170, 173, 174, 175–76, 180–81, 236t, 260, 261, 310
   ratings, 235t, 236, 236t
   regional variations in, 154–55, 158–59, 178–79, 241, 261, 342
   research on, 262
   responsiveness, 321
   shared care model of (see under shared care model)
   specialized, 157–58, 159, 169, 249, 310
   utilization of, 171, 174, 241, 261, 310, 311, 322t
   waits and treatment delays, 170, 173, 178, 276, 280, 288
mental health services, Norwegian
   access and equity, 82, 99, 111, 114–18, 127–28, 236t, 258–59
   administration of, 259, 294, 324
   cost and efficiency, 114, 121–25, 124t, 236t, 272–73
   delivery of, 99–108, 132, 316
   evaluation of, 110–35, 323, 336
   fair financing of, 114, 125–26, 236t, 293, 321
   family, substitute for, 131
   financing of, 92, 93, 96–97, 108–10, 248, 286, 324
   goal attainment, 236t, 257, 259, 320, 329, 330
   history and evolution of, 93–94, 99–103
   integration of, 118, 119, 121, 259–60
   need indicators and assessment, 87–92, 111–12, 113, 309–10
   ownership of, 84
   performance of, 319
   population relevance, 114, 130, 236t, 322t
   productivity of, 258–59, 273
   protection and participation, 114, 126–30, 236t
   quality and efficacy, 114, 118–21, 236t, 258–59, 324
   ratings, 235t, 236, 236t
   regional variations in, 117–18, 118t, 342–43
   responsiveness, 320, 330
   specialized, 85–86, 88, 90, 95, 96–97, 98, 98t, 103, 106–8, 113, 114, 121, 122–23, 135, 259, 274, 309
   statistics, 97, 97t
   transportation challenges, 82
   utilization of, 111, 116, 125, 127–28, 131, 309, 310, 314, 322t, 323
   waits and treatment delays, 115, 116, 117, 128, 240, 280, 281, 293, 309
mental health services, U.S.
   access and equity, 187, 188, 210–12, 215, 217, 220, 236t, 241, 242–43, 254, 282, 317, 320, 327
   administration of, 208
   cost and efficiency, 208, 209, 213–15, 236t, 276–77, 313
   delivery of, 185, 200–208, 242–43, 246, 316, 342
   evaluation of, 210–20, 297, 323, 336
   fair financing of, 215–17, 236t, 321

financing of, 10, 199, 208–10, 342
goal attainment, 236t, 320
insurance coverage for, 198, 199, 205, 208, 209, 210, 216, 217, 220, 222, 242–43, 246, 277, 282, 288, 291, 296, 312, 326, 344
integration of, 188, 265–67
need indicators and assessment, 190–94, 311–14
versus other nations, 189
overview of, 187–90
performance of, 319
population relevance, 220, 236t, 322–23, 322t
protection and participation, 217–20, 221, 236t
quality and efficacy, 209, 212–13, 217, 236t, 262–64, 265
ratings, 235t, 236, 236t
responsiveness, 321
specialized, 200, 201, 205, 241, 291
state variations in, 195, 216, 290, 342
utilization of, 312, 322t, 323
waits and treatment delays, 280
mental health specialists
as consultants, 334
in primary care settings, 130, 134–35, 334
mental health status, 335
Mental Health Strategies (agency), 66
mental health system (defined), 4, 256
Mental Health Systems Act, 1980, 242, 331
Mental Health Trusts, 29, 52, 52t, 57, 59, 61, 62, 65, 71, 77
mental health workers. *See* mental health professionals
mental health work *versus* medical psychiatry, 130, 131–32, 133, 134
mental hospitals and asylums
admission, involuntary into *(see* involuntary commitments to mental institutions)
versus general hospitals, 6
specialty facilities, 17
mental hospitals and asylums, British
day, 51
history of, 45–46, 99
management of, 27

staffing of, 55
mental hospitals and asylums, Canadian
capacity of, 167
closing, 275, 280
deinstitution impact on, 162–63
history of, 168
independent, 157, 261
long-term treatment in, 159
mental hospitals and asylums, Norwegian
administration and ownership of, 93
alternatives to, 100n, 101, 102
capacity of, 100–101, 102, 111, 112, 113, 116–17
closing of, 309
history of, 93, 134
specialized treatment in, 95, 104
stays, duration of, 97, 116
wards, differentiated, of, 94
mental hospitals and asylums, U.S.
alternatives to, 204
closing, 276
county, 201, 204–5
private, 201, 205–6
state-run, 187, 201, 204–5, 210, 276
treatment, coverage of, 197, 199
mental illness, attitudes toward
in Canada, 145, 170, 175–76
in Great Britain, 73
in Norway, 111
in United States, 187, 188, 189, 210, 237, 241, 314
mental illness, overclassification of, 125, 131
Mental Illness Act, 1930 (England), 39, 239
mental institutions, Norwegian, 123, 123t, 127–28
mentally handicapped, mental disorders of, 95
mentally ill
assaults by, 70
attitudes toward, 73, 171, 248, 332, 336 *(see also* social exclusion, reducing)
health care justice for, 21
legal justice for, 69, 344
protection of, 19, 217, 219, 291 *(see also* mental health services: protection and participation)

rights of, 217, 218, 219–20, 292, 297 *(see also* patients: rights of) subgroups of, 52
See also crime and criminals: mental health status of; prisoners: mentally ill as
mental retardation, 7
Mental Retardation and Community Mental Health Centers Construction Act, 1963, 202, 242, 247, 249
mental retardation facilities and services, 259, 276
mental treatment, involuntary. *See* involuntary mental treatment
MEPS (Medical Expenditure Panel Survey), 211, 212, 250
Métis (Canadian aboriginal people), 139, 244
Mexican Americans, mental health services for, 211
MH. *See* mental health
MHA (Mental Health Association), 217
MHDI (Minnesota Health Data Institute), 264
Midlife Development in the United States (MIDUS) database, 211
Mid-Missouri Community Mental Health Center (Columbia, Mo.), 203
midwives, Norwegian, 85
migraine disorders, 8, 16, 307
migrant farm workers in United States, 340
military personnel and veterans, British, mental health services for, 65, 71
military personnel and veterans, Canadian
health care services for, 151, 178
mental disorders of, 146–47, 146t, 173, 241, 244
mental health needs of, 249
mental health services for, 142, 147, 241, 244
military personnel and veterans, mental health services for, 18, 316
military personnel and veterans, U.S.
health insurance for, 189, 198, 200, 257, 263 *(see also* Department of Defense health services; Veterans Health Administration (VHA))
mental disorders of, 243

mental health needs of, 344
mental health services for, 203
MIND (National Association for Mental Health), 46, 70
Minister of Health and Welfare (Canada), 152, 172, 188, 241, 248, 249, 275
Minister of Health (Norway), 231, 248
Ministry of Health and Care Services (Norway), 86, 94, 95, 108, 110, 117, 119, 121, 127, 259, 260, 268, 272
Ministry of Health and Social Care (Norway), 248, 280, 294
Ministry of Health (Canada), 287
Minnesota
    health care reform in, 222, 325, 344
    health care service in, 283
    health insurance in, 246, 249, 263, 277, 282
    mental health care in, 16–17, 213
Minnesota Association for Children's Mental Health, 296
Minnesota Health Data Institute (MHDI), 264
Minnesota Physician-Patient Alliance, 277
Minnesota State Department of Health (MDH), 264
minorities, cultural and ethnic
    mental health needs of, 314–15, 316
    mental health services for, 18, 243, 320
minorities, cultural and ethnic, British caregivers, 66
    mental health needs of, 32, 35–37, 71, 307
    mental health services for, 41, 44, 243–44, 308
minorities, cultural and ethnic, Canadian
    demographics, 138, 139, 244
    health care services for, 142, 244
    mental health needs of, 249, 311
    mental health services for, 244–45
minorities, cultural and ethnic, Norwegian
    demographics, 82
    mental disorders of, 88
    mental health services for, 244
minorities, racial and ethnic, U.S.

death, causes of, 245
demographics, 186
health care services for, 210–11, 245–46, 340
mental disorders of, 245
mental health needs of, 312, 313
mental health services for, 211, 246, 247, 255
MMA (Medicare Modernization Act), 197, 249, 297
mobile crisis units, 159
Modernizing Mental Health Services: Safe, Sound and Supportive, 41
mood disorders
    diagnosis of, 103
    prevalence of, 114n22, 131, 143, 192
    treating, 87, 310
mood stabilizers, 133
    See also psychotropic medications
moral hazard, theory of, 277–78, 288, 342
moral obligation, theories of, 338, 340, 341
mortality. *See* deaths
multidisciplinary approach to mental health
    in Canada, 142, 159, 249
    facilitating, 334
    in Great Britain, 44, 46, 62, 72, 75, 258
    increasing, 319
    in Norway, 96
    in United States, 213
multiple sclerosis, 8, 16
Municipal Health Service Act (Norway), 87, 128, 259, 293
municipality psychologists, Norwegian, 105, 106, 260

N

National Academy of Sciences (U.S.), 185
National Alliance for the Mentally Ill, 339
National Assistance Act of 1948 (England), 43
National Association for Mental Health, 46, 70
National Association for the Mentally Ill (NAMI), 217, 296
National Association of County and City Health Officials, 189
National Association of Private Psychiatric Hospitals, 205
National Association of Psychiatric Health Systems, 205
National Board of Health (NBH)(Norway), 259
National Center for Health Statistics, Division of Data Services (NCHS), 245, 265
National Center for Policy Analysis, 197
National Clinical Practice Guideline Council, 213, 263, 326
National Coalition of Mental Health Professionals and Consumers (NCMHPC), 217
National Committee for Quality Assurance (NCQA), 213, 260, 263, 264
National Comorbidity Survey (NCS), 190–92, 193, 291, 311, 312, 333
National Comorbidity Survey-Replication (NCS-R), 192, 193, 206, 262, 265, 291, 311, 312, 322, 327, 333
National Council of Schools of Professional Psychology, 334
National Forum on Health (Health Canada, 1994), 142, 172, 175, 260
National Health Expenditure Database (Canada), 163
National Health Service Act, 1946, 239
National Health Service (England)
    administration and structure of, 27–30, 38, 271–72, 293, 294, 321
    availability of, 44
    establishment of, 27, 239
    evaluating, 329–30, 339
    financing and financial procedures, 26, 58, 59, 60, 68, 77
    funding by, 54, 58, 308
    funding of, 68, 279, 280, 284, 285
    hospital rating system of, 257
    medical specialties in, 56
    mental health services through, 47, 292, 307
    monitoring role of, 75
    overview of, 21

performance, monitoring, 258
policies, 61, 248
reforming, 40
service provision, role in, 42, 52
staffing of, 55, 57–58
universal access through, 244, 342
National Institute for Clinical Excellence, 248, 258
National Institute for Mental Health for England (NIMHE), 40, 71, 248
National Institute of Mental Health Interview Schedule for Children, 8
National Institute of Mental Health (U.S.), 190, 242, 249, 250, 262, 263
National Insurance Act (Norway), 110, 240
National Insurance Administration (Norway), 286
National Insurance Scheme (Norway), 84, 102, 109–10, 110n, 122, 123, 124, 126, 239, 240, 281, 283, 285, 286
National Library of Medicine's National Information Center on Health Services Research and Health Care Technology, 328
National Mental Health Association (U.S.), 296
national mental health policy. *See* mental health policy
National Mental Health Programme (NMHP) (Norway), 90, 94–99, 103, 105, 109, 110, 111–12, 113, 114, 115, 116, 119, 121, 125–26, 130, 132, 134, 240, 244, 248, 252, 258–59, 267, 268, 273–74, 286, 293–94, 309, 324, 329, 330
National Physician Database (Canada), 160
National Schizophrenia Fellowship (*later named Rethink*), 70
National Service Frameworks, 39–44, 44f, 51, 53, 55, 57, 61, 63, 68, 69, 74–75, 77, 239, 244, 247, 248, 257–58, 272, 292, 308, 342
Native Americans, Canadian
demographics of, 139
health care services for, 142, 241, 244
mental health and addiction services for, 169, 170, 174, 180, 181, 241, 262, 320
suicide rate of, 149, 173
Native Americans, U.S.
demographics of, 186, 245
health care services for, 200, 242, 245 (*see also* Indian Health Service (IHS))
mental health and addiction services for, 200, 245, 263, 320
suicide and homicide rates of, 245
naturopaths, Canadian, 160
NBH (National Board of Health) (Norway), 259
NCHS (National Center for Health Statistics), 245, 265
NCMHPC (National Coalition of Mental Health Professionals and Consumers), 217
NCQA (National Committee for Quality Assurance), 213, 260, 263, 264
NCS *(National Comorbidity Survey). See* National Comorbidity Survey (NCS)
NCS-R *(National Comorbidity Survey Replication). See* National Comorbidity Survey-Replication (NCS-R)
necessary or crucial care (defined), 257
neighborhood cohesion, 337
Neighborhood Health Centers Program, 202, 249
neurobiology, 133
neuroleptic medications, 168, 319
neuropsychiatric disorders
categories of, 8, 16
causes and treatment for, 52
deaths due to, 9
defined, 7
tertiary treatment for, 53
neurotic disorders
in Great Britain, 30, 31, 32
in Norway, 93, 103, 104, 131
New Jersey Health Access Study Commission, 344
Newman, Russ, 207
New Mexico, health care reform in, 325, 344
New Public Management (Norway), 286
New York City Health Security Act, 2005, 344
New Zealand, health care in, 288
New Zealand, mental health services in, 219
NHS Act of 1946 (England), 27
NHS and Community Care Act, 1990 (England), 39
NHS Direct, 51
NHS Service Delivery and Organization Research and Development, 248
NHS Trusts, 28, 29, 43, 62, 248, 293
NICE (National Institute for Clinical Excellence), 40, 66, 76
NIMHE (National Institute for Mental Health for England), 40, 71, 248
nonmedical model of mental illness and health. *See* biopsychosocial model of mental illness and health
nonmoral *versus* moral values, 15
nonphysician health care providers
Canadian, 164, 245, 287, 318
U.S., 207, 211
nonprofit hospitals, 209, 222
nonprofit organizations, British, 12, 49, 52 54
nonprofit *versus* for-profit mental health care providers, 205–6
nonpsychiatrists, 254
non-system factors in efficiency, 269
North America, health care in, 288
Northern Ireland, health care in, 26
Northern Ireland, mental health services in, 24
Norway
demographics, 10, 11t, 81–82, 316t
overview, 81–85
Norwegian Board of Health, 116, 119, 121, 260
Norwegian Health Services Research Centre, 115, 120, 120n27, 259
Norwegian Research Council, 120
NSFs (National Service Frameworks). *See* National Service Frameworks
Nuffield Hospitals, 54
nurse practitioners, U.S., 200
nurses, British
community, 49
new career categories for, 71

number of, 250, 251t
registration of, 55
senior, 57, 58
nurses, Canadian
funding for, 164
mental health issues, involvment in, 261
number of, 141, 250t, 251t
nursing care, 151
nurses, Norwegian
home, 85
mental health issues, involvment in, 94, 98, 105, 108, 132, 133, 260
number of, 250, 251t
qualifications of, 268
nurses, U.S.
mental health issues, involvement with, 201, 220
number of, 250, 250t, 251t, 277
nursing homes, British, 52
nursing homes, Canadian, 151
nursing homes, Norwegian, 85, 101n14, 115
See also psychiatric nursing homes, Norwegian
nursing homes, U.S., 187, 197

O

obsessive-compulsive disorders, national breakdown of, 8, 16
obsessive-compulsive disorders in Canada, 143
occupational activities, 47, 73
occupational health in developing countries, 340
occupational health services, 71
occupational therapy and therapists
British, 47, 56, 57, 252
Canadian, 157, 159, 249, 268, 275
offenders. See crime and criminals
Office for National Statistics (England), 30
Office of Economic Opportunity, 202
Office of National Drug Control Policy (U.S.), 312
Office of Personnel Management (OPM), 199
Office of the Deputy Prime Minister (England), 248
older people (60+ years)

demographics of, 10, 11t, 307, 316
health insurance for, 19
medications for, 257
mental disorders of, 16 (see also term in elderly under specific disorder, e.g.: dementia: in elderly)
mental health needs of, 315
mental health services for, 18, 255, 307, 320
older people (60+ years), British
co-morbidity in, 35, 43
demographics of, 307t
mental disorders of, 30, 31, 34–35, 43, 307
mental health policy for, 40, 43–44, 44f, 239, 244, 258
mental health services for, 44, 54
needs assessment of, 37, 43
protection of, 292
specialists working with, 47
suicide rate of, 33, 34, 35
older people (60+ years), Canadian
demographics of, 307, 307t
health expenditures for, 176
health insurance for, 156
mental disorders of, 143
mental health needs of, 311
mental health services for, 158, 180, 181
older people (60+ years), Norwegian
co-morbidity in, 115
demographics, 81
demographics of, 307, 307t
health care needs of, 81
mental disorders of, 89t, 115
mental health services for, 100, 103, 120, 309
services (general) for, 85, 101n14
specialized services for, 115
unmet needs of, 114–15
older people (60+ years), U.S.
demographics of, 186, 307, 307t
health insurance for, 189, 194, 197, 198, 216–17, 223, 242, 243, 246, 250, 296, 318 (see also Medicare (U.S.))
mental disorders of, 186, 193, 193t
mental health needs of, 312
mental health services for, 189, 195, 205, 250, 255
Olmstead v. L.C., 1999, 206
Ontario, health care services in, 274

Ontario, mental health services in, 162, 181, 274–75
operative agreement, 106–7, 112, 123, 124, 260, 285, 286
Oregon, health care rationing in, 279
Oregon, health care reform in, 222, 325, 344
Organization for Economic Cooperation and Development, 20, 83, 167
orgon therapy, 104
Orwell, George. *Animal Farm* (1946), 242
out-of-pocket health expenditures, 11t, 12, 13, 19, 233, 237t, 283, 284
in Canada, 152, 156, 167, 174, 177, 178, 245, 253, 276, 281, 287, 294
in Great Britain, 54, 280
in Norway, 109, 110, 122, 124, 280, 286, 293, 309
in United States, 185, 208, 214, 214t, 216, 246, 280, 288, 289t, 290, 295, 312
outpatient health care services in Norway, 286
outpatient mental health care
in Canada, 151, 159, 169, 245, 249, 261, 269, 274, 275, 276, 281, 287, 288, 294, 310, 311, 325
continuity in, 331
expenditures for, 19, 250
follow-up and after-care, 18, 111, 112, 116, 205
in Great Britain, 46, 54, 258, 280, 308
in Norway, 93, 94, 95, 96, 97, 98, 104, 106, 107, 109, 110, 112, 113, 114, 114n24, 117, 120–21, 122, 123, 125, 130, 131, 132, 244, 248, 259, 273, 286, 293, 295
trends in, 319
in United States, 197, 203, 204, 208, 209, 210, 242, 243, 250, 266, 276, 277, 282
outreach services, 168, 248

P

PADs (Psychiatric Advance Direc-

tives), 219–20
pain, risk of, 6
Pan American Health Organization, 338
panic disorders
   British statistics on, 31
   Canadian statistics on, 143, 147
   national breakdown of, 8, 16
   Norwegian statistics on, 88, 146
   U.S. studies on, 204, 220
paramedics, Canadian, 160
parasitic disease, 9
parents, support services for, 40
Parkinson's disease, 8, 16
participation (defined), 292
Partnership for Prescription Assistance (PPA), 194
pastoral counseling centers, 334
pastoral counselors, 207
patient list system, 294
Patient Ombudsman (Norway), 120, 128, 293
Patient Rights Act, 1999 (Norway), 87, 95, 127, 128, 129, 240, 293
patients
   advocacy groups for, 336
   autonomy of, 233
   protection and participation of, 19, 233, 291–92, 321–22, 330
   rights of, 16, 19, 291–92, 320, 321–22
patients, British
   participation of, 292–93
   private and paying, 59
   protection and safety of, 258, 292, 321
   rights of, 38, 292
   satisfaction surveys, 65
patients, Canadian
   participation of, 295
   protection and safety of, 182, 294–95
   rights of, 152–54, 240, 292, 294–95
   satisfaction surveys, 175, 260
patients, Norwegian
   care settings of, 99–102, 101f (*see also* mental hospitals and asylums; psychiatric nursing homes)
   employment of, 103
   hospitalization of, 99–101, 99t, 100f
   participation of, 64t, 69–70, 95, 105, 127–28, 132, 293–94
   protection and safety of, 64t, 68–69, 126–27, 293, 321
   rights of, 87, 95, 105, 126–29, 132, 240, 248, 292
   satisfaction surveys, 120
   sociodemographic characteristics of, 103
   treated, 125
patients, U.S.
   education of, 201
   participation of, 217, 266, 296–97
   protection and safety of, 196–97, 219, 250, 263, 295–96, 321
   rights of, 217, 218–20, 292, 312, 340, 343
   satisfaction surveys, 203–4, 264
Paul Wellstone Mental Health Equitable Treatment Act (2001), 218
pediatricians, U.S., 200, 265
per capita health expenditures, 13–14, 13t, 19, 232, 233, 271
   in Canada, 177, 274, 275, 322t
   in Great Britain, 322t
   in Norway, 322t
   in United States, 214, 215, 234, 281, 289, 322t, 326, 343
perinatal psychiatry, 53
period prevalence (defined), 8
personal health information, 153–54, 181, 291, 295
Personal Information Protection and Electronic Documents Act (PIPEDA), 2001 (Canada), 152–53
personality disorders
   in Canada, 143–44, 147
   in Great Britain, 30, 31, 39, 52, 53, 71
   in Norway, 88, 103–4, 129, 131
   in United States, 192
personal liberty, 338
personal responsibility, 15, 339
pharmacies, 49
pharmacists, 47, 57
pharmacological revolution, 102
pharmacotherapy, 157, 172, 173, 174, 179, 195, 263, 275, 311, 333
phobia
   in elderly, 34, 307
   prevalence of, 88, 131, 143, 149, 191
physical exercise and activity, 73, 95
physical health care, mental health services integration with, 47, 168
physical illness
   costs of, 172
   in older people, 43
   symptoms linked to mental disorders, 201
physical-neurological disorders, 16
physical pain, 35
physical psychologists, 47
physical therapies and therapists, British, 44, 49, 57, 77
physicians. *See* doctors; family doctors
Physicians for a National Health Plan, 343
Physicians for a National Health Program (PNHP), 221
Picker Institute for Mental Health Trusts, 61, 65
PICUs (psychiatric intensive care units), 42, 51, 52, 248, 292
PIPEDA (*Personal Information Protection and Electronic Documents Act*), 2001 (Canada), 152–53
podiatrists, 49
point prevalence (defined), 8
policy implementation guidelines, 41, 50, 51, 239, 241, 247–50, 258, 292, 308, 320, 335
political systems and mental health care, 316–17
pooling of resources
   in Canada, 287, 325
   defined, 284
   in Great Britain, 284
   in Norway, 285
   in United States, 288, 290
poor people, attitudes toward, 314
POS (point of service) plans, 215, 297, 327
post-traumatic stress disorders (PTSDs)
   national breakdown of, 8, 16
   prevalence of, 131, 146, 147
   risk of, 71
   treatment of, 40, 65, 204
poverty
   children in, 40, 172, 180, 194
   and mental illness, 34, 172, 180,

318
PPOs (preferred provider organizations), 215, 297, 326, 327
PPS (Prospective Payment System), 197
practice nurses, 49
Preamble to the Constitution of the United Nations, 292
pre-existing conditions, 210, 220
preferred drug lists (PDLs), 194
pregnant women, health insurance for, 197
prepaid and risk-pooling health plans, 11t, 12, 13, 284, 288, 326
prescriptions
    benefits, unfunded, 19
    cost and payment for (in Canada), 274
    cost and payment for (in Great Britain), 44, 58, 59, 285, 324
    cost and payment for (in Norway), 123
    cost and payment for (in United States), 193-94, 197, 198, 215, 222, 278
    from nonphysician health care providers, 207, 213
Presidential Advisory Commission on Consumer Protection and Quality of the Health Care Industry, 262
President's Commission on Health Needs of the Nation (1953), 339
President's Commission on Mental Health, 31, 187, 242, 246-47, 262, 331
President's Commission on the Study of Ethical Problems in Medicine and Biomedical and Behavioral Research, 338
President's Health Security Plan, 339
President's New Freedom Commission on Mental Health, 21, 188, 220, 241, 243, 266, 312, 344
prevention and early intervention
    in Canada, 142, 159, 167, 170, 171, 172, 174, 176, 178, 180, 276
    emphasizing, 332, 333, 335-36
    in Great Britain, 42, 51, 148, 267
    in Norway, 94, 106, 111, 115, 248
    promoting, 340

services, 338
    in United States, 187-88, 190, 203, 246, 262
prevention of disease, 283, 332
    in Canada, 262
    in United States, 247, 251
preventive medical care, 201, 202, 283
price controls, 279
Primary Care Groups (for GPs), 258
primary care patients, mental health issues and disorders of, 6, 30, 308
Primary Care Trusts, 29, 49, 52, 52t, 53, 57, 58-59, 61, 62, 77, 258, 284, 285, 308
primary health care
    delivery of, 6, 17
    disease prevention, role in, 251
    funding of, 71
    human resources in, 250
    mental health services integration with, 8, 18, 319, 321, 331, 332-35
    patients, mental disorders in, 8, 307
    primary practice features, 332
    professionals, 250
    reform, 332
    in rural areas, 332-33
    structural characteristics of, 322
    universal coverage, route to, 319
primary health care, British
    counselors in, 47, 268
    emphasis on, 28, 258
    free, 44
    mental health services integration with, 41, 47, 71, 258, 321, 323
    organization and administration of, 29, 76-77, 285
    professionals, 50, 251t
    promotion of, 41
    statutory, 46
primary health care, Canadian
    historically privileged, 174
    mental health services integration with, 158, 167, 170-71, 176, 179, 180, 260-61, 311
    professionals, 250t, 251t
    reform of, 159, 251t
primary health care, Norwegian
    access to, 82, 87
    local responsibility for, 85, 86, 109,

130
    mental health services integration with, 87, 94, 95, 102, 103, 106, 113, 121, 259
    professionals, 251t
    quality of, 259
    transportation challenges, 82
primary health care, U.S.
    access to, 200, 204, 246, 283
    mental health issues in, 212
    mental health services integration with, 201-2, 220, 221, 265-66, 267, 291
    quality of, 266
primary health care system (PHS) (defined), 332
primary mental health care, 321, 332, 333-34
primary mental health care, British, 48, 48f, 49-50, 54, 57, 64-65, 72, 73, 76, 252, 258, 308
primary mental health care, Canadian, 156-57
primary mental health care, Norwegian, 97, 105-6, 109, 130, 134-35, 260, 268, 286, 310
primary mental health care, U.S., 251t, 321
Principles for the Protection of Persons with Mental Illness and for the Improvement of Mental Health Care, 339
Priory Group, 54
prisoners
    mental health services for, 18, 316
    mentally ill as, 243, 331, 336
    See also crime and criminals
prisoners, British, mental health services for, 57, 65, 71
prisoners, Canadian
    health care services for, 142, 151, 178
    increase in, 176
    mental disorders of, 147, 173
    mental health needs of, 249
    mental health services for, 244
    mentally ill as, 261
prisoners, Norwegian, mental health services for, 129, 244
prisoners, U.S.
    health care services for, 242, 247
    mental disorders of, 190

mental health services for, 207–8, 247
mentally ill as, 204, 243, 247, 266, 341
privacy protection and legislation, 16, 19, 291
   in Canada, 150, 152–54, 294–95
   in Great Britain, 38, 292
   in Norway, 127
   in United States, 218–19, 277 (*see also* HIPAA (*Health Insurance Portability and Accountability Act*))
private finance initiative (PFI), 60
Private Financing Initiative, 68
private health care services in Minnesota, 16
private health care services in Norway, 85
private health expenditures
   definition and categories of, 12
   national breakdown for, 11t, 13
   versus public expenditures, 284
private health expenditures, British, 44, 54, 60, 285, 291, 324
private health expenditures, Canadian, 155–56, 164–67, 165t–166t, 177, 179, 287–88, 291
private health expenditures, Norwegian, 122, 280, 291
private health expenditures, U.S., 185, 214, 215, 282, 288–90, 289t, 291, 321
private health sector
   access, 18
   personnel in, 17, 19, 321
   reform of, 342
private mental health services
   in Canada, 276, 288, 310
   in Great Britain, 54–55
   in Norway, 85, 92–93, 96, 99, 101, 102, 125, 260, 286
   in United States, 10, 21, 205–6, 289t, 290, 321
private practitioners, Norwegian, 106–7, 114, 114n24, 117, 119, 123–24, 286
privatization in Great Britain, 324
privatization in Norway, 84
processes of care, 331–32
process indicators (defined), 256
productivity (defined), 256, 269
professional codes of conduct, 118–19, 267, 268, 319
professional codes of ethics, 340
professional groups. *See* mental health professionals and workers
Prospective Payment System (PPS), 197
protection (defined), 291–92
protection regulations, 16
provider, choice of, 233
Provincial Ministries of Health (Canada), 249
Psychiatric Advance Directives (PADs), 219–20
psychiatric care, pathway to, 47
psychiatric clinics, 6
psychiatric clinics, Norwegian, 93
psychiatric disorders. *See* mental disorders
psychiatric epidemiology, 52
psychiatric intensive care units (PICUs), 42, 51, 52, 248, 292
psychiatric nursing and nurses, 20, 321
psychiatric nursing and nurses, British, 39, 47, 50, 56, 73, 75
psychiatric nursing and nurses, Canadian, 159, 160, 268
psychiatric nursing and nurses, Norwegian, 105, 253, 260, 268
psychiatric nursing and nurses, U.S., 200, 204, 207, 254–55
psychiatric nursing homes, Norwegian, 93, 96, 98, 100, 101–2, 101f, 103, 111
psychiatric pharmacists, 57
psychiatric units and wards, Canadian, 168, 261
psychiatric units and wards, Norwegian, 93, 95, 96, 108, 110, 116, 121
psychiatric units and wards, U.S., 201, 206, 263
psychiatrists, British
   care pathway, involvement in, 47
   categories of, 55, 55t
   recruitment and working conditions of, 75
   on Regional Health Boards, 27
   sectioning process, involvement in, 39
   training of, 56
psychiatrists, Canadian
   consultations with, 146
   number of, 268
   physicians, communication with, 170, 261
   as primary mental health care providers, 159
   status of, 275, 318, 325
psychiatrists, credentialing of, 321
psychiatrists, Norwegian
   education and training of, 268
   location of, 117
   number of, 98, 107, 108, 112, 253
   private, 260
   therapy approaches of, 105
   in transition, 132
psychiatrists, U.S.
   access to, 205
   mental health care, quality of, 263
   number of, 206, 254
   on quality in health care, 262
   services by, 200
psychiatry
   evolution of, 132–33
   medical model of, 130, 131–32, 133, 134 (*see also* biopsychosocial model of mental illness and health)
   mental health system evaluation, source of, 20
psychoanalysis, 104, 105, 207, 268
psychodynamic theories and therapy, 104, 105, 268
psychoeducation, 220
psychological dysfunction, 7
psychologists
   See also clinical psychologists; forensic psychology and psychologists; school psychologists
psychologists, British, 55, 73, 77, 268
psychologists, Canadian
   number of, 159, 268
   services, cost of, 177, 178
   services, paying for, 164, 249, 275, 276
psychologists, credentialing of, 321
psychologists, Norwegian
   education and qualifications of, 98, 107
   as general practitioners, 130, 134–35
   location of, 117
   municipality, 105, 106, 260

number of, 108, 253
operational agreements of, 112
versus other mental health professionals, 96
versus physicians, 132
private, 260
services, paying for, 123–24
psychologists, U.S.
education and training of, 269, 334
prescriptions by, 213
primary care, involvement in, 220, 221
on quality in health care, 262
services by, 200
status of, 207
VA-sponsored, 203
Psychologists in Independent Practice, 213
psychology services, Canadian
funding for, 157
in hospitals, 174
private, 173
psychosis
in Canada, 159
in Great Britain, 30, 32, 42, 51, 248, 267
in Norway, 98, 99, 103, 115, 129
in United States, 209
psychosocial-economic-cultural gradient of health care, 185
See also biopsychosocial model of mental illness and health
psychosocial rehabilitation, 158, 319, 333
psychosurgery (lobotomy), 104, 168, 319
psychotherapeutic traditions in Norway, 104–5
psychotherapy and therapists
in Canada, 241, 288
in Great Britain, 47–48, 50, 53, 54, 56, 73, 308
in Norway, 93, 98, 104–5, 106, 118, 268, 321
outcomes of, 329
rise in, 319
in United States, 194, 197, 207, 212, 213, 220, 255, 263, 265, 282, 326
WHO recommendation, 333
psychotropic medications, 19, 72, 73, 105, 132, 133, 167, 172, 193, 194, 196, 204, 253, 256, 263, 265, 322
PTSD. *See* post-traumatic stress disorders (PTSDs)
public education campaigns
in Great Britain, 72, 73, 74
public health agencies and associations, 336
Public Health Agency (Canada), 149, 175
public health expenditures
funding mechanisms, 17
national breakdown for, 12–13, 13t
versus private expenditures, 284
See also social security: health expenditures
public health expenditures (and funding), British, 44, 58, 283, 285, 288, 321, 324
public health expenditures (and funding), Canadian, 161–64, 165t–166t, 166, 167, 177, 178, 179, 283, 287, 288
public health expenditures (and funding), Norwegian, 96, 167, 283, 285, 286, 288, 289, 321
public health expenditures (and funding), U.S., 167, 214, 221, 222, 242, 281, 282, 288, 289t, 290–91, 342
public health sector
access, 18
personnel in, 17, 19
reform of, 342
Public Health Service, 200
public health service
in Great Britain, 10, 27 (*see also* National Health Service (England))
in Norway, 84, 85, 86
in United States, 283
Public Health Service Act, 200
Public Health Service (U.S.), 7–8
public mental health services
in Canada, 175, 179, 249, 288, 310
continuity of care through, 331
in Great Britain, 21, 68
in Norway, 17, 21, 84, 85, 92–93, 96, 108, 124–25, 260, 286, 310
in United States, 17, 189, 195, 204–5, 289t, 320, 321
purchasing of health care services
in Canada, 287
defined, 284
in Great Britain, 284, 285
in Norway, 285
in United States, 288–89, 290
pursuit of happiness, 341

Q

quality
defined, 233, 256
indicators, 256–57
quality assurance/quality improvement (QA/QI) policies, 257–67, 335
quality of life, promoting, 95, 125, 130, 133, 134, 188, 328, 335, 340
Quebec, health insurance in, 287
Quebec Attorney General, Chaoulli v. (2005), 287

R

rationing by queue, 280, 281, 285, 326
See also health care services: waits and treatment delays; mental health services: waits and treatment delays
readmissions, inpatient and hospital recidivism rates
in Canada, 168, 176, 261, 275, 295
gathering data on, 18
in Norway, 115–16, 116n
in United States, 195, 205
Reagan, Ronald, 247
recovery process, 130, 133–34
Red Cross, 122
refugees and asylum seekers, British, mental health needs of, 36, 45, 70, 307
refugees and asylum seekers, Canadian, mental health services for, 320
refugees and asylum seekers, Norwegian
mental health needs of, 95, 115
mental health services for, 320
refugees and asylum seekers, U.S., mental health services for, 320
Regional Health Authorities (Canada),

157, 178, 249, 294
Regional Health Authorities (England), 77
Regional Health Authorities (RHAs) (Norway), 85–86, 94–95, 96, 106, 109, 110, 113, 121, 123, 124, 127, 130, 240, 248, 259, 272, 273, 293, 318
Regional Health Boards (in Great Britain), 27
Regional Health Enterprises (Norway), 109, 118t, 248
regional psychiatric centers in Norway, 17
registered mental nurses (RMNs). *See* psychiatric nursing and nurses
Regulated Health Professions Act (Ontario), 160
rehabilitation
    benefits, 203
    counselors, 207
    long-term treatment and, 95
    psychosocial, 158, 319, 333, 336
    services, 190, 198
    units and wards, 111, 117
    vocational, 194, 243, 295
Reich, Wilhelm, 104
relative performance, 233
religion and mental health, 333, 334, 340
religious minorities in Great Britain, 36
Republic of Ireland, mental health system in, 24
residential health care in Canada, 151
residential mental health care
    expenditures for, 19
    in Great Britain, 49, 51–52, 53, 74, 308
    in United States, 190, 199, 201, 204, 206, 210, 266, 276
Resnick, Bob, 207
respect for persons, 233
responsiveness (defined), 233
restraint, 205, 219, 292
Rethink (organization) (*formerly* National Schizophrenia Fellowship), 70
revenue collection
    in Canada, 287
    defined, 284

    in Great Britain, 284
    in Norway, 285
    in United States, 288, 290
revenue health care funding, 59–60
rich and poor, gap between, 314
right to life, 340, 341
role overload, 149–50, 274, 325
Romanow, Roy, 173–74
Romanow Commission on the Future of Health Care in Canada, 151, 167, 169, 174, 244, 261, 274
Ronald W. Reagan National Defense Authorization Act, 2005, 200
Royal College of Physicians and Surgeons (Canada), 160
Royal College of Psychiatrists (England), 56, 69
Royal Commission on Health Services (Canada), 160, 261
Royal Medico-Psychological Association, 55

S

SA. *See* substance abuse
safe houses in Canada, 158
Samaritans (organization), 51
SAMHSA. *See* Substance Abuse and Mental Health Services Administration (SAMHSA)
Sámi people, 82, 88
Sammons, Morgan, 207
Saskatchewan, health care services in, 155–56, 324, 325
Satcher, David, 7–8, 187
SAVE: Suicide Awareness Voice of Education, 296
Saving, Thomas R., 197
Scandinavian countries, health care in, 288
Schedule for Clinical Assessment in Neuropsychiatry (SCAN II), 89
SCHIP (State Children's Health Insurance Program), 12–13, 189, 198, 199, 208, 211–12, 222, 242, 246, 290
schizophrenia
    addiction and, 90
    associations, 70
    costs associated with, 92, 123

    diagnosis of, 103
    disability due to, 307
    involuntary hospital admission for, 99
    mental disorder classification, 7
    national breakdown of, 8, 15
    prevalence of, 34, 88, 111, 114n22, 131, 143, 149, 195
    protection for persons with, 219
    recovery, factors in, 134
    treatment of, 15, 20, 68, 87, 95, 114, 115, 195, 206, 220, 244, 265
Schjelderup, Harald, 104
school health services in Norway, 85
school health services in United States, 199
school mental health services, U.S., 201, 212
school nurses, Norwegian, 105, 260
school psychologists, 36, 254
school psychologists, Norwegian, 105–6, 260
Scotland, health care in, 26
Scotland, mental health system in, 24, 69
seclusion, 205, 219, 292
secondary mental health services in Great Britain, 48f, 71
secondary mental health services in Norway, 134
second opinion, right to, 87
Secretarial Initiative on Mental Health, 187
Secretary of State for Health (England), 25–26, 28, 29, 63, 77, 279, 293
secure services, 42, 53, 67
    See also high secure services; low secure services; medium secure services
Segal, Joel, 222
selective serotonin reuptake inhibitors (SSRIs), 209
self-acceptance, 133
self-care, 195
self-discovery, 133
self-harm
    prevention teams, 50
    protection against, 39, 69, 154
    suicide linked to history of, 34
self-help, 48, 49, 157, 159, 168, 180, 209, 239, 261, 265, 308

self-insured plans, 16–17
self-interest versus common good, 339
self-interest versus social interest, 338
self-medication, 312
self-rated mental health problems, 327
    in Canada, 145, 147
    in Great Britain, 65, 324
    in Norway, 89, 89t, 114n23, 310
    in United States, 211
severe mental illness, community-based services for, 320
severe mental illness in Canada, 168, 169, 176, 310, 311
severe mental illness in Great Britain
    policy focus of, 71
    treatment of, 39, 41, 42, 44, 49, 51, 52, 57
    unmet need, 72, 72t
severe mental illness in minorities, 314
severe mental illness in Norway
    among prisoners, 129
    involuntary hospital admissions for, 98
    prevalence of, 88, 89, 111, 114n22, 132
    recovery, factors in, 134
    treatment of, 87, 95, 104, 135, 244
    unmet need, 111, 114–15, 130, 309
severe mental illness in United States, 190, 205, 250, 341
Sexton, John, 207
shared care model of mental health care, 167, 170–71, 261
    see also primary health care: mental health services integration with
short-stay accommodations in Canada, 158
short-stay accommodations in Norway, 110
sick benefits
    in Great Britain, 45, 239
    in Norway, 239, 240
sick leaves, mental illness-related in Norway, 123
single payer health care system, 221, 223, 325, 344
single-room occupancy hotels (SROs), 204
Sinnssykeloven (1848) (Norway), 93
sleeping disturbance, 71

sleep problems, British statistics on, 31
SMI (serious mental illness), 62, 193, 195, 198, 216, 257, 278, 279, 281
social and recreational programs, 159
social capital, 337–38
social care services, British, 63, 76
social care services, Norwegian, 259, 286
social contact, 95
social contract, 340
social deprivation, 35, 37, 58, 74, 285, 308
social equality, 338
social exclusion, reducing, 69, 73
social insurance, 324–25, 338
social integration, 95
social interest *versus* self-interest, 338
social isolation, 34, 131
social justice, 20, 340, 341
social networks, 132, 134, 237
social norms, deviation from, 7
social phobia
    prevalence of, 88, 143, 144, 146, 191
    treating, 220
social policy, economic aspects of, 3
social problems, biomedical model of, 171
social resources, 338
Social Sciences and Humanities Research Council (SSHRC), 143, 260
social sciences and mental health research, 181
social security
    in Canada, 295
    in Great Britain, 29, 45, 239
    health expenditures, 11t, 12–13
    in Norway, 102, 125
Social Security Act, 195
Social Security (U.S.), 194, 196, 197, 214, 214t, 290, 343
social services, 333
social services, British, public financing of, 27
social services, Norwegian
    administration of, 119
    cooperation with, 95
    local responsibility for, 85, 86, 109
    under National Mental Health Programme (NMHP), 94

social services, U.S., 194
Social Services Inspectorate (SSI), 43, 63, 248
social support, 42, 47, 335
social support networks, 233
social systems theory, 5
Social Transfer, 287
social workers, British
    approved, 39
    on emergency teams, 51
    in mental hospitals, 55
    in multidisciplinary work, 46
    in primary care, 73
    training of, 56–57
social workers, Canadian
    number of, 159, 268
    regulation of, 160
    services, cost and funding for, 157, 177, 178, 249, 275, 276
social workers, mental health system, role in, 20, 321
social workers, Norwegian
    as child specialists, 96
    mental health issues, involvement in, 133, 260
    versus physicians, 132
    primary care, participation in, 105
    as psychotherapists, 98
    qualifications of, 268
social workers, U.S., number of, 206–7
social workers, U.S., services by, 200
Society for a Science of Clinical Psychology, 213
Society for Behavioral Medicine, 189
Society of Clinical Psychology, 213
sociologists, clinical, 207
somatic health facilities, 134
somatic treatments, 104
South America, health care in, 288
Special Health Revenue Sharing Act, 1974, 202, 249
special interest groups, 282, 297, 316, 317, 342, 344
Specialist Health Service Act (Norway), 128, 293
Specialist Health Services Act (Norway), 252
specialized community mental health teams, 48, 51
Specialized Health Care Act, 1999 (Norway), 87

specialized health services
 in Canada, 251t
 in Great Britain, 28, 29, 251t
 human resources in, 250
 in Norway, 84, 85, 86–87, 94, 113, 123, 251t, 259
 in United States, 251t
Specialized Health Services Act (Norway), 240, 268
specialty clinics, 159
speech and language therapists, 47, 57
speed (drug), 148
spina bifida, 198
SPMI (severe and persistent mental illness), 193
SSHRC (Social Sciences and Humanities Research Council), 143, 260
SSI (Social Services Inspectorate), 43, 63, 248
SSRIs (selective serotonin reuptake inhibitors), 209
St. Andrews Hospital, Northampton, 54
State Children's Health Insurance Program (SCHIP). *See* SCHIP (State Children's Health Insurance Program)
state employee health benefit plan, 199, 290
stewardship (oversight), 335, 336
stigma, 291, 332, 336
Strategic Health Authorities (SHAs) (England), 28–29, 65, 67, 71, 77, 279, 284, 285
Stratis Health (organization), 263
structural indicators (defined), 256
substance abuse
 disorders, preventing, 312
 health risks of, 6
 prevalence of, 8, 306
 studies on, 328
 treating, 19
 See also alcohol abuse; drug abuse
Substance Abuse and Mental Health Services Administration (SAMHSA), 195, 217, 221, 249, 250, 263, 289
substance abuse in Britain
 prevalence of, 32, 32t
 suicide, link to, 34
 treating, 53, 74

substance abuse in Canada
 cost of, 148, 148t, 274, 275
 funding for, 181
 help, seeking for, 145, 310
 mental health services, integration with, 261
 prevalence of, 144–45, 147–48
 preventing, 275
 treating, 160, 167, 168, 169, 170, 171, 172, 173, 180, 260, 275, 295
substance abuse in Norway
 deaths caused by, 90–92, 90t, 91t
 prevalence of, 90, 103, 115
substance abuse in United States
 agencies for, 250
 expenditures for, 289–90, 289t
 gender differences in, 192
 policy regarding, 320
 prevalence of, 193, 313
 treating, 194, 195, 200, 205, 206, 222, 245, 276
suicide
 of elderly, 33, 34, 35
 gender differences in (*see* under gender differences)
 prevention, 19
 risk factors for, 34, 37, 149
Suicide Awareness Voice of Education (SAVE), 296
suicide in Canada
 laws regarding, 155, 295
 prevention, 173, 181–82, 311
 rates, 148–49
suicide in Great Britain
 prevention, 69, 308
 rates, 30, 32–34, 33t, 35, 307
 reducing, 39, 41, 43, 257–58
suicide in Norway
 prevention, 95, 126–27
 rates, 90, 90t, 91f
suicide in United States
 causes of, 190
 rates, 245
 risk assessment for, 264
supply-side cost containment strategies, 215, 272, 275, 276, 279, 280, 282
Sure Start (social program), 49
Surgeon General's Report on Mental Health (1999), 193
surgery cost coverage, 151

system factors in efficiency, 269–70
systemic therapy, 105
system of care (SOC) approach, 266–67
systems level outcomes, 257

T

teachers in hospital schools, 57
technical quality (defined), 256–57
Temporary Assistance to Needy Families (TANF), 196, 313
TennCare, 209
tertiary mental health services in Great Britain, 47, 48f, 49, 52–53, 258, 308
Thatcher, Margaret, 324
third-party insurance, 277
third-party payers, 210, 214, 287
Thorazine, 204
three-tier health administration system, 27, 28–29
total expenditures on health, 9, 11, 11t, 12, 13t
total patient journeys, 53–54
tranquilizers, 133, 257
transportation and travel
 assistance with, 190
 to health services, 82, 283, 332–33
 to mental health services, 82, 123, 145, 174, 237
Treated as People Act, 2004, 42, 248
treatment, active *versus* custodial care
 in Canada, 168
 in Norway, 99, 102, 104, 111
 in past practice, 319
 in United States, 204
treatment, cost-effective, 105
treatment, involuntary. *See* involuntary mental treatment
treatment, risks and side effects of, 127
treatment gaps
 in Canada, 310–11, 322t, 323, 325
 causes of, 3, 4
 in Great Britain, 47, 48, 71, 73, 77, 308, 310, 322t
 identifying, 20, 21
 in Norway, 111–12, 114, 115, 116–18, 309–10, 322t
 in United States, 189–90, 211, 220, 262, 312–14, 322t, 323, 327, 344
 See also mental health services:

waits and treatment delays
treatment outcomes, improving, 340
treatment outcomes, measuring, 66, 118, 125, 213, 214–15, 257, 259, 263, 264, 328, 332
triage, 47, 57
TRICARE, 198, 200, 257, 263
Truman, Harry, 197, 221, 342
trust, measures of, 331, 332
turning points. *See* care pathways and transitions

U

underinsured persons, U.S., 189, 241, 243, 245, 291, 313, 316, 321, 341, 343
uninsured persons, U.S., 185, 189, 194, 210, 211, 215, 216, 231, 241, 242, 243, 245, 246, 250, 278, 280, 282, 283, 291, 295, 313, 314, 316, 318, 320, 321, 325, 327, 340, 341, 343
unipolar depression
    disability, cause of, 307
    national breakdown of, 8, 15
    prevalence of, 306
United Auto Workers, 278
United Nations charter, 318
United Nations Commission on Human Rights, 341
United Nations Convention on the Rights of the Child, 339
United Nations General Assembly, 339
United Nations General Assembly Resolution 46/119, 292
United Nations Millennium Declaration, 2000, 339
United States
    demographics, 10, 11t, 186, 187, 316t
    mental disorders, statistics on, 8
    overview of, 185–87, 296–97, 314, 316
United States Bureau of Health Professions, 269
United States National Health Insurance Act (HR676), 221–22
Universal Declaration of Human Rights, 339, 341
universal health care access
    achieving, factors in, 237, 319, 335
    in Canada, 142, 151, 155, 161, 231, 325, 326
    financing, 325
    in Great Britain, 26, 44–45, 239, 244, 342
    as mental health system evaluation criterion, 18, 319, 337
    in Norway, 84–85, 135, 239, 240, 324
    in United States, 15, 221–22, 223, 241, 249, 317, 320, 326, 327, 339, 340, 342, 344
universalism (ethical principle), 337
unmet need (defined), 306
    See also treatment gaps
URAC accreditation, 213, 264
Urban area helpline (England), 51
U.S. Constitution, 341
U.S. House and Senate health committees, 196
user charges, health-related. *See* out-of-pocket health expenditures
utilitarian view of distributive justice, 338

V

value-added benefits, 338
value-based practices, 328
value clarification, 332, 337–40, 337t
value judgments, 15
VAT (value added tax) (Norway), 109, 286
vertical equity, 238
veterans. *See* military personnel and veterans
Veterans Administration
    founding of, 203
    health care system, 189
    Medical Centers (VAMCs), 203
Veterans Health Administration (VHA), 196, 198, 201, 203–4, 208, 213, 242, 247, 249, 255, 263, 277, 290, 326
Veterans Hospital Administration, 166
violence, protection against, 39
vocational rehabilitation, 194, 243, 295
vocational training programs
    in Canada, 157, 159, 168
    in Norway, 110
    in United States, 194, 203
voluntary mental health services and support networks
    in Great Britain, 48, 48f, 49, 52, 77, 308
    in United States, 200

W

Waal, Nic, 96
waits and treatment delays. *See* under health care services; mental health services
Wales, health care in, 26
Wales, mental health system in, 24
welfare benefits
    in Great Britain, 43, 48, 49
    in Norway, 84, 102, 105, 239
Wellcome Trust, 63
Western Europe, health care in, 288
White, Thomas W., 207–8
White House Conference on Children (1970), 339
White House Conference on Mental Health, 187
White House Council on Domestic Policy, 339
White House Domestic Policy Council (1993), 15
WHO (World Health Organization) publications
    Constitution, 1948, 339
    as data source, 20
    Global Health Survey, 2001, 339
    on health (general), 6, 7, 122, 190, 237, 255, 256, 283, 339
    on health rankings, 232–34, 236, 240
    on mental health, 3, 4–5, 8, 9, 72, 73, 148, 176, 212, 213–14, 332
    term definitions, 7, 8, 12, 13, 14, 256, 292
World Mental Health Survey initiative, 306, 322, 327
WHO (World Health Organization) Regional Office for Europe, 20
within-service transitions, 54
women as mental patients, 42
women's mental health. *See* gender differences

work force, national breakdown of, 14
working age adults (18-59). *See* adults of working age (18-59)
work-life conflict, 149–50, 274, 325
workman's compensation, 16
workplace, mental health in, 325
work-related stress, illness due to, 30
work to family interference, 149, 150, 274, 325
World Association for Psychosocial Rehabilitation, 336
World Bank, 3, 9, 190, 337
World Health Assembly resolution, 1998, 339
World Mental Health-Composite International Diagnostic Interview (WMH-CIDI). *See* Composite International Diagnostic Interview (CIDI)

Y

young people. *See* adolescents; children

Z

Zito Trust (organization), 70